Lecture Notes in Biomathematics

Managing Editor: S. Levin

48

Tracer Kinetics and Physiologic Modeling

Theory to Practice

Proceedings of a Seminar
held at St. Louis, Missouri
June 6, 1983

Edited by R. M. Lambrecht and A. Rescigno

Springer-Verlag Berlin Heidelberg GmbH

Editors

R. M. Lambrecht
A. Rescigno
Brookhaven National Laboratory / Chemistry Department
Upton, New York 11973, USA

AMS Subject Classification (1980): 92-XX

ISBN 978-3-540-12300-2 ISBN 978-3-642-50036-7 (eBook)
DOI 10.1007/978-3-642-50036-7

Originally published by Springer-Verlag Berlin Heidelberg in 1983.

2146/3140-543210

PREFACE

These lectures were prepared by the authors for Seminars to be held on June 6, 1983, in St.Louis, Missouri, under the sponsorship of the Radiopharmaceutical Science Council of the Society of Nuclear Medicine. All manuscripts were refereed.

Tracer kinetics and the modeling of physiological and biochemical processes in vivo are the focus of a contemporary direction in biochemical research. Recent advances in instrumentation (especially positron emission tomography and digital autoradiography) and parallel developments in the production of short-lived radionuclides and rapid synthetic chemistry to prepare tracers that probe metabolism, flow, receptor-ligand kinetics, etc., are responsible for new scientific frontiers. These developments, coupled with biomathematics and computer science, make it possible to quantitatively evaluate tracer kinetic models in animals and man.(The choice of animal models in radiotracer design and tracer kinetics is the subject of a book edited by R.M.Lambrecht and W.C.Eckleman in press at Springer Verlag.)

Tracer kinetics and physiological modeling is truly multidisciplinary, as evidenced by the intellectual diversity and international representation observable in the list of contributors. The lectures outline and attempt to show the transition from the theoretical description to the practical application of modeling for understanding normal and pathological processes. It is our hope that young researchers, particularly in the physical, radiopharmaceutical, and medical sciences, will be inspired to apply tracer kinetics and physiological modeling in their work.

Quogue, NY
December 31, 1982

Richard M.Lambrecht
Aldo Rescigno

TABLE OF CONTENTS

LIST OF CONTRIBUTORS

Alavi, Abass	Departments of Neurology and Nuclear Medicine, University of Pennsylvania Hospital, Philadelphia, PA 19104
Bass, Ludvik	Department of Mathematics, University of Queensland, St. Lucia, Queensland, Australia 4067
Becker, Veit	Institute of Medicine, Nuclear Research Center, Jülich, and Department of Nuclear Medicine, University of Dusseldorf, 5170 Jülich, F.R. Germany
Bracken, Anthony J.	Department of Mathematics, University of Queensland, St. Lucia, Queensland, Australia 4067
Burden, Conrad J.	Department of Nuclear Physics, Weizmann Institute of Science, Rehovot, Israel
Carson, Richard E.	Division of Biophysics, Department of Radiological Sciences and Laboratory of Nuclear Medicine, UCLA School of Medicine, Los Angeles, CA 90024
Duncan, Charles C.	Section of Neurosurgery, Yale University School of Medicine, New Haven, CT 06510
Feinendegen, Ludwig Emil	Institute of Medicine, Nuclear Research Center, Jülich, and Department of Nuclear Medicine, University of Dusseldorf, 5170 Jülich, F.R. Germany
Freundlieb, Christian	Institute of Medicine, Nuclear Research Center, Jülich, and Department of Nuclear Medicine, University of Dusseldorf, 5170 Jülich, F.R. Germany
Gerald, Kenneth B.	Department of Biometry, University of Kansas Medical Center, Kansas City, KS 66103

Gjedde, Albert	Department of Clinical Physiology, Bispebjerg Hospital, DK-2100 Copenhagen, Denmark
Henriksen, Ole	Department of Clinical Physiology, Bispebjerg Hospital, DK-2100 Copenhagen, Denmark
Hertz, Marianne M.	Department of Psychiatry, Rigshospitalet, State University Hospital, DK-2100 Copenhagen, Denmark
Höck, Anton	Institute of Medicine, Nuclear Research Center, Jülich, and Department of Nuclear Medicine, University of Düsseldorf, 5170 Jülich, F.R. Germany
Huang, Sung-Cheng	Division of Biophysics, Department of Radiological Sciences and Laboratory of Nuclear Medicine, UCLA School of Medicine, Los Angeles, CA 90024
Lambrecht, Richard M.	Chemistry Department, Brookhaven National Laboratory, Upton, NY 11973
Lassen, Niels A.	Department of Clinical Physiology, Bispebjerg Hospital, DK-2100 Copenhagen, Denmark
Matis, James H	Institute of Statistics, Texas A & M University, College Station, TX 77840
Paulson, Olaf B.	Department of Neurology, Rigshospitalet, State University Hospital, DK-2100 Copenhagen, Denmark
Phelps, Michael E.	Division of Biophysics, Department of Radiological Sciences and Laboratory of Nuclear Medicine, UCLA School of Medicine, Los Angeles, CA 90024
Profant, Miroslav	Department of Applied Mathematics, University of Duisburg, 4100 Duisburg, F.R. Germany
Reivich, Martin	Department of Neurology, University of Pennsylvania Hospital, Philadelphia, PA 19104

Rescigno, Aldo	Chemistry Department, Brookhaven National Laboratory, Upton, NY 11973 and Yale University, New Haven, CT 06510
Schafer, David E.	Veterans Administration Medical Center, West Haven, CT 06516
Schuier, Franz	Department of Neurology, University of Dusseldorf, 4000 Dusseldorf, F.R. Germany
Smith, Carolyn B.	Laboratory of Cerebral Metabolism, National Institute of Mental Health, Bethesda, MD 20205
Sokoloff, Louis	Laboratory of Cerebral Metabolism, National Institute of Mental Health, Bethesda, MD 20205
Thal, Hans-Uwe	Department of Neurosurgery, University of Dusseldorf, 4000 Dusseldorf, F.R. Germany
Vyska, Karl	Institute of Medicine, Nuclear Research Center, Jülich, and Department of Nuclear Medicine, University of Dusseldorf, 5170 Jülich, F.R. Germany
Wagner, Henry N. Jr.	The Johns Hopkins Medical Institutions, Divisions of Nuclear Medicine and Radiation Health Sciences, Baltimore, MD 21205
Wehrly, Thomas E.	Institute of Statistics, Texas A & M University, College Station, TX 77840

THE STATISTICAL ANALYSIS OF PHARMACOKINETIC DATA

James H. Matis*, Thomas E. Wehrly*, Kenneth B. Gerald**

*Texas A&M University, College Station, TX; **University of Kansas Medical Center, Kansas City, Kansas

1. INTRODUCTION

Virtually all of the practical applications of pharmacokinetic data analysis involve two parts, one is the mathematical modelling of the underlying pharmacokinetic system and the other is the statistical analysis of pharmacokinetic data. The mathematical modelling has received great attention in the literature and has produced many practically useful and mathematically elegant models. The mathematical modelling of compartmental systems is described in (1-6). However, the statistical analysis of pharmacokinetic data has received relatively little attention in the literature. The limited attention that it has received usually addresses one of the following questions.

1) What kind of measurement error should one attach to the given mathematical model, or in other words,how should one weight the data?
2) What are the statistical techniques to fit the given mathematical, typically deterministic models to the data?

Implicit in both of these questions is a separation of the modelling process from the subsequent statistical analysis.

This chapter presents an attempt to integrate the modelling and the subsequent statistical analysis. Section 2 outlines the classical deterministic model with measurement error, and it reviews in some detail its associated statistical analysis. The section adds some recent developments of practical interest and may be regarded as a supplement to (7). Section 3 presents a stochastic foundation for the model. The inherent process error is derived for the model and incorporated into the statistical analysis. Section 4 and 5 first derive models with alternative stochastic causal mechanisms and then discuss the statistical analysis associated with such models. Section 6 derives estimates of various residence time moments and formulates a statistical analysis based on such transformed variables. Each section is structured first to derive the model and its inherent error distribution, and then to indicate an appropriate statistical analysis for the model with its assumed error structure.

The statistical analysis of stochastic models is a natural extension of previous research on the analysis of deterministic models. It is a very promising and emerging area for both the researcher and the practitioner. Of course, the statistical analysis of any real-world data set may be considered as much an art as a science, and in this light the chapter may raise more questions than it answers. However, we are not aware of any previous comprehensive review of the statistical analysis of these stochastic compartmental models. Hopefully this review will serve as a significant first step in this area and will encourage many further developments.

2. STATISTICAL ANALYSIS OF DATA FROM DETERMINISTIC MODELS

2.1 Deterministic Formulation of Model

Rescigno and Segre (4) outline the history of the development of the deterministic compartmental model, and some recent developments are noted in Rescigno (8) (Chapter 1 of this book). These linear system models have been solved historically using the theory of Laplace transforms. However, for subsequent convenience, the formulation below will be presented in a matrix framework and then solved using matrix analysis. This formulation, from Matis et al. (9), is unique in that it models the system separately for each compartment of origin. This approach will be useful later in tying together various model assumptions.

Consider the following definitions:

1) Let $X_{ij}(t)$, $i,j=1, \ldots, n$; denote the amount of substance in compartment j at time t that originated in compartment i either at the initial time, t=0, or by subsequent entry into i.
2) Let k_{ij}, $i=1, \ldots, n$; $j=0, 1, \ldots, n$; with $i \neq j$; denote the nonnegative transfer rate from i to j. Compartment 0 denotes the system exterior. The units are time^{-1}.
3) Let $k_{ii} = -\sum_{\substack{j=0 \\ j \neq i}}^{n} k_{ij}$, $i=1, \ldots, n$; be the total output rate from i.
4) Let $f_{0i}(t)$, $i=1, \ldots, n$; be the nonnegative input rate at time t from the system exterior to i. The units are mass/time.
5) Let $\underset{\sim}{X}(t) = [X_{ij}(t)]$ and $\dot{\underset{\sim}{X}}(t) = [\dot{X}_{ij}(t)]$ be the nxn matrices of amounts and their derivatives at time t, respectively.
6) Let $\underset{\sim}{K} = [k_{ij}]$ and $\underset{\sim}{F}(t) = \text{diag}\,[f_{0i}(t)]$ be the nxn matrix of flow rates and the nxn diagonal matrix of input rates at time t, respectively.

7) Let $\underset{\sim}{\Lambda} = \text{diag}\ [\lambda_i]$ and $\underset{\sim}{T} = [\underset{\sim}{T}_1, \ldots, \underset{\sim}{T}_n]$ be, respectively, the diagonal matrix of eigenvalues of $\underset{\sim}{K}$ and a corresponding matrix of right eigenvectors of $\underset{\sim}{K}$. By definition, one has $\underset{\sim}{K}\underset{\sim}{T} = \underset{\sim}{T}\underset{\sim}{\Lambda}$.

The usual (linear) compartment model may be represented by the following nxn system of linear differential equations:

$$\dot{\underset{\sim}{X}}(t) = \underset{\sim}{X}(t)\underset{\sim}{K} + \underset{\sim}{F}(t) \quad . \tag{1}$$

Let us now assume the following regularity conditions for the model in Eq. 1.

(i) Each compartment is open, i.e., for each $i \geq 1$ there exists some $j \geq 0$ such that $k_{ij} > 0$.

(ii) The system is open to the exterior, i.e., there exists some $i \geq 1$ such that $k_{i0} > 0$.

(iii) The system is at least weakly connected, i.e., the system cannot be partitioned into two sets S_1 and S_2 such that $k_{ij} = 0 = k_{ji}$ for all compartments i in S_1 and j in S_2.

(iv) The eigenvalues, λ_i are distinct.

Most biomedical system models satisfy conditions (i) to (iii) either directly or through slight model redefinitions. For example, if a system has a closed compartment, also called a sink, the closed compartment may be redefined as an exterior state and thus satisfy (i). A system which is closed to the exterior will follow the subsequent theory with slight modifications to accomodate its single eigenvalue of 0. A system which is not at least weakly connected may be partitioned into two mutually exclusive subsystems, and each subsystem may be analyzed separately. Models with equal eigenvalues in violation of (iv) are not of present interest for statistical analysis since, unless constrained otherwise, the estimates obtained by subsequent data analysis will differ with probability 1. Hence regularity conditions (i) to (iv) are reasonable to impose on system models.

The following theorem has been proven for such linear systems:

Theorem 1: Let $e^{\underset{\sim}{\Lambda}t} = \text{diag}(e^{\lambda_i t})$. The solution to Eq. 1 with regularity conditions (i) - (iv) is

a) for $f_{0i}(t) = 0$, i=1, . . . , n;

$$\underset{\sim}{X}(t) = \underset{\sim}{X}(0)\ \underset{\sim}{T}e^{\underset{\sim}{\Lambda}t}\underset{\sim}{T}^{-1} \tag{2}$$

b) for $X_{ii}(0) = 0$, i=1, . . . , n;

$$\underset{\sim}{X}(t) = \int_0^t \underset{\sim}{F}(s)\ \underset{\sim}{T}e^{\underset{\sim}{\Lambda}(t-s)}\ \underset{\sim}{T}^{-1}\ ds \quad , \tag{3}$$

The theorem is well-known in general linear systems theory (see Hearon (10)). It is useful to separate cases (a) and (b) above since in most pharmacokinetic applications they are mutually exclusive. However, if there are some i and time interval for which $f_{0i}(t) \neq 0$, and also some j for which $X_{jj}(0) \neq 0$, then $\underset{\sim}{X}(t)$ is the sum of Eq. 2 and 3. One immediate consequence of Eq. 2 and/or 3 is that all elements of the $\underset{\sim}{X}(t)$ matrix are sums of exponentials, provided $\underset{\sim}{F}(s)$ is constant.

The implementation of this theory to many specific pharmacokinetic models is outlined in several books on compartmental models (1-6). For the purposes of this chapter, we will illustrate the theory through the two-compartment open model which is sketched in Figure 1 and which is the most widely used two-compartment model in pharmacokinetics (see e.g. Metzler (11)). The $\underset{\sim}{K}$ and $\underset{\sim}{F}(t)$ matrices for this model are immediately

$$\underset{\sim}{K} = \begin{bmatrix} -(k_{12} + k_{10}) & k_{12} \\ k_{21} & -k_{21} \end{bmatrix}, \quad \underset{\sim}{F}(t) = \begin{bmatrix} f_{01}(t) & 0 \\ 0 & f_{02}(t) \end{bmatrix}. \tag{4}$$

One can show that the eigenvalues and the eigenvector matrix with its inverse are:

$$\lambda_2, \lambda_1 = -\tfrac{1}{2}\{(k_{12} + k_{21} + k_{10}) \pm [(k_{12} + k_{21} + k_{10})^2 - 4k_{21}k_{10}]^{\frac{1}{2}}\},$$

$$\underset{\sim}{T} = \begin{bmatrix} \lambda_1 + k_{21} & \lambda_2 + k_{21} \\ k_{21} & k_{21} \end{bmatrix}, \tag{5}$$

$$\underset{\sim}{T}^{-1} = \frac{1}{k_{21}(\lambda_1 - \lambda_2)} \begin{bmatrix} k_{21} & -(\lambda_2 + k_{21}) \\ -k_{21} & (\lambda_1 + k_{21}) \end{bmatrix}$$

Note that the models in Eq. 2 and 3 may be parameterized in several ways. One form is to write the model as a function, h, of the rate parameters, i.e.

$$X_{ij}(t;\underset{\sim}{\Omega}_1) = X_{ii}(0)\, h_{ij}(t;\underset{\sim}{\Omega}_1) \tag{6}$$

where $\underset{\sim}{\Omega}_1$ is the parameter vector$(k_{10}, k_{12}, \ldots k_{n,n-1})$. Another form is the parameterization of the model in terms of exponents (eigenvalues) and coefficients of exponential terms, i.e.

$$X_{ij}(t;\underset{\sim}{\Omega}_2) = X_{ii}(0) \sum_{\ell=1}^{n} a_\ell e^{\lambda_\ell t} \tag{7}$$

with parameter vector $\underset{\sim}{\Omega}_2 = (a_1, \ldots, a_n, \lambda_1, \ldots, \lambda_n)$. In most previous practical applications, the simpler form in Eq. 7 has been used for model fitting. The exponents and coefficients in $\underset{\sim}{\Omega}_2$ were estimated and these were then transformed to rate parameter estimates in $\underset{\sim}{\Omega}_1$ (see e.g. Berman & Schoenfeld (12)). However, current computer hardware and software give an experimenter the option to use either parameterization. Some discussion of the relative merits of each form follows subsequently.

In the case of a bolus input, where $f_{01}(t) = f_{02}(t) = 0$ for $t > 0$, the solutions for the two-compartment model reduce after some algebraic manipulation to:

$$X_{11}(t) = X_{11}(0)[(\lambda_1 + k_{21})e^{\lambda_1 t} - (\lambda_2 + k_{21})e^{\lambda_2 t}]/(\lambda_1 - \lambda_2) \tag{8}$$

$$X_{12}(t) = X_{11}(0)\, k_{12}(e^{\lambda_1 t} - e^{\lambda_2 t})/(\lambda_1 - \lambda_2)$$

$$X_{21}(t) = X_{22}(0)\, k_{21}(e^{\lambda_1 t} - e^{\lambda_2 t})/(\lambda_1 - \lambda_2)$$

$$X_{22}(t) = X_{22}(0)[(\lambda_1 + k_{21})e^{\lambda_2 t} - (\lambda_2 + k_{21})e^{\lambda_1 t}]/(\lambda_1 - \lambda_2).$$

Consider solution $X_{11}(t)$, which models the amount of material in compartment 1 at time t which was introduced into 1 at t=0. The $\underset{\sim}{\Omega}_1$ parameterization of Eq. 6 is given directly by Eq. 8 and the eigenvalues in Eq. 5. The $\underset{\sim}{\Omega}_2$ parameterization is given by using the simplifying transformations

$$a_1 = (\lambda_1 + k_{21})/(\lambda_1 - \lambda_2) \;;\quad a_2 = -(\lambda_2 + k_{21})/(\lambda_1 - \lambda_2) \tag{9}$$

in Eq. 8.

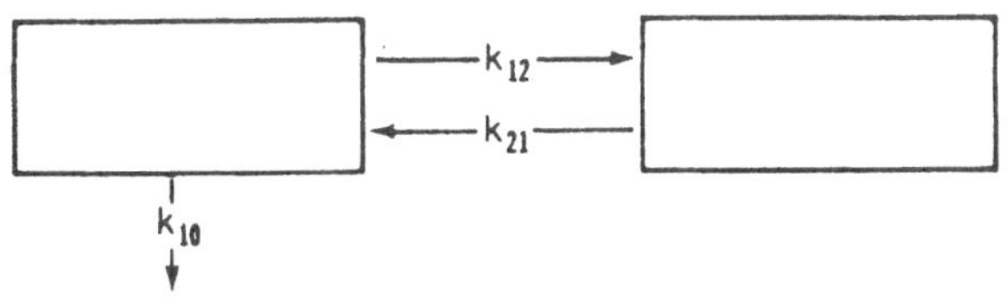

Figure 1

Two-compartment open model with elimination from the first compartment only

2.2 Analysis of Single Input, Single Output (SISO) Data

General Assumptions: Let us now consider the statistical analysis of data from a compartmental system. Clearly, with so many varied applications of compartmental modeling, the types of data generated by the different applications are very diverse. For present simplicity we first consider data from applications satisfying the following assumptions.

1) The system kinetics are sufficiently well-understood to specify the form of the compartmental model, i.e.. to identify the nonzero elements of $\underset{\sim}{K}$ and $\underset{\sim}{F}(t)$ in Eq. 1.

2) The substance of interest is pulse dosed into only one compartment, say compartment 1, at a single time only, say t=0. The amount dosed, $X_{11}(0)$, is a known constant.

3) At M prespecified times, say t_1, t_2, . . . t_M, the amount of substance in some compartment j, j=1, 2, . . . , n; is determined.

By convention, the observed values will be denoted with lower case letters and the corresponding theoretical models with capital letters. In general, the observation would be denoted $x_{1j}(t_m)$. However, for the SISO model, with input only into compartment 1, the notation will be simplified to $x_j(t_m)$.

4) The measurement process is such that the difference between the observation $x_j(t_m)$ and the theoretical solution $X_{1j}(t_m;\underset{\sim}{\Omega})$ (or $X_j(t_m;\underset{\sim}{\Omega})$ for short) is a random error, denoted $\varepsilon_j(t_m)$, which has expectation 0, known variance σ_m^2 and is stochastically independent of the measurement errors at other observation times. This gives rise to a statistical model

$$x_j(t_m) = X_j(t_m;\underset{\sim}{\Omega}) + \varepsilon_j(t_m) \quad m=1, \ . \ . \ . \ , M$$

or in vector notation

$$\underset{\sim}{x}_j = \underset{\sim}{X}_j(\underset{\sim}{\Omega}) + \underset{\sim}{\varepsilon}_j \tag{10}$$

where the random errors have expectation $E[\underset{\sim}{\varepsilon}_j] = \underset{\sim}{0}$ and variance-covariance matrix

$$E[\underset{\sim}{\varepsilon}_j \ \underset{\sim}{\varepsilon}_j^T] = \text{diag}\ (\sigma_1^2, . . . , \sigma^2_M) = \sigma^2 \underset{\sim}{D} \quad . \tag{11}$$

In the above equation, σ^2 plays the role of a scale factor. Hence, with no loss of generality, $\underset{\sim}{D}$ may be normalized so that its diagonal elements sum to M. In many applications, the variances are assumed equal, in which case one has $\underset{\sim}{D} = \underset{\sim}{I}$.

5) The model is such that the $\underset{\sim}{\Omega}$ parameter vector in Eq. 10 is identifiable.

In many practical applications, the data require slight modifications of the above assumptions. Sometimes the amount dosed, $X_{11}(0)$, is an unknown constant, in which case it could be included in expanded $\underset{\sim}{\Omega}_1$ and $\underset{\sim}{\Omega}_2$ parameter vectors. Often the basic measurement is the concentration

$$c_j(t_m) = x_j(t_m)/V_j \quad , \tag{12}$$

where V_j is the "apparent volume of distribution" in compartment j. In this case also, V_j could be included in the $\underset{\sim}{\Omega}_1$ and $\underset{\sim}{\Omega}_2$ vectors. For present simplicity, the subsequent development will focus on the $\underset{\sim}{\Omega}_i$ vectors which include only the rate coefficients or the exponents and coefficients. However, the theory applies to any expanded $\underset{\sim}{\Omega}_i$ vector of parameters.

An alternative to the model with additive errors specified by Eq. 10 is one using multiplicative errors. This model is expressed mathematically as

$$x_j(t_m) = X_j(t_m;\underset{\sim}{\Omega}) \;\; \eta_j(t_m) \quad , m=1, \ldots, M, \tag{13}$$

where

$$\varepsilon_j(t_m) = \log\,(\eta_j(t_m)) \;, \quad m=1, \ldots, M,$$

has expectation $E[\underset{\sim}{\varepsilon}j] = \underset{\sim}{0}$ and the variance-covariance matrix of $\underset{\sim}{\varepsilon}_j$ is given by Eq. 11. The multiplicative error model results in errors which are proportional to the expected response and hence provides a useful model for many experimental situations. However, for present simplicity, the subsequent discussion applies only to the additive model unless otherwise specified.

Estimation Procedures: The estimation of kinetic rate parameters, even from well-designed experiments, is a complex problem. Glass and DeGarreta (13) note that the magnitude of the error in estimating these parameters depends on a variety of factors, including appropriateness of the function to be fitted, weighting factors, correlation between variables, data accuracy, sampling frequency or spacing, number of data points, initial parameter guesses and the estimation method employed. The effect of these factors will be discussed in this and the succeeding sections.

The estimation of $\underset{\sim}{\Omega}$ is complicated considerably by the nonlinear parameterization inherent in both Eq. 6 and 7. One method developed to circumvent the nonlinear parameterization and thus simplify the problem is the so-called curve-peeling (or curve-stripping) procedure. In this procedure, one analyzes the transformed data, $\log x_j(t_m)$, which for large t_m should approximate a simple linear function. Linear regression is then used to fit the straight line in the right tail, thereby estimating the maximum λ_i and its associated a_i. This term is subtracted from Eq. 7 and successive application gives all (λ_i, a_i) pairs (see e.g. Atkins (1)). The method works in practice only in the case when the λ_i's differ substantially. Even then the fitting is subjective and the estimates have no statistical optimality property. The only use of curve-peeling, considering the current state of the art of statistical analysis, is to provide starting values for iterative algorithms. It is surprising that many experimenters still regard the curve-peeling results as acceptable final parameter estimates despite repeated demonstrations of the theoretical and empirical shortcomings of curve-peeling and also in light of the current widespread availability of computer software for alternative nonlinear estimation procedures.

Nonlinear least squares theory provides the generally accepted theoretical basis for the estimation of the $\underset{\sim}{\Omega}$ vector (see e.g. Bard (14)). The ordinary least squares (OLS) estimate, denoted $\hat{\underset{\sim}{\Omega}}_O(x_j)$, is the vector $\underset{\sim}{\Omega}$ which minimizes the sum of squared deviations

$$Q(\underset{\sim}{x}_j,\underset{\sim}{\Omega}) = [\underset{\sim}{x}_j - \underset{\sim}{X}_j(\underset{\sim}{\Omega})]^T [\underset{\sim}{x}_j - \underset{\sim}{X}_j(\underset{\sim}{\Omega})] . \tag{14}$$

The weighted least squares (WLS) estimate, $\hat{\underset{\sim}{\Omega}}_W(\underset{\sim}{x}_j,\underset{\sim}{D})$, is the vector $\underset{\sim}{\Omega}$ which minimizes the weighted sum of squared deviations,

$$Q(\underset{\sim}{x}_j,\underset{\sim}{D},\underset{\sim}{\Omega}) = [\underset{\sim}{x}_j - \underset{\sim}{X}_j(\underset{\sim}{\Omega})]^T \underset{\sim}{D}^{-1} [\underset{\sim}{x}_j - \underset{\sim}{X}_j(\underset{\sim}{\Omega})] , \tag{15}$$

where $\underset{\sim}{D}$ is a diagonal matrix of weights, but is commonly the normalized variance-covariance matrix given in Eq. 11. Many algorithms exist to minimize these quadratic forms, and some will be mentioned subsequently in the discussion of computer programs for nonlinear estimation.

No general theory exists for the small-sample properties of the individual $\hat{\omega}$ elements in $\hat{\underset{\sim}{\Omega}}$ since some, or all, of the ω_i's enter the $\underset{\approx}{X}_j$ model as nonlinear parameters. Instead, the properties of the $\hat{\underset{\sim}{\Omega}}$ estimator may be investigated either theoretically for the asymptotic case where $M \longrightarrow \infty$ or empirically through computer (Monte Carlo) simulation in the case of finite M. A discussion of each follows.

In principle, one could also use other statistical estimation approaches besides the least squares criterion to obtain estimates. Some alternatives include maximum likelihood with nonnormal errors, Bayes estimation, and robust estimation (see e.g. Metzler (7)). However, none of these alternative approaches is currently in widespread useage due to computational difficulties.

Asymptotic Properties of Least Squares Estimates: In order to study the asymptotic properties of the LS estimates, one must specify how M, the number of observations, is assumed to approach ∞. In the particular case which most closely resembles experimental protocol, one has $M \longrightarrow \infty$ by intensifying the sampling within a finite time interval either through replicate observations at a small set of observation times or by letting the time interval between observations approach 0. This asymptotic case has the following properties: (see e.g. (7) and (15)).

1) $\hat{\underset{\sim}{\Omega}}$ has a multivariate normal distribution with mean $\underset{\sim}{\Omega}$.

2) the variance-covariance matrix of $\hat{\underset{\sim}{\Omega}}$ is

$$\begin{aligned} \mathrm{Var}(\hat{\underset{\sim}{\Omega}}) &= (\underset{\sim}{Z}^T \underset{\sim}{D}^{-1} \underset{\sim}{Z})^{-1} \sigma^2 && \text{for the WLS model} \\ &= (\underset{\sim}{Z}^T \underset{\sim}{Z})^{-1} \sigma^2 && \text{for the OLS model} \end{aligned} \tag{16}$$

where $\underset{\sim}{Z} = (Z_{ab})$ is the matrix of partial derivatives

$$Z_{ab} = \partial X_j(t_a;\underset{\sim}{\Omega})/\partial\omega_b \ . \tag{17}$$

These asymptotic results are used in practice to give the following approximations for <u>finite</u> M:

1) The estimated variance of $\hat{\omega}_i$ is

$$\begin{aligned} \mathrm{var}(\hat{\omega}_i) &= b_{ii}s^2 && \text{for WLS model} \\ &= c_{ii}s^2 && \text{for OLS model} \end{aligned} \tag{18}$$

where b_{ii} and c_{ii} are respectively the ith diagonal elements of $(\underset{\sim}{Z}^T\underset{\sim}{D}^{-1}\underset{\sim}{Z})^{-1}$ and $(\underset{\sim}{Z}^T\underset{\sim}{Z})^{-1}$ evaluated at $\hat{\Omega}$, and s^2 is the error mean square estimate of σ^2 in Eq. 16.

2) Based on normal theory, the $(1-\alpha)$ confidence interval for ω_i is

$$\begin{aligned} &\hat{\omega}_i \pm t(\alpha/2,\nu)\ \sqrt{b_{ii}}\ s, \text{for WLS, and} \\ &\hat{\omega}_i \pm t(\alpha/2,\nu)\ \sqrt{c_{ii}}\ s, \text{for OLS,} \end{aligned} \tag{19}$$

where ν is the degrees of freedom in the residual error term.

3) The estimated correlation between $\hat{\omega}_i$ and $\hat{\omega}_j$ is

$$\begin{aligned} \mathrm{corr}(\hat{\omega}_i,\hat{\omega}_j) &= b_{ij}/(b_{ii}\ b_{jj})^{\frac{1}{2}} && \text{for WLS} \\ &= c_{ij}/(c_{ii}\ c_{jj})^{\frac{1}{2}} && \text{for OLS} \end{aligned} \tag{20}$$

where b_{ij} and c_{ij} are off-diagonal elements of the matrices defined in property 1) above.

One immediate problem in the application of WLS estimation is the usual experimental condition where the variances are known to be unequal, but the exact values of $\sigma_1^2, \ldots, \sigma_M^2$, and hence of $\underset{\sim}{D}$ are unknown. In this usual case, $\underset{\sim}{D}$ is also estimated from data, as discussed subsequently.

Another difficult, common problem in the estimation of parameters in compartment models is the very high correlations among the parameter estimates in Eq. 20. This is particularly true for the rate parameters which, although identifiable, may be very highly interrelated in terms of their influence on $X_j(t)$. This high correlation produces the phenomenon of a model which might fit the data exceptionally well, and hence have a very low residual error, but whose parameter estimates have enormous variances in Eq. 18. These huge variances would lead to wide, and for all practical purposes unbounded, confidence limits which might in turn limit the utility of the model despite its excellent fit to the data. Hence, the statistical analysis is often more concerned with this problem of multicollinearity than with the problem of *a priori* identifiability, and principles such as parameter parsimony become very important.

All of the above theory applies to one asymptotic case. There is also another asymptotic case, that where $M \to \infty$ with a fixed time interval between observations, hence where $t_M \to \infty$. It has been pointed out that the above asymptotic properties do not hold in this case. In particular the estimates are not consistent (see e.g. Wu (16)). However, application of this case would imply taking continued observations even after $X_j(t)$ decays to negligible levels, which is contrary to experimental practice.

Small Sample Properties of LS Estimators: No general statistical distribution theory exists for the nonlinear estimates, $\hat{\omega}_i$, from small data samples (finite M). Hence their exact properties are studied empirically using Monte Carlo simulation. The general objective of such studies is to ascertain how well the approximations outlined in the previous sections hold for certain completely specified conditions. The specifications must include 1) the underlying model assumptions with given parameter values, 2) the measurement assumptions including the error structure and the size of M, and 3) the estimation procedure. Since clearly these vary a great deal, the Monte Carlo results usually differ from study to study and they are often difficult to generalize.

The least square estimates of the λ_i and a_i parameters ($\underset{\sim}{\Omega}_2$ parameterization) have been widely used. However, few simulations studies using this parameterization appear in the literature. The problem is further compounded by the fact that most of these simulation studies have no more than 20 replicates per modeling condition which is insufficient to characterize the distributions.

Glass and De Garreta (13) performed a simulation consisting of 20 replicates for each condition of a two-compartment model. They concluded that the data should be collected over a time which adequately defines the function, otherwise large errors occur in the second pair of (λ_i, a_i) estimates involving the slow decay. They also noted that there is great difficulty in accurate estimation of the rate parameters when the λ_i's do not differ substantially.

Westlake (17) notes that usually 95% confidence regions are

constructed to examine the reliability of the parameter estimates, but because of the strong correlation between the parameter estimates, the confidence ellipsoids are greatly elongated. This implies that many very different sets of estimates fit the model equally well. Also, the λ_i and a_i parameter estimates were found to be very sensitive to small changes to the data and hence specific, estimated parameters should be used with great caution even though these estimates may give a very small residual mean square error.

A number of authors indicate the need for weighted least squares estimation of the λ_i and a_i parameters (see e.g. Boxenbaum et al.(18), Peck et al.(19), Wagner (20), and Chennavasin et al.(21)). The majority of these authors suggest weighting either by the observed amount of drug (or concentration) or by the observed amount squared. Peck et al.(19) have developed an "extended" least squares nonlinear regression program which chooses more complex weighting schemes which they claim to be superior.

Boxenbaum et al.(18) studied the accuracy of asymptotic standard deviation estimates given by the least squares algorithms. Simulations showed that the asymptotic standard deviations of the λ_i and a_i parameters frequently underestimate their true values by a factor of 2 or 3.

The difficulty of quantifying the small sample properties of the λ_i and a_i parameter estimates is illustrated in papers by Wagner (20) and Chennavasin et al.(21). Wagner collected raw data from 23 different articles that estimated pharmacokinetic parameters from intraveneous data, and found parameter estimates which differed appreciably from those reported in the original articles. Chennavasin et al. compared articles that derived parameter estimates of furosemide pharmacokinetics. They concluded that the differences between the reported estimates were due, in large part, to the different methods used by the various authors to analyze their data. Thus, any comparison of pharmacokinetic parameter estimates should be made only when each data set has been analyzed using the same estimation procedures.

The small sample properties of the LS estimates of the rate parameters ($\underset{\sim}{\Omega}_1$ parameterization) have been studied recently by Cobelli and Salvan (22), Metzler (23), Matis et al. (24), and Laskarzewski et al. (25). Cobelli and Salvan simulated data with unequal errors and found that the WLS estimates had little apparent bias. Metzler simulated data for a simple irreversible flow model with unequal errors and found that the OLS estimates had relatively small bias but very large variability. Laskarzewski et al. (25) simulated data from one-compartment and two-compartment models with errors whose variance was proportional to the drug concentration. For the one-compartment model, the WLS estimates were nearly unbiased and approximately normally distributed. For the two-compartment model, the WLS estimates were found to have considerable bias and the accuracy of the asymptotic expressions for variance and correlation was also suspect.

Matis et al. (24) simulated data from the two-compartment reversible flow model given in Figure 1 and used both additive normal errors and multiplicative lognormal errors. The study found that the OLS estimates of the k_{12} and k_{21} parameters were seriously biased, with estimated biases of up to 90%, and had enormous variability. The WLS estimates were found to be far superior, with estimated biases of only 5% or less. It was also found that the simulated results were in general agreement with the approximations given in Eq. 18-20. These studies suggest that acceptable estimation of the rate parameters of multi-compartment, reversible models with unequal measurement errors requires WLS estimation. Thus a strong case can be made for WLS estimation for either the $\underset{\sim}{\Omega}_1$ or the $\underset{\sim}{\Omega}_2$ parameterization when the weights, i.e. the $\underset{\sim}{D}$ matrix, are known.

Several empirical weighting schemes have been proposed for the case, common in experimental practice, where the σ_m^2 variances are assumed to be unequal but where the exact values are unknown. When replicate observations are available, it has been noted (26) that the asymptotic approximations in Eq. 18-20 are generally acceptable when $\underset{\sim}{D}$ is replaced by the matrix of sample variances, $\hat{\underset{\sim}{D}} = \text{diag}(s_i^2)$. Gerald and Matis (27) compare several suggested weighting schemes when replicate observations are not available. Their simulation study found that weighting by the reciprocal of the squared observation, i.e. using $\hat{\underset{\sim}{D}} = \text{diag}[x_j(t_m)^{-2}]$, provides generally acceptable, robust results, even when the true variances might be proportional to the observations, $x_j(t_m)$. Neither of the $\hat{\underset{\sim}{D}}$ matrices is difficult to implement in nonlinear least squares computer packages, and hence they are highly recommended.

One fundamental decision is whether to specify the model using the rate coefficient ($\underset{\sim}{\Omega}_1$) or the eigenvalue ($\underset{\sim}{\Omega}_2$) parameterization. Historically, experimenters have chosen the $\underset{\sim}{\Omega}_2$ parameterization due to its simpler functional form. Recently, the $\underset{\sim}{\Omega}_1$ parameterization has grown in favor as new computer software for nonlinear estimation has become available. The limited comparative studies of Cobelli and Salvan (22) support the direct use of the $\underset{\sim}{\Omega}_1$ parameterization for the optimal estimation of the k_{ij} parameters when the form of the compartmental model is known. The $\underset{\sim}{\Omega}_1$ parameterization has also been shown to provide statistically powerful response variables for testing hypotheses about designed experiments, as reported subsequently in this chapter.

Sampling Design. There is a vast recent literature to determine whether all the parameters of a model are identifiable for a given combination of inputs to and outputs from a compartment model (see e.g. DiStefano and Cobelli (28) and also papers in (29)). Identifiability for the present single input, single output (SISO) experiment was assumed previously. The assumption may be checked by determining whether the $\underset{\sim}{Z}$ matrix in Eq. 17 has full column rank, which would imply parameter estimability and hence identifiability. The lack of identifiability would necessitate observations from other compartments.

Assuming one has identifiability, the choice of particular sampling times, t_m, m=1, . . . , M, to minimize, in some sense, the variance-covariance matrix, $Var(\underset{\sim}{\hat{\Omega}})$, is a question of great importance. Landaw (30) shows that certain optimality, D-optimality, may be achieved for a particular model and error structure by finding the set of so-called points of support. The number of points of support s, would satisfy $P \leq s \leq P(P+1)/2$, where P is the number of parameters in the model. If M > s, replicate observations would be taken at the points of support if possible, otherwise the observations would be clustered as close as possible to the points of support. Computer programs have been developed to determine the optimum design, and also to give the relative efficiency of any specified suboptimal design. (see e.g. Metzler et al. (31) and Landaw (30)).

Computer Implementation of Nonlinear LS Procedures: As previously mentioned, the least squares estimator $\underset{\sim}{\hat{\Omega}}$ is obtained by minimizing the sum of squared deviations, Q, in Eq. 14 or 15, and previous sections have discussed the formulation of Q in terms of the observation times $(t_1,..,t_M)$, the weights in $\underset{\sim}{D}$, and the $\underset{\sim}{\Omega}_1$ vs. $\underset{\sim}{\Omega}_2$ parameterization. In practice, Q is minimized through iterative computer algorithms, and the implementation of these algorithms raises several questions.

An immediate question is the choice of a computer program package for nonlinear LS estimation. Metzler (7) discusses and compares three computer program packages, SAS, NONLIN, and BMDP, which are in widespread use for statistical analysis of nonlinear systems. A fourth package, SAAM, is used more extensively for complex modeling and less frequently for statistical analysis. These computer packages require the user to specify the nonlinear function, the weighting factors and the initial parameter guesses. Usually any of several nonlinear estimation methods can be selected (e.g. Gauss-Newton, Marquardt, steepest ascent or derivative-free methods). Thus the experienced user can directly control the "goodness of the fit" and hence the quality of the parameter estimates by specifying these factors.

Recent research by Cobelli and Salvan (22) indicates the importance of good initial starting values for the iterative nonlinear least squares procedures. Subsequently Gerald and Matis (27) quantify the effect of various initial values on the sampling distribution of estimates. These papers indicate that if one does not have an assurance that the initial values are close to the true estimates, and typically such assurance is lacking, it seems imperative to combine the nonlinear algorithm with an initial grid search of many sets of initial values.

The Gauss-Newton nonlinear least squares estimation procedure with modifications by Hartley (32) is by far the most widely used LS method. Many of the current nonlinear LS computer packages now offer a derivative free (or DUD) option. This option not only makes it easier to use the program but also makes it possible to solve some nonlinear systems in which differentiation of the equations with respect to the parameters is either impossible or impractical. Theoretically, the estimates obtained when the derivatives are specified (i.e. DER option) should be equal to the DUD estimates if convergence is achieved. However, this did not occur in practice for the two-compartment model in Fig. 1 (27). The DER estimates tend to remain closer to the initial guesses than the DUD estimates. In some instances the final DER estimates have been observed to remain at their initial values 70% of the time. However, the DUD estimates have been observed to be severely biased under certain system conditions. The authors are not aware of any general recommendation favoring one method over another. The current wisdom seems to favor the use of weighted least squares with the derivatives specified (if possible) and a grid search of possible sets of initial values that cover the Ω parameter space of practical interest.

Sample Simulated Data Set: A small data set was simulated from the two-compartment open model, shown in Figure 1, with bolus input to illustrate some of the above concepts. For simplicity, the parameter values were set at $k_{10} = k_{12} = k_{21} = 1$. The error was assumed to be multiplicative, as in Eq. 13, with $\eta_j(t_m)$ assumed to have a lognormal (0, .01) distribution. A previous study (24) has shown 1) that the size of such error is reasonable and 2) that the results from the multiplicative model are very similar to those from an additive model with a comparable variance. It was assumed that a unit input was introduced into compartment 1 and that the amount remaining in compartment 1 was measured at M = 10 distinct times. The experiment was replicated 10 times to simulate multiple, identical subjects. The simulated data for the first replicate, which is representative, is presented in Table 1.

The SAS NLIN (33) computer program was selected for the estimation due to its widespread usage. It is expected that other computer packages would give similar results. The $X_{11}(t)$ model in Eq. 8 was fitted to the data four times to study the influence of two factors, namely the type of weighting and the method of derivative specification, each at two levels. The four factor level combinations are: 1) DER option with OLS, 2) DER option with WLS where $\hat{\underset{\sim}{D}} = \mathrm{diag}[X_1(t_m)^{-2}]$, 3) DUD option with OLS, 4) DUD option with WLS as before. It should be noted that the assumed error structure implies an error variance which is proportional to the model value $X_1(t_m)$ squared. Thus the above WLS implementation represents a good choice for an empirical weighting scheme. The true parameter values were used as the initial guesses.

Table 1

Simulated Data Set from the Two-Compartment Open Model with Parameter Values $k_{12}=k_{21}=k_{10}=1$ and with Multiplicative Lognormal (0, .01) Error

Time t_m	Error-free Value, function $X_1(t_m,\underset{\sim}{\Omega})$	Simulated Value, observation $x_1(t_m)$
0.1	0.822968	0.77693
0.2	0.684715	0.78515
0.4	0.491156	0.53035
0.6	0.370203	0.38408
0.8	0.292725	0.29624
1.0	0.241428	0.23888
1.5	0.170103	0.14583
2.0	0.132603	0.12116
3.0	0.088157	0.08267
5.0	0.040937	0.03915

TABLE 2

SAS Computer Output for Sample Data Set

S T A T I S T I C A L   A N A L Y S I S   S Y S T E M

NON-LINEAR LEAST SQUARES SUMMARY STATISTICS   DEPENDENT VARIABLE X

SOURCE	DF	WEIGHTED SS	WEIGHTED MS
REGRESSION	3	4.94870481	3.31623494
RESIDUAL	7	0.05129519	0.00732788
UNCORRECTED TOTAL	10	10.00000000	
(CORRECTED TOTAL)	9	5.25569189	

PARAMETER	ESTIMATE	ASYMPTOTIC STD. ERROR	ASYMPTOTIC 95 % CONFIDENCE INTERVAL LOWER	UPPER
K10	1.06154625	0.12880625	0.75696442	1.36612607
K12	0.97505123	0.09518035	0.74998366	1.20011881
K21	0.92683075	0.18003861	0.50110366	1.35255784

ASYMPTOTIC CORRELATION MATRIX OF THE PARAMETERS

	K10	K12	K21
K10	1.000000	0.134729	-0.995437
K12	0.134729	1.000000	-0.114408
K21	-0.995437	-0.114408	1.000000

Table 2 contains the SAS computer output when the model is fitted to the simulated data in Table 1 using the DER option with WLS, i.e. the second factor level combination. The LS estimates which minimize Q in Eq. 15 are $\hat{k}_{10} = 1.062$, $\hat{k}_{12} = 0.975$ and $\hat{k}_{21} = 0.927$. The error mean square is estimated as $s^2 = 0073$.

These LS estimates provide an exceptional fit of the model to the data as indicated by the F-ratio, i.e. the regression mean square divided by the error mean square, of 3.316/0.00733 = 452.5. The fitted values may be obtained by substituting the parameter estimates into Eq. 8. The approximate standard errors of the parameter estimates calculated from Eq. 18 are .129, .095, and .180 respectively. The asymptotic 95% confidence intervals are found by multiplying the standard errors by the t percentage point $t(.025, 7) = 2.365$. The product is then added and subtracted from the parameter estimate as given in Eq. 19. Note that the stated 95% level of confidence applies to each individual confidence interval. To find simultaneous confidence intervals with an overall level of confidence, one should use a family of confidence intervals such as those obtained using Bonferroni's inequality (34) or else a confidence region based on a multivariate distribution. As expected, all three of the confidence intervals contain the true parameter values of 1.0. The estimated correlations between the parameter estimates are given in the correlation matrix. The correlation coefficient between $\hat{k}_{21}$ and $\hat{k}_{10}$ is -0.995. Such large correlation coefficients between parameter estimates are typical of compartment models. In general, compartment models usually fit the data very well, but problems with multicollinearity reduce the precision of individual parameter estimates. This leads to wide confidence intervals for the parameters despite a possibly exceptional fit of the model to the data.

Table 3 lists the parameter estimates and their asymptotic standard error approximations, denoted $s(\hat{k}_{ij})$, for each of the 10 replicates of the four combinations. The means and the standard deviations of the $\hat{k}_{ij}$ estimates, denoted $\overline{k_{ij}}$ and $\hat{\sigma}(k_{ij})$, and the means of the standard error approximations, $\overline{s(\hat{k}_{ij})}$, are also given. The following qualitative conclusions are apparent in the study, and are supported by much more extensive simulation studies:

1) The DER method has smaller estimated biases, i.e. $(\overline{k_{ij}}-1)$
2) The DER method often does not deviate from the given initial parameter guesses.
3) WLS reduces the bias. It also tends to reduce the standard error $\hat{\sigma}(\hat{k}_{ij})$ and improve the standard error approximation, $s(\hat{k}_{ij})$, particularly for the DUD option.

These findings are quantified in (24,27), which also characterize the skewness of the distribution of rate parameter estimates. Such skewness suggests the use of nonparametric procedures for subsequent hypothesis tests relative to possible treatment effects among the individuals. The dependency of the DER method, as well as many other algorithms, on the initial starting values is an important point. Recent study (27) has shown that a similar

TABLE 3

Simulation Results for Four Combinations of Weighting and Derivative Specification with Initial Value Vector [1,1,1].

	SAS DER WT=1			SAS DER WT=1/x^2			SAS DUD WT=1			SAS DUD WT=1/x^2		
Exp #	$\hat{k}_{12}$	$\hat{k}_{21}$	$\hat{k}_{10}$	$\hat{k}_{12}$	$\hat{k}_{21}$	$\hat{k}_{10}$	$\hat{k}_{12}$	$\hat{k}_{21}$	$\hat{k}_{10}$	$\hat{k}_{12}$	$\hat{k}_{21}$	$\hat{k}_{10}$
	$s(\hat{k}_{12})$	$s(\hat{k}_{21})$	$s(\hat{k}_{10})$	$s(\hat{k}_{12})$	$s(\hat{k}_{21})$	$s(\hat{k}_{10})$	$s(\hat{k}_{12})$	$s(\hat{k}_{21})$	$s(\hat{k}_{10})$	$s(\hat{k}_{12})$	$s(\hat{k}_{21})$	$s(\hat{k}_{10})$
1	0.678	1.004	1.094	.975	.927	1.062	.753	.493	.932	.800	.727	1.009
	.182	.271	.145	.095	.180	.129	.310	.492	.357	.095	.120	.023
2	1.000	1.000	1.000	1.000	1.000	1.000	1.286	1.615	1.062	1.209	1.475	1.06
	.154	.148	.107	.169	.303	.240	.141	.395	.081	.236	.282	.029
3	1.027	.965	1.023	1.000	1.000	1.000	1.065	.948	.983	1.416	1.604	1.070
	.291	.236	.169	.165	.321	.254	.278	.686	.249	.310	.396	.030
4	.999	1.001	.999	1.006	.967	1.027	1.005	1.175	1.041	.918	.787	.982
	.175	.169	.123	.121	.227	.171	.189	.554	.148	.137	.165	.037
5	1.000	1.000	1.000	1.000	1.000	1.000	.683	.581	.906	.715	.756	.953
	.314	.301	.218	.135	.244	.191	.232	.561	.260	.086	.133	.026
6	1.003	.993	1.005	1.000	1.000	1.000	1.000	1.000	1.001	1.223	1.232	1.038
	.444	.413	.298	.139	.271	.213	.473	1.222	.409	.245	.273	.036
7	.956	1.086	.937	.968	1.063	.939	5.338	22.45	1.271	.842	.846	.940
	.262	.385	.296	.226	.292	.244	3.752	20.86	.094	.181	.240	.045
8	1.200	1.014	.949	1.000	1.000	1.000	1.317	1.788	1.071	1.034	1.244	1.094
	.300	.269	.222	.234	.430	.339	.359	1.021	.181	.274	.369	.055
9	1.000	1.000	1.000	1.000	1.000	1.000	1.435	1.725	1.073	1.392	1.538	1.056
	.265	.254	.184	.133	.245	.194	.312	.756	.158	.222	.248	.025
10	.989	.962	1.036	1.014	.914	1.080	.862	.673	.990	.946	.851	1.040
	.295	.240	.168	.127	.228	.164	.320	.639	.339	.150	.177	.038
Mean $\hat{k}$	.9852	1.0025	1.0043	.9963	.9871	1.0108	1.4744	3.2448	1.033	1.0495	1.106	1.0245
$\hat{\sigma}(\hat{k})$	.1266	.0330	.0436	.0139	.0423	.0388	1.3794	6.7644	.1013	.2478	.3506	.0549
$\bar{s}(\hat{k})$	.268	.269	.193	.154	.274	.214	.637	2.719	.2276	.186	.240	.0344
Mean $\hat{k}$ excluding Exp #7							1.0451	1.1109	1.0966			
$\bar{s}(\hat{k})$ excluding Exp #7							.2904	.7031	.2424			

dependency occurs even when the starting values are not the true parameter values, which leads to the strong recommmendation for a preliminary grid search of possible starting values as an integral part of the parameter estimation procedure.

The above analysis has obtained a separate set of parameter estimates for each replicate, and then summarized them with sample statistics. Some researchers have used alternative procedures of pooling all replicates into one large data set and then analyzing them as though they came from a single individual. Sheiner and Beal (35) call this the naive pooled data approach. Section 5 discusses the desireability of analyzing each replicate separately.

2.3 Analysis of Data with Other Inputs and/or Outputs

General Assumptions: For present simplicity, the previous statistical theory was developed in the context of a particular single input, single output (SISO) experiment. However, the theory holds for broad generalizations of input and output as noted below. We consider now data that meet the following assumptions:

1) The form of the underlying compartmental model is known.
2) The substance of interest consists of either pulse doses into specified compartments, yielding an initial diagonal matrix $\underset{\sim}{X}(0)$, or continuous infusion into specified compartments, which gives the diagonal input matrix $\underset{\sim}{F}(t)$. Let C, $1 \leq C \leq n$, denote the number of compartments which receive material from the system exterior.
3) At each of M prespecified times, measurements are taken in L, $1 \leq L \leq n$, different compartments. Each time series of observations $\underset{\sim}{x}_\ell$, $\ell = 1, \ldots, L$, is then an M-vector with model

$$\underset{\sim}{x}_\ell = \underset{\sim}{X}_\ell(\underset{\sim}{\Omega}) + \underset{\sim}{\varepsilon}_\ell \quad , \quad \ell = 1, \ldots, L \qquad (21)$$

with $E[\underset{\sim}{\varepsilon}_\ell] = 0$.

4) The measurement process is such that observations are independent for different times and for different time series, i.e.

$$E\left[\underset{\sim}{\varepsilon}_\ell \; \underset{\sim}{\varepsilon}_{\ell'}^{T}\right] = \begin{cases} \underset{\sim}{0} & \ell \neq \ell' \\ \underset{\sim}{D}_\ell & \ell = \ell' \end{cases} \qquad (22)$$

where $\underset{\sim}{D}_\ell$ is a diagonal matrix.

5) The parameter vector is identifiable.

Alternative Input Specifications: The generalization to multiple inputs and/or a continuous infusion input follows the same theory as given. Frequently multiple inputs are used either to achieve complete identifiability or to enhance the precision of parameter estimation. If one can use unique labels for each of C different inputs and if observations occur subsequently in compartment j, then one has C different x_{ij} observation vectors. The vectors may be joined (concatenated) into one combined MxC vector, say $\underset{\sim}{x}_T$, which has model

$$\underset{\sim}{x}_T = \underset{\sim}{X}_T(\underset{\sim}{\Omega}) + \underset{\sim}{\varepsilon}_T \qquad (23)$$

where $\underset{\sim}{\varepsilon}_T$ satisfies all conditions given in section 2.2. Hence one may estimate Ω using the theory given previously. Pond (36) gives an example where a compartment model is used to describe the breakdown of forage particles in ruminant animals. Forage particles of different initial sizes were labelled with various activated rare earth elements and observed in subsequent compartments. The multiple labelling greatly increased the precision of the final estimates.

Often multiple labelling is used but the identity of the different input sources is not preserved. In such cases, the multiple labelling is useful to achieve identifiability. The appropriate model is a weighted sum of $\underset{\sim}{X}_{ij}(\underset{\sim}{\Omega})$'s, and the weighted sum of error vectors satisfies all conditions given previously. Models with continuous infusion follow the same theory; the only change occurs in the specific form of the $\underset{\sim}{X}_{ij}(\underset{\sim}{\Omega})$ model which, of course, is still a sum-of-exponentials function for constant $\underset{\sim}{F}(t)$.

Alternative Output Specifications: Frequently several compartments are accessible for observation. In this case, given a single input, one would have L time series of vectors $\underset{\sim}{X}_{1j}$. These vectors could also be joined together, as above, to yield one combined MxL vector, denoted again as $\underset{\sim}{X}_T$, with the model in Eq. 23. One example of this procedure, though with a different error structure is given in Kodell and Matis (37).

In some instances, one might not have access to specific compartments but might be able to observed various linear combinations of the amounts in the compartments. One example of this is given in (38) where only the total amount which exits the system was observable. In such cases, the appropriate model is a linear combination of the $\underset{\sim}{X}_{ij}(\underset{\sim}{\Omega})$'s and the previous theory is again satisfied. It is also easy to generalize the theory to the case where some of the L observations for multiple outputs, or some of the C observations for multiple inputs, might be missing for one or more of the M sampling times.

3. STATISTICAL ANALYSIS OF DATA FROM STOCHASTIC PARTICLE MODELS

3.1 Stochastic Formulation of a Particle Model

One basic assumption in the previous statistical analysis fitting a deterministic model to data is that the system has no process, or stochastic, error and hence it is plausible to assume that the observations are independent over time. Many generalizations are introduced by modeling the process error which is inherent in the system. One class of generalizations is provided by the stochastic particle model and its extensions which are developed in the following sections. Other generalizations are discussed in (39).

The need to incorporate stochasticity into the model was recognized early in the development of compartmental modeling, and most of the writings on the foundations of the theory discussed in general qualitative terms the probabilistic movement of individual "particles" between compartments (see e.g. Rescigno and Beck (40)). One early paper outlining a quantitative structure for such stochasticity is Bartholomay (41). Matis and Hartley

(38) proposed the so-called stochastic particle model. This stochastic model is closely linked to the deterministic model presented in section 2, and provides a strong, explicit, probabilistic foundation for compartmental models. To illustrate the linkage, we preserve the notation of section 2 but redefine the terms as follows:

1) Let $x_{ij}(t)$, $i,j=1, \ldots, n$; denote the random count of particles which originated in i and are in j at time t.
2) Let k_{ij}, $i=1, \ldots, n$; $j=0, 1, \ldots, n$; with $i \neq j$; denote the probability intensity coefficient, in units of time^{-1}. It is defined such that

   Prob {any given particle in i at time t goes to j in $(t,t+\Delta t) \mid x_{11}(t), \ldots, x_{nn}(t)\} = k_{ij}\Delta t+o(\Delta t)$. (24)
3) Let $k_{ii} = - \sum_{\substack{j=0 \\ j\neq 1}}^{n} k_{ij}$.
4) Let $f_{0i}(t)$, $i=1, \ldots, n$; be the Poisson immigration rate at time t from the system exterior to i. It is defined such that

   Prob {compartment i gains a particle from the system exterior in $(t, t+\Delta t) \mid x_{11}(t), \ldots, x_{nn}(t)\} =$
   $f_{0i}(t)\ \Delta t + o(\Delta t)$. (25)
5) Let $\underset{\sim}{x}(t) = [x_{ij}(t)]$ be the random nxn matrix of $x_{ij}(t)$ counts.

Let also the $\underset{\sim}{K}$, $\underset{\sim}{F}(t)$, $\underset{\sim}{\Lambda}$ and $\underset{\sim}{T}$ matrices be defined as in 6) and 7) previously in Section 2.1.

For this particle model, we assume the following in addition to the previous conditions (i) - (iv) in section 2.1:

(v) The particle transfers are independent.
(vi) The initial counts, $x_{ii}(0)$, are fixed and the $f_{0i}(t)$ and k_{ij} rates are non-stochastic.

The above formulation has many important implications. One basic implication of the "chance mechanisms" defined in Eq. 24 and 25 and in assumption (v), is that the system is probabilistic, or stochastic. In general terms, a stochastic system has an "uncertain output", which in the present context, implies that the counts, $x_{ij}(t)$, are random variables. Thus even in the absence of measurement error, the individual $x_{ij}(t)$ counts are random variables with probability distributions, say $f_{ij}[x;t,\underset{\sim}{\Omega}]$ and hence means (or expected values) and variances denoted respectively by $\mu_{ij}(t;\underset{\sim}{\Omega})$ and $\sigma_{ij}^2(t;\underset{\sim}{\Omega})$. Moreover, the $x_{ij}(t)$'s in general are not independent for different i,j, or t, and hence the multivariate distributions of random vectors of $x_{ij}(t)$'s may involve considerable covariance structure. One general procedure with such a stochastic process is to solve for the mean value functions, $\mu_{ij}(t;\underset{\sim}{\Omega})$, and the variance-covariance structure in order to estimate the parameter vector, $\underset{\sim}{\Omega}$, through the linear model

$$\underset{\sim}{x}_{ij} = \underset{\sim}{\mu}_{ij}(\underset{\sim}{\Omega}) + \underset{\sim}{\varepsilon}_{ij} \quad . \tag{26}$$

In Eq. 26, the random errors $\underset{\sim}{\varepsilon}_{ij}$ have expectation $E[\underset{\sim}{\varepsilon}_{ij}] = \underset{\sim}{0}$, by definition, and the same variance-covariance matrix as $\underset{\sim}{x}_{ij}$. Therefore, whereas before the formulation for the deterministic model involved finding the exact model predictions $X_{ij}(t)$, the complete formulation for the stochastic model requires the multivariate probability distributions of the $x_{ij}(t)$ counts. The statistical moments of interest, i.e., the means, variances and covariances, may then be obtained from the probability distributions.

Other implications of the above stochastic formulation are more technical. Eq. 24 implies that all particles in a given compartment have identical and time-invariant transfer probabilities. Section 4 develops the notion that the time-invariance implies exponential retention times of the particles in the compartments, and the section presents some generalizations. The assumption of identical probabilities is discussed and partially relaxed in section 5. Assumption (v) implies that the system is devoid of clustering and/or binding, and some alternatives to this assumption are presented in section 5 also. In brief, the stochastic formulation provides a very rich theoretical foundation for the micro level of particle transfers. This detailed foundation, which is missing in the corresponding deterministic formulation, can be carefully examined and generalized, where appropriate, in many different ways.

The above conditions are sufficient to prove the following, which are restatements of results in (9) and (42):

<u>Lemma</u>: Let $p_{ij}(0,t)$ denote the probability that a particle in i at t=0 will be in j at time t, and let $\underset{\sim}{P}(0,t) = [p_{ij}(0,t)]$. The above assumptions (i) - (vi) are sufficient to show

$$\underset{\sim}{P}(0,t) = e^{\underset{\sim}{K}t} = \underset{\sim}{T}e^{\underset{\sim}{\Lambda}t}\underset{\sim}{T}^{-1} \quad . \tag{27}$$

<u>Theorem 2</u>. Consider the particles which were initially in i at t=0. The random vector describing their distribution at time t is an (n+1) - fold multinomial with parameters $x_{ii}(0)$ and $p_{ij}(0,t)$, j=1, . . . , n, i.e.

$$\left[x_{i1}(t),\ldots, x_{in}(t)\right] \sim \text{Multinomial } [x_{ii}(0), p_{i1}(0,t),\ldots,p_{in}(0,t)] \tag{28}$$

where the $p_{ij}(0,t)$ are given in Eq. 27.

Theorem 3. Consider the particles which immigrate to i after t=0. The random variables describing their distribution at time t are independent Poisson random variables with parameters $\phi_{ij}(t)$, j=1, . . . , n, respectively. Therefore

$$\left[x_{i1}(t), \ldots, x_{in}(t)\right] \sim \text{Poisson}[\phi_{i1}(t), \ldots, \phi_{in}(t)] , \tag{29}$$

where

$$\underset{\sim}{\phi} = [\phi_{ij}(t)] = \int_0^t \underset{\sim}{F}(s)\, \underset{\sim}{T} e^{\underset{\sim}{\Lambda}(t-s)} \underset{\sim}{T}^{-1}\, ds . \tag{30}$$

In most practical applications, all particles of interest are either started at t=0 or are introduced after t=0. Also, the particles usually are started in only one location. However, for the sake of generality, let $x_{.j}(t) = \sum_{i=1}^{n} x_{ij}(t)$ represent the total count in compartment j of particles introduced at t=0 and through subsequent immigration. It follows then that the distribution of the random vector $\left[x_{.1}(t), \ldots, x_{.n}(t)\right]$ is a convolution of the multinomials in Eq. 28 and the independent Poissons in Eq. 29.

The moments of the $x_{ij}(t)$'s are readily found from the distribution above. The distribution of $x_{ij}(t)$ for particles initially in the system at t=0, corresponding to the pulse dosing, is the binomial which is the marginal distribution of Eq. 28. Therefore, the expectation of $x_{ij}(t)$ has the form

$$\mu_{ij}(t) = x_{ii}(0)\; p_{ij}(t) \tag{31}$$

(see e.g. (43)), from whence the matrix of expectations is

$$E[\underset{\sim}{x}(t)] = \underset{\sim}{x}(0)\underset{\sim}{T}e^{\underset{\sim}{\Lambda}\underset{\sim}{t}}\underset{\sim}{T}^{-1} \tag{32}$$

where $\underset{\sim}{x}(0)$ is a diagonal matrix. Note that this coincides with the deterministic model in Eq. 2, which implies that one would fit the same mathematical functions to the data even though the foundation and interpretations have changed somewhat. However, different weighting schemes are required in the least squares estimation.

The distribution of $x_{ij}(t)$ describing those particles immigrating to the system after t=0, according to Eq. 25, is a Poisson with parameter $\phi_{ij}(t)$. It follows that the expectation of $x_{ij}(t)$ is $\phi_{ij}(t)$, and hence the matrix of expectations is

$$E[\underset{\sim}{x}(t)] = \int_0^t \underset{\sim}{F}(s)\ \underset{\sim}{T}e^{\underset{\sim}{\Lambda}(t-s)}\underset{\sim}{T}^{-1}\ ds, \tag{33}$$

which coincides with the deterministic model in Eq. 3. The variance-covariance matrices for the $x_{ij}(t)$ counts at any given time t are also easy to find from the distributions given in Eq. 28 and 29.

3.2 Analysis of Data from the Stochastic Particle Model

General Assumptions: Let us now consider the statistical analysis of data from a stochastic particle model under assumptions similar to those imposed for data from the deterministic model in section 2.2. Specifically, we assume the following:

1) The form of the compartmental model is known.
2) The substance of interest is introduced into one compartment, say compartment 1, at t=0. This initial number of particles, $x_{11}(0)$, is a known constant.
3) The count in some compartment j, j=1, . . ., n, is measured at M prespecified times. The random count, $x_{1j}(t_m)$, m=1,. . ., M, will be denoted $x_j(t_m)$ for present convenience.
4) The counting is error-free, i.e. there is no measurement error. Hence one has the linear model in Eq. 26, i.e.

$$\underset{\sim}{x}_j = \underset{\sim}{\mu}_j(\underset{\sim}{\Omega}) + \underset{\sim}{\varepsilon}_j \tag{34}$$

where $\underset{\sim}{\varepsilon}_j$ represent only the process errors resulting from the inherent stochastic variability introduced by Eq. 24. It follows through properties of expectations that $E(\underset{\sim}{\varepsilon}_j) = \underset{\sim}{0}$. The variance-covariance matrix for this process error, denoted

$$E[\underset{\sim}{\varepsilon}_j\ \underset{\sim}{\varepsilon}_j^T] = \underset{\sim}{\Sigma}_p(\underset{\sim}{\Omega})\ , \tag{35}$$

must be derived from the model.
5) The $\underset{\sim}{\Omega}$ parameter vector in Eq. 34 is identifiable.

The slight modification for concentration data may be handled as before in section 2.2. The generalization to include counting error will be considered subsequently. Although most applications do involve counting error, there are many problems where $x_{11}(0)$ is relatively small and the counting is exact, as in (38). The present assumption is useful also to identify the general effect of process error alone.

Estimation Procedure for a Model without Measurement Error:
Chiang (44) has shown that the estimator $\hat{\Omega}(\underset{\sim}{x}_j)$ which minimizes the quadratic form

$$Q(\underset{\sim}{x}_j, \Sigma, \Omega) = [\underset{\sim}{x}_j - \underset{\sim}{\mu}_j(\Omega)]^T \underset{\sim}{\Sigma}_p^{-1}(\Omega) \ [\underset{\sim}{x}_j - \underset{\sim}{\mu}_j(\Omega)] \tag{36}$$

is asymptotically normal as $x_{11}(0) \longrightarrow \infty$, with variance-covariance matrix given in Eq. 16 where $\underset{\sim}{\Sigma}_p$ is substituted for $\underset{\sim}{D}$. Therefore, one can use least squares procedures to estimate $\underset{\sim}{\Omega}$ and then apply the approximations given in Eq. 18-20 for the case of finite $x_{11}(0)$.

In order to minimize Q in Eq. 36, one must first find the elements of the $\underset{\sim}{\Sigma}_p$ matrix. The diagonal elements correspond to the variances of the counts and from properties of the binomial distribution they are

$$\sigma^2_{jj}(t_m) = \text{Var}[x_j(t_m)] = x_{11}(0) \ p_{1j}(t_m) \ [1-p_{1j}(t_m)] \tag{37}$$

where $p_{1j}(t_m)$ is given in Eq. 27. The off-diagonal elements are the covariances which may be shown from properties of the chain-binomial distribution (see e.g. (45)) to be

$$\sigma^2_{jj}(t_m, t_m') = \text{Cov}[x_j(t_m), x_j(t_m')] = x_{11}(0) p_{1j}(t_m)[1-p_{1j}(t_m')]$$

$$\text{for } t_m \leq t_{m'} \ . \tag{38}$$

In practice, Q is minimized in a two-step process. A trial value of $\underset{\sim}{\Omega}$ is specified which determines the initial $\underset{\sim}{\Sigma}_p$ matrix. Q is then minimized to find the generalized LS estimate of Ω for the given initial $\underset{\sim}{\Sigma}_p$ matrix. Although most computer programs do not provide generalized LS procedures directly, an equivalent procedure is to find the spectral decomposition of $\underset{\sim}{\Sigma}_p$, transform the data, and then use WLS procedures on the transformed data as outlined in (37). The estimate of $\underset{\sim}{\Omega}$ is then used to update $\underset{\sim}{\Sigma}_p$, and the process is repeated until the procedure converges to give $\hat{\underset{\sim}{\Omega}}$.

A recent variation on this analysis is the conditional least squares approach (46). The conditional least squares procedures transforms the model and simplifies the estimation process to one involving a diagonal Σ matrix, as in section 2.2.

Generalization to Other Outputs: When output is determined from several compartments, the above procedures may be modified as previously in section 2.3. The case where only the sum of all outputs is known is considered in (38) which also derives its appropriate $\underset{\sim}{\Sigma}_p$ matrix and applies it to sample data. A χ^2 goodness-of-fit test is also derived. The case where two compartments are observed simultaneously is discussed in (37).

Implications of the Stochastic Particle Model: There are two practical qualitative differences between the analysis of data assuming the stochastic model and that assuming the deterministic model. Both of the differences are related to the variance-covariance matrix, since the regression equations to be fitted are identical in form. The first difference is the functional linkage between the moments, e.g. between the means and variances, in the stochastic particle model. Several papers have observed that the coefficient of variation for a count $x_{ij}(t)$, defined as

$$CV[x_{ij}(t)] = Var[x_{ij}(t)]^{\frac{1}{2}} / E[x_{ij}(t)] \ , \tag{39}$$

is inversely proportional to $x_{11}(0)^{\frac{1}{2}}$, as noted when equations such as Eq. 31 and 37 are substituted into Eq. 39. Since the number of particles (molecules) in applications involving drug and tracer kinetics is of the order 10^{20}, McInnis et al. (47) observe that the coefficient of variation (also called the relative variation) of $x_{ij}(t)$ in such applications is small and they therefore question the usefulness of the stochastic particle model. However, Rescigno and Matis (48) note the above argument but point out cases where the coefficient of variation is sizeable despite the large number of particles. In general, when data exhibit larger relative variation than that predicted by the stochastic particle model, one should consider whether 1) the data have measurement error also and/or 2) whether the system has binding or clustering. Both of these are discussed subsequently.

The second practical qualitative difference between the analyses is the non-zero off-diagonal elements of $\underset{\sim}{\Sigma}$ under the stochastic model. As pointed out in (37) this serial correlation between observations has the conceptual effect of reducing the information of the sample, which would widen the confidence regions of the parameter estimates. Stated in another way, if the observations were correlated over time due to stochastic variation and one were to ignore the correlation by using the improper WLS procedure in Eq. 15, the confidence intervals for the parameter estimates given in Eq. 19 would be too narrow.

As an illustration of this, (37) contains data simulated according to the probabilistic assumptions in section 3.1 with $k_{12} = 0.50$ and $k_{21} = 0.25$. The 95% confidence intervals for the parameters using WLS with the correct $\underset{\sim}{\Sigma}$ matrix were (0.4586, 0.6410) and (0.1914, 0.6024) and the corresponding intervals using the usual OLS procedures were (0.5266, 0.6036) and (0.3961, 0.5671). Hence both intervals using the OLS procedures, which are inappropriate for the particle model, are apparently too narrow since they failed to contain the true parameter point, whereas the analysis procedures of section 3.2 gave wider, more realistic intervals.

Estimation Procedure for Stochastic Models with Measurement Error: In many cases, particularly those involving large initial $x_{11}(0)$, the measurement errors are not negligible relative to the process errors. In such cases, it is usually reasonable to assume that the two error components are additive and independent. Thus the total variance-covariance matrix, denoted $\Sigma_T(\Omega)$, would be the sum of the variance-covariance matrix of the process error, $\Sigma_p(\Omega)$, in section 3 and that of the measurement errors, Σ_M, in section 2, i.e.

$$\Sigma_T(\Omega) = \Sigma_p(\Omega) + \Sigma_M \tag{40}$$

The $\hat{\Omega}$ estimates are then obtained by substituting $\Sigma_T(\Omega)$ in place of $\Sigma_p(\Omega)$ in Eq. 36.

4. STATISTICAL ANALYSIS OF DATA FROM STOCHASTIC MODELS WITH AGE- AND TIME-VARYING RATES

4.1 Stochastic Particle Model with Age-and Time-Varying Rates

General Framework: One key assumption of the previous stochastic particle model is the age- and time-invariance of the probability intensity coefficient, k_{ij}, as given in Eq. 24. To focus on this assumption, let us assume that the particle was introduced to the system at t=0 and to compartment i at time t'. Let a=t-t' denote the present "age", or retention time, of the particle in i since its most recent entry. Then one could restate Eq. 24 as

$$\text{Prob}\{\text{a given particle of age } a \text{ in compartment } i \text{ at time } t \text{ transfers to compartment } j \text{ by time } t+\Delta t\} = k_{ij}\Delta t+o(\Delta t), \quad \text{for } i,j = 1, \ldots, n. \tag{41}$$

The above transfer probability implies that the likelihood of particle transfer from i to j is independent both of the time t which the particle has spent in the total system and of the age which the particle has spent in compartment i. The particle is said to "lack a memory" both of time and of age. Consequently, the assumption implies that the particle in i which entered the compartment (or the system) most recently is as likely to transfer as the particle which has been in i (or in the system) for the longest period of time.

It has been shown (49) that an equivalent characterization of the assumption in Eq. 24 and 41 is the assumption of exponentially distributed retention times in compartment i of these particles passing to j. In mathematical terms, the assumption is as follows:

Assumption: Let R_{ij} denote the retention time in i of a particle which transfers from i to j. Let R_{ij} have probability density function with parameter k_{ij},

$$f_R(a;k_{ij}) = k_{ij} \exp(-k_{ij}a), \quad a \geq 0, \quad k_{ij} \geq 0. \qquad (42)$$

The deterministic analog of time- and age-invariance is the notion of a "homogeneous" compartment. Wise(50) has challenged for many years the assumption of homogeneous compartments. As an alternative, he has formulated the power law model which has been successfully fitted to describe the kinetics of many substances in certain physiological compartments. One such substance is bone, where a particle of the substance is envisioned to "drift" through a medium rather than being instantly mixed with all other particles. The Wise power law models have a stochastic formulation related to first-passage times in a random walk with drift. Wise's generalization thus describes a relatively detailed causal mechanism as the alternative to homogeneous compartments.

A second approach to generalizing Eq. 41 is to assume simple parametric forms for the time- and age-varying rates without a detailed linkage to specific causal mechanisms. This approach specifies the time-varying rates as follows,

$$\text{Prob \{a given particle of age a in i at time t transfers to j by } t+\Delta t\} = k_{ij}(t)\Delta t + o(\Delta t) \qquad (44)$$

and the age-varying rates as follows,

$$\text{Prob \{a given particle of age a in i at time t transfers to j by } t+\Delta t\} = k_{ij}(a)\,\Delta t + o(\Delta t)\ . \qquad (45)$$

In practice, Eq. 44 is incorporated by using simple functional forms, such as periodic functions, for $k_{ij}(t)$. Age-dependency can either be implemented directly by assuming functional forms of $k_{ij}(a)$ or by assuming various non-exponential retention time distributions which, of course, imply age-varying rates.

Stochastic Solutions with Age-Varying Rates: The general solution for compartment models with non-exponential retention times is given by Weiner and Purdue (51) and by Marcus and Becker (52). The solution is based on the theory of semi-Markov processes (53). The solution is given in general terms and its complexity rules out a general analytical solution for the distribution of the $x_{ij}(t)$ counts.

One simplifying assumption which has been proposed in (54) is to assume that one or more compartments have gamma retention time distributions. This assumption yields a rich family of distributions which is very flexible in describing nonnegative, unimodal lifetime variables such as might be encountered in compartmental passage. The particular family of gamma distributions in common useage is further assumed to have an integer-valued shape parameter, n. This probability density function, also called the Erlang density, of the retention time R_{ij} is

$$f_R(a;\lambda_{ij},n) = \lambda_{ij}^{\,n}\, a^{n-1} \exp\{-\lambda_{ij}a\}/(n-1)! \qquad (46)$$

$$\text{with } a \geq 0,\ \lambda_{ij} > 0,\ n=1,2,\ldots$$

The λ_{ij} parameter is called the scale parameter. Johnson & Kotz (55) illustrate the wide variety of unimodal shapes which the gamma distribution can produce. Note that the exponential distribution in Eq. 42 is a special case of the gamma with n=1.

The age-varying transfer rate, also called the hazard rate, can be obtained from a density function through the relationship

$$k_{ij}(a) = f_R(a)/\left[1 - \int_0^a f_R(t)\,dt\right] . \qquad (47)$$

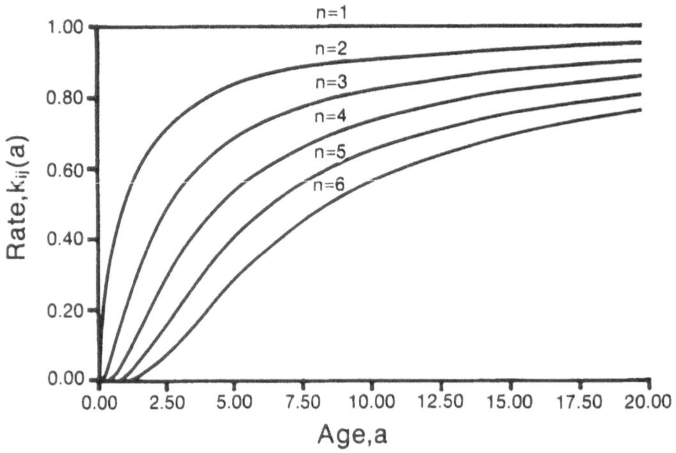

FIGURE 2

Age-varying rate functions for gamma retention time distributions with λ_{ij} = 1 and several small, integer n.

Therefore, the age-varying rate corresponding to a gamma retention time is found by substituting Eq. 46 into Eq. 47 to yield (see e.g. (56)).

$$k_{ij}(a) = \frac{\lambda_{ij}^{\,n}\, a^{n-1}/(n-1)!}{\sum_{\ell=0}^{n-1} (\lambda_{ij}a)^{\ell}/\ell!} \quad . \tag{48}$$

The age-varying rate function is illustrated in Figure 2 for $\lambda_{ij}=1$ and for several small n.

Note that for n=1, the gamma gives the constant rate λ_{ij}. The form of the hazard rate for n > 1 has been found to have wide application in natural processes which either lack instant mixing and/or have an inherent initialization or retardation period. The first is often apparent in data where the actual physical sampling site is not the exact site of material introduction, which indeed is usually the case in practice. The second occurs in processes such as digestion where an initial coating inhibits digestive breakdown but which then asymptotes to a constant rate λ_{ij}.

The solution of a system with gamma (Erlang) compartments may be obtained as a limiting case of a system with exponential compartments. Mathematically, a gamma (n,α) compartment may be created by a sequence of n consecutive exponential (α) compartments. Hence, the previous solutions given in Theorems 2 and 3 hold for the gamma compartment models except that one has n equal eigenvalues, whereas before they were assumed unequal. The limiting case of the previous solution when the eigenvalues approach equality gives the desired new solution. Matis (54) gives the following particular solution for a two-compartment irreversible model where the first compartment is a "gamma" compartment with parameters λ_1 and n, and the second is an exponential compartment with parameter k_2:

$$E\left[x_{11}(t)\right] = e^{-\lambda_1 t} \sum_{\ell=1}^{n} (\lambda_1 t)^{\ell-1}/(\ell-1)!$$

$$E\left[x_{12}(t)\right] = e^{-k_2 t}\left(\frac{-\lambda_1}{k_2-\lambda_1}\right)^{n} - e^{-\lambda_1 t} \sum_{\ell=1}^{n} \left(\frac{-\lambda_1}{k_2-\lambda_1}\right)^{\ell} \frac{(\lambda_1 t)^{n-\ell}}{(n-\ell)!} \tag{49}$$

The above functions are relatively simple for small n. Hughes and Matis (57) give the solution for two consecutive gamma compartments. We are not aware of any analytical solutions for multicompartment models using age-varying rates other than those in Eq. 48 derived from the gamma.

Stochastic Solutions with Time-Varying Rates: The closed form solution for a general system with time-varying rates has proven intractible. However, the solution for an irreversible system with time-varying rates is given in (58) and the solution for a system where all rates have the same parametric form with possibly different coefficients is given in (59).

4.2 Statistical Analysis of Data

Once the $\mu_{ij}(t;\underset{\sim}{\Omega})$ regression functions have been obtained, the model may be fitted to data using the estimation theory given in section 3. However, several points are unique to these models. Previously one had the option of using either the rate parameter ($\underset{\sim}{\Omega}_1$) or the eigenvalue ($\underset{\sim}{\Omega}_2$) parameterization with the exponents and their coefficients. Clearly, the $\underset{\sim}{\Omega}_2$ parameterization loses its attraction with gamma retention time compartments since the $\underset{\sim}{\Omega}_1$ parameterization involves only two coefficients, n and λ_{ij} for each compartment, whereas the $\underset{\sim}{\Omega}_2$ parameterization involves n+1 coefficients, one for each power of t.

In practice, when there is only one gamma compartment, a series of models is produced, one for each integer, n. The models are fitted starting with n=1 and then increasing n in steps of 1. The error sum of squares, which determines the fit of the model, reaches a minimum for small n, usually n=2,3, or 4, and then increases monotonically as n increases. Therefore, the usual practice is to fit models with increasing n until the error sum of squares begins to increase. When there are several gamma compartments, models with various combinations of small n_i are fitted until the minimum is located in the same way (57).

In many applications, the principal interest of the experiment is on the estimation of a key rate coefficient and the other, usually prior, compartmental structure is of interest only inasmuch as it describes how material passes to the compartment in question. One example of such applications is the modeling of forage passage in ruminant animals. In this application, the initial compartments and rates may be interpreted as describing the rumen mixing and the key rate is the turnover rate from the final compartment which may be interpreted as the rate of passage from the rumen (see e.g. (60)). The initial mixing generates so-called "nuisance" parameters which must be estimated in order to reduce the model error sum of squares and thus enhance the precision with which the passage rate is estimated. Two approaches are possible to model the initial mixing. The first is to describe it by adding exponential compartments until the error mean square is minimized. This traditional approach generates models which fit the data well, as measured by the error mean square or by the coefficient of determination, R^2, yet paradoxically it produces a very poor precision for the estimation of the key parameter, the passage rate. This results from the fact that the proliferation of parameters increases the multicollinearity problem mentioned in section 2.2 with its resulting wide confidence intervals for any particular parameter. The alternative approach is to use a gamma compartment to describe the initial mixing. This second approach has far fewer parameters, and its model may not fit the data as well as the traditional approach as measured by the error mean square or R^2. However, the precision of the rate parameter may be increased substantially since there are fewer nuisance parameters.

The above considerations hold even when the structure of the model is well-formulated. Rodda (61) discusses the desirability of the minimum model and the importance of parameter parsimony for subsequent statistical inference with parameter estimates.

The following data given in (36) may be used to illustrate many of these principles. In this experiment, cows were fed a diet of coarsely ground straw particles, and one labelled meal of unknown size was given to the cows. The number of labelled particles recovered per gram of fecal output was recorded at various elapsed times since feeding. The data for one representative cow are given in Table 4.

Several models were fitted to the data. The stochastic theory was used to generate the models, however, the magnitude of the measurement (and sampling) errors was much larger than that of the stochastic error. Therefore, the OLS procedures of section 2 were used to fit the models to the data.

The first model was a two-compartment, irreversible model with exponential residence times and with elimination from the second compartment only. A fixed time delay was added to the model. The expected number of particles remaining in the system under this model, denoted $\mu_1(t)$, may be found by adding $E[x_{11}(t-\tau)]$ and $E[x_{12}(t-\tau)]$ in Eq. 49 with n=1. This yields (see also (36))

$$\mu_1(t) = x_{11}(0)\left[\lambda_1 e^{-k_2 t^*} - k_2 e^{-\lambda_1 t^*}\right]/(\lambda_1 - k_2), \text{for } t^* \geq 0$$
$$= x_{11}(0) \qquad ,\text{for } t^* < 0$$

with $t^* = t - \tau$.

TABLE 4

Number of labelled straw particles recovered per gram at various sampling times

time (hrs)	0	12	24	32	36	40	44	48	52	56	60
# particles	0	4	101	340	468	536	677	723	543	417	475

time (hrs)	71	95	119	143	167	191	215	234	287	335	359
# particles	469	235	126	99	104	90	45	30	17	14	6

However, since the available data describe the rate of particle elimination, the model appropriate for fitting to the data is the derivative of $\mu_1(t)$ and is given by

$$-\mu_1'(t) = x_{11}(0)\ \lambda_1 k_2\left(e^{-k_2\ t^*} - e^{-\lambda_1\ t^*}\right)/(\lambda_1 - k_2), \text{ for } t^* \geq 0$$
$$= 0 \qquad , \text{for } t^* < 0 \tag{50}$$

indicating the rate at which particles are expected to depart. When Eq. 50 is fitted to the data, the LS estimates are $\hat{x}_{11}(0) = 41{,}023$, $\hat{\lambda}_1 = 0.0744$, $\hat{k} = 0.0239$, and $\hat{\tau} = 21.01$. The mean squared error is $s^2 = 4155.3$ and the F-ratio is 154.0.

The second model assumes that the first compartment has gamma $(2,\lambda_1)$ residence times. The model to be fitted to the data, $\mu_2'(t)$, is found by summing the expectations in Eq. 49 with n=2 and then differentiating the sum. The model so obtained giving the rate of decrease in the expected number of particles is

$$-\mu_2'(t) = x_{11}(0)\ k_2\left\{e^{-k\ t^*}\left(\frac{\lambda_1}{k_2-\lambda_1}\right)^2 + e^{-\lambda_1 t^*}\left[\left(\frac{\lambda_1^2}{k_2-\lambda_1}\right)t^* - \left(\frac{\lambda_1}{k_2-\lambda_1}\right)^2\right]\right\} \quad \text{for } t^* \geq 0$$
$$= 0 \text{ for } t^* < 0$$

where $t^* = t - \tau$.

(51)

When fitted to the data in Table 4, the model has OLS estimates $\hat{x}_{11}(0) = 40{,}062$, $\hat{\lambda}_1 = 0.229$, $\hat{k}_2 = 0.0207$ and $\hat{\tau} = 23.95$. The mean squared error for model 2 is $s^2 = 3404.9$ with an F-ratio of 188.9.

The third model assumes a single compartment with gamma $(2,\lambda_1)$ residence times. It may be derived from $E[x_{11}(t-\tau)]$ in Eq. 49 with n=2, or as a limit of Eq. 50 or 51. Its rate of decrease in the expected value is

$$-\mu_3'(t) = x_{11}(0)\lambda_1^2\ t^*\ \ e^{-k\ t^*}, \text{ for } t^* \geq 0 \tag{52}$$
$$= 0 \qquad , \text{ for } t^* < 0\ .$$

Its OLS parameter estimates are $\hat{x}_{11}(0) = 34{,}197$, $\hat{\lambda}_1 = 0.0474$ and $\hat{\tau} = 23.73$ with $s^2 = 4433.9$ and an F-ratio of 191.7.

In comparing these models, clearly the second provides a better fit to the data than does the first. Its estimated particle residence time distribution and estimated age-varying transfer rate may be found by substituting the OLS estimates into Eq. 46 and 48 respectively. The second model also provides a better fit than the third on the basis of s^2 . However, as noted in (36), the third often provides a more powerful basis for subsequent statistical analysis to detect treatment effects since it has fewer parameters and hence greater precision of key parameter estimates.

5. STATISTICAL ANALYSIS OF DATA FROM MODELS WITH INTERSUBJECT VARIABILITY AND/OR PARTICLE CLUSTERING

5.1. Introduction

Consider an experiment that is replicated on U subjects, and let ${}_u x_{ij}(t;{}_u\underset{\sim}{\Omega})$ denote the data on the uth subject, u=1, ..., U, where ${}_u\underset{\sim}{\Omega}$ represents the parameter vector of subject u. Two cases are encountered in practice. Sometimes data are available on each subject individually, in which case the individual vectors, ${}_1\underset{\sim}{\Omega}, \ldots, {}_U\underset{\sim}{\Omega}$ could be estimated separately using the theory developed previously. Often, however, data are not available on separate subjects, but instead one has mean data of the form

$$\bar{x}_{ij}(t;{}_1\underset{\sim}{\Omega}, \ldots, {}_U\underset{\sim}{\Omega}) = \sum_{u=1}^{U} {}_u x_{ij}(t;{}_u\underset{\sim}{\Omega})/U \quad . \tag{52}$$

Cocchetto et al. (62) give many examples in the fields of toxicology and pharmacokinetics of studies where only such mean data, pooled over many subjects, are available. In either case, whether analyzing mean data or separate data sets, the primary objective is to make statistical inferences concerning the underlying distribution of the ${}_u\underset{\sim}{\Omega}$'s. This raises questions concerning both appropriate models and analyses.

Consider first the case where the individual ${}_u x_{ij}(t;{}_u\underset{\sim}{\Omega})$'s and hence the estimated ${}_u\underset{\sim}{\Omega}$ vectors are available. Sheiner and Beal (35) point out numerous problems in pooling the ${}_u\underset{\sim}{\Omega}$ estimates due to variability in the amount and quality of data and in the experimental design used for the different subjects. In particular, it has been noted that the arithmetic average of the ${}_u\underset{\sim}{\Omega}$ estimates may deviate substantially from and be biased estimates of the true population values. Sheiner and Beal (35) suggest an alternative approach. The general problem is considered for this case where separate data sets are available in the analysis section 5.3 below.

The case where only mean data are available requires careful consideration of the model as well as of the subsequent statistical analysis. If there were no variability in the parameter vector, i.e. if ${}_1\underset{\sim}{\Omega} = \ldots = {}_U\underset{\sim}{\Omega}$, then the mean data could be modeled by the previous $x_{ij}(t;\underset{\sim}{\Omega})$ solution for a single subject and the problem is primarily one of statistical inference with incomplete or inaccurate error term specification. However, it is self-evident in most applications that intersubject variability, usually sizeable in nature, exists among the ${}_u\underset{\sim}{\Omega}$ vectors in the rate coefficients, in the apparent volumes of distribution, and/or in the sizes of the initial doses. Such intersubject variability leads to new models given below which are different from the ones given in previous sections. These models are called models for heterogeneous subjects.

Another class of generalizations occurs when a given system has heterogeneous particles, i.e. particles with differing k_{ij} transfer coefficients in violation of the assumption in Eq. 24. Such particle variability is a very useful construct for many problems. Typically only the aggregate data measuring the cumulative count of all particles are available. Heterogeneous particles generate new models also.

A third class of generalizations arises when the particles within a subject transfer either as clusters or bound to one another. Such clustering/binding invalidates the assumption of independent particles given in assumption (v) of section 3.1. Bernard (63) describes processes with such phenomena. The dependency between particle transfers leads to modified models and analyses.

5.2 Stochastic Models with Mixing and/or Clustering

Models with Intersubject Variability: To illustrate the effects of intersubject variability, consider a deterministic one-compartment open model

$$X(t;k) = X(0)e^{-kt} \tag{53}$$

where k is a random rate coefficient which varies among subjects. Let k have probability density function $f(k;\underset{\sim}{\phi})$, where $\underset{\sim}{\phi}$ is a vector of parameters. Suppose now that 1) a sample of subjects is chosen at random, 2) each subject has the same experimental design and measurement error variability, and 3) the data are pooled, or aggregated, over all subjects. It follows that the model which should be fitted to the aggregate data, $\overline{X}(t;k)$, is the expectation

$$E[\bar{X}(t;k)] = \int_0^{\infty} X(t;k)\ f(k;\underset{\sim}{\phi})\ dk \tag{54}$$

$$= X(0)M_k(-t;\underset{\sim}{\phi}) \quad .$$

The function M_k is called the moment-generating function of the random variable k, with argument (-t) and parameter vector $\underset{\sim}{\phi}$. As an example, let us assume that the variable k has a gamma distribution with parameters α and β. One could write $f(k;\underset{\sim}{\phi})$ as

$$f(k;\underset{\sim}{\phi}) = k^{\alpha-1} \exp\{-k/\beta\}/\beta^{\alpha}\Gamma(\alpha) \qquad (55)$$

which is an alternative form of Eq. 46 where the gamma was used for a different purpose. The model to fit $\bar{X}(t;k)$ is found by substituting Eq. 55 into Eq. 54 to yield

$$E\left[\bar{X}(t;k)\right] = X(0)(1+\beta t)^{-\alpha} \qquad (56)$$

This model and models for many other common unimodal distributions of k are given in (64).

These models have some far-reaching consequences. It is immediately apparent that one no longer has the sum-of-exponentials model for the data. Indeed, it is shown in (64) that the expectation of the average data always exceeds the model for a single individual evaluated at the average rate, E(k), i.e.

$$M(-t) > \exp\{-E(k)t\} \ , \quad t > 0$$

for any nontrivial distribution of k. As an illustration of this, Cocchetto et al. (62) simulated 100 values of k from a normal distribution, determined the theoretical model X(t) for each k, and averaged these to obtain the idealized, error-free data $\bar{X}(t)$. When fitting these aggregate data to a simple monoexponential model, the estimate of k seriously underestimated the true mean value whenever the variability in k was sizeable (coefficient of variability $\geq$ 15%).

Another consequence is that an experimenter using a sum-of-exponentials model is likely to find that the biexponential model provides a better fit than the monoexponential model. Therefore care should be taken to differentiate in this particular case an underlying two-compartment model from a underlying single compartment model for aggregate data with intersubject variability.

In general, models with many different chance mechanisms may share the same mean value function. However, their covariance kernels are unique and in principle the covariances could be used for model identification. Many such covariance structures are given in (64).

The above illustration of variability in the random rate k may be extended to include variation in the apparent volumes of distribution, V, and in the initial doses, X(0). The modeling has also been extended in the articles above to describe the one-compartment stochastic model. We are not aware at the present time of any analytical solutions of multi-compartment models with bivariate distributions other than the relatively simple one in (65), which, as discussed in (66), contains an assumption that is inadmissible for real data. However, the bivariate distributions for given parametric families can be estimated numerically as discussed below.

Models with Heterogeneous Particles: Models of this type arise in one of two ways. The first is a model where all particles share the same destination and general operative forces but have different sizes or shapes and thus possess varying rate coefficients, k. An example of this is the passage of indigestible material through the gastrointestinal tract of ruminants. Particles of different size would inherently have different passage probabilities through the rumen orifice, as noted in (54), yet only the aggregate recovery data are available.

A variation of this is to have material which may be conceptually divided into fractions with different sources and/or destinations, but where only the aggregate is observed. For example, in a one-compartment model, let the ith fraction of proportional size p_i, $\Sigma p_i = 1$, have rate k_i. Then the deterministic passage model is

$$X(t) = X(0) \sum_i e^{-k_i t} p_i \quad .$$

Waldo et al. (67) give one illustration of such application by describing a simple model of cellulose disappearance involving 2 fractions. A more general passage model would involve many more than 2 fractions in which case the separate pairs (k_i, p_i) are not estimable in practice. However, the model could be approximated with a distribution of k_i, as noted in (68).

Whether the "particle heterogeneity" arises inherently in the process or as an approximation as described above, the model to fit the aggregate data within a single subject has the same mean value as that given in the preceeding section, i.e.

$$E[X(t;k)] = X(0)\ M_k\ (-t) \quad . \tag{57}$$

However, the variability of $X(t;k)$ is now related to particle variation and is of a smaller order of magnitude, as outlined in (64).

Models with Particle Clustering: The assumption of independent particle transfers has been questioned on both theoretical and empirical grounds. One theoretical fact developed in section 3.2 is that all stochastic models with independent particle transfers have coefficients of variation for any $x_{ij}(t)$ of order $[x_{11}(0)]^{-\frac{1}{2}}$. This implies that the coefficient of variation is negligible for the large $x_{11}(0)$'s associated with numbers of molecules. However, in many processes, nonnegligible coefficients of variation are observable which make the assumption of particle independence questionable. Based on such logic, Bernard and associates (63) have constructed a theoretical model where particle transfers occur in groups.

The nonindependence of particle transfers is also motivated by empirical reasons. Matis and Wehrly (69) discuss an example of the passage of a water soluble marker through the gastrointestinal tract of a ruminant. The marker particles are adsorbed and irrevocably bound to hay particles during passage. The expected number of molecules adsorbed per particle is assumed to be proportional to the particle size, and the particle sizes vary tremendously in size (see e.g. (70) and (60)). Thus, instead of independent movement of tracer particles, passage occurs as clusters of particles.

Several general one-compartment clustered models are presented in (69). To illustrate the models, consider the above problem concerning passage of a water-soluble marker. Let $x(t)$ denote the number of particles, $b(t)$ the random number of clusters, and d_i, $i=1, \ldots, b(t)$, the random number of particles in cluster i, hence

$$x(t) = \sum_{i=1}^{b(t)} d_i \quad . \tag{58}$$

For present simplicity, we assume the following very special case:

i) The initial number of clusters, $b(0)$, is a Poisson (α).
ii) The d_i's are independent, identical Poisson (β)'s.
iii) The time-invariant transfer rate for all the clusters is k.

Then it can be shown that the expectation and variance of $x(t)$ are

$$E[x(t)] = \alpha\beta e^{-kt} \quad \text{and}$$
$$Var[x(t)] = \alpha\beta(1+\beta)\, e^{-kt} \tag{59}$$

from whence the coefficient of variation due to process variability is

$$CV[x(t)] = [(1+\beta)/\alpha\beta\, e^{-kt}]^{\frac{1}{2}} \quad . \tag{60}$$

Since the initial number of clusters, $b(0)$, in this and many other applications may not be very large, it is clear that α may be small and that the coefficient of variation is non-negligible. Matis and Wehrly (69) generalize the above to include many different one-compartment clustering models, among them models with age-varying rates and with subject or particle heterogeneity. A general theorem for such clustered models states that

$$CV\,[x(t)] \geq CV[b(0)]$$

which establishes a lower bound for the relative variability. Multi-compartment models are expected to have similar bounds.

5.3 Statistical Analysis of Data

Case where Data are Available for Individual Subjects: Consider the case where an experiment is replicated on U subjects, chosen at random from a population, and where data ${}_uX_{ij}(t;{}_u\underset{\sim}{\Omega})$ are available for each subject u=1,. . . , U. It is reasonable to assume that ${}_u\underset{\sim}{\Omega}$ is a random variable which varies among individuals, and the objective is to estimate parameters of the ${}_u\underset{\sim}{\Omega}$ distribution. Sheiner and Beal (35) note that the standard approach consists of estimating the parameter vector ${}_u\underset{\sim}{\Omega}$ for each subject separately, and then using simple summary statistics, e.g. simple arithmetic averages, to estimate the population parameters of the ${}_u\underset{\sim}{\Omega}$ distribution. They point out some shortcomings of the approach when the replicates have varying amounts of data per subject, varying data quality and/or varying experimental designs. Their alternative to the standard approach is to use an extended least squares procedure which pools all data together. We propose that another alternative to the standard approach is to first estimate each parameter ${}_u\omega_i$ of the ${}_u\underset{\sim}{\Omega}$ vector. Each parameter estimate ${}_u\hat{\omega}_i$ could be assigned a weight which is the reciprocal of the asymptotic variance estimate, i.e. $[s^2({}_u\hat{\omega}_i)]^{-1}$, where the $s^2({}_u\hat{\omega}_i)$'s are obtained as illustrated in section 2. The population moments of the ω_i distribution could then be estimated through weighted sample estimates. As an illustration, the estimate of the mean value of the ω_i variable would be

$$\hat{\mu}(\omega_i) = \sum_{u=1}^{U} [{}_u\hat{\omega}_i/s^2({}_u\hat{\omega}_i)]/ \sum_{u=1}^{U} [s^2({}_u\hat{\omega}_i)]^{-1} \qquad (61)$$

The estimator in Eq. 61 is simple to obtain and takes into account the differences in design and data quality. The properties of the above estimators should be a subject of further study.

Case where Data are Combined Over Individuals: In the case where only aggregate data are available, i.e., the data have been pooled over individual subjects, one would fit the model in Eq. 54 to the data. At present, explicit solutions for such random rate coefficients exist only for one-compartment models. In principle one could extend the procedure to multiple compartments. Closed-form solutions are not available for multiple compartments, but one could use nonlinear least squares algorithms which employ numerical integration to determine the theoretical model. One such example is (57) which used the ZXMIN algorithm of the IMSL computer package (71) to solve a similar problem.

The one-compartment case is illustrated in (64). Data were available describing the combined depuration of vanadium from several marine species. Several _a priori_ forms of the density function $f(k;\underset{\sim}{\phi})$ were selected, one of them being the gamma given in Eq. 55. The parameter vector $\underset{\sim}{\phi}$ was estimated for the aggregate data, and the estimate of $\underset{\sim}{\phi}$ is sufficient to give estimates of any moment of the k random variables.

This illustration is a relatively simple application of the above theory involved with aggregate data since the experimental protocol involved the serial sacrifice of organisms. Hence each organism was measured only once which ruled out serial correlation over time. In cases where multiple observations over time are involved and where measurement error is relatively small, the optimum estimation requires the solution for the $\underset{\sim}{\Sigma}_p$ variance-covariance matrix of the process error. The $\underset{\sim}{\Sigma}_p$ matrix is given in (64) for the case where all individuals are weighted equally. In such cases, the estimation would proceed along the lines given in Eq. 36. An example of such calculations involving the survivorship of fish in heated water is given in (64).

Case of Data for Heterogeneous Particles: As noted in section 5.2, the regression functions for models involving heterogeneous particles, as given in Eq. 57 may be identical to those for models involving aggregated data over heterogeneous subjects, as given in Eq. 54. In practical terms, the chief difference between the models is in the size of their inherent $\underset{\sim}{\Sigma}_p$ matrices. As noted in (64), the $\underset{\sim}{\Sigma}_p$ matrix for data involving heterogeneous individuals has elements which are multiples of $[x(0)]^2$. Therefore, the $\underset{\sim}{\Sigma}_p$ matrix usually has an important effect on the estimates. However, the $\underset{\sim}{\Sigma}_p$ matrix for data involving heterogeneous particles has elements which are multiples of x(0), and their corresponding coefficients of variation may be small relative to the measurement error. In such cases $\underset{\sim}{\Sigma}_p$ does not have a large influence on the estimation and it is often deleted for computational simplicity. Typically in models involving heterogeneous particles, the stochastic theory is important in formulating the model in Eq. 57, which of course differs from the usual deterministic model. However, the stochastic theory does not have much of an effect on the statistical analysis and the procedures outlined in section 2 are used.

An example of fitting a model involving heterogeneous particles to data is described in (72). Two masticated hay samples, one of whole leaf fragments (frac 1602) and the other of ground leaf fragments (frac 1603) were removed from the esophagus of a cow. The samples were then incubated _in vitro_ to determine the chemical degradation into potentially digestible fiber. The concentration of undegraded fiber in the masticate, involving particles of different sizes, was then measured _in vitro_. Two one-compartment models were fitted to the data. One model involved a signle degradation rate k with a time delay, giving expectation

$$E[c(t)] = C(0)\, e^{-k(t-\tau)}, \text{ for } t > \tau \quad . \tag{62}$$

The second model had a gamma distribution of rates and gave the following expectation, which is similar to Eq. 56:

$$E[c(t)] = C(0)[1+\beta(t-\tau)]^{-\alpha} \quad . \text{ for } t > \tau \quad . \tag{63}$$

The OLS parameter estimates and the mean squared error s^2 are given in Table 5. Note that the model with heterogeneous particles, Eq. 63, provided a better fit in both cases than the model in Eq. 62. The estimated distributions of k are graphed in Figure 3 along with the corresponding estimates of the constant k. As a comparison, the estimated mean rates for the gamma distributions, which may be found by the $\hat{\alpha}\hat{\beta}$ products, are 3.33 and 5.78 and the estimates of the constant k are 3.10 and 5.10, respectively. Since the gamma distribution is skewed, the median is a useful measure of location. For the fitted gamma distributions, the medians were 3.03 and 5.20, respectively.

TABLE 5

OLS Estimates for the Hay Masticate Samples from (72).

Sample	Model with Constant k		Model with Gamma k		
	$\hat{k}$	s^2	$\hat{\alpha}$	$\hat{\beta}$	s^2
1602	3.10	1.91	3.58	0.93	1.37
1603	5.10	1.54	3.30	1.75	1.34

6. STATISTICAL ANALYSIS BASED ON RESIDENCE TIME MOMENTS

6.1 Derivation of Residence Time Moments for Stochastic Particle Models

The stochastic particle model outlined in section 3 provides a strong foundation for compartmental theory. It also provides a basis for many important generalizations, as given in sections 4 and 5, which describe counting distributions under various alternative assumptions of practical interest. Our interest in this section is no longer on describing the random counts (or amounts) of particles in the various compartments but rather on the random lengths of time which the particles spend in the compartments. These times are called by various writers residence times, retention times, lifetimes, or sojourn times. It was noted in section 4 that a compartmental structure may be characterized

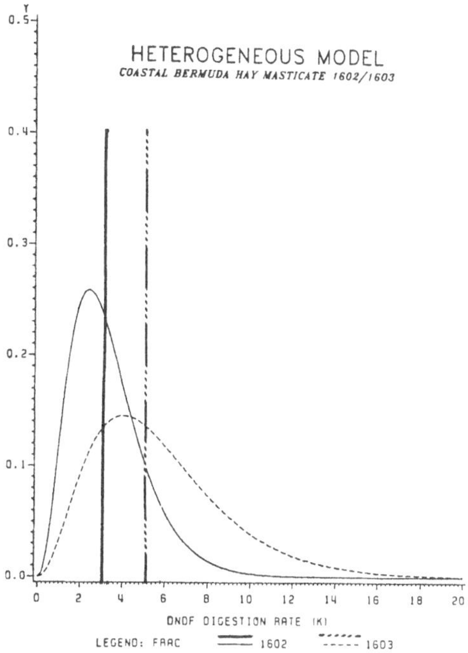

FIGURE 3

Distributions of the rate coefficient k for heterogeneous particle models fitted to masticated hay samples. Solid and dashed curves are estimated gamma distributions of k for samples 1602 and 1603, respectively. Straight lines are the corresponding estimates of the constant k.

in terms of residence time distributions such as those in Eq. 42 and 46, as an alternative to specifying the rate coefficients, such as those in Eq. 41, 44 and 45, which describe how the counts might change over time. In section 4, however, the residence time distributions were used only to give alternative assumptions for the purpose of generating discrete counting distributions of interest. In this section, the principal focus will be on finding the statistical moments, e.g. the means and variances, for the continuous residence time distributions of particles in various compartments.

The duality between counting distributions and waiting time distributions is well-known in the theory of stochastic processes (49). Our present interest is to exploit the duality for a special purpose, namely that of obtaining the moments for use as response variables for subsequent statistical analysis.

Consider the following definitions in addition to those given in section 3, for the stochastic particle model:

8) Let S_{ij} be the total residence (or sojourn) time in j prior to leaving the system of a particle which started in i at t=0.

9) Let V_{ij} be the total number of visitations to j prior to leaving the system of a particle which started in i at t=0.

10) Let $\underset{\sim}{S} = [S_{ij}]$ and $\underset{\sim}{V} = [V_{ij}]$ be the respective nxn random matrices.

11) Let $\underset{\sim}{\theta} = E[\underset{\sim}{S}]$, $\underset{\sim}{\theta}' = E[\underset{\sim}{V}]$, $\underset{\sim}{\Gamma} = Var[\underset{\sim}{S}]$ and $\underset{\sim}{\Gamma}' = Var[\underset{\sim}{V}]$ be the nxn matrices of means and variances of the $\underset{\sim}{S}$ and $\underset{\sim}{V}$ matrices.

12) Let the following operators be defined for a square matrix $\underset{\sim}{A} = (a_{ij})$: the diagonal operator $\underset{\sim}{A}_d = diag(a_{ii})$, the squared element operator $\underset{\sim}{A}_{(2)} = (a_{ij}^2)$, and the normalization matrix $\underset{\sim}{A}^* = (a_{ij}^*)$ where $a_{ii}^* = 0$ and $a_{ij}^* = -a_{ij}/a_{ii}$ for i≠j.

The following theorem may now be proven:

Theorem 4: In the stochastic particle model previously described with conditions (i)-(vi) as in Theorem 2, one has

i) $\underset{\sim}{\theta} = \int_0^\infty \underset{\sim}{P}(0,t)dt = -\underset{\sim}{\dot{K}}^{-1}$ (64)

ii) $\underset{\sim}{\Gamma} = 2\underset{\sim}{\theta}\underset{\sim}{\theta}_d - \underset{\sim}{\theta}_{(2)}$ (65)

iii) $\underset{\sim}{\theta}' = (\underset{\sim}{I} - \underset{\sim}{K}^*)^{-1}$ (66)

iv) $\underset{\sim}{\Gamma}' = 2\underset{\sim}{\theta}'\underset{\sim}{\theta}'_d - \underset{\sim}{\theta}'_{(2)}$ (67)

Eq. 64 describing the mean residence times is a well-known result and is proven in (73). We are not aware of any proof of Eq. 65, which describes the variances of the residence times, other than that given in (9). Eq. 66 and 67, which give the means and variances of the number of visitations, can be proven by using finite Markov chain theory in (74). A complete proof is given in (75).

The moments given in Theorem 4 may be very useful in practice for several reasons. Firstly, they may be biologically important measures for experimenters. For example, in one common application of the two-compartment model, the parameter θ_{12}, which gives the expected residence time in the target organ (comp 2) of a drug injected into the plasma (comp 1), is usually of more inherent interest than k_{12}, the flow rate from 1 to 2. The expected residence times are of particular importance in specified multicompartment models where the number of rate coefficients is large. Secondly, the estimated residence time moments are very robust to changes in the compartmental structure whereas the estimated rate parameters are very dependent upon the specified compartmental model. One simple illustration of this is given by the three models fitted to the data in section 4. The parameters vary in size and the rate functions are difficult to compare between models. However, the expected total residence time of a particle in the system provides a convenient framework for model comparisons. For the previous parameter estimates, the expected residence times under the three models are

$$S_1 = (.0744)^{-1} + (.0239)^{-1} + 21.01 = 76.29 \text{ hrs.},$$

$$S_2 = 2(.229)^{-1} + 23.95 = 80.99 \text{ hrs., and}$$

$$S_3 = 2(.0474)^{-1} + 23.73 = 65.92 \text{ hrs.}$$

Thirdly, the estimates of the above moments may enhance the statistical power of experiments to detect treatment differences. This has been observed in several specific examples (9 ,76) and will be investigated subsequently in this section via computer simulation.

Note that all of the above residence time moments are relatively easy to calculate from the k_{ij} constants and indeed may be given as explicit functions of the k_{ij} 's for most common pharmacokinetic models. As an illustration, consider these moments for the present two-compartment open model with coefficient matrix in Eq. 4, i.e.

$$\underset{\sim}{K} = \begin{bmatrix} -(k_{12} + k_{10}) & k_{12} \\ k_{21} & -k_{21} \end{bmatrix} .$$

It can be shown that when $\underset{\sim}{K}$ is substituted into Eq. 4-7, one has

$$\underset{\sim}{\theta} = \begin{bmatrix} k_{10}^{-1} & k_{12}/k_{10}k_{21} \\ k_{10}^{-1} & (k_{12} + k_{10})/k_{10}k_{21} \end{bmatrix} ,$$

$$\underset{\sim}{\Gamma} = \begin{bmatrix} k_{10}^{-2} & k_{12}(k_{12} + 2k_{10})/(k_{10}k_{21})^2 \\ k_{10}^{-2} & (k_{12} + k_{10})^2/(k_{10}k_{21})^2 \end{bmatrix},$$

$$\underset{\sim}{\theta}' = \begin{bmatrix} 1 + k_{12}/k_{10} & k_{12}/k_{10} \\ 1 + k_{12}/k_{10} & 1 + k_{12}/k_{10} \end{bmatrix},$$

$$\underset{\sim}{\Gamma}' = \begin{bmatrix} (1 + k_{12}/k_{10})^2 & k_{12}(k_{12} + 2k_{10})/k_{10})^2 \\ (1 + k_{12}/k_{10})^2 & (1 + k_{12}/k_{10})^2 \end{bmatrix}.$$

The simple structure of the $\underset{\sim}{K}$ coefficient matrix for the present model leads to some simple structure of the above matrices of means and variance. Note for example that equality of the (1,1) and the (2,1) elements for each of the above matrices is due to the structural constraint that particles may exit only from compartment 1. Many other functional relationships are built into the above matrices as properties of the particular model.

The moment calculations in Theorem 4 are based upon the $\underset{\sim}{K}$ matrix, or in other words upon the $\underset{\sim}{\Omega}_1$ rate-coefficient parameterization. The methodology may be called model-dependent since it relies implicitly upon the assumption that the structure of the compartmental system is known. Rescigno and his coworkers (77) have developed an alternative, "model-free" approach which is based on the $\underset{\sim}{\Omega}_2$ parameterization. It can be shown for the case of idealized, error-free data from a known compartmental structure that the two methods lead to equivalent results. We are not aware of any simulation study that has compared the small sample properties of the two methods for a specified error structure. However, based on general statistical principles, we conjecture that the methodology in Theorem 4 is more powerful if the structure is known since it imposes theoretical constraints on the parameter space. On the other hand, the model-free methodology would seem more powerful if the structure is not known since it virtually eliminates the error due to model misspecification.

6.2 Statistical Analysis of Data Using Estimated Residence Time Moments

Estimated Moments and Their Asymptotic Properties: Theorem 4 provides the means and variances of the residence time random variables when the rate parameters are known. In practice, however, the k_{ij} rates are not known but rather are estimated from data. It is proposed in (9) that estimates of the matrices in Theorem 4, namely $\hat{\theta}$, $\hat{\Gamma}$, $\hat{\theta}'$, and $\hat{\Gamma}'$, be found by substituting $\hat{K}$, the LS estimate of K, into Eq. 64-67.

It was shown in sections 2.2 and 3.2 for measurement and for process error, respectively, that under very broad conditions the LS estimator $\hat{K}$ is a consistent estimator of K as $M \rightarrow \infty$ and as $X_{11}(0) \rightarrow \infty$, respectively. Since θ, Γ, θ', and Γ', are continuous functions of K and since $\hat{K}$ is consistent, it can be shown ((78) p. 124) that $\hat{\theta}$, $\hat{\Gamma}$, $\hat{\theta}'$, and $\hat{\Gamma}'$ are consistent estimators of their corresponding parameter matrices.

One can also show under the above conditions leading to consistent $\hat{K}$ that the estimators $\hat{\theta}$, $\hat{\theta}'$, $\hat{\Gamma}$, and $\hat{\Gamma}'$ are asymptotically normal. The asymptotic variances of these estimators can be derived from those of the $\hat{k}_{ij}$'s using formula (6a.2.6) of Rao (78). For instance, we consider $\hat{\theta}_{12}$. Let Δ be the asymptotic variance-covariance matrix of $\hat{\Omega}_1 = (\hat{k}_{10}, \hat{k}_{12}, \hat{k}_{21})'$. Then the asymptotic variance of $\hat{\theta}_{12}$ is $G'\Delta G$ where

$$G' = \left(-\frac{k_{12}}{k_{10}^2 \, k_{21}} \; , \; \frac{1}{k_{10} \, k_{21}} \; , \; -\frac{k_{12}}{k_{10} \, k_{21}^2} \right).$$ Since the estimate of Δ is available from any standard nonlinear least squares program, one can obtain the estimated asymptotic variance of $\hat{\theta}_{12}$ by substituting the estimated values of k_{10}, k_{12}, and k_{21} into G. Approximate confidence intervals for the θ_{ij}'s and the γ_{ij}'s may be constructed using the approximate variances. In summary, one can find analogous results for residence time moments to those given in Eq. 15-19 for rate parameters.

Small Sample Properties of Moment Estimators: The small sample properties of the $\hat{\theta}_{ij}$ estimators are investigated in (24) for the two-compartment open model involving different error structures and different parameter values. The study indicates the following: 1) the qualitative results were the same for the additive and the multiplicative error models, 2) the WLS estimates of θ_{ij} had a much smaller mean squared error than the OLS estimators, as noted for the $\hat{k}_{ij}$'s, 3) the mean squared errors of the WLS estimates of θ_{ij} compare favorably with the WLS estimates of k_{ij} and 4) the asymptotic, approximate confidence intervals were very close to their nominal (95%) level of confidence. Another specific finding is the pronounced skewness of the $\hat{\theta}_{ij}$ distributions which would suggest nonparametric inference for subsequent statistical analysis of the estimates. The general conclusion is that the $\hat{\theta}_{ij}$ estimates, calculated by substituting WLS estimates of k_{ij} into Eq. 65, form a suitable, well-behaved response variable for subsequent statistical analysis, at least for the specified model. It is assumed that the $\hat{\theta}'_{ij}$, $\hat{\gamma}_{ij}$, and $\hat{\gamma}'_{ij}$ estimates would possess similar benign properties.

Some Applications: Relatively few studies have used estimated residence time moments in their analysis, at least insofar as they are calculated through the $\hat{\Omega}_1$ parameterization in Theorem 4. One early exception is Saffer et al. (76) who uses the estimated mean number of visitations, $\hat{\theta}_{ij}'$, to analyze Rose Bengal transport through the hepatobiliary system. These estimated means were found to provide results consistent with the projected and actual clinical status. Another application is Cobelli et al. (79) who calculate $\hat{\theta}_{ij}$'s as estimates of inherent biological interest. Recently (9) used both $\hat{\theta}_{ij}$'s and $\hat{k}_{ij}$'s to analyze experimental data on the cholesterol turnover in rats, and the study observed that the $\hat{\theta}_{ij}$'s found many significant treatment differences which were not detected with the $\hat{k}_{ij}$'s. The apparently large increase in the power of the statistical hypothesis tests in this one example leads to further studies to compare the power of analyses based on estimated residence time moments to those using other response variables. The results of this study are presented in Section 6.3.

6.3 Comparative Power of Analyses Based on Estimates of Various Parameters

This subsection reports a simulation study (80) which compares the powers of analyses based on estimates of rate parameters, residence time parameters, and other parameters of biological interest. The exact conditions of the simulation are first described, the variables are then outlined, and lastly the results are given.

Specification of Simulation: The following set of assumptions and procedures were used for the study:

1) On the overall design, each "experiment" had a completely randomized (CR) design with 2 groups (treatment and control) and with 10 experimental units per group.

2) On the underlying compartment model, the two-compartment open model in Figure 1 was chosen for the study. It was assumed that $X_{11}(0) = 1.0$ and that data on the first compartment, $X_1(t_m)$, were available at M=10 times (t=.1, .2, .4, .6, .8, 1.0, 1.5, 2.0, 3.0, 5.0).

3) On measurement conditions, an independent, multiplicative lognormal (0,.01) error was assumed. It was assumed that the number of individual molecules in the unit dose was so large that the process error was negligible.

4) On the estimation procedures, the model was fitted using WLS. The matrix of weights was $\hat{\Sigma}_{\tilde{T}} = \text{diag}[\hat{X}_1(t_m)^2]$ where the $\hat{X}_1(t_m)$'s are the predicted model values from a preliminary OLS analysis. The SAS NLIN procedure was used with the DUD option, and the control parameter vector was used as the initial starting values for both the control and the treatment data.

5) On the statistical analysis, a total of 18 variables defined subsequently were used. Let y_i, i=1, . . ., 18 denote the variables. The values for each of the variables were calculated for each of the 10 experimental units in each of the 2 groups. For each experiment, the null hypothesis

$$H_0\text{: } E[y_i] \text{ for control} = E[y_i] \text{ for treatment} \quad (68)$$

was tested for each of the 18 variables using the non-parametric Wilcoxon rank-sum test (81) with $\alpha = .01$.

6) On the power study, the experiment was replicated 50 times to estimate the power, i.e. the probability of detection of a treatment effect for each experimental condition and each of the 18 variables. The experiment was repeated for all combinations of five control vectors, namely $c\tilde{\Omega}$ = [1, ½, ¼], [1, $2^{-\frac{1}{2}}$, ½], [1, 1, 1], [1, $2^{\frac{1}{2}}$, 2] and [1, 2, 4] and of five treatments, namely (i) 25% increase in k_{10}, (ii) 50% increase in k_{12}, (iii) 50% increase in k_{21}, (iv) combined (ii) and (iii), and (v) combined (i) and (iv).

These assumptions seem a reasonable description of current practice, as noted also in (24).

<u>Description of Variables</u>: The simulated $X_1(t_m)$ data were first used to find the WLS estimates $\hat{k}_{10}$, $\hat{k}_{12}$ and $\hat{k}_{21}$, which are now denoted y_1 to y_3, respectively. The other variables, y_4 to y_{18}, are identified in Table 6. Note that y_4 to y_{10} describe various

TABLE 6

Variables Used in Simulation Study

New Designation	Formula	Description
y_1	$\hat{k}_{10}$	elimination rate from 1
y_2	$\hat{k}_{12}$	transfer rate from 1 to 2
y_3	$\hat{k}_{21}$	transfer rate from 2 to 1
y_4	$\hat{\theta}_{11} = (\hat{k}_{10})-1$	mean time in 1 given start in 1
y_5	$\hat{\theta}_{12} = \hat{k}_{12}/\hat{k}_{10}\hat{k}_{21}$	mean time in 2 given start in 1
y_6	$\hat{\theta}_{22} = (\hat{k}_{12} + \hat{k}_{10})/\hat{k}_{10}\hat{k}_{21}$	mean time in 2 given start in 2
y_7	$\hat{\gamma}_{12} = [\hat{k}_{12}(\hat{k}_{12} + 2\hat{k}_{10})]/\hat{k}_{10}\hat{k}_{21})^2$	variance of time in 2 given start in 1
y_8	$\hat{\theta}'_{12} = \hat{k}_{12}/\hat{k}_{10}$	mean number of visits to 2 given start in 1
y_9	$\hat{\gamma}_{12} = [\hat{k}_{12}(\hat{k}_{12} + 2\hat{k}_{10})]/\hat{k}_{10}^2$	variance of number of visits to 2 given start in 1
y_{10}	$\hat{p} = \hat{k}_{12}/(\hat{k}_{10} + \hat{k}_{12})$	prob of at least 1 visit to 2
y_{11}	$\hat{\lambda}_1$ in equation (5)	slow decay coefficient
y_{12}	$\hat{\lambda}_2$ in equation (5)	rapid decay coefficient
y_{13}	$\hat{c}_1 = (\hat{\lambda}_1 + \hat{k}_{21})/(\hat{\lambda}_1 - \hat{\lambda}_2)$	coefficient of exp $(\lambda_1 t)$
y_{14}	$\hat{c}_2 = (\hat{\lambda}_2 + \hat{k}_{21})/(\hat{\lambda}_2 - \hat{\lambda}_1)$	coefficient of exp $(\lambda_2 t)$
y_{15}	$\hat{\beta}_{\frac{1}{2}} = -\ell n2/\hat{\lambda}_1$	biologic half-life (2)
y_{16}	$\hat{K}_{\frac{1}{2}} = \ell n2/(\hat{k}_{10} + \hat{k}_{12})$	half-life for total elimination
y_{17}	$\hat{t}_{max} = [\ell n(-\lambda_2) - \ell n(-\lambda_1)]/\lambda_1 - \lambda_2$	time of max $X_{12}(t)$
y_{18}	$\hat{c}_{max} = e^{-\lambda_1 t_{max}} - e^{-\lambda_2 t_{max}}$	scaled max concentration in comp. 2

moments and probabilities which are concepts unique to the stochastic formulation. Variables y_{11} to y_{18} also have stochastic interpretations, but they are interpretable for and derivable from the deterministic models as well, and therefore they are in common useage in the literature.

Results: The results for one of the treatment effects, a 25% increase in k_{10}, are listed in Table 7 for all five control vectors. Since each estimated power is based on 50 points, the standard error of an estimate could be as large as $.5/\sqrt{50} = .07$.

Several variables were grouped together since they gave identical results. One general conclusion for the model is that the power of many of these measures is related to $p=k_{12}/(k_{10}+k_{12})$, which is the probability that a particle will visit compartment 2 at least once. For the control vectors, p varies from 1/3 for the vector [1, ½, ¼] to 2/3 for the vector [1,2,4].

The estimated power function of $\hat{\theta}_{11}$ (and $\hat{k}_{10}$) is virtually 1.0 over the present range of p. The estimated power of $\hat{\theta}_{12}$ and of $\hat{\lambda}_1$ increases with p and is virtually 1.0 for $p > .585$; whereas the estimated power of $\hat{K}_{\frac{1}{2}}$ decreases with p and is virtually 1.0 for $p < .415$. The five estimated power functions with the greatest average power are plotted in Figure 4 as a function of p.

The study was repeated for two other treatments, namely a 50% increase in k_{12} and a 50% increase in k_{21}. Figure 5 gives the four variables with the greatest average power to detect the 50% increase in k_{21}.

The two outstanding conclusions from these three cases where a treatment effect occurs in a single parameter are 1) the $\hat{k}_{ij}$ rate estimators as a group are not very powerful in detecting certain treatment effects (e.g. for k_{21}) and 2) the best single variable, and in fact the only one with relatively high power for all three cases, is $\hat{\theta}_{12}$. In the regions of the parameter space where $\hat{\theta}_{12}$ has relatively low power, the best complementary variables seem to be either $\hat{\theta}_{11}$, $\hat{\theta}_{12}'$ or $\hat{K}_{\frac{1}{2}}$.

Clearly, many other sets of treatment effects could be proposed with various combinations of increases and decreases in the k_{ij}'s. The two combinations chosen for this study, namely a 50% increase in both k_{12} and k_{21} and the increase in both k_{12} and k_{21} combined with a 25% increase in k_{10}, were chosen since the identical

TABLE 7

Estimated Power of Experiment to Detect a 25% Increase in k_{10} for the Different Variables and Control Vectors

Variable	Underlying Parameter Vector				
	$[1,\frac{1}{2},\frac{1}{4}]$	$[1,2^{\frac{1}{2}},\frac{1}{2}]$	$[1,1,1]$	$[1,2^{\frac{1}{2}},2]$	$[1,2,4]$
$\hat{k}_{10}$, $\hat{\theta}_{11}$	.96	1.00	1.00	1.00	1.00
$\hat{k}_{12}$	.02	.00	.00	.02	.02
$\hat{k}_{21}$	.00	.00	.00	.02	.00
$\hat{\theta}_{12}$	.00	.12	.70	.96	.98
$\hat{\theta}_{22}$	.00	.02	.04	.28	.26
$\hat{\gamma}_{12}$	.00	.04	.20	.64	.52
$\hat{\theta}_{12}'$, $\hat{\gamma}_{12}'$, $\hat{p}$	.32	.80	.66	.14	.18
$\hat{\lambda}_1$, $\hat{\beta}_{\frac{1}{2}}$	.00	.04	.54	1.00	1.00
$\hat{\lambda}_2$	1.00	.44	.02	.06	.00
$\hat{c}_1$, $\hat{c}_2$	.42	.30	.30	.12	.10
$\hat{K}_{\frac{1}{2}}$	1.00	.98	.44	.14	.02
$\hat{t}_{max}$	.12	.14	.18	.10	.02
$\hat{C}_{max}$	.06	.20	.32	.08	.04

percentage increases in k_{12} and k_{21} should neutralize the power of $\hat{\theta}_{12}$. They therefore represent the worst possible cases for $\hat{\theta}_{12}$ and are designed to detect which variables can be used to supplement $\hat{\theta}_{12}$. Figure 6 gives the estimated power curves for treatment effect consisting of a 50% increase in both k_{12} and k_{21}.

The following recommendations summarize the findings for all five cases of the model:

1) $\hat{\theta}_{12}$ is overall the most powerful variable for detecting treatment differences.

2) $\hat{\theta}_{12}'$, $\hat{\theta}_{11}$ and $\hat{K}_{\frac{1}{2}}$ are the best complementary variables to use in conjunction with $\hat{\theta}_{12}$.

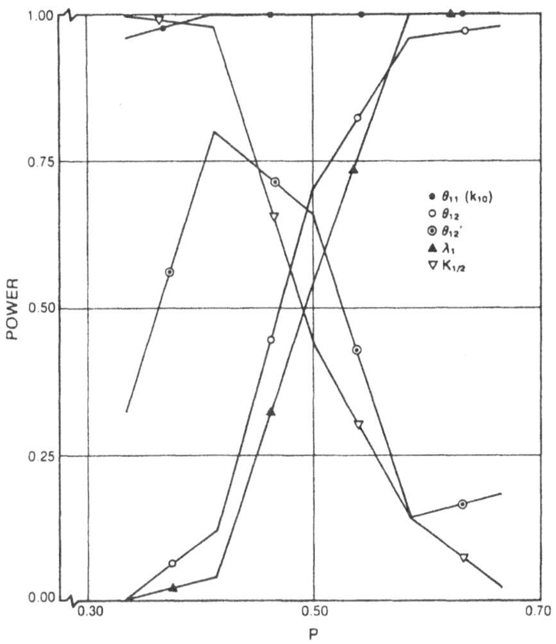

FIGURE 4

Estimated power curves to detect a 25% increase in k_{10} as a function of p, the probability of at least one visit to 2.

Of course, these recommendations hold in a strict sense only for the present two-compartment model with all the particular assumptions and procedures listed at the beginning of the subsection concerning the parameter space, error structure, sampling conditions, estimation procedures, etc. Clearly the simulation study needs to be broadened to include other conditions, and particularly a preliminary grid search of initial values. Nevertheless, we expect that the above measures, particularly the $\hat{\theta}_{ij}$ mean residence times and the $\hat{\theta}_{ij}'$ mean number of visitations, would perform well under the present general condition of having a specified compartment model with rate parameter ($\underset{\sim}{\Omega}_1$) parameterization. Further research is in progress to extend the simulation to include mean residence times available through the alternative, model-free procedures such as 1) the $\underset{\sim}{\Omega}_2$ parameterization in (77) and 2) the numerical integration of area under the curve (AUC) methods in (82, 83).

In summary, perhaps the greatest contribution of the stochastic model lies in its inherent residence time random variables. The estimated residence time moments form a new powerful basis for the statistical analysis of pharmacokinetic data. The estimated

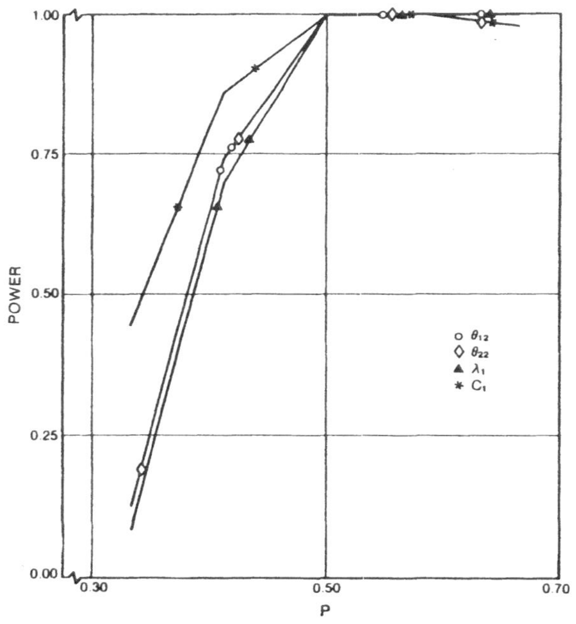

FIGURE 5

Estimated power curves to detect a 50% increase in k_{21} as a function of p, the probability of at least one visit to 2.

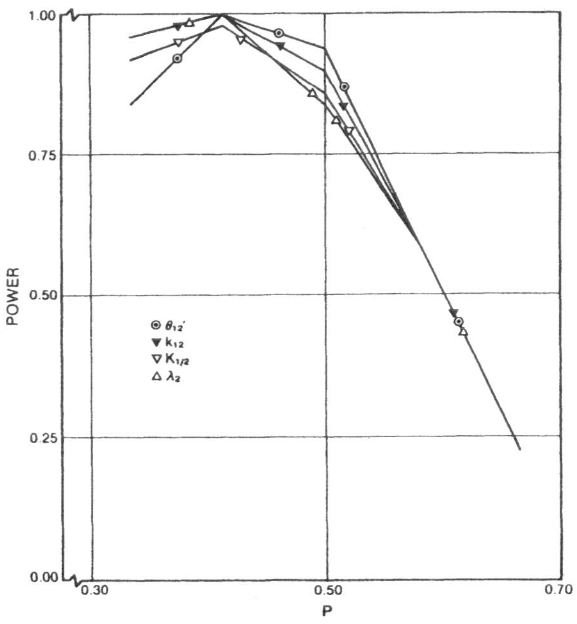

FIGURE 6

Estimated power curves to detect a 50% increase in k_{12} and k_{21} as a function of p, the probability of at least one visit to 2.

moments are easy to calculate from the estimated rate coefficients for any specified model. Moreover, the estimated moments are 1) of great inherent biological interest, 2) convenient to use in comparing results of different models, and 3) relatively powerful in detecting treatment effects.

ACKNOWLEDGEMENTS

It is a pleasure to acknowledge W. C. Ellis, Texas A&M University for providing unpublished data in section 5 and Helen Schiffhauer for typing the manuscript.

REFERENCES

1. Atkins GL: Multicompartment Models in Biological Systems. London, Methuen, 1969

2. Gibaldi M, Perrier D: Pharmacokinetics. New York, Marcel Dekker, 1975

3. Jacquez JA: Compartmental Analysis in Biology and Medicine. New York, Elsevier, 1972

4. Rescigno A, Segre G: Drug and Tracer Kinetics. Waltham MD, Blaisdell, 1966

5. Thakur AK: Some statistical principles in compartmental analysis. In Robertson J, Ed. Mathematical Techniques in Pharmacokinetics, to appear.

6. Wagner JG: Biopharmaceutics and Relevant Pharmacokinetics. Hamilton IL, Drug Intelligence Publ., 1971

7. Metzler CM: Estimation of pharmacokinetic parameters: Statistical considerations. Pharmac Ther 13: 543-556, 1981

8. Rescigno A: Mathematical methods in the formulation of pharmacokinetic models. In Lambrecht RM and Rescigno A, Eds. Tracer Kinetics and Physiologic Modelling--Theory to Practice

9. Matis JH, Wehrly TE, Metzler CM: On some stochastic formulations and related statistical moments of pharmacokinetic models. J Pharmacokin Biopharm, to appear

10. Hearon JZ: Theorems on linear systems. Ann N Y Acad Sc 108: 36-68, 1963

11. Metzler CM: Usefulness of the two-compartment open model in pharmacokinetics. J Am Stat Assoc 66: 49-53, 1971

12. Berman M, Schoenfeld R: Invariants in experimental data on linear kinetics and the formulation of models. J Appl Phys 27: 1361-1370, 1956

13. Glass HI, de Garreta AC: The quantitative limitations of exponential curve fitting. Phys Med Biol 16: 119-130, 1971

14. Bard Y: Nonlinear Parameter Estimation. New York Academic, 1974

15. Gallant AR: Nonlinear regression. Am Stat 29: 73-81, 1975

16. Wu CF: Asymptotic theory of nonlinear least squares estimation. Ann Stat 9: 501-513, 1981

17. Westlake WJ: Use of statistical methods in evaluation of in vivo performance of dosage forms. J Pharm Sci 62: 1579-1589, 1973

18. Boxenbaum HG, Riegelman S, Elashoff RM: Statistical estimators in pharmacokinetics. J Pharmacokin Biopharm 2:123-148, 1974

19. Peck CC, Sheiner L, Beal S, Nichols A: Pharmacokinetic data analysis using extended least-squares nonlinear regression. Clin Pharmacol Ther 27: 277-278, 1980

20. Wagner JG, et al. : Pharmacokinetic parameters estimated from intravenous data by uniform methods and some of their uses. J Pharmacokin Biopharm 5: 161-182, 1977

21. Chennavasin P, Johnson RA, Brater DC: Variability in derived parameters of furosemide pharmacokinetics. J Pharmacokin Biopharm 9: 623-633, 1981

22. Cobelli, C, Salvan A: Parameter estimation in a biological two compartment model - II. A computer experimental study of the influence of the initial estimate in the parameter space of some sampling protocols and of weighting factors. Math Biosci 33: 267-274, 1977

23. Metzler CM: Statistical properties of kinetic estimates. In Endreny L, Ed. Kinetic Data Analysis. New York, Plenum, 1981, pp 25-37

24. Matis JH, Olson DR, Gerald KB:On the statistical moments transformation in pharmacokinetic models: A study of the rate parameter and the mean residence time estimates. Math Comp Sim 24: 515-524, 1983

25. Laskarzewski PM, Weiner DL, Ott L: A simulation study of parameter estimation in the one and two compartment models. J Pharmacokin Biopharm 10: 317-334, 1982

26. Ottaway JH: Normalization in the fitting of data by iterative methods. Biochem J 134: 729-736, 1973

27. Gerald KB, Matis JH: A comparison of weighted and unweighted nonlinear least squares in compartmental modelling. Manuscript

28. DiStefano III JJ, Cobelli C: On parameter and structural identifiability: Nonunique observability/reconstructibility for identifiable systems, other ambiguities and new definitions. IEEE Trans Autom Control 25: 830-833, 1980

29. Eisenfeld J, Rideout VC, Eds: Special Issue on Modeling of Biomedical Systems. Math Comp Sim 24: in press, 1983

30. Landaw EM: Optimal multi-compartmental sampling designs for parameter estimation--Practical aspects of the identification problem. Math Comp Sim 24: in press, 1983

31. Metzler CM, Elfring GL, McEwen AJ: A User's Manual for NONLIN and Associated Programs. Kalamazoo MI, Upjohn Co, 1974

32. Hartley HO: The modified Gauss-Newton method for the fitting of nonlinear regression functions by least squares. Technometrics 3: 269-280, 1961

33. SAS Institute Inc: SAS User's Guide: Statistics, 1982 ed. Cary NC, SAS Institute Inc, 1982

34. Miller Jr. RG: Simultaneous Statistical Inference. 2 ed. New York, Springer Verlag, 1981

35. Sheiner LB, Beal SL: Evaluation of methods for estimating population pharmacokinetic data. J Pharmacokin Biopharm 9: 635-651, 1981

36. Pond KP: The fragmentation and flow of forage residues through the gastrointestinal tract of cattle. Ph.D. Dissertation. College Station TX, Texas A&M Univ, Dept An Sci, 1982

37. Kodell RL, Matis JH: Estimating the rate constant in a two-compartment stochastic model. Biometrics 32: 377-380, 1976

38. Matis JH, Hartley HO: Stochastic compartmental analysis: Model and least squares estimation from time series data. Biometrics 27: 77-102, 1971

39. Cobelli C, Morato LM: On the identification by filtering techniques of a biological n-compartment model in which the transport rate parameters are assumed to be stochastic processes. Bull Math Biol 40: 651-660, 1978

40. Rescigno A, Beck JS: Compartments. In Rosen R, Ed. Foundations of Mathematical Biology. New York, Academic, 1972

41. Bartholomay AF: Stochastic models for chemical reactions: I. Theory of the unimolecular reaction process. Bull Math Biophys 20: 179-190, 1958

42. Matis JH: Stochastic compartmental analysis: Model and least squares estimation from time series data. Ph.D. Dissertation. College Station TX, Texas A&M Univ., Inst Stat, 1970

43. Johnson NL, Kotz S: Discrete Distributions. Boston, Houghton Mifflin, 1969

44. Chiang CL: On regular best asymptotically normal estimates. Ann Math Stat 27: 336-351, 1956

45. Chiang CL: Introduction to Stochastic Processes in Biostatistics. New York, Wiley, 1968

46. Kalbfleisch JD, Lawless JF, Vollmer VM: Estimation in Markov models from aggregate data. Submitted manuscript, 1983

47. McInnis BC, El-Asfouri SA, Kapadia SA: On stochastic compartmental modeling. Bull Math Biol 41: 611-613, 1979

48. Rescigno A, Matis JH: On the relevance of stochastic compartmental models to pharmacokinetic systems. Bull Math Biol 43: 245-247, 1981

49. Parzen E: Stochastic Processes. San Francisco, Holden-Day, 1962

50. Wise ME: The need for rethinking on both compartments and modeling. In Matis JH, Patten BC and White GC, Eds. Compartmental Analysis of Ecosystem Models. Burtonsville MD, Int Co-op Publ., 1979, pp 279-293

51. Weiner D, Purdue P: A semi-Markov approach to stochastic compartmental models. Comm Stat Th Meth A6: 1231-1243, 1977

52. Marcus AH, Becker A: Power laws in compartmental analysis II. Math Biosc 35: 27-45, 1977

53. Cinlar E: Markov renewal theory. Adv Appl Prob 1: 123-187, 1969

54. Matis JH: Gamma time-dependency in Blaxter's compartmental model. Biometrics 28: 597-602, 1972

55. Johnson NL, Kotz S: Continuous Univariate Distributions - 1. New York, Wiley, 1970

56. Gross AJ, Clark VA: Survival Distributions: Reliability Applications in the Biomedical Sciences. New York, Wiley, 1975

57. Hughes TH, Matis JH: An irreversible two-compartment model with age-dependent turnover rates. Biometrics, to appear, 1983

58. Epperson JO, Matis JH: On distribution of the general irreversible n-compartmental model having time-dependent transition probabilities. Bull Math Biol 41: 737-749, 1979

59. Cardenas M, Matis JH: On the time-dependent reversible stochastic compartmental model--II. A class of n-compartment systems. Bull Math Biol 37: 555-564, 1975

60. Ellis WC, Matis JH, Lascano C: Quantitating ruminal turnover. Fed Proc 38: 3702-3710, 1979

61. Rodda BE: Analysis of sets of estimates from pharmacokinetic studies. In Endreny, Ed. Kinetic Data Analysis. New York, Plenum, 1981, pp 285-298

62. Cocchetto DM, Wargin WA, Crow JW: Pitfalls and valid approaches to pharmacokinetic analysis of mean concentration data following intravenous administration. J Pharmacokin Biopharm 8: 539-552, 1980

63. Bernard SR: An urn model study of variability within a compartment. Bull Math Biol 39: 463-470, 1977

64. Matis JH, Wehrly TE: Stochastic models of compartmental systems. Biometrics 35: 199-220, 1979

65. Soong TT, Dowdee JW: Pharmacokinetics with uncertainties in rate constants-III. The inverse problem. Math Biosci 19: 343-353, 1974

66. Matis JH, Wehrly TE: An approach to a compartmental model with multiple squares of stochasticity for modeling ecological systems. In Matis JH, Patten BC and White GC, Eds. Compartmental Analysis of Ecosystem Models. Burtonsville MD, Int. Co-op Publ. 1979, pp 195-222

67. Waldo DR, Smith LW, Cox EL: Model of cellulose disappearance from the rumen. J Dairy Sci 15: 125-129, 1972

68. Matis JH, Tolley HD: Compartmental models with multiple sources of stochastic variability: The one-compartment, time invariant hazard rate case. Bull Math Biol 41: 491-515, 1979

69. Matis JH, Wehrly TE: Compartmental models with multiple sources of stochastic variability: The one-compartment models with clustering. Bull Math Biol 43: 651-664, 1981

70. Troelsen JE, Campbell JB: Voluntary consumption of forage by sheep and its relation to the size and shape of particles in the digestive tract. Anim Prod 10: 289-296, 1968

71. International Mathematical & Statistical Libraries, Inc: The IMSL Library Reference Manual, Vol 1, ed 7. Houston, IMSL Inc, 1979

72. Ellis WC, Matis JH, Pond KR, Schelling GT, Mahlooji M: Degradation of forage fiber as a stochastic process. J An Sci 53: Supplement 1, 273, 1981

73. Eisenfeld J: Relationship between stochastic and differential models of compartmental system. Math Biosci 43: 289-305, 1979

74. Kemeny JG, Snell JL: Finite Markov Chains. New York, Springer-Verlag, 1976

75. Matis JH, Patten BC: Environ analysis of linear compartmental systems: The static, time invariant case. Int Stat Inst Bull 48, to appear

76. Saffer SI, Mize CE, Bhat UN, Szygenda SA: Use of nonlinear programming and stochastic modeling in the medical evaluation of normal-abnormal liver function. IEEE Trans Biomed Eng BME-23: 200-207, 1976

77. Rescigno A, Gurpide E: Estimation of average times of residence, recycle and interconversion of blood-borne compounds using tracer methods. J Clin Endocrinal Metab 36: 263-276, 1973

78. Rao CR: Linear Statistical Inference and Its Applications 2 ed. New York, Wiley, 1973

79. Cobelli C, Toffolo G, Nosadin R: Mathematical models of ketone bodies kinetics in the human. Experiment design and their identification/validation. In IFAC Symp, Identification and System Parameter Estimation. Washington, McGregor and Werner, 1982

80. Matis JH, Wehrly TE, Gerald KB: Statistical analysis of specified, compartmental models through residence time moments and related parameters: A paper in honor of H.O. Hartley. Manuscript

81. Conover WJ: Practical Nonparametric Statistics, 2 ed. New York, Wiley, 1980

82. Yamaoka K, Nakagawa T, Uno T: Statistical moments in pharmacokinetics. J Pharmacokin Biopharm 6: 547-558, 1978

83. Riegelman S, Collier P: The application of statistical moment theory to the evaluation of in vivo dissolution time and absorption time. J Pharmacokin Biopharm 8: 509-534, 1980

MATHEMATICAL METHODS IN THE FORMULATION OF PHARMACOKINETIC MODELS

Aldo Rescigno, Richard M. Lambrecht, and Charles C. Duncan

Brookhaven National Laboratory and Yale University

1. HISTORICAL CONSIDERATIONS

The first quantitative analysis in pharmacokinetics was made by Widmark (1), who studied both theoretically and experimentally the kinetics of distribution of several narcotics, in particlar acetone. He studied the concentration curve of acetone in the blood after a single dose administration, and assumed that the fall of the curve was due principally to elimination from the lungs and chemical metabolism. The mathematical model used by Widmark was

$$dx/dt = -\beta x - \gamma x \qquad x(0) = x_0$$

$$dy/dt = \beta x \qquad y(0) = 0$$

$$dz/dt = \gamma x \qquad z(0) = 0$$

where x,y,z are the amount of acetone in the body, exhaled, and metabolized, respectively; x_0 is the amount administered initially. From the knowledge of the time behavior of the concentration c(t) of the acetone in the blood and of the so-called "reduced body volume" m, where $m = x/c$, Widmark computed the time behavior of x,y,z in several experimental conditions.

Later Widmark and Tandberg (2) derived the equation of a model where there is a constant rate administration, and also when the drug is administered with rapid intravenous injections repeated at uniform intervals of time.

Another important contribution has been given by Gehlen (3) who derived some theoretical expressions for what we would now call a two-compartment system.

Widmark (4) studied also the elimination of ethanol and developed in this context what we would now call a zero-order compartment model.

The first systematic study of the kinetics of drugs introduced into the mammalian body in various ways was performed by Teorell (5). As in the dynamical analysis of exchange of inert gases and of the distribution of narcotics, the assumptions about the transport and the definition of the regions or compartments wherein measurements are to be made lead to a set of linear differential equations with constant coefficients. Beyond that, however, two other interesting considerations appear in these papers. One is the idea of chemical transformation as a route between compartments where the latter term has a more general meaning in the sense evidenced by Widmark. Teorell's concern was the disappearance of a drug from blood or tissue in a more general framework and the generalization of the term compartment is made to include possible inactivation of the drug via transformation to another chemical form. The other idea is the distinction between what one may call Fick kinetics and one may call stochastic kinetics. For the resorption of a drug from a subcutaneous depot, Teorell considers that each particle has the same probability of being transported; therefore the instantaneous rate of loss is proportional to the number of particles present at that instant. In our notation this assumption leads to the set of equations

$$dX_i/dt = \sum_{j\neq i}^{1\ldots n} k_{ji}X_j - K_iX_i, \quad i=1,2,\ldots,n, \qquad (1\text{-}1)$$

where X_i is the amount of substance present in compartment _i_, the constant k_{ji} is the fraction of the substance in compartment _j_ transported to compartment _i_ per unit time, and the constant K_i is the total fractional efflux from compartment _i_. On the other end, for transport between blood and tissues, Teorell assumed what may be called Fick (6) kinetics; this may be expressed by equation

$$\phi = A(\psi_j - \psi_i),$$

where ϕ is the net flux from compartment _j_ to compartment _i_, ψ_i and ψ_j are the activities in compartments _i_ and _j_ respectively, and A is a constant. Here the driving force for transport is _activity_, a thermodynamic quantity, rather than an amount of _substance_. Then with the assumption that the activity of a chemical entity is adequately approximated by its concentration, and that the rate of change of concentration in a homogeneous constant volume is proportional to the net flux across its boundary, we have the equations

$$dC_i/dt = \sum_{j\neq i}^{1\ldots n} h_{ij}(C_j - C_i), \quad i=1,2,\ldots,n, \qquad (1\text{-}2)$$

where h_{ij} is the _permeability constant_ for the barrier of _constant thickness and area between_ compartments _i_ and _j_. These equations represent the kinetics of the system of compartments governed by Fick kinetics. Eqs. 1-1 are more general than Eqs.

1-2; this is to be expected, as Eqs. 1-2 follow from physical conditions that narrow their applicability. Now define

$$C_i = Y_i/V_i, \quad i=1,2,\ldots,n$$

where V_i is a parameter independent on time; then Eqs. 1-2 become

$$dY_i/dt = \sum_{j\neq i}^{1\ldots n} h_{ij}V_i(Y_j/V_j - Y_i/V_i),$$

formally identical with Eqs. 1-1 if we put

$$h_{ij}\ V_i/V_j = k_{ji}, \quad \sum_{j\neq i}^{1\ldots n} h_{ij} = K_i. \qquad (1\text{-}3)$$

Fick kinetics is thus formally a special case of stochastic kinetics, where definition (1-3) holds. Again formally, whatever X_i is, k_{ji} is the instantaneous time rate of increase of X_i due to X_j, expressed as a fraction of X_j. Given the physical interpretation of C_i and h_{ij}, one may choose to regard V_i as a volume, which then leads to the interpretation of X_i as an amount; then k_{ji} becomes the fractional transfer rate, the fraction of X_j contributed to X_i per unit time. Though Eqs. 1-2 are very restrictive, the special case of Fick kinetics is an important one, having wide use as a model for biological transport processes.

Another important step on the use of compartment equations in physiological models was made by Artom, Sarzana and Segrè (7). To study the formation of phospholipids as affected by dietary fat, they administered inorganic phosphate containing radioactive ^{32}P to rats and measured the radioactivity present in inorganic phosphate of blood, in the lipid of liver and in the skeleton at known times after administration. The physical correlate of compartment, then, is a state determined by the simultaneous existence of a particular location in space and a particular chemical state. For example, the variable representing the amount of ^{32}P in inorganic form in blood is a compartment and is distinct from the variable representing inorganic ^{32}P in the liver and distinct as well as from that representing lipid ^{32}P in blood.

As a basis for their analysis, Artom et al. (7) specify four assumptions:

(a) that the organism is incapable of distinguishing between ^{32}P and ^{31}P;

(b) that the quantity of P fixed in any form whatever (for example, as lipid P) by a tissue per unit time is proportional to the amount of inorganic P in the blood; and, similarly, that the amount of inorganic P which, in the same time, is returned to the blood from the considered form is proportional to the amount of P present in that form in that tissue;

(c) that the total amount of P in the tissues remains constant during the experiment;

(d) that the quantity of P administered is sufficiently small that it does not modify the metabolism of the animal.

They then define the following symbols:

1. N_s, N_f, N_w represent the number of atoms of ^{31}P of the form of interest in blood, liver, and skeleton, respectively.

2. n_s, n_f, n_w represent the analogous numbers of atoms of ^{32}P.

3. f/N_s represents the probability per unit time of fixation in the form of interest of a given atom of inorganic P by the liver.

4. w/N_s represents the analogous probability for fixation by bone.

From these assumptions and definitions and the additional assumption that no other appreciable exchange of P occurs, three differential equations follow:

$$dn_s/dt = -(f+w)n_s/N_s + fn_f/N_f + wn_w/N_w,$$

$$dn_f/dt = fn_s/N_s - fn_f/N_f, \qquad (1\text{-}4)$$

$$dn_w/dt = wn_s/N_s - wn_w/N_w.$$

These three equations are analogous with Eqs. 1-1, where, say $k_{fs} = f/N_f$, and so forth. The solutions as functions of time, Artom et al. go on to say, are in general sums of three exponentials. The constants of the exponents are characteristic of the system, that is, they depend upon f, w, N_s, N_f, N_w; the coefficients on the other hand are constants dependent upon these parameters and the initial conditions of the experiment.

It is of interest to note here that the parameters f,w play a two-way role in this case as does the permeability parameter h_{ij} in the case of Fick kinetics; the reason is quite different, however. In this case f,w are numbers of atoms per unit time transported between compartments. Hence the number of atoms per unit time transported from blood inorganic P to liver lipid P, say, is f. The probability per unit time of transport for a single atom, then, if f/N_s and the number per unit time of radioactive atoms transported is fn_s/N_s. That the same parameter f appears in the term for transport from liver lipid P to blood inorganic P is required by the assumption (c) quoted above. It should be clear that the probabilities per unit time of transport between liver lipid and blood phosphate $(f/N_f, f/N_s)$ are not necessarily equal in the two directions. Furthermore, if there were a path for transport from liver to bone not including blood inorganic P, then this steady-state assumption would not imply the single parameter f for both directions.

2. DEFINITIONS OF COMPARTMENTS

Probably Sheppard (8) used the term compartment for the first time: "There are numerous instances in biological and chemical research where multiple compartment systems are encountered. This is undoubtedly true in other fields as well. In such a system, real compartments may exist whose contents are homogeneous and which are separated from one another by real boundaries. However, the concept may be generalized so that a substance, such as a chemical element, can be considered to be in a different compartment when it is in a different state of chemical combination." Later Sheppard and Householder (9) made this concept more precise: "In isotope studies compartments may be regions of space in which the absolute specific activity (fractional amount of the substance that is tagged) is uniform such as erythrocytes and plasma in vitro or states of uniform chemical composition such as copper ions and copper chelate compounds."

Other definitions, substantially equivalent to Sheppard's, can be found in Rescigno and Segre (10), Brownell et al. (11), Berman (12), Jacquez (13), Gùrpide (14). This last author suggested the use of the term pool instead of compartment, "to avoid the purely spatial implication that might be assigned to the latter term"; despite its evident merits, this suggestion has not been followed by later authors.

For our present purposes we shall use an operational definition of compartment, as proposed by Rescigno and Beck (15): "A variable x(t) of a system is called a compartment if it is governed by the differential equation

$$dx/dt = -Kx + f(t) \qquad (2\text{-}1)$$

with K constant." For a physical interpretation of Eq. 2-1, consider x the amount of a certain substance in a particular subdivision of a system, through which its concentration is uniform at any given time; that substance leaves that subdivision at a rate proportional to its total amount there, i.e. with a process of first order, with relative rate K; f(t) measures the rate of entry of that substance in that subdivision of the system from other subdivisions or from outside the system. Thus Eq. 2-1 represents the relationship between the behavior of the precursor f(t) and the behavior of its successor x(t).

Going back to the paper by Artom et al. (7), it is worth observing that they were aware of the necessity of defining a compartment operationally, though they did not use the term compartment explicitly. (See page 257 of Artom et al. (7)).

From a different point of view, a compartment can be defined stochastically, as done for instance by Rescigno and Segre (10): "A compartment can be considered as being made up of an ensemble of particles, molecules or parts of molecules which have the same probability of passing from their state to other possible states."

More precise stochastic definitions were given by Matis and Hartley (16), Thakur et al. (17), Purdue (18) and many other authors. The stochastic approach to compartmental analysis will be described in detail in Section 11.

3. ORDINARY DIFFERENTIAL EQUATIONS

Before returning to the operational definition of compartment, let us introduce some additional definitions.

The entity whose distribution we are interested in is called tracee, and it may be a substance, or a component of a substance, like a radical or an atom, or a material; in any case the tracee implies the existence of a tracer. Tracee and tracer are defined by the three characteristic properties:

(1) Tracer and tracee should have the same physical, chemical, and biological properties of interest inside the system;

(2) The tracer should be detectable by the observer when introduced with the system in the presence of the tracee;

(3) The tracer should be introduced into the system in quantities small enough as not to alter the normal behavior of the tracee.

Define now

Q_i = mass of tracee i,

R_i = mass turnover rate of tracee i, i.e. amount of tracee i transformed in another tracee per unit time,

R_{ij} = mass transfer rate from tracee i to tracee j, i.e. amount of tracee i transformed in tracee j per unit time,

R_{oi} = mass formation rate of tracee i from external sources; the conservation of mass of tracee i is expressed by the equation

$$dQ_i/dt = -R_i + \sum_{j\neq i}^{1\ldots n} R_{ji} + R_{oi}; \tag{3-1}$$

this equation can be written for all possible values of i, and it is valid in general, no matter how the tracee is eliminated. With the additional definitions

$$K_i = R_i/Q_i,$$

$$k_{ij} = R_{ij}/Q_i,$$

Eq. 3-1 becomes

$$dQ_i/dt = -K_iQ_i + \sum_{j\neq i}^{1\ldots n} k_{ji}Q_j + R_{oi}. \tag{3-2}$$

This equation, like Eq. 3-1 is valid in general, but it is useful only when K_i and k_{ji} are constant; in this last case they represent the relative turnover rate and relative transfer rates as defined in Section 2. This is true of course when the tracee follows only reactions of first order, i.e. when it behaves like a compartment; it is also true when all R's and Q's are constant, i.e. when the system is in a steady state.

Consider now the tracer instead of the tracee; its conservation equation may be written

$$dq_i/dt = -r_i + \sum_j r_{ji} + r_{oi}, \tag{3-3}$$

where q_i, r_i, r_{ji}, r_{oi} are defined for the tracer as the corresponding symbols with capital letters were defined for the tracee. From the fundamental properties of a tracer it follows that we can write the proportions

$$r_i/R_i = q_i/Q_i,$$

$$r_{ij}/R_{ij} = q_i/Q_i,$$

thence Eq. 3-3 becomes

$$dq_i/dt = -R_i q_i/Q_i + \sum_j R_{ji} q_j/Q_j + r_{oi},$$

and

$$dq_i/dt = -K_i q_i + \sum_j k_{ji} q_j + r_{oi}; \tag{3-4}$$

this equation is analogous to Eq. 3-2, with the same values for the coefficients K_i and k_{ji}. These coefficients are constants, as said before, when the tracee undergoes only reactions of the first order, but also when the tracee is at steady state. In other words, the steady state of the tracee implies first order reactions of the tracer, and the reaction rates of the tracer are equal to the relative rates of the tracee at steady state, irrespective of their order.

While the amount of tracer could be expressed in grams or moles (or submultiples thereof), those units are impractical due to the minute amounts of tracer used; more often the units used are microcuries or disintegrations per unit time (if the tracer is radioactive), or fraction of a given dose; in all cases we can call activity the amount of tracer of a given compartment.

Other units can be used. For instance if V_i is the volume of tracee i, then define the concentration c_i of the tracer in a compartment as

$$c_i = q_i/V_i,$$

and, if V_i is constant, Eq. 3-4 becomes

$$dc_i/dt = -K_i c_i + \sum_j k_{ji} V_j/V_i \cdot c_j + r_{oi}/V_i; \tag{3-5}$$

if we define the specific activity a_i as

$$a_i = q_i/Q_i,$$

then, if Q_i is constant,

$$da_i/dt = -K_i a_i + \sum_j k_{ji} Q_j/Q_i \cdot a_j + r_{oi}/Q_i. \qquad (3\text{-}6)$$

Each of the three equations 3-4, 3-5, 3-6 can be conveniently used according to the quantities that can be measured. Returning now to Eq. 2-1, we see that it includes, as special cases, Eqs. 3-2, 3-4, 3-5, 3-6, where x_i may represent amount of first order tracee, or amount of tracer, or concentration of tracer, or specific activity, respectively.

Note that dimensional homogeneity of all those equations requires that the dimension of K_i be t^{-1}.

Let us write now Eqs. 3-2, 3-4, 3-5, 3-6 in the general form

$$dx_i/dt = -K_i x_i + \sum_{j \neq i} k_{ji} x_j + f_i(t); \qquad (3\text{-}7)$$

dimensional homogeneity again requires that $K_i x_i$ have the same dimensions of the generical term $k_{ji} x_j$, without x_i being necessarily homogeneous with x_j; in fact the different x's may measure different kinds of variables, some extensive, like activity, some intensive, like concentration; for example if x_i is mass measured in gram, x_n is concentration measured in mole·liter^{-1}, and time is measured in second, then the requirements that $K_i x_i$ and $k_{ni} x_n$ be homogeneous implies that k_{ni} have the dimensions of liter gram mole^{-1} sec^{-1}; the physical meaning of such parameters may seem obscure, but by writing

$$k_{ni} = k_{ni}' \cdot k_{ni}'' \cdot k_{ni}'''$$

one may think of k_{ni}' as the volume of the compartment, in liter, of k_{ni}'' as the molecular weight of the tracee (dimensions gram·mole^{-1}), and of k_{ni}''' as a fractional transfer rate, in sec^{-1}.

4. MATRICES

The differential equations of a system of compartments can be written in matrix form

$$\dot{\underset{\sim}{x}} = \underset{\sim}{x} \cdot \underset{\sim}{K} + \underset{\sim}{f}, \qquad (4\text{-}1)$$

where

$$\underset{\sim}{K} = [k_{ij}]$$

is the nxn matrix of the transfer rates, with

$$k_{ii} = -K_i$$

the transfer rate out of compartment i, $\underset{\sim}{x}$ is the row vector of the n variables of the system, $\dot{\underset{\sim}{x}}$ its time derivative, and $\underset{\sim}{f}$ the row vector of input functions into the system. Eq. 4-1 must be completed by the initial conditions

$$\underset{\sim}{x}(0) = \underset{\sim}{x}_0,$$

where $\underset{\sim}{x}_0$ is the initial value of row vector $\underset{\sim}{x}$.

An important observation must be made at this point. I have indicated with k_{ij} the relative transfer rate from i to j, while a number of authors use that symbol for the rate to i from j; in fact a casual survey of the literature has shown that each of the two definitions is preferred by approximately 50% of the authors. The reasons for my choice are three:

(1) The physical meaning of k_{ij} becomes more evident if the transfer of material from one compartment to another is shown by reading the subscripts from left to right;

(2) If material is transferred through a succession of compartments, the product of the transfer constants involved, written as a string with the second subscript of a constant equal to the first subscript of the following constant, has a particularly useful physical and mathematical meaning;

(3) This definition is consistent with the notation used in the theory of Markov processes, as shown by Thakur et al. (17).

On the other hand the symbol k_{ij} has been used by some authors for the transfer to i from j because in that case the constant k_{ij} will appear in row i and column j when the matrix $[k_{ij}]$ is postmultiplied by the column vector $\underset{\sim}{x}$; I have shown above that premultiplication of matrix $[k_{ij}]$ by row vector $\underset{\sim}{x}$ is consistent with the present definition of k_{ij}.

The integral of Eq. 4-1 is

$$\underset{\sim}{x} = \underset{\sim}{x}_0 \cdot e^{\underset{\sim}{K}t} + \int_0^t \underset{\sim}{f}(\tau) \cdot e^{\underset{\sim}{K}(t-\tau)}\, d\tau, \tag{4-2}$$

where by definition

$$e^{\underset{\sim}{K}t} = \underset{\sim}{I} + \underset{\sim}{K}t + \underset{\sim}{K}^2 t^2/2! + \underset{\sim}{K}^3 t^3/3! + \ldots,$$

$\underset{\sim}{I}$ being the nxn identity matrix. The properties of the exponential matrix $e^{\underset{\sim}{K}t}$ depend on the eigenvalues of $\underset{\sim}{K}$, therefore we shall spend the next few pages on the analysis of these eigenvalues.

Physical realizability of the system requires that

$$k_{ij} \geqq 0 \quad \text{for any } i \text{ and } j, \tag{4-3}$$

$K_i \geq \sum_j k_{ij}$ for any i, and the sum extended to all values of $j \neq i$; (4-4)

Hadamard (19) has shown that these properties imply that all real eigenvalues of $\underset{\sim}{K}$ are non-positive, and all complex eigenvalues have a negative real part. For the presence of zero eigenvalues a further analysis of $\underset{\sim}{K}$ is necessary.

Matrix $\underset{\sim}{K}$ is said to be decomposable if with a number of permutations of its rows and corresponding columns it can be put in quasi-diagonal form, i.e. in the form

$$\underset{\sim}{K} = \begin{bmatrix} \underset{\sim}{K}_1 & \underset{\sim}{0} \\ \underset{\sim}{0} & \underset{\sim}{K}_2 \end{bmatrix},$$

where $\underset{\sim}{K}_1$ and $\underset{\sim}{K}_2$ are two square matrices. When this is the case, if $m \times m$ is the size of $\underset{\sim}{K}_1$, then the n compartments can be partitioned in two different systems, one of m and the other of $n-m$ compartments, completely independent one on the other. Unless otherwise explicitly stated, we shall only consider non-decomposable matrices.

Matrix $\underset{\sim}{K}$ is said to be reducible if, with appropriate permutations of its rows and corresponding columns, it can be put in the form

$$\underset{\sim}{K} = \begin{bmatrix} \underset{\sim}{K}_1 & \underset{\sim}{B} \\ \underset{\sim}{0} & \underset{\sim}{K}_2 \end{bmatrix}, \qquad (4\text{-}5)$$

where $\underset{\sim}{K}_1$ is $m \times m$, $\underset{\sim}{K}_2$ is $(n-m)\times(n-m)$, and $\underset{\sim}{B}$ is $(n-m)\times m$. When this is the case, then the n compartments can be relabeled in such a way that the first m of them are independent from the remaining $n-m$.

Hearon (20) has proved that, if $\underset{\sim}{K}$ is irreducible then it is singular if and only if condition 4-4 is a strict equality, i.e. if

$$K_i = \sum_j k_{ij}$$

for any values of i and for the sum extended to all values of $j \neq i$. When this is the case, then the system is closed, i.e. material is transferred from one compartment to another, but nothing to the outside. It is also easy to prove that if $\underset{\sim}{K}$ is irreducible, then it is of rank n or $n-1$, i.e. zero cannot be a multiple eigenvalue.

Suppose now that $\underset{\sim}{K}$ is singular and reducible; we can put it in the form 4-5; if either $\underset{\sim}{K}_1$ or $\underset{\sim}{K}_2$, or both, are further reducible, we can transform them in the same way, and proceed until we have

$$\underset{\sim}{K} = \begin{bmatrix} \underset{\sim}{K}_1 & \underset{\sim}{B}_{12} & \underset{\sim}{B}_{13} & --- & \underset{\sim}{B}_{1m} \\ \underset{\sim}{0} & \underset{\sim}{K}_2 & \underset{\sim}{B}_{23} & --- & \underset{\sim}{B}_{2m} \\ \underset{\sim}{0} & \underset{\sim}{0} & \underset{\sim}{K}_3 & --- & \underset{\sim}{B}_{3m} \\ \hline \underset{\sim}{0} & \underset{\sim}{0} & \underset{\sim}{0} & --- & \underset{\sim}{K}_m \end{bmatrix},$$

where $\underset{\sim}{K}_1, \underset{\sim}{K}_2, \ldots, \underset{\sim}{K}_m$ are all irreducible square matrices. If any of these last matrices, say $\underset{\sim}{K}_i$, is singular, then 0 is a simple eigenvalue of it, and the corresponding subsystem is closed; this implies that all matrices on the same column as $\underset{\sim}{K}_i$ are zero, and the system is decomposable. It follows that if $\underset{\sim}{K}$ is not decomposable, only matrix $\underset{\sim}{K}_m$ can be singular.

Returning now to Eq. 4-2, consider the case

$$\underset{\sim}{f}(t) \equiv \underset{\sim}{0};$$

if all eigenvalues of $\underset{\sim}{K}$ are real and distinct, then there exist a non-singular matrix $\underset{\sim}{P}$ such that

$$\underset{\sim}{K} = \underset{\sim}{P}^{-1} \cdot \underset{\sim}{\Lambda} \cdot \underset{\sim}{P},$$

where $\underset{\sim}{\Lambda}$ is the diagonal matrix of the eigenvalues of $\underset{\sim}{K}$; Eq. 4-2 can be written

$$\underset{\sim}{x} = \underset{\sim}{x}_0 \cdot \underset{\sim}{P}^{-1} \cdot e^{\underset{\sim}{\Lambda} t}\, \underset{\sim}{P} \qquad (4\text{-}6)$$

where

$$e^{\underset{\sim}{\Lambda} t} = \begin{bmatrix} e^{\lambda_1 t} & 0 & 0 & 0 \\ 0 & e^{\lambda_2 t} & 0 & 0 \\ \hline 0 & 0 & 0 & e^{\lambda_n t} \end{bmatrix},$$

with $\lambda_1, \lambda_2, \ldots, \lambda_n$ the eigenvalues of $\underset{\sim}{K}$. Then Eq. 4-6 shows that the elements of vector $\underset{\sim}{x}$ are linear combinations of the exponentials $e^{\lambda_1 t}$, $e^{\lambda_2 t}, \ldots, e^{\lambda_n t}$, the coefficients of which depend on the elements of $\underset{\sim}{x}_0$; all exponential terms have a negative exponent, i.e. they decrease when t increases, except possibly one, and no more than one, that can be constant.

If some eigenvalues of $\underset{\sim}{K}$ are multiple, then we can find two matrices $\underset{\sim}{S}$ and $\underset{\sim}{N}$ such that

$$\underset{\sim}{K} = \underset{\sim}{S} + \underset{\sim}{N},$$

$$\underset{\sim}{S} \cdot \underset{\sim}{N} = \underset{\sim}{N} \cdot \underset{\sim}{S},$$

where $\underset{\sim}{S}$ is diagonalizable, and $\underset{\sim}{N}$ is nilpotent, i.e. all its powers above a certain one are void. In this case Eq. 4-2 can be written

$$\underset{\sim}{x} = \underset{\sim}{x}_0 \cdot e^{\underset{\sim}{N}t} \cdot e^{\underset{\sim}{S}t} \quad ;$$

now matrix $\underset{\sim}{S}$ can be diagonalized and leads to a sum of exponentials with all the eigenvalues of $\underset{\sim}{K}$, while

$$e^{\underset{\sim}{N}t} = \underset{\sim}{I} + \underset{\sim}{N}t + \underset{\sim}{N}^2 \cdot t^2/2! + \ldots + \underset{\sim}{N}^m \cdot t^m/m!$$

is a sum of a finite number of terms, since $\underset{\sim}{N}$ is nilpotent, and m is certainly not larger than n; therefore the elements of $\underset{\sim}{x}$ are a sum of exponential terms, each one multiplied by a polynomial in t of degree equal to the multiplicity of the corresponding eigenvalue minus one.

The case when some eigenvalues of $\underset{\sim}{K}$ are complex will be treated in Section 10.

5. DIRECTED GRAPHS

One important problem in the analysis of compartment systems is the study of the properties related to the structure of the model, i.e. of the properties depending upon the presence or absence of a connection between any two compartments and not upon the values of such connections.

The topological properties of a system of compartments have been studied by Rescigno and Segre (21) using a directed graph (22). A directed graph was called réseau orienté by Sainte-Laguë (23) and graphe by Berge (24); we shall use the term graph for brevity in this section when referring to a directed graph. A graph consists of a set of nodes, representing the compartments, together with a set of arms connecting the nodes and representing the transfers between compartments.

To each graph containing n nodes, we can associate a square matrix of order n, called the connectivity matrix; the element a_{ij} of row i, column j of the connectivity matrix is equal to 1 if there is an arm from node i to node j, is equal to 0 if not. The sum of two connectivity matrices $\underset{\sim}{A} = [a_{ij}]$ and $\underset{\sim}{B} = [b_{ij}]$ of the same order is the matrix

$$\underset{\sim}{A} + \underset{\sim}{B} = [a_{ij} + b_{ij}],$$

where the elements are added according to the rules of Boolean algebra; the product of $\underset{\sim}{A}$ and $\underset{\sim}{B}$ is

$$\underset{\sim}{A} \cdot \underset{\sim}{B} = \left[\sum_{\ell=1}^{n} a_{i\ell} \cdot b_{\ell j} \right],$$

where again addition and multiplication of elements follow the rules of Boolean algebra; the power $\underset{\sim}{A}^r$ of a connectivity matrix is defined by

$$\underset{\sim}{A}^{r} = \underset{\sim}{A} \cdot \underset{\sim}{A}^{r-1}; \quad r=2,3,\ldots$$

finally the transpose $\underset{\sim}{A}^{T}$ of $\underset{\sim}{A}$ is defined by

$$\underset{\sim}{A}^{T} = [a_{ji}].$$

In a connectivity matrix a column of zeros means that the corresponding node is an initial node, a row of zeros means that the corresponding node is a terminal node. For convenience we shall consider only graphs with only one initial node; this kind of graph corresponds to systems of compartments where the tracer is introduced only at one point; of course the linearity of the system implies that if the tracer enters through several compartments, that system can be considered to be the sum of several systems, each one with one initial node.

We shall call the initial node, node 0. Node 0 does not correspond to a real compartment of the system, but rather to the ideal point from where the tracer enters the system (25).

A succession of arms such that the node entered by each of them (except the last) is the node at which the next arm begins, is called a path. If the starting node of the first arm coincides with the ending node of the last arm of a path, that path is called a cycle. The length of a path is equal to the number of its arms. A path, including a cycle, is called simple if every arm of it appears only once; it is called elementary if every node of it is entered only once.

A graph is called connected if there is at least a path from its initial node to any other node; in this section we consider only connected graphs. A graph is called strongly connected, or a strong graph, if there is at least a path from every node, including node 0, to every other node, excluding node 0. In a strong graph there is at least a cycle.

A subgraph is a connected graph obtained by suppressing some nodes and their connecting arms from a given graph; the subgraph obtained by suppressing the initial node and the arms leaving it, from a given graph, is called its G_0 subgraph. A subgraph in which each node occurs in exactly one cycle is called a linear subgraph. Each set of cycles in which each node of the subgraph occurs in exactly one cycle is called a strong component. A Hamiltonian cycle of a graph or subgraph is an elementary cycle that joins all the nodes of that graph or subgraph. For instance the graph of Fig. 1 has one Hamiltonian cycle (1→2→3→4→5→6→7→8→1), two strong components (1→2→3→4→5→6→7→8→1; 1→2→7→8→1 and 3→4→5→6→3), three elementary cycles (1→2→3→4→5→6→7→8→1; 1→2→7→8→1; 3→4→5→6→3).

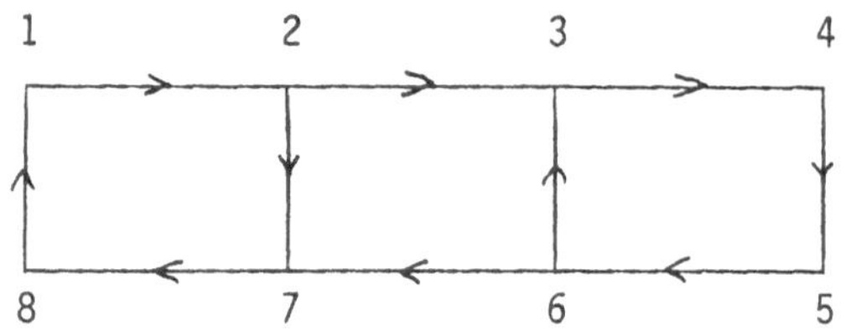

Fig. 1

The graph of Fig. 2 too is strongly connected, but it is not the linear subgraph of any graph; it does not have Hamiltonian cycles or strong components, but it has two elementary cycles ($1\to2\to5\to6\to1$; $2\to5\to4\to3\to2$).

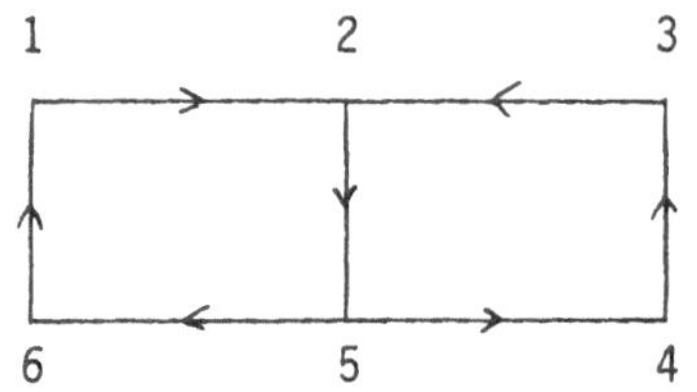

Fig. 2

A graph is symmetric if for any arm connecting a non-initial node to another node, there is an arm in the opposite direction; the connectivity matrix of the G_0 subgraph of a symmetric graph is symmetric, i.e. $\underset{\sim}{A}_0 = \underset{\sim}{A}_0^T$.

A graph is asymmetric if there is no more than one arm between any two nodes; if an asymmetric graph is strongly connected, it admits one Hamiltonian cycle. Define the element by element product $\underset{\sim}{A}x\underset{\sim}{B}$ of two matrices $\underset{\sim}{A} = [a_{ij}]$ and $\underset{\sim}{B} = [b_{ij}]$ by

$$\underset{\sim}{A}x\underset{\sim}{B} = [a_{ij} \cdot b_{ij}];$$

then for an asymmetric graph,

$$\underset{\sim}{A}x\underset{\sim}{A}^T = \underset{\sim}{0};$$

if in a graph some of the connections between nodes are symmetric, the set of such connections is given by the non-zero elements of the element by element product $\underset{\sim}{A}x\underset{\sim}{A}^T$.

A lineal or catenary graph is a graph with all nodes entered by no more than one arm and left by no more than one arm; it has one initial node, one terminal node, and one path; its connectivity matrix has no more than one non-zero element in each column and in each row.

A tree is a graph in which all nodes, except the initial

one, are entered by exactly one arm, and at least one node from which more than one arm starts; these nodes are called roots. The connectivity matrix of a tree has no more than one non-zero element in each column and at least one row with more than one; the rows with more than one non-zero element correspond to the roots of the tree.

A mammillary graph (26) has a central node connected with all other nodes, in one direction or in both directions, while all other nodes are not connected among them. Its connectivity matrix has all elements not on the row or column corresponding to the central compartment, equal to zero.

The successive powers of the connectivity matrix show the existence of paths in the corresponding graph; in fact the element of row i and column j of matrix A^r is one if there is a path of length r from i to j; of course the diagonal elements of A^r show the existence of cycles of length r.

If a graph with n nodes does not contain any cycle, then there is a number $r < n$ such that $A^r = 0$, and matrix A is said to be nilpotent. If $A^r = 0$ but $A^{r-1} \neq 0$, then $r-1$ is the length of the longest path of the graph. Marimont (27) has proved that a matrix is nilpotent if and only if every principal submatrix has at least one zero row or zero column; as a practical rule for finding whether a matrix is nilpotent, i.e. the corresponding graph has no cycles, we can delete successively the rows (or columns) whose elements are all zero, and the corresponding columns (or rows); if some non-zero elements are left, the original matrix is not nilpotent.

The sum of successive powers

$$R_k = A + A^2 + \ldots + A^k$$

shows the paths of length up to k. If A is nilpotent and $A^{k+1} = 0$, then R_k shows the paths of any length. If A is not nilpotent, and k is the length of the longest simple path in the graph, then adding higher powers of A does not change R_k because it includes all possible connections between nodes. If we call R, the reachability matrix, the limit of the sum above for k sufficiently large, then a non-zero element r_{ij} of R shows that there exist a path from node i to node j, i.e. that compartment j can be reached from compartment i. Harary (28) has shown that the element by element product of R and its transpose, $R \times R^T$, indicates in row i the nodes belonging to the same cycle as node i.

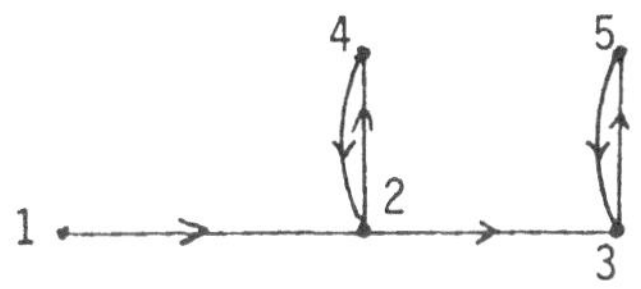

Fig. 3

For instance, from the graph of Fig. 3,

$$\underset{\sim}{A} = \begin{bmatrix} 0&1&0&0&0 \\ 0&0&1&1&0 \\ 0&0&0&0&1 \\ 0&1&0&0&0 \\ 0&0&1&0&0 \end{bmatrix}, \quad \underset{\sim}{A}^2 = \begin{bmatrix} 0&0&1&1&0 \\ 0&1&0&0&1 \\ 0&0&1&0&0 \\ 0&0&1&1&0 \\ 0&0&0&0&1 \end{bmatrix}, \quad \underset{\sim}{A}^3 = \begin{bmatrix} 0&1&0&0&1 \\ 0&0&1&1&0 \\ 0&0&0&0&1 \\ 0&1&0&0&1 \\ 0&0&1&0&0 \end{bmatrix},$$

$\underset{\sim}{A}^4 = \underset{\sim}{A}^2$, $\underset{\sim}{A}^5 = \underset{\sim}{A}^3, \ldots$; therefore

$$\underset{\sim}{R}=\underset{\sim}{A}+\underset{\sim}{A}^2+\underset{\sim}{A}^3 = \begin{bmatrix} 0&1&1&1&1 \\ 0&1&1&1&1 \\ 0&0&1&0&1 \\ 0&1&1&1&1 \\ 0&0&1&0&1 \end{bmatrix}; \quad \underset{\sim}{R}\times\underset{\sim}{R}^T = \begin{bmatrix} 0&0&0&0&0 \\ 0&1&0&1&0 \\ 0&0&1&0&1 \\ 0&1&0&1&0 \\ 0&0&1&0&1 \end{bmatrix};$$

this last matrix shows that nodes 2 and 4 are on one cycle and nodes 3 and 5 on another.

Another important application of graphs to compartmental analysis is the classification of the precursor-successor relationship (29). If in a graph there is a path from i to j, then i is a precursor of j, and j is a successor of i; the length of the shortest path from i to j is called the order of the precursor. For instance in the graph of Fig. 3, node 1 is the precursor of order one of node 2, of order two of nodes 3 and 4, and of order three of node 5. Precursors of order one can be further classified in different types:

(a) Absolute precursor: the arm from i to j is the only one leaving i and the only one entering j;

(b) Complete precursor: there is only one arm leaving i; no cycle may enter j except from i;

(c) Complete precursor with recycling: there is only one arm leaving i; j belongs to a cycle not including i;

(d) Unique precursor: there is only one arm entering j;

(e) Total precursor: there are no paths from i to j of length more than one; if j belongs to a cycle, i belongs to the same cycle;

(f) Total precursor with recycling: there are no paths from i to j of length more than one; there is a cycle in j not through i;

(g) Partial precursor: there is a path from i to j of length more than one; if j belongs to a cycle, no node of the cycle except i has an arm entering j;

(h) Partial precursor with recycling: there is a path from i to j of length more than one; there is a cycle in j not through i.

The following table shows how the different types of precursors of order one can be classified according to the values of the matrices $\underset{\sim}{A}$ and $\underset{\sim}{R}$.

$a_{ij}=1$		$a_{kj}=0$, any $k\neq i$	$a_{kj}=1$, some $k\neq i$	
			$r_{jk}a_{kj}=0$, any $k\neq i$	$r_{jk}a_{kj}=1$, some $k\neq i$
$a_{ih}=0$, any $h\neq j$		a	b	c
$a_{ih}=1$, some $h\neq j$	$a_{ih}r_{hj}=0$, any h	d	e	f
	$a_{ih}r_{hj}=1$, some h	-	g	h

If $a_{ij} = 0$ but $a_{ih}a_{hj} = 1$ for some h, then i is a precursor of order two of j; classification of second order precursors according to different types is done as above. More details on the precursor-successor relationship will be given in Section 9.

It is easy to find the relationships between the matrix $\underset{\sim}{K}$ of a system, as defined in Section 4, and the graph G of the same system. For instance if $\underset{\sim}{K}$ is decomposable, then G is not connected; if $\underset{\sim}{K}$ is irreducible, then G is strongly connected; if $\underset{\sim}{K}$ is reducible and can be put in the triangular form 4-5, then $\underset{\sim}{K}_1$ and $\underset{\sim}{K}_2$ correspond to two strong subgraphs, and $\underset{\sim}{B}$ to the arms going from the nodes of the first subgraph to the nodes of the second.

Due to the importance of the strong components of a G_0 subgraph, it is useful to describe a special notation devised by Caley (30) to represent them. The symbol $|ijk...|$ represent an elementary cycle through the nodes i,j,k,..., and the symbol $|abc...|ijk...|vwx...|$ represents the set of elementary cycles $|abc...|$, $|ijk...|$, $|vwx...|$; then the strong component of a graph with n nodes can be represented by a string with a permutation of the first n natural numbers, interrupted by an appropriate number of bars. For instance the graph of Fig. 1 has the strong components $|12345678|$ and $|1278|3456|$. In general with four nodes the strong components have one of the two forms $|i_1i_2i_3i_4|$ or $|i_1i_2|i_3i_4|$; with five nodes one of the two forms $|i_1i_2i_3i_4i_5|$ or $|i_1i_2i_3|i_4i_5|$. A graphical rule for the construction of the strong components of a G_0 subgraph was described by Rescigno and Segre (31).

6. OPERATIONAL CALCULUS

We return now for a moment to the operational definition of compartment given in Section 2. Integration of Eq. 2-1 gives

$$x = x_0 e^{-Kt} + \int_0^t e^{-K(t-\tau)} f(\tau) d\tau,$$

where x_0 is the initial value of x; the exponential function e^{-Kt} plays a very important role in both terms of the right hand side of the above identity, and it is a characteristic of a given compartment; of course if f(t) is not an arbitrary function chosen by the experimenter, but is the result of the transfer of the tracer from other compartments, then in the integral above the characteristic function e^{-Kt} of this compartment combines with the characteristic functions of other compartments, yielding a more complex function characteristic of the whole system. A very simple way to study the synthesis of such functions is by means of the operational calculus (32). More details can be found elsewhere (15), while here I give only the fundamental concepts.

We shall consider here functions of time, defined for all values $t \geqq 0$, and we shall use the brackets { } to distinguish between the function itself and its values; for instance f(t) represents the value of <u>f</u> at time <u>t</u>, while {f} represents the whole function; similarly, say, 2 represents the natural number <u>two</u> while {2} represents the function with the constant value 2 for all values of t.

Define the two operations

$$\{f\} + \{g\} = \{f+g\},$$

$$\{f\} \cdot \{g\} = \{\int_0^t f(\tau)\, g(t-\tau)\, d\tau\};$$

the first definition shows that the symbol {f} + {g} represents a function whose values are given by the sum of the values of the functions <u>f</u> and <u>g</u>; this operation has all the properties of the addition of natural numbers, in particular it is commutative and associative, therefore we can conveniently call it <u>addition of functions</u>. The second definition shows that the symbol {f}·{g} represents a function whose values are given by a certain integral called <u>convolution</u>; it is not as obvious as before, but this operation also can be proved to be commutative and associative; it is also distributive with respect to the addition of functions, exactly as the multiplication of natural numbers; we can therefore call this operation multiplication of functions. Thus, by definition,

$$2 \cdot 3 = 6,$$

while

$$\{2\} \cdot \{3\} = \{\int_0^t 2 \cdot 3 \cdot d\tau\}$$

$$= \{6t\};$$

on the other hand

$$2+3 = 5$$

and

$$\{2\} + \{3\} = \{5\}.$$

The product of a function by itself can be defined as with natural numbers, thus

$$\{f\} \cdot \{f\} = \{f\}^2,$$

$$\{f\} \cdot \{f\}^2 = \{f\}^3,$$

and so forth.

A very special function is the constant function {1}; in fact

$$\{1\} \cdot \{f\} = \{\int_0^t f(\tau)d\tau\}$$

for any $f(t)$; i.e. multiplication of a function by {1} is equivalent to integration between 0 and t. Other interesting functions are

$$\{1\}^2 = \{t\},$$

$$\{1\}^3 = \{t^2/2\},$$

and in general

$$\{1\}^n = \{t^{n-1}/(n-1)!\}.$$

The division of functions can be defined as the division of natural numbers, thus: given two functions {f} and {g}, with $\{g\} \neq \{0\}$, a third function {h} is called their quotient, and we write

$$\{f\}/\{g\} = \{h\},$$

if a function $\{h\}$ exists such that

$$\{f\} = \{g\}\cdot\{h\}.$$

Exactly as with natural numbers, not all pairs of functions have a quotient; to make the division of functions always possible, with the only restriction that the divisor be different from $\{0\}$, we define the operators. In analogy with rational numbers we define the equality of operators,

$$\{f\}/\{g\} = \{\phi\}/\{\psi\} \text{ if and only if } \{f\}\cdot\{\psi\} = \{g\}\cdot\{\phi\};$$

the addition of operators,

$$\{f\}/\{g\} + \{\phi\}/\{\psi\} = (\{f\}\cdot\{\psi\} + \{g\}\cdot\{\phi\})/(\{g\}\cdot\{\psi\});$$

the multiplication of operators,

$$\{f\}/\{g\}\cdot\{\phi\}/\{\psi\} = (\{f\}\cdot\{\phi\})/(\{g\}\cdot\{\psi\}).$$

From the above definitions it follows that

$$\frac{\{f\}\cdot\{\phi\}}{\{g\}\cdot\{\phi\}} = \frac{\{f\}}{\{g\}}$$

and

$$\frac{\{f\}\cdot\{\phi\}}{\{\phi\}} = \{f\},$$

equivalent to the elementary operations of reduction of fractions.

The last expression is particularly important because it shows that any function can be written as the quotient of two functions, i.e. as an operator. As a consequence we can regard any function as a special kind of operator; therefore even though strictly speaking we cannot, for instance, add a function to an operator, we can look at such hibrid operation as the sum of a special operator with another operator.

Another special operator, called numerical operator, is $\{\alpha\}/\{1\}$, where α is a constant; for the numerical operators we have

$$\frac{\{\alpha\}}{\{1\}} + \frac{\{\beta\}}{\{1\}} = \frac{\{\alpha\}\cdot\{1\} + \{1\}\cdot\{\beta\}}{\{1\}\cdot\{1\}}$$

$$= \frac{\{1\}\cdot(\{\alpha\} + \{\beta\})}{\{1\}\cdot\{1\}}$$

$$= \frac{\{\alpha + \beta\}}{\{1\}}$$

and

$$\frac{\{\alpha\}}{\{1\}} \frac{\{\beta\}}{\{1\}} = \frac{\{\alpha\}\cdot\{\beta\}}{\{1\}\cdot\{1\}}$$

$$= \frac{\{\int_0^t \alpha\beta d\tau\}}{\{1\}\cdot\{1\}}$$

$$= \frac{\{1\}\cdot\{\alpha\beta\}}{\{1\}\cdot\{1\}}$$

$$= \frac{\{\alpha\beta\}}{\{1\}} ;$$

therefore the sum and the product of numerical operators is a numerical operator, whose dividend is the sum or product of the dividends of the given numerical operators. As a consequence we can operate on numerical operators as on natural numbers, and use for brevity the symbol

$$\frac{\{\alpha\}}{\{1\}} = \alpha .$$

Using the definitions above,

$$\alpha \cdot \{f\} = \frac{\{\alpha\}}{\{1\}} \cdot \frac{\{f\}\cdot\{\psi\}}{\{\psi\}}$$

$$= \frac{\{\alpha\}\cdot\{f\}\cdot\{\psi\}}{\{1\}\cdot\{\psi\}}$$

$$= \frac{\{\int_0^t \alpha f(\tau) d\tau\}}{\{1\}}$$

$$= \frac{\{1\}\cdot\{\alpha f\}}{\{1\}} = \{\alpha f\},$$

i.e. the numerical operator can be imported into or exported out of the brackets.

For the numerical operator 0,

$$0 = \frac{\{0\}}{\{1\}} = \frac{\{0\}\cdot\{1\}}{\{1\}} = \{0\},$$

i.e. this is the only numerical operator equal to its

corresponding function.

We can now define the <u>inverse</u> of an operator $\{f\}/\{g\}$ as the operator $\{g\}/\{f\}$, provided <u>that $\{f\}$</u> $\neq 0$. The product of an operator by its inverse is obviously equal to the numerical operator 1. Let us represent with the letter <u>s</u> the inverse of the operator $\{1\}$; then

$$s\,\{1\} = 1. \tag{6-1}$$

Consider now a function f(t) with a derivative f'(t); obviously

$$\{\int_0^t f'(\tau)d\tau\} = \{f(t)\}-\{f(0)\},$$

or

$$\{1\}\cdot\{f'\} = \{f\}-\{f(0)\};$$

divide both sides by $\{1\}$,

$$\{f'\} = s\{f\}-f(0) \tag{6-2}$$

or

$$s\{f\} = \{f'\} + f(0).$$

This last expression justifies the name of <u>differential operator</u> given to <u>s</u>. By induction we can show that

$$\{f''\} = s^2\{f\}-sf(0)-f'(0),$$

$$\{f'''\} = s^3\{f\}-s^2f(0)-sf'(0)-f''(0),$$

and so forth.

We can now use identity 6-2 to represent some functions as operators. In fact from

$$\frac{d}{dt}e^{-\alpha t} = -\alpha e^{-\alpha t},$$

$$e^0 = 1$$

we get

$$-\alpha\{e^{-\alpha t}\} = s\,\{e^{-\alpha t}\}-1,$$

and

$$\{e^{-\alpha t}\} = \frac{1}{s+\alpha}; \tag{6-3}$$

also from

$$\frac{d}{dt}\cos \omega t = -\omega \sin \omega t$$

$$\frac{d}{dt}\sin \omega t = \omega \cos \omega t$$

$$\cos 0 = 1$$

$$\sin 0 = 0$$

we get

$$-\omega\{\sin \omega t\} = s\{\cos \omega t\} - 1$$

$$\omega\{\cos \omega t\} = s\{\sin \omega t\}$$

and

$$\{\cos \omega t\} = \frac{s}{s^2+\omega^2}$$

$$\{\sin \omega t\} = \frac{\omega}{s^2+\omega^2}\ .$$

From

$$\frac{d}{dt}(e^{-\alpha t}\cos \omega t) = -\alpha e^{-\alpha t}\cos \omega t - \omega e^{-\alpha t}\sin \omega t$$

$$\frac{d}{dt}(e^{-\alpha t}\sin \omega t) = -\alpha e^{-\alpha t}\sin \omega t + \omega e^{-\alpha t}\cos \omega t$$

$$e^0 \cos 0 = 1$$

$$e^0 \sin 0 = 0$$

we get

$$-\alpha\{e^{-\alpha t}\cos \omega t\} - \omega\{e^{-\alpha t}\sin \omega t\} = s\{e^{-\alpha t}\cos \omega t\} - 1$$

$$-\alpha\{e^{-\alpha t}\sin \omega t\} + \omega\{e^{-\alpha t}\cos \omega t\} = s\{e^{-\alpha t}\sin \omega t\}$$

$$\{e^{-\alpha t}\cos \omega t\} = \frac{s+\alpha}{(s+\alpha)^2+\omega^2} \tag{6-4}$$

$$\{e^{-\alpha t}\sin \omega t\} = \frac{\omega}{(s+\alpha)^2+\omega^2}\ . \tag{6-5}$$

From 6-1 we have

$$\{1\} = 1/s$$

$$\{t\} = 1/s^2$$

$$\{t^2\} = 2/s^3$$

and so forth.

In a similar way many other functions can be written in operational form. An extensive list of such correlates was compiled by Bateman (33), but for all practical purposes the short list appended in Rescigno and Segre's book (10) is sufficient.

We can now write Eq. 3-7 in operational form

$$\{dx_i/dt\} = \{-K_i x_i\} + \sum_{j \neq i} \{k_{ji} x_j\} + \{f_i(t)\},$$

or, using the properties of operators just seen,

$$s\{x_i\} - x_i(0) = -K_i\{x_i\} + \sum_{j \neq i} k_{ji}\{x_j\} + \{f_i\},$$

thence

$$\{x_i\} = \frac{1}{s+K_i} [x_i(0) + \{f_i\}] + \sum_{j \neq i} \frac{k_{ji}}{s+K_i} \{x_j\}. \qquad (6\text{-}6)$$

Another important property of operators, often referred to as the Final Value Theorem, is:

If

$$\{f\} = \frac{p(s)}{q(s)}$$

and

$$\lim_{t \to \infty} f(t)$$

exists, then

$$\lim_{t \to \infty} f(t) = \left. \frac{s \cdot p(s)}{q(s)} \right|_{s=0},$$

where the symbol on the right-hand side represents the value obtained when the operator $s \cdot p(s)/q(s)$ is written with 0 instead of s.

In fact we can distinguish two cases. If $q(s)$ does not contain the factor s, it can be written as a product of terms of the form $(s+\alpha)^2+\omega^2$ and $s+\alpha$, and the operator $p(s)/q(s)$ as a sum of operators of the form 6-3, 6-4, 6-5, all corresponding to functions with a limit of $\underline{0}$ for $\underline{t}$ approaching infinity; and in this case of course the operator $\underline{s}$ $p(s)/q(s)$ becomes $\underline{0}$ when $\underline{s}$ is substituted by $\underline{0}$. The other possibility is that $q(s)$ contains the factor $\underline{0}$, but no more than once for the reasons seen in Section 4; in this case we can write

$$\{f\} = \frac{a+bs+...}{s(c+ds+...)} = \frac{a/c}{s} + \frac{(b-ad)/c+...}{c+ds+...} ,$$

therefore,

$$\lim_{t\to\infty} f(t) = a/c,$$

while

$$\frac{s\cdot p(s)}{q(s)} = \frac{a+bs+...}{c+ds+...}$$

becomes a/c when $\underline{s}$ is substituted by $\underline{0}$.

7. LINEAR GRAPHS

Eq. 6-6 shows how the operator $\{x_i\}$ of compartment i depends on the numerical operator $x_i(0)$ of its initial condition, on the feeding function $\{f_i\}$, and on the operators $\{x_j\}$ of all other compartments. That equation can be represented graphically with a node for $x_i(0) + \{f_i\}$, a node for each function $\{x_j\}$, and a node for $\{x_i\}$, plus an arm from each of the former nodes to this last node, these arms equal to the coefficients of the respective terms on the right hand side of Eq. 6-6. Thus node $\{x_i\}$ is equal to the sum of all arms entering it times their nodes of departure. For instance to equation

$$\{x_1\} = \frac{1}{s+K_1} x_1(0) + \frac{k_{21}}{s+K_1} \{x_2\} + \frac{k_{31}}{s+K_1} \{x_3\} \qquad (7\text{-}1)$$

corresponds to the graph

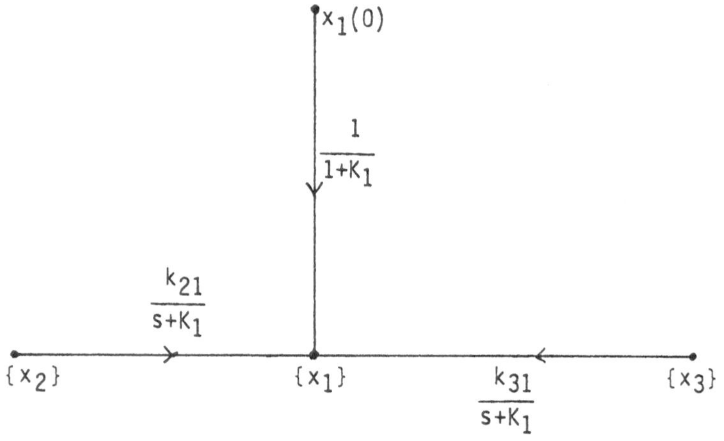

Of course an equation like 6-6 can be written for each compartment of a system, and to each equation corresponds a graph; all those graphs can be combined together, because the arms entering a node of one graph will not change the values of the nodes determined by another equation. If Eq. 7-1 is holding with the two additional equations, for instance

$$\{x_2\} = \frac{k_{12}}{s+K_2}\{x_1\} + \frac{k_{32}}{s+K_2}\{x_3\},$$

$$\{x_3\} = \frac{k_{13}}{s+K_3}\{x_1\},$$

then their two corresponding graphs

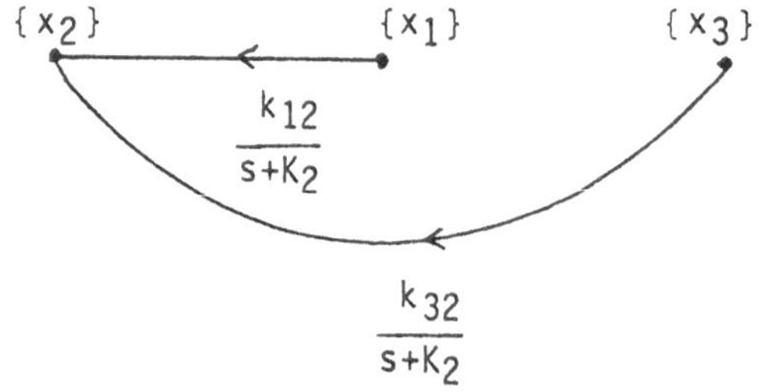

and

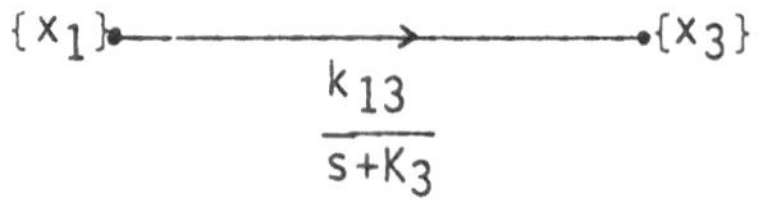

can be combined with the first one thus

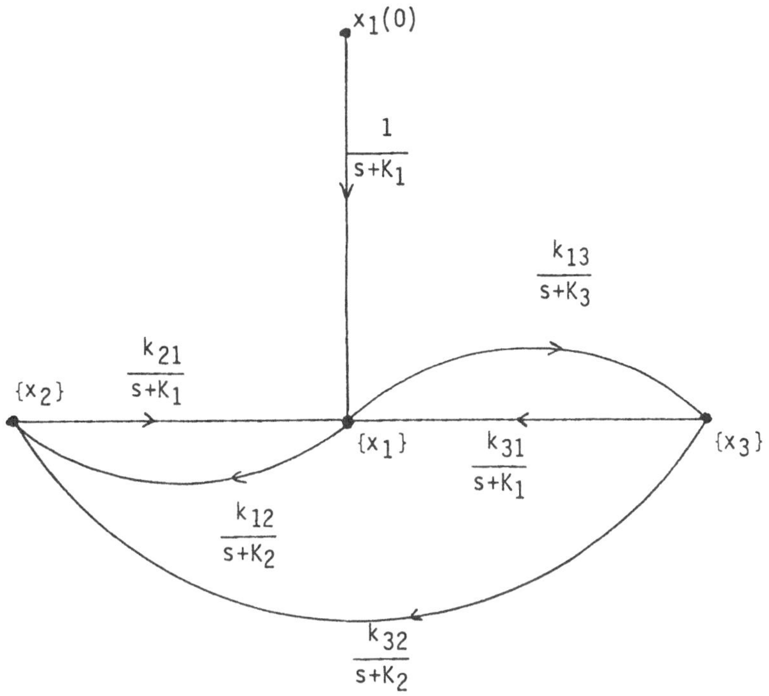

This graph includes all information contained in the given differential equations plus the initial conditions. This kind of graph was introduced in 1953 by Mason (34) who called it signal-flow graph; it has been used in compartmental analysis since 1960 (25). We prefer the name linear graph as more indicative of its function, even though this term was used by Kirchhoff (35) in a slightly different context.

Almost all definitions given for directed graphs are valid for linear graphs too. In particular a path has a length, as in a directed graph, but also a value, equal to the product of its arms.

The fundamental property of a linear graph, as an immediate consequence of its definition, is: "Each node is equal to the sum of the products of the arms entering it times their departing nodes." A number of transformations can be made, including the suppression of some nodes, without changing the fundamental properties of the nodes left. These four transformations were described by Mason (34):

(a) Two tandem arms can be substituted by a single arm equal to their product, and the intermediate node suppressed.

(b) Two parallel arms can be substituted by a single arm equal to their sum.

(c) An arm entering a node can be substituted by arms entering all nodes immediately following it, each new arm being equal to the product of the original arm and the arm connecting the previous to the new end.

(d) An arm starting and ending at the same node can be suppressed by dividing all arms entering that node by one minus the value of the suppressed arm.

Repeated application of these four rules leads to a much simpler linear graph that helps interpreting some of the properties of the system of compartments it represents. More details can be found in the literature (36,37,38); here we intend to show only some simple properties of the linear graphs.

Going back to Eq. 6-6, observe that the term

$$x_i(0) + \{f_i\}$$

represents the contribution to compartment i from outside the system of compartments, either as material put in it at time 0, or fed to it successively; we can call this term the input to compartment i. For simplicity consider the case when only one compartment, say compartment i, has an input different from zero; then its linear graph has only one initial node, as defined in Section 5. If the graph does not contain any cycle, then there are only a finite number of paths between its initial node and any other node; repeated application of the first three Mason's rules leads to a graph containing exactly one arm between the source and each other node. For instance the graph

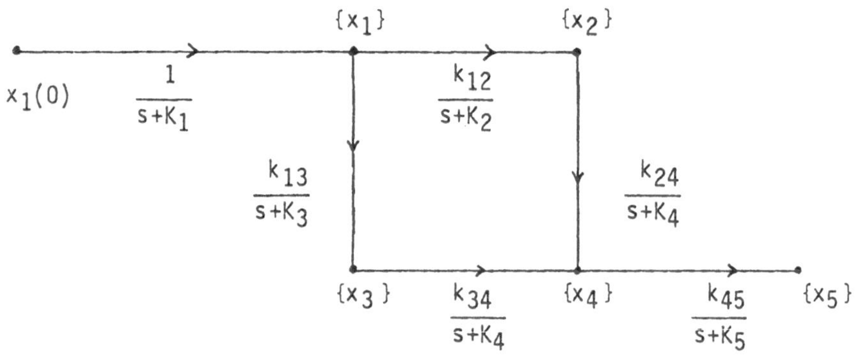

has one path from $x_1(0)$ to $\{x_1\}$, equal to $\frac{1}{s+K_1}$, one path from $x_1(0)$ to $\{x_2\}$, equal to $\frac{k_{12}}{(s+K_1)(s+K_2)}$, two paths from $x_1(0)$ to $\{x_4\}$, respectively equal to $\frac{k_{12}k_{24}}{(s+K_1)(s+K_2)(s+K_4)}$ and $\frac{k_{13}k_{34}}{(s+K_1)(s+K_3)(s+K_4)}$, and so forth. This graph is therefore equivalent to the graph

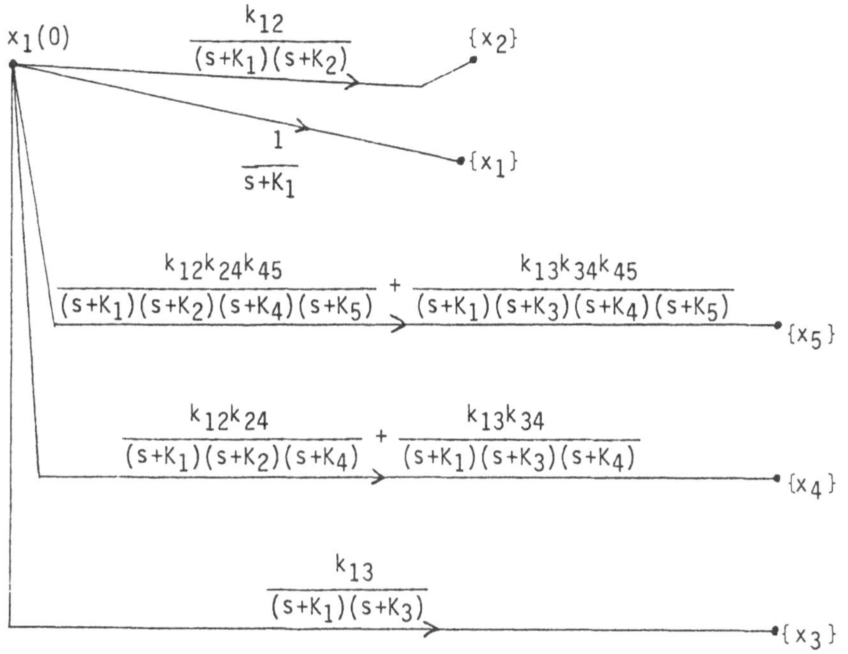

In this new graph there is one initial node, the source; all other nodes are terminal nodes, therefore any of them can be suppressed without altering the properties of the rest of the graph. This is important, because when the behavior of only one compartment is of interest, the graph can be reduced to only one arm, between the source and that particular node.

The problem is slightly more complicated when the original graph contains some cycles, because in this case the number of paths between some nodes is infinite. A first step in the simplification of such graph is to look for essential nodes, i.e. nodes that must be removed to interrupt all cycles; their choice is not unique, but in any case it should be such that the number of essential nodes is minimum. Once the essential nodes are chosen, the simplified graph contains:

a) an arm from the source to the terminal node of interest,
b) an arm from the source to each essential node,
c) an arm from each essential node to the terminal node,
d) an arm from each essential node to each other essential node,
e) an arm from each essential node to itself.

The value of each of these arms is equal to the sum of the values of the elementary paths between the nodes they connect, excluding all other nodes of the simplified graph. Some of the arms listed above may be missing, and the terminal node itself may be an essential node. Figure 4 shows a simplified graph with one essential node:

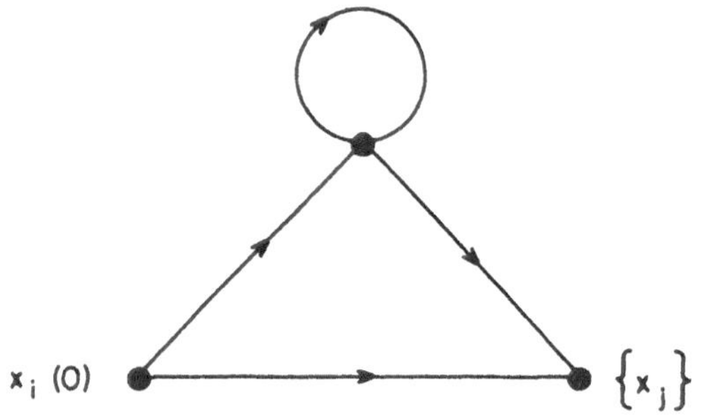

Fig. 4 A simplified graph with one essential node

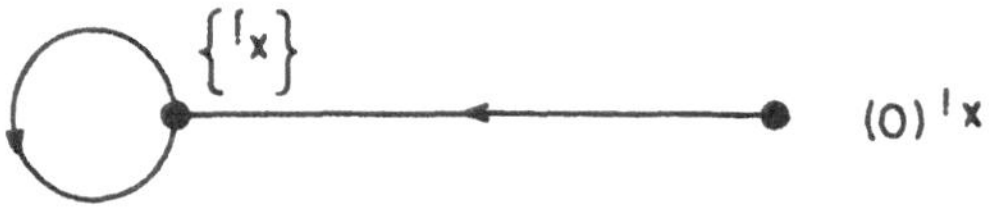

Fig. 5 A simplified graph where the essential node is the terminal node

Fig. 5 shows a simplified graph where the terminal node is an essential one; Figs. 6 and 7 show simplified graphs with two essential nodes; in all cases $x_i(0) + \{f_i\}$ is the source and $\{x_j\}$ the terminal node.

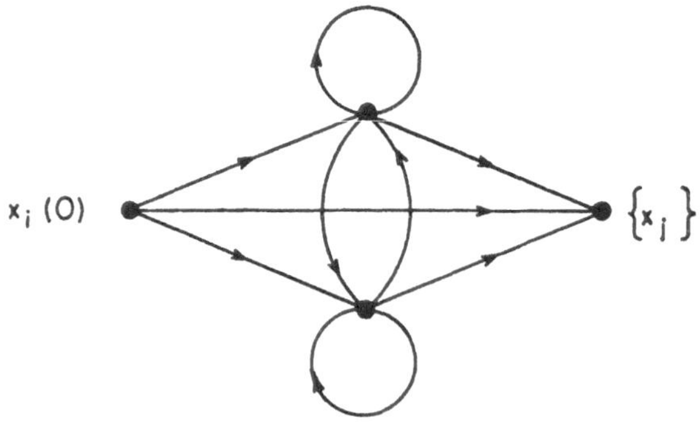

Fig. 6 A simplified graph with two essential nodes, general case

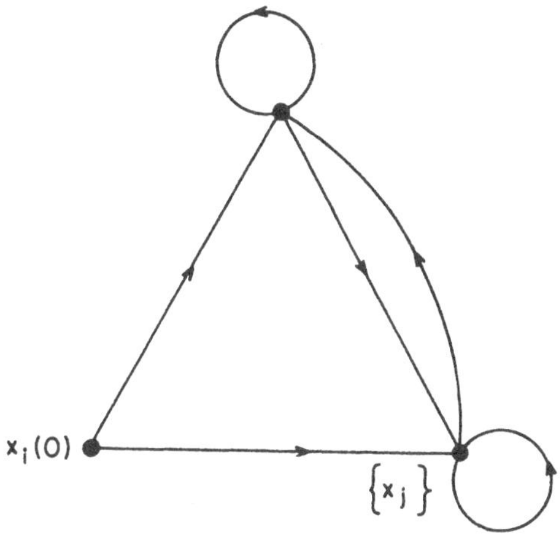

Fig. 7 A simplified graph with two essential nodes, one of them being the terminal node

From the simplified graph the closed arms can be eliminated using Mason's fourth rule, then the new graph can be further simplified as before, until only an initial and a terminal node are left.

Now write Eq. 4-2 in operational form,

$$\{\underset{\sim}{x}\} = \underset{\sim}{x}_0 \{e^{\underset{\sim}{K}t}\} + \{\underset{\sim}{f}\} \{e^{\underset{\sim}{K}t}\}$$

or

$$\{\underset{\sim}{x}\} = [\underset{\sim}{x}_0 + \{\underset{\sim}{f}\}] \{e^{\underset{\sim}{K}t}\},$$

where $\{\underset{\sim}{x}\}$, $\underset{\sim}{x}_0$ and $\{\underset{\sim}{f}\}$ are row vectors of operators, and $\{e^{\underset{\sim}{K}t}\}$ is a square matrix of operators.

Remember now that we are considering the case when only one compartment has an input different from zero, therefore the row vector $\underset{\sim}{x}_0 + \{\underset{\sim}{f}\}$ has only one non-zero element, equal to $x_i(0) + \{f_i\}$; it follows that $\{\underset{\sim}{x}\}$is equal to this last operator times the $\underline{i}$-th row of $\{e^{\underset{\sim}{K}t}\}$, and the $\underline{j}$-th element of $\{\underset{\sim}{x}\}$ is

$$\{x_j\} = [x_i(0) + \{f_i\}] \{f_{ij}\}, \tag{7-2}$$

where $\{f_{ij}\}$ is the element of row $\underline{i}$ and column j of $\{e^{\underset{\sim}{K}t}\}$.

Function $\{f_{ij}\}$ is called the transfer function from the source of compartment $\underline{i}$ to compartment $\underline{j}$, and it is equal to the value of the single arm left when the graph is simplified as described above.

The rules shown here are conveniently applied when a graph

does not contain many cycles; if the simplification of the graph involves more than one or two essential nodes, it is more convenient to use the method based on the strong components of a graph (31).

8. INTEGRAL EQUATIONS

We have seen that the element $\{f_{ij}\}$ of row i and column j of matrix $\{e^{\underline{K}t}\}$ is called the transfer function from the source of compartment i to compartment j. We can rewrite Eq. 7-2 in the form,

$$x_j(t) = x_i(0)\ f_{ij}(t) + \int_0^t f_i(\tau)\ f_{ij}(t-\tau)d\tau; \qquad (8\text{-}1)$$

this is a Volterra integral equation of the second type. If $x_i(0)$ and $f_i(t)$ are given and $x_j(t)$ is measured, the transfer function can be computed.

A simple physical interpretation of the transfer function is obtained by considering Eq. 8-1 with $f_i(t) \equiv 0$ and $x_i(0) = 1$; then

$$x_j(t) = f_{ij}(t),$$

i.e. the transfer function from the source of i to j is equal to the function describing compartment j when compartment i is fed with a unitary instantaneous dose at time 0. If instead $x_i(0) = 0$ but $f_i(t) \not\equiv 0$, then

$$x_j(t) = \int_0^t f_i(\tau)\ f_{ij}(t-\tau)d\tau,$$

i.e. the behavior of compartment j is the convolution between the feeding function of compartment i and the transfer function from the source of i to j when compartment i is initially empty.

The integral equation approach for the description of metabolizing systems was introduced by Branson (39,40,41,42) as early as 1948 and reformulated in 1963 (43); Stephenson (44) too used integral equations for the description of transport through linear biological systems.

Eq. 7-2, or its correlate 8-1, can be made more general; suppose that compartment i is not directly controllable, i.e. it is not possible to introduce a tracer directly into it, but that a tracer introduced in a precursor of i can be measured in i and in j, and that no tracer can reach j without passing first through i; or alternatively suppose that, even though the tracer can be fed directly into i, the feeding function $f_i(t)$ cannot be measured, but $x_i(t)$ can. In either case, from the linear graph we see that

$$\{x_j\} = \{x_i\}\{g_{ij}\},$$

where

$$\{g_{ij}\} = \{f_{ij}\}(s+K_i)$$

is called the <u>transfer function from compartment i to compartment j</u>. This equation is equivalent to

$$x_j(t) = \int_0^t x_i(\tau)\ g_{ij}(t-\tau)d\tau,$$

and a partial solution of it may be obtained with a graphical method (45). By sampling x_i and x_j at different times we can plot a number of values of $x_j/(tx_i)$ versus t and extrapolate those values for t = 0; if $x_i(0) = 0$ but $x_i'(0) \neq 0$, using L'Hospital rule,

$$\lim_{t\to 0} \frac{x_j(t)}{t\ x_i(t)} = \lim_{t\to 0} \frac{\int_0^t x_i(\tau)\ g_{ij}(t-\tau)d\tau}{t\ x_i(t)}$$

$$= \lim_{t\to 0} \frac{\int_0^t x_i(\tau)\ g_{ij}'(t-\tau)d\tau + x_i(t)\ g_{ij}(0)}{x_i(t) + tx'(t)}$$

$$= \lim_{t\to 0} \frac{\int_0^t x_i(\tau)\ g_{ij}''(t-\tau)d\tau + x_i(t)\ g_{ij}'(0) + x_i'(t)\ g_{ij}(0)}{2x_i'(t) + tx_i''(t)}$$

$$= 1/2 \cdot g_{ij}(0);$$

if $x_i(0) = x_i'(0) = 0$ but $x_i''(0) \neq 0$ we apply L'Hospital rule once more and get

$$\lim_{t\to 0} \frac{x_j(t)}{t\ x_i(t)} =$$

$$\lim_{t\to 0} \frac{\int_0^t x_i(\tau)\ g_{ij}'''(t-\tau)d\tau + x_i(t)\ g_{ij}''(0) + x_i'(t)\ g_{ij}'(0) + x_i''(t) g_{ij}(0)}{3x_i''(t) + t\ x_i'''(t)}$$

$$= \frac{1}{3}\ g_{ij}(0);$$

in general, if m is the lowest order of derivative of $x_i(t)$ different from 0 for t=0, then

$$\lim_{t\to 0} \frac{x_j(t)}{t\ x_i(t)} = \frac{1}{m+1}\, g_{ij}(0).$$

Suppose now it has been found that

$$g_{ij}(0) = 0;$$

we can plot $x_j/(t^2 x_i)$ versus t and extrapolate those values for t=0; again if $x_i(0)=0$ but $x_i'(0)\neq 0$,

$$\lim_{t\to 0} \frac{x_j(t)}{t^2\, x_i(t)} = \lim_{t\to 0} \frac{\int_0^t x_i(\tau)\, g_{ij}(t-\tau)d\tau}{t^2\, x_i(t)}$$

$$= \lim_{t\to 0} \frac{\int_0^t x_i(\tau)\, g_{ij}'(t-\tau)d\tau}{2t\, x_i(t)+t^2 x_i'(t)}$$

$$= \lim_{t\to 0} \frac{\int_0^t x_i(\tau)\, g_{ij}''(t-\tau)d\tau + x_i(t)\, g_{ij}'(0)}{2x_i(t)+4tx_i'(t)+t^2 x_i''(t)}$$

$$= \lim_{t\to 0} \frac{\int_0^t x_i(\tau)\, g_{ij}'''(t-\tau)d\tau + x_i(t) g_{ij}''(0) + x_i'(t)\, g_{ij}'(0)}{6x_i'(t)+6tx_i''(t)+t^2 x_i'''(t)}$$

$$= \frac{1}{6}\, g_{ij}'(0).$$

Proceeding in the same way it is easy to prove that, if

$$x_i(0) = x_i'(0)=\ldots=x_i^{(m-1)}(0)=0,\quad x_i^{(m)}\neq 0$$

$$g_{ij}(0) = g_{ij}'(0)=\ldots=g_{ij}^{(n-1)}(0)=0, \tag{8-2}$$

then

$$g_{ij}^{(n)}(0) = \frac{(m+n+1)!}{m!} \lim_{t\to 0} \frac{x_j(t)}{t^{n+1} x_i(t)} \tag{8-3}$$

Conditions 8-2 are not very restrictive, for if they do not hold for a specific transfer function $g_{ij}(t)$, we define the function

$$\overline{g}_{ij}(t) = g_{ij}(t)-g_{ij}(0)-tg'_{ij}(0)-\frac{t^2}{2!}g''_{ij}(0)-\dots-\frac{t^{n-1}}{(n-1)}g_{ij}^{(n-1)}(0),$$

and conditions 8-3 hold for $\overline{g}_{ij}(t)$; and since

$$\frac{d^n}{dt^n}\overline{g}_{ij}(t)\bigg|_{t=0} = \frac{d^n}{dt^n}g_{ij}(t)\bigg|_{t=0},$$

from 8-3 we get

$$g_{ij}^{(n)}(0) = \frac{(m+n+1)!}{m!} \lim_{t\to 0} \frac{\overline{x}_j(t)}{t^{n+1} x_i(t)}, \tag{8-4}$$

where

$$\overline{x}_j(t) = \int_0^t x_i(\tau)\, g_{ij}(t-\tau)d\tau,$$

and using the formalism of the operational calculus,

$$\{\overline{x}_j\} = \{x_i\}\ \{\overline{g}_{ij}\}$$

$$= \{x_i\}\ (\{g_{ij}\}-\{g_{ij}(0)\}-\{tg'_{ij}(0)\}-\dots-\{\frac{t^{n-1}}{(n-1)!}g_{ij}^{(n-1)}(0)\})$$

$$= \{x_i\}(\{g_{ij}\}-g_{ij}(0)\{1\}-g'_{ij}(0)\{1\}^2-\dots-g_{ij}^{(n-1)}(0)\{1\}^n)$$

$$= \{x_j\}-g_{ij}(0)\{\int_0^t x_i\}-g_{ij}(0)\{\int_0^t\int_0^t x_i\}-\dots-g_{ij}^{(n-1)}(0)\{\int_0^t\int_0^t\dots\int_0^t x_i\} \tag{8-5}$$

Thus relations 8-4 and 8-5 permit the determination of initial values of derivatives of all orders of the transfer function $g_{ij}(0)$. The physical meaning of those initial values will be explained in the next section.

9. PRECURSOR-SUCCESSOR RELATIONSHIP

In Section 5 we described qualitatively the precursor-successor relationship; now we can reconsider this relationship from a quantitative point of view.

Consider a linear graph without cycles; we can reduce it to a single arm simply by adding the values of all paths from the two chosen nodes; each of those paths is a product of factors of the form $k_{ab}/(s+K_b)$, i.e. it is a fraction whose numerator is formed by a string of small k's, while the denominator is a polynomial in s of degree equal to the length of that path. When adding the values of the different paths, a fraction is formed whose denominator contains terms of the form $s+K_b$ corresponding to the compartments on any path between precursor and successor, including the successor but excluding the precursor. The numerator of that fraction will be a sum of strings of small k's, each string multiplied by the factor $s+K_b$ corresponding to arms not on the path from where that particular string comes from; of all the terms on the numerator, the one with the highest degree in s will be the one coming from the shortest path; in fact the difference of degree in s between the denominator and the numerator will be exactly equal to the number of arms on the shortest path, i.e. to the order of the precursor. Furthermore the coefficient of the highest term in s of the numerator is the string of small k's along this shortest path; this product is called the precursor's principal term (29). If cycles are present the formation of the transfer function from the factors $k_{ab}/(s+K_b)$ is more complicated, but the last two statements still hold. In fact each time a closed arm is eliminated, the value of some arms is multiplied by one minus the value of a path; this last value is an operator with the degree in s of the numerator smaller than the degree in s of the denominator; one minus that value generates a fraction with exactly the same degree in s on numerator and denominator, and with exactly the same coefficient for the highest term of numerator and denominator.

For instance from the graph

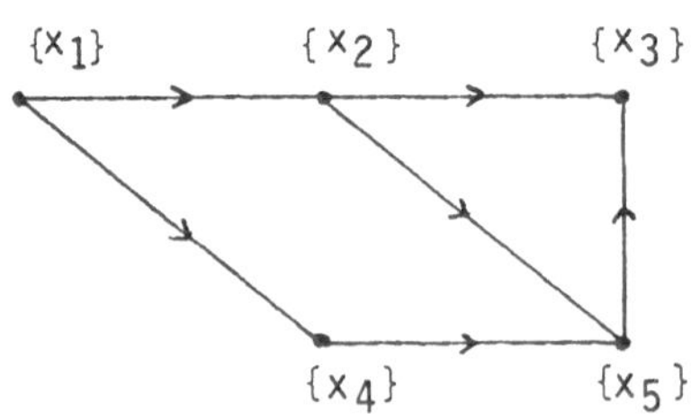

we get

$$\{x_3\} = \left[\frac{k_{12}k_{23}}{(s+K_2)(s+K_3)} + \frac{k_{12}k_{25}k_{53}}{(s+K_2)(s+K_5)(s+K_3)} + \frac{k_{14}k_{45}k_{53}}{(s+K_4)(s+K_5)(s+K_3)}\right]\{x_1\}$$

$$\{x_3\} = \frac{k_{12}k_{23}(s+K_4)(s+K_5)+k_{12}k_{25}k_{53}(s+K_4)+k_{14}k_{45}k_{53}(s+K_2)}{(s+K_2)(s+K_3)(s+K_4)(s+K_5)}\{x_1\};$$

compartment 1 is a precursor of order two of compartment 3, and the difference of degree in s between denominator and numerator of $\{g_{13}\}$ is two; the coefficient of s^2 in the numerator is $k_{12}k_{23}$, the product of the transfer coefficients on the shortest path from $\{x_1\}$ to $\{x_3\}$. Now consider the graph

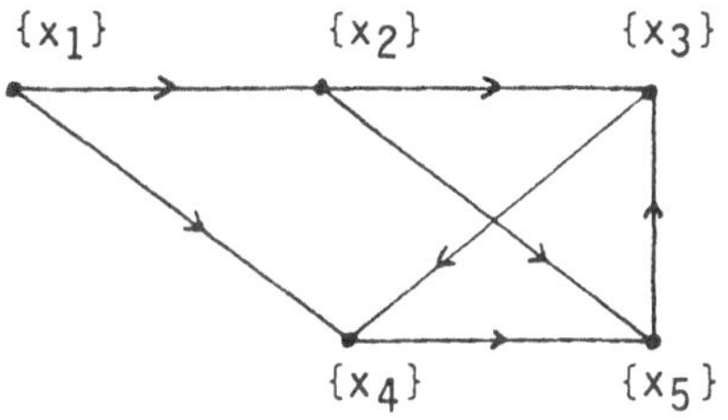

$\{x_3\}$ is an essential node, therefore this graph can be simplified thus

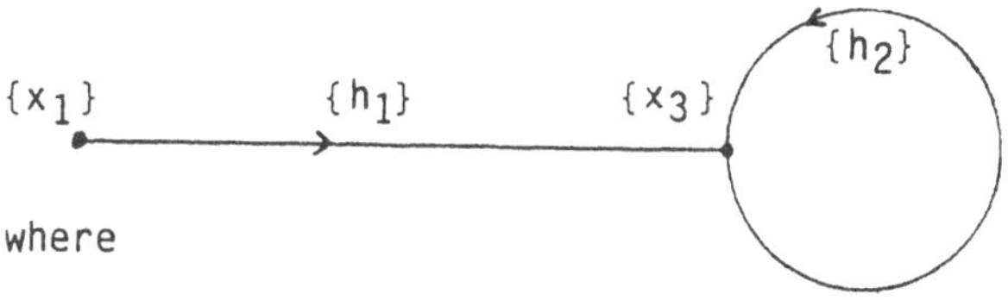

where

$$\{h_1\} = \frac{k_{12}k_{23}(s+K_4)(s+K_5)+k_{12}k_{25}k_{53}(s+K_4)+k_{14}k_{45}k_{53}(s+K_2)}{(s+K_2)(s+K_3)(s+K_4)(s+K_5)}$$

$$\{h_2\} = \frac{k_{34}k_{45}k_{53}}{(s+K_4)(s+K_5)(s+K_3)};$$

using Mason's fourth rule we get

$$\{x_3\} = \frac{\{h_1\}}{1-\{h_2\}}\{x_1\}$$

$$\{x_3\} = \{h_1\}\frac{(s+K_3)(s+K_4)(s+K_5)}{(s+K_3)(s+K_4)(s+K_5)-k_{34}k_{45}k_{53}}\{x_1\}$$

$$\{x_3\} = \frac{k_{12}k_{23}(s+K_4)(s+K_5)+k_{12}k_{25}k_{53}(s+K_4)+k_{14}k_{45}k_{53}(s+K_2)}{(s+K_2)[(s+K_3)(s+K_4)(s+K_5)-k_{34}k_{45}k_{53}}\{x_1\};$$

in this new graph the order of the precursor is the same, and even though the denominator of the new transfer function is different, the difference of degree between denominator and numerator, and the coefficient of s^2 in the numerator, are the same as in the previous graph.

We have seen that in general if n+1 is the precursor order of $\{x_i\}$ with respect to $\{x_j\}$, then the transfer function $\{g_{ij}\}$ is a fraction of two polynomials in s, with denominator of degree n+1 higher than the numerator; therefore the operator

$$s^n\{g_{ij}\} = \{g_{ij}^{(n)}\}$$

has exactly one as difference between degrees of denominator and numerator. Then

$$\{g_{ij}^{(n)}\} = \frac{as^{\alpha-1} + bs^{\alpha-2}+\dots}{s^{\alpha} + cs^{\alpha-1}+\dots}$$

$$= \frac{a}{s} + \frac{1}{s}\,\frac{(b-ac)s^{\alpha-1}+\dots}{s^{\alpha}+cs^{\alpha-1}+\dots}$$

$$= \{a\} + \{\int_0^t f(\tau)d\tau\},$$

where

$$\{f\} = \frac{(b-ac)s^{\alpha-1}+\dots}{s^{\alpha}+cs^{\alpha-1}+\dots}$$

is a certain function and a is the precursor's principal term; but the integral above vanishes for t=0, therefore

$$g_{ij}^{(n)}(0)=a.$$

We have thus proved that if

$$g_{ij}(0) = g'_{ij}(0) =\dots= g_{ij}^{(n-1)}(0) = 0,\ g_{ij}^{(n)}(0) = a \neq 0,$$

then n+1 is the order of the precursor, and a is the principal term.

10. OSCILLATIONS

We have seen in Section 4 that some eigenvalues of matrix $\underset{\sim}{K}$

can be complex; we shall examine here what are the conditions for this to happen, and what its physical consequences.

We first observe that with two compartments $\underset{\sim}{K}$ cannot have complex eigenvalues; in fact the eigenvalues of

$$\begin{bmatrix} -K_1 & k_{12} \\ k_{21} & -K_2 \end{bmatrix}$$

are the roots of equation

$$\lambda^2 + (K_1+K_2)\lambda + K_1K_2-k_{12}k_{21} = 0,$$

but the discriminant of this equation is

$$(K_1-K_2)^2 + 4\ k_{12}k_{21},$$

never negative.

With more than two compartments $\underset{\sim}{K}$ can have complex eigenvalues; let us consider as an example the case of three compartments. Matrix

$$\underset{\sim}{K} = \begin{bmatrix} -K_1 & k_{12} & k_{13} \\ k_{21} & -K_2 & k_{23} \\ k_{31} & k_{32} & -K_3 \end{bmatrix}$$

has complex eigenvalues if and only if equation

$$(\lambda+K_1)(\lambda+K_2)(\lambda+K_3) = k_{12}k_{21}(\lambda+K_3)+k_{13}k_{31}(\lambda+K_2)+k_{23}k_{32}(\lambda+K_1)+$$
$$+\ k_{12}k_{23}k_{31}+k_{13}k_{32}k_{21}$$

has two complex roots. This last equation can be graphically represented by the intersection of a cubic with a straight line; the cubic intersects the abscissa at the points $-K_1$, $-K_2$, $-K_3$, and the ordinate at the point $K_1K_2K_3$; the straight line intersects the ordinate at the point

$$r = k_{12}k_{21}K_3+k_{13}k_{31}K_2+k_{23}k_{32}K_1+k_{12}k_{23}k_{31}+k_{13}k_{32}k_{21},$$

with conditions 4-4 requiring

$$r \leqq K_1K_2K_3;$$

the slope of the straight line is

$$\alpha = k_{12}k_{21}+k_{13}k_{31}+k_{23}k_{32},$$

while the slope of the tangent to the cubic at the point where it intersects the ordinate is

$$\beta = K_1K_2+K_1K_3+K_2K_3,$$

and again conditions 4-4 require

$$\alpha \leqq \beta \cdot$$

Consider the extreme case when $\alpha = \beta$; this implies

$$k_{12}(k_{23}+k_{31}+k_{32})+k_{13}(k_{21}+k_{23}+k_{32})+$$

$$+k_{21}(k_{31}+k_{32})+k_{23}k_{31} = 0$$

$$K_1 = k_{12}+k_{13}$$

$$K_2 = k_{31}+k_{23}$$

$$K_3 = k_{31}+k_{32}$$

and, if the system is not decomposable, this is possible only if the system is a tree, i.e.

$$K_1 = k_{12}+k_{13}$$

$$K_2 = 0$$

$$K_3 = 0,$$

or an equivalent structure obtained by rotating the subscripts; but this also implies

$$\alpha=\beta=0,$$

and $\underset{\sim}{K}$ has the eigenvalue $\underline{0}$ of multiplicity 3.

Now any change in the transfer rates makes the difference $\beta-\alpha$ larger, with both α and β positive; the cubic and the ordinate will intersect on the left of the ordinate, in general at three different points, the three real eigenvalues of $\underset{\sim}{K}$. A sufficient, though not necessary, condition to have just one such intersection, therefore just one real eigenvalue, is to minimize the foldings of the cubic; i.e. to make

$$K_1 = K_2 = K_3,$$

and at the same time to maximize r and minimize α, i.e. to make

$$k_{12}k_{21}+k_{13}k_{31}+k_{23}k_{32} = 0$$

$$k_{12}k_{23}k_{31}+k_{13}k_{32}k_{21} = \max;$$

these three conditions are satisfied by making

$$k_{21} = k_{13} = k_{32} = 0$$

$$K_1 = k_{12}$$

$$K_2 = k_{23}$$

$$K_3 = k_{31},$$

thence

$$\underset{\sim}{K} = \begin{bmatrix} -K_1 & K_1 & 0 \\ 0 & -K_1 & K_1 \\ K_1 & 0 & -K_1 \end{bmatrix}$$

has eigenvalues

$$0,\ -\frac{1}{2}(3+\sqrt{-3})K_1,\ -\frac{1}{2}(3-\sqrt{-3})K_1.$$

With $x_1(0)=1$, $f_1(t)\equiv 0$, $K_1=1$ we have

$$\{x_1\} = \frac{s^2+2s+1}{s^3+3s^2+3s}$$

$$= \frac{1}{3}\frac{1}{s} + \frac{2}{3}\frac{s+3/2}{(s+3/2)^2+3/4}$$

$$= \{\frac{1}{3} + \frac{2}{3}\exp(-\frac{3}{2}t)\cos(\sqrt{3}\,t/2)\}.$$

This function approaches the asymptotic value 1/3 through some weak oscillations, as shown by Fig. 8.

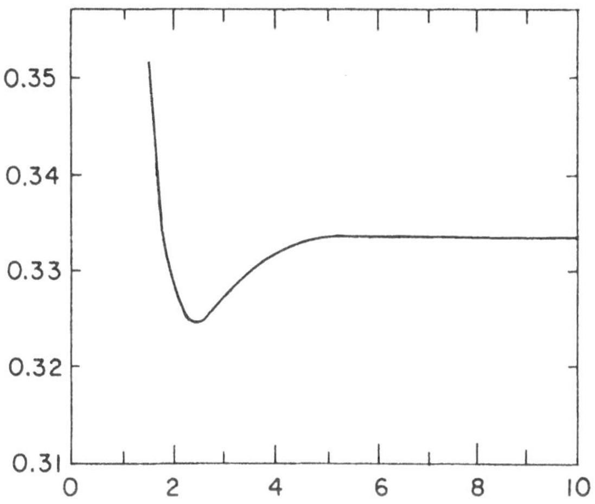

Fig. 8

With four compartment we have complex eigenvalues by making

$$\underset{\sim}{K} = \begin{bmatrix} -K_1 & K_1 & 0 & 0 \\ 0 & -K_1 & K_1 & 0 \\ 0 & 0 & -K_1 & K_1 \\ K_1 & 0 & 0 & -K_1 \end{bmatrix};$$

Fig. 9 shows that in this case also we have oscillations, not as weak as with three compartments. But observe that any relaxation of the conditions imposed on the system make those oscillations weaker, and then disappear altogether.

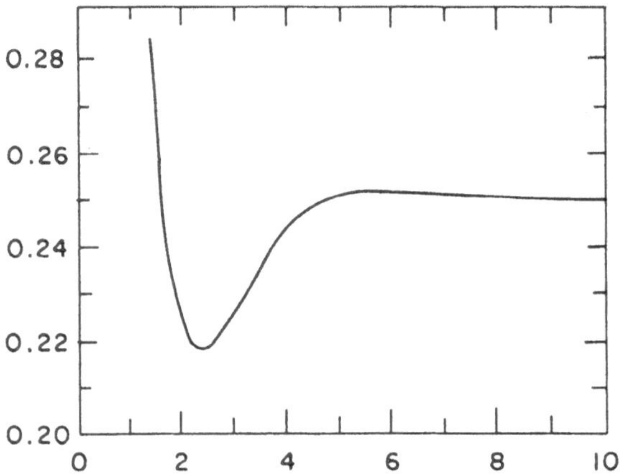

Fig. 9

11. STOCHASTIC COMPARTMENTS

The general problem of stochastic compartments is treated in a more general way in this volume by Matis, Wehrly and Gerald (46); here we plan to consider only one aspect of the problem, useful for redefining some important concepts (47).

We define a compartment as a pool of particles all having the same probability of transition from their present state to another identifiable state. Call μdt the probability that a given particle present in a specified compartment leaves from that compartment in the interval of time t,t+dt; for the time being we consider μ a constant, i.e. the said probability depends on the length of time considered but not on the absolute time; this hypothesis is not strictly necessary, but it simplifies our treatment considerably. Also call

$P(t)$ = probability that a given particle is present in a given compartment at time $\underline{t}$,

t^* = actual time of entrance of a particle into that compartment;

then

$$P(t^*) = 1,$$
$$P(t) = 0 \quad \text{for } t < t^*,$$
$$P(t+dt) = P(t)\cdot(1-\mu dt);$$

this last equation can be written

$$\frac{dP}{dt} = -\mu P$$

and by integration

$$P(t) = 0 \qquad \text{for } t < t^*$$
$$= e^{-\mu(t-t^*)} \qquad \text{for } t \geqq t^*.$$

The probability that a given particle leaves from a given compartment in the interval τ, $\tau+d\tau$, is therefore

$$P(\tau)\mu d\tau,$$

and the expected time of this event is

$$\int_0^\infty \tau P(\tau)\mu d\tau = \int_{t^*}^\infty \mu\tau e^{-\mu(\tau-t^*)} d\tau$$
$$= t^* + 1/\mu.$$

If from the expected time of exit we subtract the time of entrance t^*, we have the expected interval of time $1/\mu$ spent by each particle in a passage through a given compartment.

Now we return to Eq. 2-1 used to define a deterministic compartment; by integration from 0 to ∞,

$$\int_0^\infty \frac{dx}{dt}\, dt = -K\int_0^\infty x\, dt + \int_0^\infty f(t)dt,$$

and if the system is open, i.e. if

$$\lim_{t\to\infty} x = 0, \tag{11-1}$$

then

$$-x(0) = -K\int_0^\infty x\, dt + \int_0^\infty f(t)dt$$

or

$$\frac{1}{K} = \frac{\int_0^\infty x\,dt}{x(0) + \int_0^\infty f(t)dt} \quad .$$

The denominator of the fraction on the right hand side is the number of particles present in the compartment at time 0 plus the number of particles that entered it later, counting again all particles that reenter that compartment because of recirculation; thus that fraction is the expected time spent by each particle that goes through that compartment in each passage through it. This is what was called μ at the beginning of this section. We can therefore say that K, as defined in Eq. 2-1, is the inverse of the transit time through a compartment.

When the tracee is at steady state, 1/K is the interval of time necessary for the renewal of an amount of tracee equal to the amount present, and it may be properly called turnover time; in fact if X is the amount of tracee, the steady state requires that

$$\frac{dX}{dt} = 0,$$

and the tracer is eliminated at a fractional rate K; the tracee is eliminated and introduced at exactly the same rate, therefore KX is the amount of tracee renewed per unit time, and the amount renewed during the interval 1/K is

$$KX/K = X,$$

equal to the amount present. For a more detailed discussion on the definition of turnover time see Rescigno and Beck (15).

Back again at Eq. 2-1, we write it in the form

$$\frac{dx}{dt} = -K'x + g(t),$$

where

α = fraction of particles recirculated,

$K' = (1-\alpha)K$

$g(t) = f(t)-\alpha Kx;$

by integration from 0 to ∞ we get

$$-x(0) = -K' \int_0^\infty x\,dt + \int_0^\infty g(t)dt$$

and

$$\frac{1}{K'} = \frac{\int_0^\infty x\,dt}{x(0) + \int_0^\infty g(t)dt} .$$

The denominator of this new fraction is the number of particles present in the compartment at time 0 plus the number of particles that enter it later, but counted only if they did not enter the compartment before; therefore $1/K'$ is the expected time spent by a particle in all passages through a compartment, and is called residence time (47).

The ratio between residence time and transit time is the average number of times a given particle goes through the same compartment (48):

$$\nu = \frac{1/K'}{1/K} .$$

Also observe that if all particles are recirculated, the system is closed and hypothesis 11-1 does not hold anymore. If the system is open, then

$$0 \leq \alpha < 1;$$

from the definition of α,

$$\nu = \frac{1}{1-\alpha}$$

and

$$\frac{1}{K'} = \frac{1}{1-\alpha}\frac{1}{K}$$

$$= (1+\alpha+\alpha^2+\ldots)\,\frac{1}{K} ,$$

i.e. the permanence time is equal to the transit time plus this same time weighed for the particles that recirculate the first time, plus the same time weighed for the particles that recirculate a second time, and so forth.

Of course, if $\alpha=0$, i.e. if there is no recirculation, transit time and permanence time are identical.

Another useful quantity to define is the transfer time. The probability that any particle leave a specified compartment in the interval $t,t+dt$ is

$$K\ x(t)dt,$$

where x(t) is the expected number of particles present in that compartment; therefore the ratio

$$\frac{\int_0^\infty \tau K\ x(\tau)d\tau}{\int_0^\infty K\ x(\tau)d\tau}$$

is the expected time of this event, i.e. of the exit of a particle from that compartment. Observe that it does not matter whether a particle leaves that compartment for the last time or not, as the probability of exit does not depend on the past history of the particle; it does matter though whether the system is open or closed, because in a closed system the integral above does not converge. Now if x_i and x_j measure respectively the expected number of particles present in the precursor *i* and the successor *j*, then the difference

$$T_{ij} = \frac{\int_0^\infty \tau x_j(\tau)d\tau}{\int_0^\infty x_j(\tau)d\tau} - \frac{\int_0^\infty \tau x_i(\tau)d\tau}{\int_0^\infty x_i(\tau)d\tau},$$

called the transfer time from *i* to *j*, is the expected interval of time from the exit of a particle from *i* to the exit of the same particle from *j*. Note that the effective time spent by a particle when moving from *i* to *j* is equal to the transfer time from *i* to *j* minus the transit time in *j*.

12. MOMENTS

We return once more to Eq. 4-1 for the case f=0 and write in in the form

$$\dot{\underset{\sim}{x}} = \underset{\sim}{x}\cdot\underset{\sim}{A}; \qquad (12\text{-}1)$$

by successive differentiations we have

$$\underset{\sim}{x}^{(p)} = \underset{\sim}{x}^{(p-1)}\cdot\underset{\sim}{A}, \quad p=1,2,\ldots$$

thence

$$\underset{\sim}{x}^{(p)}(0) = \underset{\sim}{x}_0\cdot\underset{\sim}{A}^p$$

for any non-negative integer $\underline{p}$.
   Also from Eq. 12-1 we get

$$\int_0^t \dot{\underline{x}} \, dt = \int_0^t \underline{x} \, dt \cdot \underline{A}$$

$$\int_0^t t^p/p! \dot{\underline{x}} \, dt = \int_0^t t^p/p! \cdot \underline{x} \, dt \cdot \underline{A}, \quad p=1,2,\ldots$$

thence

$$x - x_0 = \int_0^t \underline{x} \, dt \cdot \underline{A}$$

$$t^p/p! \cdot \underline{x} - \int_0^t t^{p-1}/(p-1)! \cdot \underline{x} \, dt = \int_0^t t^p/p! \cdot \underline{x} \, dt \cdot \underline{A}$$

and by induction, with the hypothesis that the system is open,

$$\int_0^\infty t^{p-1}/(p-1)! \cdot \underline{x} \, dt = \underline{x}_0(-\underline{A})^{-p}, \quad p=1,2,\ldots$$

For convenience we put

$$-\underline{A}^{-1} = \underline{V},$$

and the last equation becomes

$$\int_0^\infty t^{p-1}/(p-1)! \cdot \underline{x} \, dt = \underline{x}_0 \cdot \underline{V}^p$$

Matrix $\underline{V}$ and all its powers are non-negative.

   In fact, as a consequence of inequality 4-4 matrix $-\underline{A}$ is diagonal dominant, i.e. each diagonal element is larger than or equal to the absolute value of the sum of the other elements of the same row. The determinant of such a matrix has been called unisignant by Muir (49), and it has been shown to be non-negative. In our case $\underline{A}$ is non-singular, therefore this determinant is strictly positive.
   The elements of $\underline{V}$ have the sign of the cofactors of the elements of $-\underline{A}$. The cofactors of the diagonal elements are principal minors of $-\underline{A}$; these principal minors are also diagonal dominant, therefore they are non-negative. The cofactor of $-a_{ij}$ in $-A$, with $i \neq j$, is $(-1)^{i+j}(-A)_{i,j}$, where this last symbol represents determinant $-A$ without row i and column j. Developing this determinant according to the elements of row j,

then developing the resulting non-principal minors in the same way, until only principal minors are left, this cofactor is equal to

$$a_{ji}(-A)_{ij,ij} + \sum_{\ell_1} a_{j\ell_1}(-A)_{ij\ell_1,ij\ell_1}$$

$$+ \sum_{\ell_1,\ell_2} a_{j\ell_1} a_{\ell_1\ell_2} a_{\ell_2 i}(-A)_{ij\ell_1\ell_2,ij\ell_1\ell_2} + \dots ; \tag{12-2}$$

obviously none of these terms is negative, according to inequality 4-3.

All elements of $\underset{\sim}{V}$, and consequently of all its powers, are strictly positive if and only if $\underset{\sim}{A}$ is irreducible.

In fact if $\underset{\sim}{A}$ is reducible, there is at least a value of j and a value of i such that all products a_{ji}, $a_{j\ell_1}a_{\ell_1 i}$, $a_{j\ell_1}\ a_{\ell_1\ell_2}a_{\ell_2 i}, \dots$, for any $\ell_1, \ell_2, \dots$, contained in sum 12-2, are void. On the other hand suppose an element of $\underset{\sim}{V}$ is zero; if it is an element of the principal diagonal, then the sum of the elements of each of its rows is zero, and consequently the elements of the same rows and the missing column in $\underset{\sim}{A}$ are zero, and $\underset{\sim}{A}$ is reducible; if the void element of $\underset{\sim}{V}$ is not on the diagonal, then the corresponding sum 12-2 is zero; if any principal minor $(-A)_{ij\ell_1\dots,ij\ell_1\dots}$ in that sum is void, the elements of its rows and the missing columns in $\underset{\sim}{A}$ are zero, therefore the coefficient multiplying that minor in 12-2 is zero; when all coefficients in 12-2 are zero, $\underset{\sim}{A}$ is reducible, q.e.d.

We shall call $a_{ij}{}^{(p)}$ and $v_{ij}{}^{(p)}$ the elements of matrices $\underset{\sim}{A}^p$ and $\underset{\sim}{V}^p$, respectively; their physical meaning becomes clear if one thinks of an experiment in which all compartments are initially empty except compartment i whose state variable has the initial value 1; in this case the products

$$\underset{\sim}{x}_0 \cdot \underset{\sim}{A}^p, \quad \underset{\sim}{x}_0 \cdot \underset{\sim}{V}^p$$

are equal to the i row of $\underset{\sim}{A}^p$ and $\underset{\sim}{V}^p$, respectively. Calling x_{ij} the state variable of compartment j in such experiment, then

$$a_{ij}{}^{(p)} = x_{ij}{}^{(p)}(0), \tag{12-3}$$

$$v_{ij}{}^{(p)} = \int_0^\infty t^{p-1}/(p-1)! \cdot x_{ij}\ dt, \tag{12-4}$$

for all integer values of p; the above identities can be completed by the obvious one,

$$\delta_{ij} = x_{ij}(0), \tag{12-5}$$

where δ_{ij} is the Kronecker delta.

For p=1 identity 12-4 becomes

$$v_{ij}^{(1)} = \int_0^\infty x_{ij}\, dt$$

which can also be written

$$v_{ij}^{(1)} = 1/K_j \cdot \int_0^\infty K_j x_{ij}\, dt,$$

where $1/K_j$ is the transit time through compartment j, while

$$\int_0^\infty K_j x_{ij}\, dt$$

is the fraction of particles introduced into compartment i that exit from compartment _j_; it follows that $v_{ij}^{(1)}$ is the expected total time spent in compartment _j_ by particles introduced into compartment _i_. For i=j we see that $v_{ii}^{(1)}$ is the permanence time in compartment _i_.

For p > 1 we can write

$$\frac{v_{ij}^{(p)}}{v_{ij}^{(1)}} = \frac{\int_0^\infty t^{p-1}/(p-1)! \cdot x_{ij}\, dt}{\int_0^\infty x_{ij} dt}$$

$$\frac{\int_0^\infty t^{p-1}/(p-1)! \cdot K_j x_{ij}\, dt}{\int_0^\infty K_j x_{ij}\, dt} ;$$

if we define the random variable T_{ij} as the interval of time between the introduction of a particle into compartment i and its exit from compartment j, then

$$p!\ v_{ij}^{(p+1)}/v_{ij}^{(1)}$$

is the p-moment of T_{ij}, and

$$\int_0^\infty \exp(ts)\, x_{ij}\, dt \Big/ \int_0^\infty x_{ij}\, dt$$

is the moment generating function of T_{ij}.

If all compartments of a system can be controlled and all observed, then from n experiments and n measurements for each experiment, all elements $v_{ij}^{(1)}$ of $\underset{\sim}{V}$ can be computed, hence by inversion $\underset{\sim}{A}$ is obtained, which describes completely the compartment system. More often than not only very few compartments are controllable and few observable, so that only a few elements of $\underset{\sim}{V}$, and the corresponding elements of its powers, can be computed. The problem is the reconstruction of $\underset{\sim}{A}$ from those known elements.

Call

$$p(\lambda) = \lambda^m + c_1\lambda^{m-1} + c_2\lambda^{m-2} + \ldots + c_m, \quad m \leq n,$$

the minimum polynomial of $\underset{\sim}{A}$; this polynomial is equal to the characteristic polynomial of $\underset{\sim}{A}$ or is one of its divisors. By definition $p(\lambda)$ annihilates $\underset{\sim}{A}$, that is,

$$\underset{\sim}{A}^m + c_1\underset{\sim}{A}^{m-1} + c_2\underset{\sim}{A}^{m-2} + \ldots + c_m\underset{\sim}{I} = \underset{\sim}{0}; \tag{12-6}$$

multiply each term of this equation by $\underset{\sim}{V}^m, \underset{\sim}{V}^{m+1}, \underset{\sim}{V}^{m+2}, \ldots$

$$\begin{aligned} &\underset{\sim}{I} - c_1\underset{\sim}{V} + c_2\underset{\sim}{V}^2 - \ldots + (-1)^m c_m\underset{\sim}{V}^m = \underset{\sim}{0} \\ &\underset{\sim}{V} - c_1\underset{\sim}{V}^2 + c_2\underset{\sim}{V}^3 - \ldots + (-1)^m c_m\underset{\sim}{V}^{m+1} = \underset{\sim}{0} \\ &\underset{\sim}{V}^2 - c_1\underset{\sim}{V}^3 + c_2\underset{\sim}{V}^4 - \ldots + (-1)^m c_m\underset{\sim}{V}^{m+2} = \underset{\sim}{0} \\ &\text{-------------------------------} \end{aligned} \tag{12-7}$$

Now multiply each term of equation 12-6 by $\underset{\sim}{V}^{m-1}$, $\underset{\sim}{V}^{m-2}$, $\underset{\sim}{V}^{m-3}, \ldots$

$$\begin{aligned} -c_1\underset{\sim}{I} + c_2\underset{\sim}{V} - c_3\underset{\sim}{V}^2 + \ldots + (-1)^m c_m\underset{\sim}{V}^{m-1} &= \underset{\sim}{A} \\ c_2\underset{\sim}{I} - c_3\underset{\sim}{V} + \ldots + (-1)^m c_m\underset{\sim}{V}^{m-2} &= -\underset{\sim}{A}^2 - c_1\underset{\sim}{A} \\ -c_3\underset{\sim}{I} + \ldots + (-1)^m c_m\underset{\sim}{V}^{m-3} &= \underset{\sim}{A}^3 + c_1\underset{\sim}{A}^2 + c_2\underset{\sim}{A} \\ &\text{-------------------------------} \end{aligned} \tag{12-8}$$

As we said before, not all elements of $\underset{\sim}{V}$ and its powers are known, but if $x_{ij}(t)$ has been measured for a particular set of values i,j, then we can rewrite Eqs. 12-7 for row $\underline{i}$ and column $\underline{j}$

only, using 12-4 and 12-5,

$$\delta_{ij} - c_1 v_{ij}^{(1)} + c_2 v_{ij}^{(2)} + \ldots + (-1)^m c_m v_{ij}^{(m)} = 0$$

$$v_{ij}^{(1)} - c_1 v_{ij}^{(2)} + c_2 v_{ij}^{(3)} + \ldots + (-1)^m c_m v_{ij}^{(m+1)} = 0$$

$$v_{ij}^{(2)} - c_1 v_{ij}^{(3)} + c_2 v_{ij}^{(4)} + \ldots + (-1)^m c_m v_{ij}^{(m+2)} = 0$$

$$\text{-----------------------------------}$$

These equations have a unique non-trivial solution for $c_1, c_2, \ldots, c_m$ if matrix

$$\begin{bmatrix} \delta_{ij} & v_{ij}^{(1)} & v_{ij}^{(2)} & \ldots & v_{ij}^{(m)} \\ v_{ij}^{(1)} & v_{ij}^{(2)} & v_{ij}^{(3)} & \ldots & v_{ij}^{(m+1)} \\ \text{---} & \text{---} & \text{---} & \text{---} & \text{---} \\ v_{ij}^{(m)} & v_{ij}^{(m+1)} & v_{ij}^{(m+2)} & \ldots & v_{ij}^{(2m)} \end{bmatrix}$$

has rank $\underline{m}$. Thus $\underline{m}$ is determined by checking which of the matrices

$$\begin{bmatrix} \delta_{ij} & v_{ij}^{(1)} \\ v_{ij}^{(1)} & v_{ij}^{(2)} \end{bmatrix}, \quad \begin{bmatrix} \delta_{ij} & v_{ij}^{(1)} & v_{ij}^{(2)} \\ v_{ij}^{(1)} & v_{ij}^{(2)} & v_{ij}^{(3)} \\ v_{ij}^{(2)} & v_{ij}^{(3)} & v_{ij}^{(4)} \end{bmatrix}, \ldots$$

is singular; then the coefficients of the minimum polynomial p( ) of A are given by the product

$$\begin{bmatrix} -c_1 \\ +c_2 \\ \text{---} \\ (-1)^m c_m \end{bmatrix} = - \begin{bmatrix} v_{ij}^{(1)} & v_{ij}^{(2)} & \ldots & v_{ij}^{(m)} \\ v_{ij}^{(2)} & v_{ij}^{(3)} & \ldots & v_{ij}^{(m+1)} \\ \text{---} & \text{---} & \text{---} & \text{---} \\ v_{ij}^{(m)} & v_{ij}^{(m+1)} & \ldots & v_{ij}^{(2m-1)} \end{bmatrix}^{-1} \begin{bmatrix} \delta_{ij} \\ v_{ij}^{(1)} \\ \text{------} \\ v_{ij}^{(m-1)} \end{bmatrix}$$

Now from equations 12-8, with the same values of i,j,

$$-c_1\delta_{ij} + c_2 v_{ij}^{(1)} - c_3 v_{ij}^{(2)} + \ldots + (-1)^m c_m v_{ij}^{(m-1)} = a_{ij}$$

$$c_2\delta_{ij} - c_3 v_{ij}^{(1)} + \ldots + (-1)^m c_m v_{ij}^{(m-2)} = -a_{ij}^{(2)} - c_1 a_{ij}^{(1)}$$

$$-c_3\delta_{ij} + \ldots + (-1)^m c_m v_{ij}^{(m-3)} = a_{ij}^{(3)} + c_1 a_{ij}^{(2)} + c_2 a^{(1)}$$

----

and from these equations the elements $a_{ij}^{(1)}$, $a_{ij}^{(2)}, \ldots$ can be computed sequentially.

If the minimum polynomial of $\underset{\sim}{A}$ has $\underline{m}$ distinct real zeros $\lambda_1, \lambda_2, \ldots, \lambda_m$, then equation 12-1 by integration becomes

$$\underset{\sim}{x} = \underset{\sim}{x}_0 \cdot \underset{\sim}{P} \cdot \exp(t\underset{\sim}{\Lambda}) \cdot \underset{\sim}{P}^{-1},$$

where $\underset{\sim}{P}$ is an appropriate non-singular mxm matrix and $\underset{\sim}{\Lambda}$ is the diagonal matrix of the eigenvalues of $\underset{\sim}{A}$; with the same hypothesis on $\underset{\sim}{x}_0$ as before, the product above gives

$$x_{ij} = \sum_{\ell=1}^{m} u_\ell \exp(\lambda_\ell t), \qquad (12\text{-}9)$$

hence

$$\delta_{ij} = \sum_{\ell=1}^{m} u_\ell,$$

$$x_{ij}^{(p)}(0) = \sum_{\ell=1}^{m} \lambda_\ell^p u_\ell, \; p=1,2,\ldots$$

and remembering 12-3,

$$\begin{bmatrix} \delta_{ij} \\ a_{ij}^{(1)} \\ a_{ij}^{(2)} \\ ------ \\ a_{ij}^{(m-1)} \end{bmatrix} = \begin{bmatrix} 1 & 1 & \ldots & 1 \\ \lambda_1 & \lambda_2 & \ldots & \lambda_m \\ \lambda_1^2 & \lambda_2^2 & \ldots & \lambda_m^2 \\ --- & --- & --- & --- \\ \lambda_1^{m-1} & \lambda_2^{m-1} & \ldots & \lambda_m^{m-1} \end{bmatrix} \cdot \begin{bmatrix} u_1 \\ u_2 \\ u_3 \\ -- \\ u_m \end{bmatrix} \qquad (12\text{-}10)$$

In the present hypothesis the coefficients $u_1, u_2, \ldots, u_m$ can be computed from the equation above; if the λ_ℓ's are not all different, or if some of them are complex, this equation must be slightly modified.

If $\alpha \pm \beta\sqrt{-1}$ are complex conjugate eigenvalues of $\underset{\sim}{A}$, then the corresponding terms in sum 12-9 are substituted by

$$(\mu \cos\beta t + \nu \sin \beta t) \cdot \exp(\alpha t);$$

the corresponding columns of the square matrix in equation 12-10 are substituted by the real part and the imaginary part, respectively, of the successive powers of the complex zero, i.e.

$$\begin{array}{ll} 1 & 0 \\ \alpha & \beta \\ \alpha^2-\beta^2 & 2\alpha\beta \\ \alpha^3-3\alpha\beta^2 & 3\alpha^2\beta-\beta^3 \\ --- & --- \end{array}$$

If λ_ℓ is a zero of multiplicity k, then k terms in sum 12-9 are substituted by

$$(\mu_{\ell_1} t^{k-1} + \mu_{\ell_2} t^{k-2} + \ldots + \mu_{\ell_k}) \cdot \exp(\lambda_\ell t)$$

and in the matrix in equation 12-10 the column with the successive powers of λ_ℓ will be followed by columns with the 1st, 2nd,...,(k-1)th derivative of that column with respect to λ_ℓ.

13. GENERALIZATION OF THE MOMENT EQUATION

The results presented in Section 12 are valid with the hypothesis $\underset{\sim}{f}=\underset{\sim}{0}$; this restriction may now be lifted. In fact, Eq. 12-1 in operational form is

$$s\{\underset{\sim}{x}\} - \underset{\sim}{x}_0 = \{\underset{\sim}{x}\} \cdot \underset{\sim}{A},$$

where s is the differential operator. With an obvious transformation,

$$\{\underset{\sim}{x}\} = \underset{\sim}{x}_0 (s\underset{\sim}{I}-\underset{\sim}{A})^{-1};$$

but,

$$(s\underset{\sim}{I}-\underset{\sim}{A})^{-1} = \sum_{\ell+r=0}^{m-1} c_\ell \underset{\sim}{A}^r s^{m-\ell-r-1} / \sum_{\ell=0}^{m} c_\ell s^{m-\ell} .$$

In fact

$$(s\underset{\sim}{I}-\underset{\sim}{A}) \sum_{\ell+r=0}^{m-1} c_\ell \underset{\sim}{A}^r s^{m-\ell-r-1} =$$

$$= \sum_{\ell+r=0}^{m-1} c_\ell \underset{\sim}{A}^r s^{m-\ell-r} - \sum_{\ell+r=0}^{m-1} c_\ell \underset{\sim}{A}^{r+1} s^{m-\ell-r-1}$$

$$= \sum_{\ell=0}^{m-1} c_\ell \underset{\sim}{I} s^{m-\ell} + \sum_{\substack{\ell+r=1 \\ r>0}}^{m-1} c_\ell \underset{\sim}{A}^r s^{m-\ell-r} - \sum_{\substack{\ell+r=1 \\ r>0}}^{m} c_\ell \underset{\sim}{A}^r s^{m-\ell-r} =$$

$$= \sum_{\ell=0}^{m} c_\ell s^{m-\ell} \underset{\sim}{I} - c_m \underset{\sim}{I} - \sum_{\ell=0}^{m-1} c_\ell \underset{\sim}{A}^{m-\ell} =$$

$$= \sum_{\ell=0}^{m} c_\ell s^{m-\ell} \underset{\sim}{I} - \sum_{\ell=0}^{m} c_\ell \underset{\sim}{A}^{m-\ell};$$

where the last sum sum is zero according to Eq. 12-6.

Therefore

$$\{x_{ij}\} = \sum_{\ell+r=0}^{m-1} c_\ell a_{ij}^{(r)} s^{m-\ell-r-1} / \sum_{\ell=0}^{m} c_\ell s^{m-\ell},$$

where for convenience we have put

$$a_{ij}^{(0)} = \delta_{ij}.$$

Suppose now that $\underset{\sim}{f}$ in Eq. 4-1 is not $\underset{\sim}{0}$, but that $\underset{\sim}{x}_0 = \underset{\sim}{0}$. Eq. 4-2 in this case becomes

$$\underset{\sim}{x} = \int_0^t \underset{\sim}{f}(t-\tau) \exp(\tau\underset{\sim}{A})d\tau.$$

With the same hypotheses as before, from eq. 4-1 we get

$$\int_0^\infty \underset{\sim}{x}\, dt = - \int_0^\infty \underset{\sim}{f}\, dt \cdot \underset{\sim}{A}^{-1},$$

$$\int_0^\infty t^{p-1}/(p-1)!\cdot \underset{\sim}{x}\ dt = -\int_0^\infty t^p/p!\cdot \underset{\sim}{x}\ dt\cdot \underline{A} + \int_0^\infty t^p/p!\cdot \underset{\sim}{f}\ dt$$

$$(p=1,2,\ldots)$$

and by induction,

$$\int_0^\infty t^{p-1}/(p-1)!\cdot \underset{\sim}{x}\ dt$$

$$= \sum_{\ell=0}^{p-1} \int_0^\infty t^\ell/\ell!\cdot \underset{\sim}{f}\ dt\cdot(-A)^{-(p-\ell)}, \quad (p=1,2,\ldots) \qquad (13\text{-}1)$$

Using the notation

$$\underset{\sim}{F}_\ell = \int_0^\infty t^\ell/\ell!\cdot \underset{\sim}{f}\ dt,$$

eq. 13-1 can be written

$$\int_0^\infty \underset{\sim}{x}\ dt = \underset{\sim}{F}_0\cdot \underset{\sim}{V}$$

$$\int_0^\infty t\ \underset{\sim}{x}\ dt = \underset{\sim}{F}_0\cdot \underset{\sim}{V}^2 + \underset{\sim}{F}_1\cdot \underset{\sim}{V}$$

$$\int_0^\infty t^2/2!\cdot \underset{\sim}{x}\ dt = \underset{\sim}{F}_0\cdot \underset{\sim}{V}^3 + \underset{\sim}{F}_1\cdot \underset{\sim}{V}^2 + \underset{\sim}{F}_2\cdot \underset{\sim}{V}$$

and so on. To understand the physical meaning of vectors $\underset{\sim}{V}_\ell$, think of an experiment in which only compartment $\underline{i}$ is fed according to function $f_i(t)$; the product $\underset{\sim}{F}_\ell\cdot \underset{\sim}{V}^{-(p-\ell)}$ is equal to the $\underline{i}$ row of $V^{-(p-1)}$ multiplied by $\int_0^\infty t^\ell/\ell!\cdot f_i(t)dt$, and eq. 13-1 in this case becomes

$$\int_0^\infty t^{p-1}/(p-1)!\cdot x_{ij}\ dt = \sum_{\ell=0}^{p-1} \int_0^\infty t^\ell/\ell!\cdot f_i dt\cdot v_{ij}{}^{(p-\ell)},$$

which shows that the sequence

$$\int_0^\infty x_{ij}dt,\ \int_0^\infty t\ x_{ij}dt,\ \int_0^\infty t^2/2!\cdot x_{ij}dt,\ldots$$

is the convolution of the sequences

$$\int_0^\infty f_i dt, \int_0^\infty t f_i dt, \int_0^\infty t^2/2!\, f_i dt, \ldots$$

and

$$v_{ij}, v_{ij}^{(2)}, v_{ij}^{(3)}, \ldots$$

Thus if we define the random variable T_i as the time of introduction of a particle into compartment $\underline{i}$, then

$$p! \int_0^\infty t^p/p! \cdot f_i dt / \int_0^\infty f_i dt$$

is its $\underline{p}$-moment.

By measuring $x_{ij}(t)$ and $f_i(t)$, the elements of row $\underline{i}$ and column $\underline{j}$ of matrices $\underline{V}$, $\underline{V}^2$, $\underline{V}^3$,... can be computed, and the reconstruction of $\underline{A}$ follows as in the previous case.

Actually eq. 13-1 is the special case of a more general Theorem of the Moments.

Define the moments of function A(t):

$$A_n = \int_0^\infty t^n/n! \cdot A(t)dt, \quad (n=0,1,2,\ldots)$$

and the convolution of functions A(t) and B(t):

$$A*B = \int_0^t A(\tau)B(t-\tau)d\tau.$$

Theorem: If

$$A*B = C,$$

then

$$C_n = A_n B_0 + A_{n-1}B_1 + \ldots + A_0 B_n. \qquad (13\text{-}2)$$

Proof:

For any non-negative integer $\underline{n}$, by definition

$$C_n = \int_0^\infty t^n/n! \cdot \left[\int_0^t A(\tau)B(t-\tau)d\tau\right]dt,$$

and by inverting the order of integration,

$$C_n = \int_0^\infty A(\tau)[\int_\tau^\infty t^n/n!\cdot B(t-\tau)dt]d\tau;$$

with a change of variable,

$$C_n = \int_0^\infty A(\tau)[\int_0^\infty \frac{(\tau+\sigma)^n}{n} B(\sigma)d\sigma]d\tau$$

$$= \int_0^\infty A(\tau)[\tau^n/n!\cdot B_0 + \tau^{n-1}/(n-1)!\cdot B_1 +\ldots+ B_n]d\tau$$

$$= A_n B_0 + A_{n-1}B_1 +\ldots+ A_0 B_n, \text{ q.e.d.}$$

Eq. 13-1 represents the case, where one of the functions in the convolution is the exponential function $\exp(t\underset{\sim}{A})$; for this function

$$\int_0^\infty \exp(t\underset{\sim}{A})dt = -\underset{\sim}{A}^{-1}$$

$$\int_0^\infty t\exp(t\underset{\sim}{A})dt = \underset{\sim}{A}^{-2}$$

$$\int_0^\infty t^n/n!\cdot\exp(t\underset{\sim}{A})dt = (-\underset{\sim}{A})^{-(n+1)}$$

Eq. 13-2 can be used whenever two of the three functions of a convolution are known.

14. CONCLUSION

Starting from the papers by Widmark, by Gehlen and by Teorell, we described a few mathematical methods used in the quantitative analysis of the behavior of drugs (including radiopharmaceuticals) introduced into a living organism. The analysis presented here is far from complete; the number of papers that have been written on the subject of pharmacokinetics is very large and still growing. In fact a number of journals are dedicated to this single subject.

In this chapter the aim was simply to give an idea of the range of possibilities that are open to the investigator willing to put on more quantitative grounds the results of his investigations. We have not attempted to present an exhaustive bibliography; an up-to-date list of references may be found in the series "Radiotracers in Biology and Medicine," and in particular in the volume "Compartmental Distribution of Radiotracers," edited by J. S. Robertson and presently in the process of being published by C.R.C. Press.

ACKNOWLEDGEMENTS

This research was performed at Brookhaven National Laboratory under contract with the U. S. Department of Energy and supported by its Office of Health and Environmental Research. Partial support from the National Institutes of Neurological Communicative Disease and Stroke Grant No. NS 16801-02 is also acknowledged.

REFERENCES

1. Widmark EMP: Studies in the concentration of indifferent narcotics in blood and tissues. Acta Med. Scand. 52:87-164, 1920

2. Widmark EMP and Tandberg J: Über die Bedingungen für die Akkumulation indifferenter Narkotiken. Theoretische Berechnungen. Biochem. Z. 147:358-369, 1924

3. Gehlen W: Wirkungsstärke intravenös verabreichter Arzneimittel als Zeitfunction. Ein Beitrag zur mathematischen Behandlung pharmakologischer Probleme. Arch. Exptl. Pathol. Pharmakol. 171, 541-554, 1933

4. Widmark EMP: Die wissenschaftliche Grundlagen und die praktische Verwendbarkeit der Gerichtlich-Medizinschen Alkoholbestimmung. Urban und Schwarzenberg, Berlin, 1932

5. Teorell T: Kinetics of distribution of substances administered to the body. Arch. Internat. Pharmacodynamic Thérapie 57:205-240, 1937

6. Fick A: Über Diffusion. Pogg. Ann. 94:59-86, 1855

7. Artom C, Sarzana G and Segrè E: Influence des grasses alimentaires sur la formation des phospholipides dans les tissues animaux. Arch. Internat. Physiol. 147:245-276, 1938

8. Sheppard CW: The theory of the study of transfers within a multi-compartment system using isotopic tracers. J. Appl. Physics 19:70-76, 1948

9. Sheppard CW and Householder AS: The mathematical basis of the interpretation of tracer experiments in closed steady-state systems. J. Appl. Physics 22:510-520, 1951

10. Rescigno A and Segre G: La cinetica dei farmaci e dei traccianti radioattivi. Boringhieri, Torino, 1961. Drug and Tracer Kinetics. Blaisdell, Waltham, Mass., 1966

11. Brownell GL, Berman M, Robertson JS: Nomenclature for tracer kinetics. Int. J. Appl. Rad. Isotopes 19:249-262, 1968

12. Berman M: Iodine kinetics. In Methods of Investigative and Diagnostic Endocrinology, North-Holland Publishing Co. Amsterdam, 1972

13. Jacquez JA: Compartmental Analysis in Biology and Medicine. Elsevier, Amsterdam, 1972

14. Gùrpide E: Tracer Methods in Hormone Research. Springer-Verlag, Berlin, 1975

15. Rescigno A and Beck JS: Compartments. In Rosen R, Ed. Foundations of Mathematical Biology, Vol. 2. Academic Press, New York, 1972, p. 255-322

16. Matis JH and Hartley HO: Stochastic compartmental analysis: Model and least square estimation from time series data. Biometrics 27:77-102, 1971

17. Thakur AK, Rescigno A, Schafer DE: On the stochastic theory of compartments. Bull. Math. Biol. 34:53-63, 1972; 35:263-271, 1973

18. Purdue P: Stochastic theory of compartments. Bull. Math. Biol. 36:305-309; 577-587, 1974

19. Hadamard J: Leçons sur la propagation des ondes et les équations de l'hydrodynamique. Herman, Paris, 1903

20. Hearon JZ: Theorems on linear systems. Annals N. Y. Acad. Sci. 108:36-68, 1963

21. Rescigno A and Segre G: On some topological properties of the systems of compartments. Bull. Math. Biol. 26:31-38, 1964

22. Ore O: Theory of Graphs. Am. Math. Soc., Providence, Rhode Island, 1962

23. Sainte-Laguë MA: Les Réseaux. Gauthier-Villars, Paris, 1926

24. Berge C: Théorie des Graphes et ses Applications. Dunod, Paris, 1958

25. Rescigno A: Synthesis of a multicompartmented biological model. Biochim. Biophys. Acta 37:463-468, 1960

26. Matthews CME: The theory of tracer experiments with ^{131}I-labelled plasma proteins. Phys. Med. Biol. 2:36-53, 1957

27. Marimont RB: A new method of checking the consistency of precedence matrices. J. Assoc. Comp. Machinery 6:164-171, 1959

28. Harary F: A graph theoretic method for the complete reduction of a matrix with a view toward finding its eigenvalues. J. Math. Physics 38:104-111, 1959

29. Rescigno A and Segre G: The precursor-product relationship. J. Theoret. Biol. 1:498-513, 1961

30. Cayley A: Note on the theory of determinants. Philos. Magazine 21:180-185, 1861.

31. Rescigno A and Segre G: On some metric properties of the systems of compartments. Bull. Math. Biol. 27:315-323, 1965

32. Mikusinski J: Operational Calculus. Pergamon Press, New York, 1959

33. Bateman H: Tables of Integral Transforms, Vol. 1, Chapter 4. McGraw-Hill, New York, 1954

34. Mason SJ: Feedback theory - some properties of signal flow graphs. Proc. Inst. Radio. Eng. 41:1144-1156, 1953

35. Kirchhoff G: Über die Anflösung der Gleichungen auf welche man bei der Untersuchung der linearen Vertheilung galvanischer Ströme geführt wird. Am. Phys. Chem. 72:497-514, 1847

36. Robichaud LPA, Boisvert M, Robert J: Signal Flow Graphs and Applications. Prentice-Hall, Englewood Cliffs, New Jersey, 1962

37. Chow Y and Cassignol E: Graphs and Applications. Wiley, New York, 1962

38. Laue R: Elemente der Graphentheorie und ihre Anwendung in den biologischen Wissenschaften. Geest and Portig, Leipzig, 1970

39. Branson H: A mathematical description of metabolizing systems. Bull. Math. Biol. 8:159-165, 1946; 9:93-98, 1947

40. Branson H: The use of isotopes to determine the rate of a biochemical reaction. Science 106:404, 1947

41. Branson H: The use of isotopes in an integral equation description of metabolizing systems. Cold Spring Harbor Symposium Quant. Biol. 13:35-42, 1948

42. Branson H: Metabolic pathways from tracer experiments. Arch. Biochem. Biophysics 36:60-70, 1952

43. Branson H: The integral equation representation of reactions in compartment systems. Annals N. Y. Acad. Sci. 108:4-14, 1963

44. Stephenson JL: Theory of transport in linear biological systems. Bull. Math. Biol. 22:1-17; 113-138, 1960

45. Beck JS and Rescigno A: Determination of precursor order and particular weighting functions from kinetic data. J. Theoret. Biol. 6:1-12, 1964

46. Matis, JH, Wehrly TE, Gerald KB: The statistical analysis of pharmacokinetic data. This volume

47. Rescigno A: On transfer times in tracer experiments. J. Theoret. Biol. 39:9-27, 1973

48. Rescigno A and Gùrpide E: Estimation of average times of residence, recycle and interconversion of blood-borne compounds using tracer methods. J. Clin. Endocrinol. Metab. 36:263-276, 1973

49. Muir T: A Treatise on the Theory of Determinants. Longmans, Green and Co., London, 1933

NEW APPROACHES TO UPTAKE BY HETEROGENEOUS PERFUSED ORGANS: FROM LINEAR TO SATURATION KINETICS

Ludvik Bass, Anthony J. Bracken, and Conrad J. Burden*

University of Queensland, Brisbane, Australia

1. INTRODUCTION: UPTAKE KINETICS IN PHYSIOLOGICAL SETTINGS

The central problem of modeling biochemical kinetics in intact organs is to put the corresponding test-tube kinetics (known or postulated) into the appropriate physiological setting, and hence to deduce relations between quantities observable on the organ. Some normal or pathological features of the physiological setting can then be quantified from experimental data. Such work must navigate between the Scylla of losing the physiology in over-simplifications, and the Charybdis of so complicating the modeling for the sake of realism that the multitude of adjustable parameters can get no grip on the data (see especially Sections 7 and 10).

As an introductory problem, consider steady elimination (by irreversible metabolic transformation) of a blood-borne substrate by cellular enzymes of the intact liver. Let the hepatic blood flow of rate F carry the substrate convectively into the liver at the observed concentration c_i, and out of it at the observed concentration c_o. The steady rate of elimination of the substrate by the intact liver is then

$$V = F(c_i - c_o) . \tag{1}$$

For any saturation kinetics, increasing c_i (and hence c_o) to sufficiently high values makes V tend to the maximum (saturated) rate V_{max}, so that V_{max}/F is the greatest possible magnitude of the input-output (arterial-venous) concentration difference $c_i - c_o$.

Next, let Michaelis-Menten kinetics hold at each enzyme molecule. Then, if the substrate - enzyme system in the liver could be homogenized without change in the kinetic constants V_{max} and K_m of the totality of the enzyme in the organ, the resulting substrate concentration c and the elimination rate V_{hom} would be related by Eq. 2.

$$V_{hom} = V_{max} \frac{c}{c+K_m} \quad . \tag{2}$$

Since V_{hom} will in general be different from V in Eq. 1 (except at saturation), our problem is to replace Eq. 2 by an equation pertaining to the intact liver. The modeling may be introduced by asking whether one can construct from measurements an effective concentration such that if it is put in Eq. 2 in place of c, the result will be V (in place of V_{hom}).

As a first attempt (1), consider a substrate rapidly equilibrated between blood and liver cells which contain the enzyme, and envisage the many liver cells being held in the hepatic blood flow by the scaffolding of the hepatic parenchyma (2) so that they provide a spatially distributed sink of the substrate. Putting the x-axis along the blood flow, with the inlet at x=0 and the outlet at x=L, the depletion of the predominantly convective (1) substrate flux Fc by uptake in the interval x,x+dx is modeled by using Eq. 2 locally:

$$Fdc = -\rho(x)dx \frac{c}{c+K_m} \quad , \tag{3}$$

where now c(x) varies with x between the observed boundary values $c(0)=c_i$, $c(L)=c_o$, and $\rho(x)dx$ is the fraction of the organ V_{max} in the interval x,x+dx, so that

$$\int_0^L \rho(x)dx = V_{max} \, . \tag{4}$$

Separating and integrating Eq. 3 from x=0 to x=L and using Eq. 4, we get the connection between c_i and c_o:

$$F(c_i-c_o) + FK_m \ln(c_i/c_o) = V_{max} \, . \tag{5}$$

Note that here the form of $\rho(x)$ is immaterial: uptake by the organ is affected by the number of cells contacted by a travelling element of blood, but not by their spatial distribution along the blood flow. We shall see in Section 8 that this "blindness" of the observable concentrations to any longitudinal organisation of uptake in the steady state persists only as long as substrates are not interconverted in transit through the organ. We note further that when $c \gg K_m$ throughout the organ, then $c/(c+K_m)$ in Eq. 3 tends to unity, the logarithmic term in Eq. 5 becomes negligible as compared with $F(c_i-c_o)$,and we arrive at the saturated limit of Eq. 1:

$$V_{max} = F(c_i-c_o) \, . \tag{5a}$$

In the opposite limit $c \ll K_m$ we arrive at first-order kinetics in Eq. 3, $F(c_i-c_o)$ becomes negligible as compared with the logarithmic term in Eq. 5 and, solving for c_o/c_i, we obtain the first-order limit of Eq. 5:

$$c_o = c_i e^{-V_{max}/(FK_m)} . \tag{5b}$$

Using Eq. 1 to eliminate F from Eq. 5, we can rewrite Eq. 5 in the Michaelis-Menten form

$$V = V_{max} \frac{\hat{c}_1}{\hat{c}_1 + K_m} , \tag{6}$$

where

$$\hat{c}_1 = \frac{c_i - c_o}{\ln(c_i/c_o)} . \tag{7}$$

Here is a first answer to the foregoing question: V is obtained in place of V_{hom} in Eq. 2 if c is replaced by $\hat{c}_1$, which is constructed according to Eq. 7 from the concentrations observed at the inlet and outlet. The substrate is, of course, not actually present throughout the liver with the concentration $\hat{c}_1$; that concentration is merely an effective mean value in the context of uptake. In fact, $\hat{c}_1$ is the harmonic mean of the linear interpolation of c_i and c_o along the flow:

$$\frac{1}{\hat{c}_1} = \frac{1}{L} \int_0^L \frac{dx}{c_i - \frac{c_i - c_o}{L} x} , \tag{8}$$

which yields Eq. 7 on integration. It is to be noted that $\hat{c}_1$ is in general different from the spatial average $\langle c \rangle$ of the concentration,

$$\langle c \rangle = \frac{1}{L} \int_0^L c(x) dx . \tag{8a}$$

$\hat{c}_1$ coincides with $\langle c \rangle$ only in the limiting case of first-order kinetics ($c \ll K_m$) if, moreover, the enzyme is distributed uniformly along the blood flow: $\rho(x) = V_{max}/L = \text{const}$. Under these special circumstances we obtain $F(c_i - c_o) = (V_{max}/K_m)\langle c \rangle$ by integrating the first-order limit of Eq. 3 directly from inlet to outlet; substituting for V_{max}/K_m from Eq. 5b, $\hat{c}_1 = \langle c \rangle$ follows.

So far physiology has contributed only the unidirectional blood flow of rate F, but that is enough to prevent enzyme molecules from operating independently of each other. For some fixed V_{max} and K_m of an organ, the determination of V requires measurements of concentrations in two locations (c_i and c_o); if one of them is eliminated using Eq. 1, then V is determined by a concentration in one location and by F, that is, by the magnitude of the causal agent which connects spatially separated events along the flow. If now c_i and hence $\hat{c}_1$ is varied experimentally and V is measured at constant F, a first estimate of organ values of V_{max} and K_m can be obtained from standard biochemical plots (3): see Sections 4 and 7.

These considerations can be extended (4) to more general (cooperative) saturation kinetics (5):

$$V_{hom} = V_{max}\frac{c^n}{c^n+K^n}, \quad n>0, \tag{9}$$

where n is Hill's cooperativity constant. With the same assumptions and mathematical steps as above for n=1, we find

$$V = V_{max}\frac{(\hat{c}_n)^n}{(\hat{c}_n)^n+K^n} \tag{10}$$

where now

$$\hat{c}_n = \left[\frac{(n-1)(c_i-c_o)}{c_o^{1-n}-c_i^{1-n}}\right]^{\frac{1}{n}}, \quad n\neq 1 \tag{11}$$

from which $\hat{c}_1$, given by Eq. 7, is recovered in the limit $n\to 1$ using l'Hopital's rule. Again, one can show that $(\hat{c}_n)^n$ is the harmonic mean of the n'th power of the linear interpolation of c_i and c_o. Practical uses of these relations discussed below include the identification of particularly informative experimental maneuvers called null experiments (Section 7).

The foregoing considerations provide a starting point from which we shall advance in several directions, constrained throughout by existing sets of experimental data. First of all, a more detailed study of hepatic architecture shows the liver organized as an ensemble of many (10^7-10^8) conduits of blood flow (fenestrated capillaries called hepatic sinusoids) just wide enough to pass red blood cells, and each lined with liver cells. Hepatic blood flow is manifolded through these sinusoids from their common inlet and reunites at the outlet into the liver vein. If the liver is modeled as an ensemble of N such sinusoids acting in parallel, the foregoing calculations apply to uptake by any one of them because, on the time-scale of the convective transit time of blood through any sinusoid, the transverse equilibration of the substrate is very rapid and its longitudinal diffusion is very slow (1). To model uptake by a single sinusoid we thus need only to replace the organ values V_{max}, V and F by their microscopic counterparts v_{max}, v and f, leaving the constants K_m, K unchanged because they pertain to substrate-enzyme interactions at the molecular level.

Conversely, Eqs. 1, 3-7, 10-11 would describe uptake by the intact liver modeled as an ensemble of N sinusoids on the assumption, evidently implausible in this biological context, that all sinusoids have the same values $v_{max}=V_{max}/N$ and f=F/N: since then $v_{max}/f=V_{max}/F$ and as c_i is common to all sinusoids, Eq. 5 implies that c_o is the same for all sinusoids, whence Eq. 1 follows. The resulting undistributed model of organ uptake (1) neglects the functional heterogeneity of the sinusoids, that is, the dispersions of sinusoidal v_{max} and f values from their ensemble means V_{max}/N, F/N. The degree of quantitative failure of the undistributed model gives an opportunity to quantify the functional heterogeneity of the sinusoids in terms of the distributed model of uptake (6-8) discussed in Section 4, which takes such heterogeneity into account. Since the sinusoids act in parallel, we call the heterogeneity so detected transverse to the blood flow. An extreme example of such heterogeneity is the intrahepatic shunt (commonly seen in liver cirrhosis) which is kinetically equivalent (6) to a fraction of sinusoids with $v_{max}=0$ and $f\neq 0$. Such a shunt is harmful because it allows toxic substances from the intestines to reach the brain and other organs without the prior detoxifying intervention by liver enzymes; its quantification is therefore of clinical interest.

Other toxic substances are not infused into the liver through the inlet, but are produced within it as by-products (toxic metabolites:(9)) of some of the many useful biochemical reactions going on in the liver. To prevent such endogenous toxic substances from reaching unhindered the general circulation, it would be advantageous if the liver had a detoxifying zone located downstream of any zone in which toxic metabolites might be produced (10). This may be the physiological reason for the zonal distribution of liver function which is being increasingly detected by enzymological methods (11). Because these zones appear to be arranged sequentially in relation to the direction of blood flow, they exemplify longitudinal heterogeneity of the organ. The kinetic detection (12) of such zones, discussed and generalized in Section 8, involves interconverting substrates for which the steady state input-output relations are no longer insensitive to longitudinal distributions of enzyme densities, in contrast to the foregoing relations for single substrates. The minimization of the outflux of an endogenous toxic metabolite by such zonal arrangements gives rise to a novel kind of optimization problem which cannot be solved by classical Euler-Lagrange methods; a solution will be outlined in Section 9.

When the uptake problems sketched above in relation to liver metabolism are extended to time-dependence of input concentrations and of flow rates, and modeled by partial differential equations as in Section 3, they become mathematically similar (isomorphic) to an important and much wider set of problems arising in all those organs in which blood flow is manifolded through many parallel capillaries in order to optimize blood-tissue contact(brain, lung, muscle). In this larger context, "uptake" can also mean the escape of a labeled indicator from capillary blood into extravascular spaces by passive or facilitated transport across capillary walls. Facilitated transport can have the same mathematical form of concentration-dependence as enzymatic conversion (such as the Michaelis-Menten form); if the blood-borne indicator never returned into the capillaries, the effect of its depletion within the capillary on the relation between c_i and c_o would thus be indistinguishable from that caused by equivalent wall-removal by metabolic conversion. However, when the labeled indicator returns (back-diffuses) into the capillaries after some characteristic time, the mathematical isomorphism of the two kinds of uptake comes to an end. Before this happens, the input-output relations yield important information about capillary permeability of organs to various substances, especially when each substance of interest is used in conjunction with a reference substance which is confined to the blood (13). As in the case of uptake by irreversible metabolic transformation, there is here a corresponding problem of understanding the effects of transverse heterogeneity in organ uptake of indicators: the flows and uptake parameters of individual capillaries are distributed about their mean values taken over the organ, and the magnitudes of these dispersions affect uptake in a calculable way (14); but now time-dependence is an essential feature of the method and so effects of heterogeneity are unfolded in the time-course of the compositions of venous samples. We discuss this in Section 6.

When organ blood flow is varied, the possibility of changes in the number N of perfused capillaries adds another degree of freedom to the foregoing considerations. We shall see in Section 5 that observed deviations from the flow-dependence of uptake predicted by the undistributed model, can be attributed either to such changes in N (15), or to effects of transverse heterogeneity at fixed N (8). The latter alternative is important because changes in N (recruitment of capillaries) are often conjectured from analyses of uptake data.

These are difficult problems, especially when we insist on trying to keep a grip on experimental data obtained with great ingenuity by methods ranging from tracer kinetics (15,16) through enzymatic analysis (3) to the use of microelectrodes (17). Our general approach will have some resemblance to the statistical mechanics of physics and chemistry (18): quantitative hypotheses are made about the single elements of the ensemble of capillaries comprising an organ, but observable quantities are usually predicted only after summation over the organ (18,14). New methods arising in this context and discussed below include null experiments, upper and lower bounds on the quantities of interest, and appropriate sample-splitting for statistical significance tests.

But are all these devices really necessary in order to draw interesting conclusions from the data? Have older methods been fully exploited? In response to these questions we begin with a retrospect: a review and fuller development of the compartmental analysis of the elimination of a test-substrate by the saturated liver, when sampling is made from a single site in the intact body(19).

2. RETROSPECT: COMPARTMENTAL ANALYSIS OF SATURATED UPTAKE IN THE BODY

Compartmental analysis emphasizes time-dependence of organ concentrations, while drastically simplifying (lumping) their spatial variations. Such analysis replaces partial differential equations (with time and space as independent variables) by sets of ordinary differential equation, with each equation describing an effective concentration in one compartment as a function of time. In such simplifications the need for a clear physiological meaning of each compartment is evident (20).

The limited aims of compartmental analysis do not extend to processes affected substantially by internal structures of the compartments, which are left to other methods of analysis: "One man's black box is another man's problem" (21). Uptake by perfused organs is not, in general, a suitable subject for compartmental analysis because the interplay between local uptake and unidirectional blood flow generates concentration gradients which affect the rate of uptake, especially profoundly in saturation kinetics (cf. Introduction). In the context of uptake, unidirectional flow thus generates an internal structure of each compartment. However, there are limiting circumstances in which flow does not affect uptake, whereby the applicability of compartmental analysis is restored. We begin by examining in detail how these limiting circumstances can be attained in the simplest case of steady Michaelis-Menten uptake by the undistributed model of the liver (or each of its constituent sinusoids).

As the single characteristic concentration we choose the inlet (arterial) concentration c_i which can be monitored conveniently in clinical practice. Eliminating c_o from Eqs. 1 and 5 we get a transcendental equation for the uptake rate V:

$$V = Fc_i\left(1 - e^{-\frac{V_{max}-V}{FK_m}}\right). \tag{12}$$

We note in passing that this may also be rewritten in terms of the extraction fraction E,

$$E = (c_i - c_o)/c_i = V/(Fc_i) : \tag{13}$$

$$E = 1 - e^{-(V_{max}/F - Ec_i)/K_m}. \tag{14}$$

We now expand the exponential in Eq. 12 :

$$V/(Fc_i) = 1 - e^{-\frac{V_{max}-V}{FK_m}} = \frac{V_{max}-V}{FK_m} - \tfrac{1}{2}\left(\frac{V_{max}-V}{FK_m}\right)^2 + \dots \tag{15}$$

and observe that whenever $(V_{max}-V)/(FK_m)$ is sufficiently small to retain only its first power in Eq. 15, F drops out; solving for V we then obtain

$$V = V_{max}\,\frac{c_i}{c_i+K_m} \tag{16}$$

which has the test-tube form of Eq. 2, so that the organ takes up substrate as if it was an unstructured compartment. Now, there are three ways of attaining this limiting case of small $(V_{max}-V)/(FK_m)$. Since V_{max} is greater than V, it is evidently sufficient to make $V_{max}/(FK_m)$ small. The effect of increasing the flow rate

F is seen directly from Eq. 1 for any form of saturation kinetics: since

$$c_i - c_o = V/F \leq V_{max}/F \ ,$$

the arterial-venous difference can be reduced arbitrarily by choosing a sufficiently high value of F; but this is rarely possible in practice because of physiological limitations on rates of blood flow. A second way to reduce $V_{max}/(FK_m)$ is to choose a substrate with a very low ratio V_{max}/K_m, such as antipyrine, and observe its depletion in the blood pool of the body over a time sufficiently long to determine V. The third approach uses a saturating infusion of a non-toxic substrate such as galactose (22). Here $V_{max}/(FK_m)$ need not be small; instead, the compartmental behaviour of the eliminating organ is attained by making V approach V_{max} (by choosing c_i as high as needed: $c_i \gg K_m$). This approach is used in the following piece of compartmental analysis which underlies a clinical liver function test (19): one estimates the V_{max} of the patient's liver for the phosphorylation of galactose, and regards that V_{max} as a measure of the functional mass of the liver. Because of the concentration-independence of the uptake rate, one speaks of zero-order kinetics.

In the intact body, envisage a blood compartment of volume V_B containing substrate at a representative concentration c_B; and an extravascular compartment of volume V_E with corresponding concentration c_E. The two compartments exchange substrate by passive diffusion, and the blood compartment is in contact with the liver eliminating the substrate at the saturated rate V_{max}. The blood compartment may also be receiving an infusion of the substrate at the rate I. The primary purpose is to estimate V_{max}, but several other interesting quantities are estimated in the process.

The model equations are evidently

$$V_B \dot{c}_B = I - V_{max} - k(c_B - c_E) \tag{17}$$

$$V_E \dot{c}_E = k(c_B - c_E) \tag{18}$$

where dot denotes differentiation with respect to time, and the constant k (with the dimension of flow rate or clearance) characterizes the specific rate of exchange of the substrate between the compartments. One controls I, and measures c_B as a function of time. By contrast, c_E is not observed and plays the role of a "hidden variable". It is not difficult to eliminate c_E (by differentiation) and then solve the resulting second-order equation for $c_B(t)$. However, in rapid time-dependence c_E is surely far from uniform within V_E, and this suspect concentration needs to be watched rather than swept under the carpet. Indeed, it is impossible to believe that the simplistic Eqs. 17-18 are valid physiologically except in specially favourable kinetic circumstances which we regard as strategic regions, in the time-course of c_B, for the determination of parameters of interest. The delimitation of these regions will be facilitated by working with the original first order Eqs. 17-18.

Adding Eqs. 17 and 18 we get

$$V_B\dot{c}_B + V_E\dot{c}_E = I - V_{max} \tag{19}$$

for the time-change of the total amount of the substrate in the body. Dividing Eq. 17 by V_B and Eq. 18 by V_E and subtracting, we get

$$\dot{c}_B - \dot{c}_E = \frac{I-V_{max}}{V_B} - \frac{1}{\tau}(c_B - c_E) , \tag{20}$$

where

$$\tau = \frac{V_B V_E}{k(V_B+V_E)} \tag{21}$$

is a characteristic relaxation time of the system.

For simplicity we assume from now on that whenever I is not zero, it is a constant, as is usual experimentally. The solution of Eq. 20 is

$$c_B - c_E = \tau\frac{I-V_{max}}{V_B} + Ce^{-t/\tau} \tag{22}$$

with an arbitrary constant C of integration. Hence, on differentiating Eq. 22,

$$\dot{c}_B - \dot{c}_E = -\frac{C}{\tau}\, e^{-t/\tau} . \tag{22a}$$

The integration constant is determined by initial concentrations specified at a time from which there has been no change in I.

Eq. 22a shows that the difference between the slopes of $c_B(t)$ and $c_E(t)$ decays to zero exponentially with the relaxation time τ, while the difference of the two concentration tends to the constant first term in Eq. 22. In that limit Eq. 19 gives

$$(V_E+V_B)\dot{c}_B = I - V_{max} \tag{23}$$

so that $\dot{c}_B(t)$ and hence $\dot{c}_E(t)$ are then constants: the time courses of the two concentrations have become parallel and <u>rectilinear</u>. Thus the lapse of some number of relaxation times (which depends on the magnitude of C) brings us arbitrarily close to a state of <u>quasi-equilibrium</u> in which there is a steady transfer of the substrate between the compartments, such that it just balances the constant source or sink $I-V_{max}$ of substrate in the blood compartment. It is this kinetic regime that is most favourable to modeling the uptake process by only two compartments: the rectilinear segment of $c_B(t)$ is thus the strategic region for determining the parameters of interest. Eq. 23 gives already one relation between two of them, V_{max} and V_B+V_E.

We now outline the calculations which quantify the experiment (Fig.1) underlying the galactose liver function test (19).

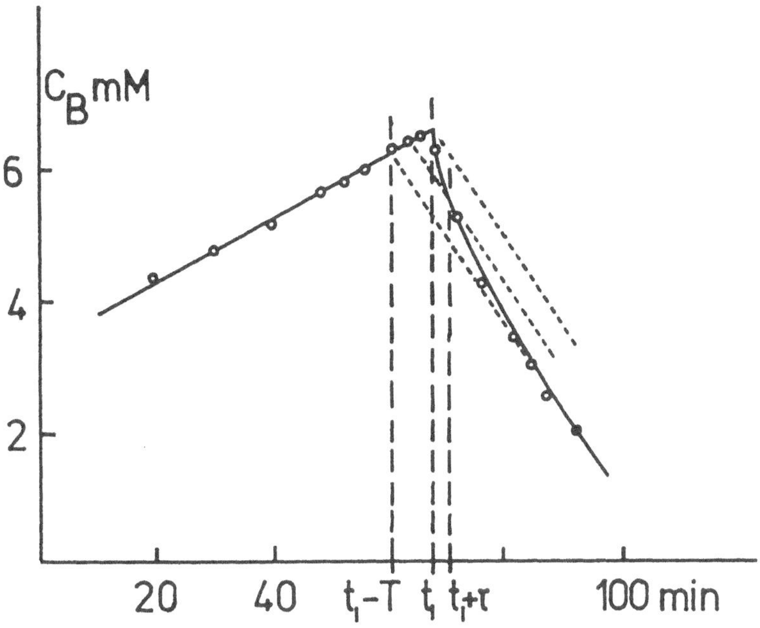

FIG.1

Time course of galactose concentration c_B in blood. A steady infusion is stopped at $t=t_1$. Data points inserted from Fig.2 of (19).

Initially there is no substrate in the body. From t=0 to $t=t_1$ a constant infusion of rate $I>V_{max}$ is delivered into the blood compartment, and stopped thereafter. During the infusion, Eq. 19 has the integral

$$V_B c_B + V_E c_E = (I-V_{max})t \, , \tag{24}$$

and the determination of C transforms Eq. 22 into

$$c_B - c_E = \tau \frac{I-V_{max}}{V_B} (1-e^{-t/\tau}) \, . \tag{25}$$

Eliminating c_E from Eqs. 24,25 we find the time-course of c_B :

$$(V_E+V_B)c_B = (I-V_{max}) \left[t+\tau\frac{V_E}{V_B}(1-e^{-t/\tau}) \right] . \tag{26}$$

We note here a minor imperfection of the theory: while c_B is rising from zero, the uptake rate cannot be saturated until sufficiently high values of c_B have been reached.

For the period $t>t_1$, when $I=0$, Eqs. 24 and 25 give the relevant initial values on setting $t=t_1$. In place of Eq. 26 we find by corresponding steps:

$$(V_B+V_E)c_B = It_1-V_{max}\left(t+\tau\frac{V_E}{V_B}\right)+\tau\frac{V_E}{V_B}\left[I-(I-V_{max})e^{-t_1/\tau}\right]e^{-(t-t_1)/\tau} . \quad (27)$$

To display the essentials of this result, we write

$$D = It_1 \quad (28)$$

for the total dose infused;

$$T = \tau\frac{V_E}{V_B} = \frac{V_E^2}{k(V_B+V_E)} \quad (29)$$

for another characteristic time, and

$$K = \frac{T}{V_B+V_E}\left[I-(I-V_{max})e^{-t_1/\tau}\right] \quad (30)$$

to abbreviate the last term of Eq. 27. That equation now becomes:

$$c_B = \frac{D-V_{max}(t+T)}{V_B+V_E}+Ke^{-(t-t_1)/\tau} . \quad (31)$$

When the time $t-t_1$ since the stop of the infusion is long enough to reduce the last term of Eq. 31 to zero with any desired accuracy, the rectilinear region of $c_B(t)$ is reached. If we then extrapolate the straight line to $c_B=0$ at some $t_{c=0}$, we have the basic formula used in the clinical method (19):

$$V_{max} = D/(t_{c=0}+T) . \quad (32)$$

Any part of the dose which is known to have been eliminated outside the liver, such as galactose found in urine, may be subtracted from D for greater physiological accuracy.

That much can be obtained from the straight line region after the stop of the infusion; but we still do not know V_{max} because we do not know T. In order to estimate T and τ, we now have to turn to non-strategic regions of curvilinear $c_B(t)$, in which the simple two-compartment model is less plausible. Going back to $t=t_1$, we see from Eq. 31 that the actual c_B is higher by K (Eq. 30) than the value obtained by backward extrapolation of the straight line (Fig.1). In order to estimate T, we must now require also that the duration $t_1=D/I$ of the infusion was sufficient to make the exponential term in Eq. 30 negligible. Then $c_B(t)$ becomes a straight line before the end of the infusion according to Eq. 26 (Fig.1), and at $t=t_1$ we obtain from Eqs.30,31:

$$c_B - \frac{D-V_{max}(t_1+T)}{V_B+V_E} = K = \frac{TI}{V_B+V_E} = T\left(\frac{V_{max}}{V_B+V_E} + \frac{I-V_{max}}{V_B+V_E}\right) . \tag{33}$$

Since the two terms in the bracket are the slopes of the two limiting straight-line segments of $c_B(t)$, it is seen that the intersection of the straight lines is at t_1-T, as shown in Fig. 1. This construction gives an estimate of T (19). Hence V_{max} is estimated from Eq. 32, and V_B+V_E from Eq. 23. Moreover, Eq. 31 shows that the excess of c_B over the extrapolated straight line falls exponentially from its initial value K at t_1, with the relaxation time τ. The half-life of that excess, or a semilogarithmic plot of its time-course, yields an estimate of τ. Next, since $T/\tau = V_E/V_B$ from Eq. 29, and V_B+V_E is now known, V_B and V_E can each be estimated. Then an estimate of k follows from Eq. 29.

Proceeding in this way from data such as are illustrated in Fig.1, one obtains for a typical normal human subject: V_{max} = 2 mmol/min, V_E = 10 l, V_B = 4 l, k = 1 l/min, τ = 3 min and T = 7 min. We observe in Fig.1 that $t_{c=0}$ is greater than 100 min, so that the precise value of T is of little importance in Eq. 32. This fortunate circumstance justifies our departure from the straight line region when determining T; it also makes it possible to use a typical human value of T, in place of individual patients' values, in the standard clinical test (19) to which we now turn.

In clinical practice t_1=5 min, so that a typical dose of 150 mmol of galactose is delivered at the rate I=30 mmol/min. Using the aforementioned typical values to calculate K from Eq. 30, we obtain K = 12.3 mmol/l, while at $t = t_1$ the first term in Eq. 31 (that is, the backward extrapolation of the limiting straight line) gives 9 mmol/l. Four relaxation times (4τ = 12 min) suffice to reverse the balance of the two terms in Eq. 31: at $t_1+4\tau$ = 17 min the first term is still 7.3 mmol/l, while the second term has dropped to 0.23 mmol/l, and we can assume the validity of the limiting straight line thereafter. Thus the strategic region for determining V_{max} starts some 20 min after the commencement of the infusion. On the other hand, K_m for <u>in vivo</u> galactose phosphorylation is (3) about 0.2 mmol/l, so that appreciable unsaturation of the elimination rate begins below 10 K_m = 2 mmol/l which corresponds to V_{hom}=0.91 V_{max} according to Eq. 2. If we require at least that degree of saturation <u>throughout</u> the liver, we must have c_o=10K_m while c_B as measured (19) is essentially $c_i = c_o + V_{max}/F$. In normal man, F is typically 1.5 l/min, so that the smallest acceptable c_B is 2+1.3 = 3.3 mmol/l. How long a run does this leave for the straight-line segment? Traversing the concentration range 7.3-3.3 = 4 mmol/l with the slope $V_{max}/(V_B+V_E)$=2/14 mmol/l.min gives us 28 min. With a safety margin, we thus have some 20 minutes in the strategic region: and that is why the method works. We note that the fortunate conjunction of orders of magnitude, several of them unconnected with the liver, might not be repeated for another substrate.

The foregoing <u>a priori</u> estimates of the limits of the strategic region of the clinical method are all the more necessary because even in that region $c_B(t)$ is in reality somewhat convex to the time axis: in practice a straight line is sometimes interpolated, rather than recognized, in the strategic region. This is due in large part to the intervention of the kidney, which eliminates galactose by first-order kinetics: one needs to add the term $-rc_B$ to $-V_{max}$ on the right-hand side of Eq. 17. We know from analyses of urine that the constant r is typically about 0.05 l/min (19). As c_B falls after the stop of the infusion, the actual elimination rate $V_{max}+rc_B$ is reduced, and so is the magnitude of the slope $\dot{c}_B$. Since in the strategic region the term rc_B is small as compared with V_{max}, we can estimate its effect on the curvature of $c_B(t)$ by retaining the foregoing calculations as a first approximation, and superposing the effect of the additional term. If we add $-rc_B$ on the right-hand side of Eq. 23 (with I=0), apply the modified equation at the beginning and end of the strategic region, and subtract, we get

$$(V_B+V_E)\Delta\dot{c}_B = -r\Delta c_B \qquad (34)$$

for the increments of slope and concentration across the region. Using Eq. 23 again we obtain, to first order in r, the relative change of slope across the region:

$$\Delta\dot{c}_B/\dot{c}_B \cong r\Delta c_B/V_{max}\,, \qquad (35)$$

which is about 0.1 at c_B=4 mmol/l. This effect precludes the use of very high galactose concentrations in the clinical method. In contrast to the convexity caused by unsaturation at the low-concentration limit of the range, the convexity expressed by Eq. 35 is due to two organs, and it is increased in patients who have reduced liver function but normal kidney function.

The foregoing considerations present an antidote to unduly ready use of curve-fitting by exponentials, with the attendant partiality to half-life and to semilogarithmic plots in pharmacokinetics. The complete time-course of $c_B(t)$ after the end of the infusion might well be fitted by a falling exponential (23). However, none of the convexities that might make such fitting appear successful have anything to do with liver function. The early (indeed, exponential) convexity is due entirely to the redistribution of substrate between the compartments; the convexity in the intermediate (strategic) range is due to extrahepatic factors exemplified by the kidney; and the late convexity due to unsaturation is determined by the value of K_m which is independent of functional liver mass (3).

It seems difficult to escape the conclusion that this exceptionally simple and physiologically and kinetically well-founded model operates in practice near the limits of its resolving power. The application of its central idea (the state of quasi-equilibrium) is hemmed in by limitations on concentrations from above and from below, and on time between early and late periods, leaving us with a somewhat precarious practical hold on the strategic part of the blood concentration curve. These limitations are due largely to sampling from a single site in the intact body (evidently desirable for a standard clinical test). It is apparent that methods with enough power to illuminate aspects of organ architecture must involve sampling at least from upstream and downstream of the organ of interest, so that the influences emanating from the rest of the body are summarized in the time-dependence of the input concentration of the substrate, as in Sections 3 and 6. The resulting study of input-output relations, and of their dependence on organ blood flow (cf. Introduction), then takes the problem out of the domain of applicability of compartmental analysis.

3. UNSTEADY MICHAELIS-MENTEN UPTAKE FROM BLOOD

We return to Eq. 3 in order to generalize it to time-dependence. We note first that the flux depletion term in Eq. 3 is more generally d(Fc), but that F has been assumed independent of position along the conduit. Since the fluid is practically incompressible, this assumption holds even if the cross-sectional area of the conduit varies with position. It is only when the solvent is also taken up through the walls of the conduit, as for example water from kidney tubules, that the extra term cdF = c(dF/dx)dx becomes important in the kinetics of uptake of solutes (24,25). Here we shall not pursue this interesting set of problems, but confine outselves to F independent of x, though possibly varying with time t.

When concentration c is not steady, there is a time-change $\dot{c}(Adx)$ in the amount of substrate between cross-sections of area A placed at x and x+dx (volume Adx); and now this term plus the flux increment Fdc balance the rate of wall uptake given on the right-hand side of Eq. 3. That equation is thus generalized to

$$A\frac{\partial c}{\partial t} + F\frac{\partial c}{\partial x} = -\rho\frac{c}{c+K_m}, \tag{36}$$

provided that the previously assumed transverse equilibration of the substrate can keep up with the time-changes which we are modeling here (25). Again, Eq. 4 holds for $\rho(x)$. Given the functions $F(t)$, $\rho(x)$ and $A(x)$, this non-linear partial differential equation of the first order governs the concentration $c(x,t)$ throughout each sinusoid (capillary), or equivalently throughout the undistributed organ model.

When c is very small compared with K_m throughout the interval $0 \leq x \leq L$, the right-hand side of Eq. 36 becomes $-\rho(x)c/K_m$ and the equation becomes linear. When F is constant, a more powerful method of linearization is to superpose an unsteady tracer concentration $c(x,t)$ on a steady concentration profile $c_M(x)$ of its mother substance. Substituting $c+c_M$ for c in Eq. 36 and again neglecting c as compared with K_m, we obtain

$$A\frac{\partial c}{\partial t} + F\left(\frac{\partial c}{\partial x} + \frac{dc_M}{dx}\right) = -\rho\left[\frac{c}{c_M+K_m} + \frac{c_M}{c_M+K_m}\right]. \tag{37}$$

Since $c_M(x)$ satisfies the steady-state Eq. 3, the last terms on both sides of Eq. 37 cancel and we are left with a linear equation for the tracer concentration $c(x,t)$. The new linear equation differs from the previous one only in that $\rho(x)c/K_m$ is replaced with $\rho(x)c/(c_M+K_m)$. With $c_M(x)$ varied experimentally (and often approximated by its spatial average), this method permits tracer investigations of uptake at different levels of saturation of the uptake process (26).

Linear problems of this kind, with constant F, ρ and A, but including a slowly equilibrating extravascular layer along each capillary, have been solved (27) and then used powerfully (28) in the interpretation of experiments; a metabolic sink in the extravascular layer has extended the linear model further (29). By contrast, in what follows we shall keep to Eq. 36 which is limited by its assumption of rapid transverse equilibration, but which is suitable for the study of nonlinear uptake kinetics under conditions of time-dependent input concentrations and of unsteady flow rates.

Eq. 36 can in fact be linearized, without any approximations, by choosing a new dependent variable $u(x,t)$ in place of $c(x,t)$ (25):

$$u = c + K_m \ln c . \tag{38}$$

Since then $du=dc(1+K_m/c)$, Eq. 36 becomes

$$A\frac{\partial u}{\partial t} + F\frac{\partial u}{\partial x} = -\rho . \tag{39}$$

It is thus apparent that the study of such kinetics is greatly simplified by considering u in place of c. As c varies from 0 to $+\infty$, u increases monotonically from $-\infty$ to $+\infty$: u and c are in one-to-one correspondence. Given any value of u, the corresponding c is obtained readily by numerical or graphical methods.

We shall assume that the substrate concentration is given (observed) at the inlet x=0 at all times $t : c(0,t)=c_i(t)$. We wish to calculate $c(x,t)$, and especially the observable outflow concentration $c(L,t)=c_o(t)$. The corresponding boundary values $u_i(t),u_o(t)$ follow from Eq. 38. For a solution including initial conditions on the interval $0 \leq x \leq L$, see (25). We shall assume in the present Section that A is independent of x, and lift this restriction in Appendix I. We now show that if also F is independent of time, then the observable relation between $c_i(t)$ and $c_o(t)$ is independent of the form of $\rho(x)$, as it was in the steady state. Then we show that this indifference of input-output relations to the longitudinal organization of uptake is lost in unsteady flow (when F depends on t). Experiments with unsteady flow could therefore be used to infer salient features of $\rho(x)$, and we shall show in Section 8 how that could be done using pulsating flow with a range of periodic times.

The general solution of Eq. 39 is the sum of the general solution of Eq. 39 with the right-hand side set to zero, and of any particular solution of the complete equation. It is easy to check that when A and F are constants, then any function f of the argument t-Ax/F satisfies Eq. 39 without the right-hand side. For the particular solution we choose the time-independent function

$$-\frac{1}{F}\int_0^x \rho dx ,$$

which obviously satisfies Eq. 39. Thus the general solution of Eq. 39 is

$$u(x,t) = f(t-Ax/F) - \frac{1}{F}\int_0^x \rho dx \qquad (40)$$

with an arbitrary (differentiable) function f. Now, at the inlet x=0 we are given $u(0,t)=u_i(t)$ which is equal to f(t) according to Eq. 40. This shows that the functional form of f is the same as that of u_i; hence, reverting to the argument t-Ax/F, Eq. 40 gives the solution satisfying the boundary condition:

$$u(x,t) = u_i(t-Ax/F) - \frac{1}{F}\int_0^x \rho dx , \qquad (41)$$

and this may be rewritten in terms of c(x,t) using Eq. 38. Thus u at any place and time in the capillary is obtained by referring back to the inlet value, as it was at a time earlier by Ax/F, and subtracting 1/F times the maximum uptake capacity present between the inlet and the position under consideration. In particular, at the outlet x=L we obtain, using Eq. 4,

$$u_o(t) = u_i(t-AL/F) - V_{max}/F , \qquad (42)$$

so that the form of $\rho(x)$ is indeed immaterial. Using Eq. 38, we see from Eq. 42 that the relation between c_o and c_i is the same as in the steady state according to Eq. 5, except that c_i has to be taken earlier than c_o by the time AL/F.

These considerations are clarified by using one of the equations of characteristics associated with Eq. 36 or 39 (Appendix I):

$$dx/dt = F/A , \qquad (43)$$

which describes the motion of an element of substrate through the capillary. If F/A is constant as hitherto, t=Ax/F is the travel time of the element from the inlet to the position x, and AL/F is the transit time through the whole capillary. It should be emphasized that F/A can be interpreted as the convective velocity of the blood only for substances taken up at the very surface of the conduit. If the substance is rapidly equilibrated with a layer of cells lining the conduit, as in the case of uptake by hepatic sinusoids, then the cross-sectional area A includes parts through which there is no convective flow. When this important point was elucidated (30), it became apparent how volumes of distribution of indicator substances in an organ can be estimated from differences in their times of arrival in the vein, following their injection in a common arterial bolus.

As a practical application of the foregoing results, we supplement the clinical method of estimating galactose V_{max} (Section 2) by an estimate of the corresponding Michaelis constant K_m in the intact patient whose liver vein is also sampled (1). Consider the time-courses of c_i and c_o in Fig.2, where the early part of $c_i(t)$ corresponds to the late part of $c_B(t)$ in Fig.1: we now follow the galactose concentrations down to values which do not saturate liver uptake. What is the relation between $c_i(t)$ and $c_o(t)$ at constant hepatic blood flow? In particular, what is the meaning of the apparent kink in the patient's venous outflow concentration $c_o(t)$ in Fig.2?

Writing Eq. 42 in terms of c_i and c_o using Eq. 38, and then differentiating with respect to time, we obtain

$$\dot{c}_o(t)[1+K_m/c_o(t)] = \dot{c}_i(t-T)[1+K_m/c_i(t-T)] \qquad (44)$$

where the transit time T is given by

$$T = AL/F \ , \qquad (45)$$

since A/F is constant. In this application of the undistributed model, AL is the volume of distribution of galactose in the liver, and F is the total hepatic blood flow. In man, AL is of the order of 1 l and F is of the order of 1 l/min, so that T is about 1 min. We now consider the neighbourhood of the sharp turn of $c_o(t)$

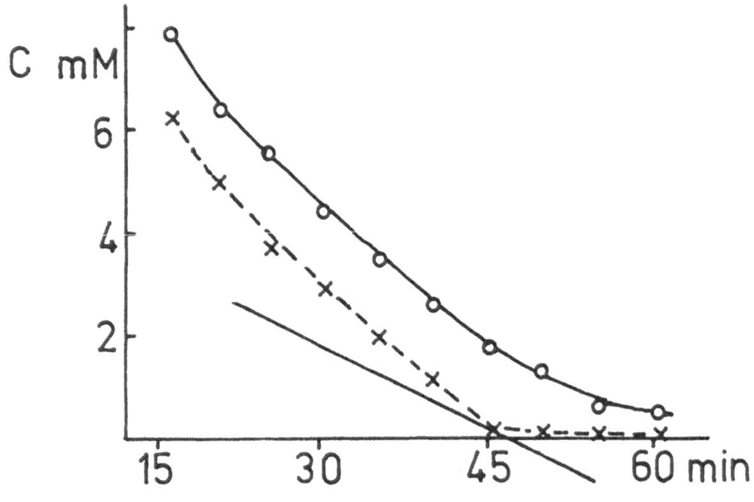

FIG.2

Time course of galactose concentration in the artery (c_i, upper curve) and hepatic vein (c_o, lower curve) in a human subject after a single injection. Data points inserted from (22).

in Fig.2, which occurs at about 46 min. The simultaneous value of c_i is about 1.8 mmol/l, and the value of a minute earlier is nearly 2 mmol/min because the slope $\dot{c}_i$ at that time (still in the straight-line strategic region of Section 2) is about 0.14 mmol/l. min. Since K_m for galactose is an order of magnitude smaller than 2 mmol/l, we neglect $K_m/c_i(t-T)$ against unity in Eq. 44 in the neighbourhood of t=46 min, and regard $\dot{c}_i$ as a constant still given by $-V_{max}/(V_B+V_E)$ according to Eq. 23 (with I=0):

$$\dot{c}_o = \frac{\dot{c}_i}{1+K_m/c_o}, \quad \dot{c}_i = \text{const.} \quad . \tag{46}$$

We note first that when $c_o=K_m$, $\dot{c}_o=\frac{1}{2}\dot{c}_i$: the tangent to $c_o(t)$ drawn with half the slope of $c_i(t)$ at the corresponding time, touches the $c_o(t)$ curve at $c_o=K_m$ (Fig.2). We thus obtain the value K_m=0.16 mmol/l for this patient directly from the venous outflow data, in good agreement with steady-state measurements _in vitro_ (31) and _in vivo_ (3). Next we consider how sharp the turn of $c_o(t)$ can be according to the model. Differentiating Eq. 46 with respect to time at constant $\dot{c}_i$ and using Eq. 46 again, we obtain

$$\ddot{c}_o = \frac{K_m c_o(\dot{c}_i)^2}{(c_o+K_m)^3}, \tag{47}$$

and it is easy to show by further differentiation that $\ddot{c}_o$ has the maximum value $4(\dot{c}_i)^2/(27K_m)$ at $2c_o=K_m$. In a time-interval dt we then have the relative change of slope, $d\dot{c}_o/\dot{c}_o$, equal to $4\dot{c}_i dt/(9K_m)$ from Eqs. 46,47. For our patient we thus obtain the maximum rate of change of the slope of c_o equal to about 39% per minute, which is consistent with the appearance of a kink in the curve. We note that since the magnitude of $\dot{c}_i$ is estimated from Eq. 23 to be $V_{max}/(V_E+V_B)$, large patients with reduced liver function have much slower c_o-turns, as is apparent from Eq. 47.

According to the distributed liver model (6-8) discussed in Section 4, there is a distribution of sinusoidal c_o's arising from a common c_i because the sinusoidal counterparts of V_{max} and F have a statistical distribution over the liver. The resulting refinement of the foregoing considerations (32) will not be discussed here, except for a note on the effect of an intrahepatic shunt. Suppose that a shunted flow of rate F_s bypasses the enzymatic system of the liver, which is otherwise undistributed. Then the observed venous concentration of the substrate, say c_o^{mix}, is given by the flux conservation formula

$$Fc_o^{mix} = F_s c_i + (F-F_s)c_o \tag{48}$$

in which c_o, calculated from the foregoing undistributed theory, is not observed. Since $\dot{c}_i$ is approximately constant in the region of interest, $\ddot{c}_o^{mix}=(1-F_s/F)\ddot{c}_o$ and so the turn is slowed by the shunt. Moreover, $c_o^{mix} > c_o$ and so the foregoing estimation of K_m from the tangent of the venous outflow curve yields only an upper bound on K_m in the presence of shunting. It is because our patient had a normal liver (22) that we have approached closely the true value of K_m in his case.

At any time t, there is an instantaneous rate of uptake V of substrate by the organ; V is an observable, measured by the disappearance of substrate from the blood pool (3). In the steady state V is connected simply with c_i and c_o by Eq. 1 and it is thus sometimes used as an inferred (rather than independently observed) quantity; however, steady states are rarely perfectly steady (see below). In time-dependence V remains simple only under saturation, $V=V_{max}$, in which case Eq. 1 still holds provided that c_i-c_o is replaced by $c_i(t-T)-c_o(t)$, where the transit time T is given by Eq. 45 when A/F is constant. This result follows from Eq. 42 because at very large values of c, u tends to c according to Eq. 38. In general,

$$V(t) = \int_0^L \rho(x)\frac{c(x,t)}{c(x,t)+K_m}dx \quad , \tag{49}$$

and the straightforward (but intractable) procedure would be to substitute for c(x,t) the solution of Eq. 36 which is given by Eqs. 41,38 for any time-dependent input concentration $c_i(t)$. The problem is difficult because we have to sum over uptake from elements of substrate which had spent different times in the capillary, and had entered it with different concentrations.

We prefer to return to Eq. 36, integrate through from 0 to L and use Eq. 49:

$$A\int_0^L \frac{\partial c(x,t)}{\partial t}dx + F[c_o(t)-c_i(t)] = -V \ . \tag{50}$$

The integrand of the first term is found by differentiating Eq.41 with respect to time, and using Eq. 38:

$$\frac{\partial c(x,t)}{\partial t} = \frac{c(x,t)}{c(x,t)+K_m}\left[\dot{c}_i\left(1+\frac{K_m}{c_i}\right)\right]_{t-Ax/F} \quad , \tag{51}$$

where the suffix on the square bracket denotes the time at which the quantities in the bracket are to be evaluated. The square bracketed term is thus also a function of position. Eq. 51 is the generalization of Eq. 44, valid at all x.

We now simplify the calculation of V by two restrictive assumptions (for a deeper treatment, see (25)). Firstly, we take $\rho(x)$=const.$=V_{max}/L$. Secondly, we suppose that $c_i(t)$ and $\dot{c}_i(t)$ change so little during one transit time T, that the suffix on the right-hand side of Eq. 51 can be dropped (replaced by t), and the square bracket becomes a function of t alone: we take the state to be quasi-steady. In evaluating the first term of Eq. 50, we can now use Eq. 49, and we obtain after some rearrangement

$$V = \frac{F(c_i-c_o)}{1+(AL\dot{c}_i/V_{max})(1+K_m/c_i)} \tag{52}$$

where now all the quantities refer to the same time t. When c_i is rising ($\dot{c}_i>0$), V is lower than $F(c_i-c_o)$ because some of that flux difference is due to an increase in the amount of substrate in the organ. The qualitative effect of falling c_i can be understood similarly.

We apply this result to the interpretation of data on the steady uptake of galactose by isolated pig livers perfused in a recirculating solution (3). In this work, V_{max} and K_m were inferred from Eqs. 6,7 using the undistributed model (1) of hepatic uptake, so that the validity of Eq. 1 was assumed.(Section 1). However, c_i was not quite steady during some of the experimental periods, and we shall now use Eq. 52 to assess deviations from Eq. 1 in these experiments. While $\dot{c}_i$ was nearly constant in each experimental period, no magnitude $|\dot{c}_i|$ exceeded 0.05 mmol/l.min. Since appreciable magnitudes $|\dot{c}_i|$ occurred only at large c_i ($c_i > 2$ mmol/l) as a result of the requisite high rates of infusion, relative changes in c_i were small during T=AL/F, which was about 0.5 min. The conditions for a quasi-steady state were therefore satisfied in all the experiments. The average values V_{max}=0.43 mmol/min, K_m=0.23 mmol/l for the experimental group of pig livers, obtained by steady-state analysis (3), can therefore serve as a first approximation in Eq. 52, where we can now also replace $\dot{c}_i(1+K_m/c_i)$ by $\dot{c}_i$. Taking AL=0.6 l as an upper bound for the volume of distribution of galactose in the pig livers, we have from Eq. 52:

$$\frac{F(c_i-c_o)-V}{V} = AL\dot{c}_i/V_{max} < 0.6\text{x}0.05/0.43 < 0.07 \; , \tag{53}$$

so that the relative error in using Eq. 1 did not exceed 7% even in the least steady states (cf. Fig.2 in (3)).

We now turn to the case of unsteady flow. In contrast to the preceding cases with F=const., the relation between $c_i(t)$ and $c_o(t)$ will no longer be insensitive to the form of $\rho(x)$. Suppose for example that $\rho(x)$ is sharply peaked at some x_o, F(t) is sharply peaked at some t_o, and $c_i(t)$ is a concentrated pulse (bolus) of the substrate. If the bolus passes x_o at the time t_o, depletion of the substrate will be minimized because the bolus will spend as little time as possible in the highly extracting region.

To make the problem definite and simple, we shall assume that

$$\left.\begin{aligned} \rho(x) &= \text{const.} = V_{max}/L \;, \quad 0 < x < L \;, \\ \rho(x) &= 0 \qquad\qquad\qquad\;\;, \quad x < 0 \text{ and } x > L \;. \end{aligned}\right\} \tag{54}$$

Now the organ may have its inlet at $x < 0$, and outlet at $x > L$; it is in such non-extracting regions ($\rho=0$) that sampling of input and output concentrations occurs in practice. The concentrations so sampled are connected with $c_i(t)=c(0,t)$ and $c_o(t)=c(L,t)$ by simple time-shifts due to travel through the non-extracting regions (cf. Section 8). Next we assume that A is constant. With these restrictions on ρ and on A (which will be lifted in Appendix I) we can solve Eq. 39 more simply than before. Consider an element of substrate moving according to Eq. 43, now with $F=F(t)$, and introduce the total derivative du/dt (material derivative) which denotes differentiation following the motion:

$$\frac{du}{dt} = \frac{\partial u}{\partial t} + \frac{\partial u}{\partial x}\frac{dx}{dt} = \frac{\partial u}{\partial t} + \frac{F}{A}\frac{\partial u}{\partial x} . \tag{55}$$

Dividing Eq. 39 through with A, we see that the left-hand side is just du/dt given by Eq. 55. Using also Eqs. 54 we have

$$\frac{du}{dt} = -V_{max}/(AL) . \tag{56}$$

The moving element passes x=0 with the value $u_i(t-T)$ at the time t-T, and reaches x=L with the value $u_o(t)$ at the time t, where T is the appropriate transit time. Integrating Eq. 56 with respect to time, we therefore obtain

$$u_o(t) = u_i(t-T) - \frac{V_{max}}{AL}T \tag{57}$$

which would coincide with Eq. 42 if the transit time was AL/F according to Eq. 45. But Eq. 45 no longer holds because F depends on t. Instead, integrating Eq. 43 from $x(t-T)=0$ at the time of entry to $x(t)=L$ at the time of exit, we obtain

$$AL = \int_{t-T}^{t} F(v)dv , \tag{58}$$

where v is a dummy variable. Whenever F/A can be interpreted as convection velocity (cf. the remark following Eq. 43), Eq. 58 has the simple meaning: between times t-T and t, F(t) sweeps out the volume AL. Eq. 58 expresses the time-dependence of the transit time, T(t), brought about by the unsteadiness of the flow rate F(t). Much of the following mathematical work arises from making explicit the effects of this (inevitably implicit) definition of T. Using Eq. 38, we can rewrite Eq. 57 more explicitly:

$$c_o(t) + K_m \ln c_o(t) = c_i(t-T) + K_m \ln c_i(t-T) - \frac{V_{max}}{AL}T , \tag{59}$$

where T is still given only implicitly by Eq. 58 at each time t.

As a first application of these new results, we calculate uptake by Michaelis-Menten kinetics from blood pulsating with a periodic flow rate, and in particular from intermittent flow which is often seen in capillaries of perfused organs. In Section 8 we shall use some of these results to propose an experimental study, by kinetic means, of aspects of the longitudinal organization of hepatic uptake. Consider a capillary, such as a liver sinusoid, extracting a substrate when the unidirectional flow pulsates with a period τ:

$$F(t) = F(t+\tau) > 0 \ . \tag{60}$$

We shall consider only the case of steady inlet concentration $c(0,t)=c_i=\text{const}$. Then $c(x,t)$ is periodic throughout the capillary with the same period τ (but not with the same phase at all x) as $F(t)$, since the form of Eq. 36, and the boundary condition, are unchanged in terms of a new time variable $t+\tau=t'$ (say). If venous outflow samples over many periods are pooled and then analyzed, the observed concentration is equal to the flow-weighted time-average $\bar{c}_0$ over one period:

$$\bar{c}_o = \overline{Fc_o}/\bar{F} = \int_t^{t+\tau} F(v)c_o dv \Big/ \int_t^{t+\tau} F(v)dv \ . \tag{61}$$

The corresponding uptake rate is then

$$\bar{V} = \bar{F}(c_i - \bar{c}_o) \ . \tag{62}$$

To bring out the effect of pulsation on such long-term uptake, we compare $\bar{c}_0$ with the concentration $c_0(\bar{F})$ which would be observed at the outlet if the flow was steady at the rate $\bar{F}$; $c_0(\bar{F})$ is thus the solution of Eq. 5 with F replaced by $\bar{F}$.

Several observable results follow from the periodicity (Eq. 60) regardless of the detailed form of $F(t)$. Without loss of generality we can write T at any time t in the form

$$T = n\tau + q\tau \ , \ 0 \leq q < 1 \tag{63}$$

where the constant n is zero or a positive integer, and q depends on time. This is seen by considering the area under the curve $F(v)$ according to Eq. 58. Using Eq. 63 and the periodicity of $F(t)$, Eq. 58 becomes

$$AL = \int_{t-n\tau-q\tau}^{t} F(v)dv = n\tau\bar{F} + \int_{t-q\tau}^{t} F(v)dv \ . \tag{64}$$

Using Eqs. 63 and 64, the quantity T/AL which multiplies V_{max} in Eq. 59 becomes

$$\frac{T}{AL} = \frac{n+q}{n\bar{F}+q\bar{F}_{t-q\tau,t}} \tag{65}$$

where

$$\bar{F}_{t-q\tau,t} = \frac{1}{q\tau}\int_{t-q\tau}^{t} F(v)dv \tag{66}$$

is the mean flow rate between the times $t-q\tau, t$. The following cases are of particular interest.

(i) When $q=0$, $AL=n\tau\bar{F}$ from Eq. 64 and $T/AL=1/\bar{F}$ from Eq. 65; hence $c_o=c_o(\bar{F})=\text{const.}=\bar{c}_o$ from Eq. 59 with $c_i=\text{const.}$ Therefore, whenever an integral number of volumes $\bar{F}\tau$ just fits into the volume of distribution AL, the pulsation has no effect on the time-averaged uptake.

(ii) When n is large ($T\gg\tau$), T/AL tends to $1/\bar{F}$ for any value of q ($0\leq q<1$) according to Eq. 65 since $\bar{F}_{t-q\tau,t}$ cannot exceed the peak value of F(t); hence $\bar{c}_o$ tends to $c_o(\bar{F})$ and pulsation again does not influence the time-averaged uptake rate. Here the many complete periods within T make the effect of an additional incomplete period relatively insignificant.

(iii) When $n=0$ ($T<\tau$), $T/AL=1/\bar{F}_{t-q\tau,t}$ according to Eq. 65. If moreover $q\ll 1$ ($T\ll\tau$), then $\bar{F}_{t-q\tau,t}$ tends to F(t) according to Eq. 66, and the uptake is quasi-steady in the sense that $c_o(t)$ is a succession of values calculated from Eq. 59 with $c_i=\text{const.}$ by inserting the simultaneous value $1/F(t)$ for T/AL. Since c_i is independent of time, the $\bar{c}_o$ produced by pooling the outflux $F(t)c_o(t)$ over one period τ (Eq. 61) is the same as if we mixed steady outfluxes from an ensemble of parallel conduits perfused at the steady flow rates $F(v)dv/\tau$ ($0\leq v\leq\tau$), and all having the same c_i and the same fraction of V_{max}. We shall prove in Section 4 that $c_o(\bar{F}) < \bar{c}_o$ for any shape of F(v), and we shall exemplify this below in connection with Eqs. 73-75.

We thus have $c_o(\bar{F}) \leq \bar{c}_o$ in all the cases (i)-(iii); from Eq. 62 we deduce $V(\bar{F}) \geq \bar{V}$.

We exemplify the magnitude of these effects by considering first-order uptake when the flow rate has the form of a square wave with amplitude $\delta \leq \bar{F}$, and by comparing the limits of high and low pulsation frequency. As shown in (ii), T approaches $AL/\bar{F}$ and $\bar{c}_o$ approaches $c_o(\bar{F})$ when $T\gg\tau$ so that, in the first-order regime $c\ll K_m$, Eq. 59 attains the simple form of Eq. 5b:

$$\bar{c}_o = c_o(\bar{F}) = c_i\, e^{-V_{max}/(\bar{F}K_m)}, \quad T \gg \tau . \tag{67}$$

In the opposite limit $T\ll\tau$ discussed in (iii), T(t) approaches $AL/F(t)$ so that, at every instant t,

$$c_o(t) = c_i e^{-V_{max}/(F(t)K_m)}, \quad T \ll \tau . \tag{68}$$

In this limit then, for the square wave,

$$\bar{c}_o = \overline{Fc_o}/\bar{F} = \frac{c_i}{2\bar{F}}\left[(\bar{F}+\delta)\exp\left(-\frac{V_{max}}{(\bar{F}+\delta)K_m}\right) + (\bar{F}-\delta)\exp\left(-\frac{V_{max}}{(\bar{F}-\delta)K_m}\right)\right], \tag{69}$$

where the longest transit time, $AL/(\bar{F}-\delta)$, must still be short as compared with τ for our approximation to be valid. The second term in Eq. 69 is evidently smaller than the first, and it becomes negligible compared with the first term when $V_{max}/\bar{F}K_m$ is sufficiently large.

In the physiologically interesting case of periodic intermittency, $\bar{F}-\delta=0$, only the first term in Eq. 69 remains, but this does not follow legitimately from Eq. 69 because the limit $T<<\tau$ is no longer available when F is intermittently zero. Instead, we note that uptake depletes the substrate during the half-period of stopped flow; when the flow re-commences, the previously stagnant contents of the capillary is ejected in the time $T=AL/2\delta$. If this time is short as compared with $\tau/2$, that contribution to the time-averaged outflux $\overline{Fc_o}$ is negligible as compared with the outflux during the following half-period with flow rate 2δ, which gives just the first term of Eq. 69:

$$\bar{c}_o = c_i e^{-V_{max}/(2\bar{F}K_m)}, \quad AL/\delta << \tau \tag{70}$$

where we have set $\bar{F}=\delta$, and where now $AL/\delta<<\tau$ expresses the condition $T<<\tau$ for the periodic time to be long. The effect of such intermittency on the average venous outflow concentration is the same as if the flow was steady at double the mean flow rate. Thus $\bar{c}_o/c_i$ in the limit $AL/\delta<<\tau$ is the square root of the corresponding ratio in the limit $T>>\tau$. Suppose for example that when pulsation is rapid, a substrate is so strongly extracted in one pass through the organ that the extraction fraction defined by Eq. 13 is $1-\bar{c}_o/c_i=0.99$. Then at the same value of $\bar{F}$, but at very long τ, the extraction fraction drops to 0.90, allowing appreciable (10%) transmission of the substrate through the organ. Using the long-term uptake rate $\bar{V}$ defined by Eq. 62, the difference in the limiting extraction fractions in intermittency is

$$\Delta E = (\bar{V}_{T>>\tau}-\bar{V}_{T<<\tau})/(\bar{F}c_i) = e^{-V_{max}/(2\bar{F}K_m)} - e^{-V_{max}/(\bar{F}K_m)} \tag{71}$$

using Eqs. 13,67,70. The increment ΔE is always positive; at small $V_{max}/(\bar{F}K_m)$ it varies as $V_{max}/(2\bar{F}K_m)$, it rises to the maximum of 0.25 at $V_{max}/(\bar{F}K_m) = 2\ln 2 = 1.386$, and at large $V_{max}/(\bar{F}K_m)$ it falls off rapidly as $\exp(-V_{max}/2\bar{F}K_m)$.

Such large changes in $\bar{c}_o/c_i$ and in E are evidently measureable, so that the form of the transition between the two limiting cases is of practical interest. In Appendix II we calculate $\bar{c}_o$ at all periodic times τ of a flow rate pulsating with a small amplitude F_1:

$$F(t) = \bar{F} + F_1\cos(2\pi t/\tau) \; . \tag{72}$$

Working to order $(F_1/\bar{F})^2$, we show there that

$$\bar{c}_o/c_o(\bar{F}) = 1 + \tfrac{1}{4}\left(\frac{V_{max}}{\bar{F}K_m}\right)^2\left(\frac{F_1}{\bar{F}}\right)^2\left[1+\frac{c_o(\bar{F})}{K_m}\right]^{-3}\left[\frac{\sin\left(\pi\frac{AL}{\bar{F}\tau}\right)}{\pi\frac{AL}{\bar{F}\tau}}\right]^2 \; . \tag{73}$$

The last factor exemplifies the dependence on τ, of which some salient features were obtained in (i)-(iii) above for any periodic form of F(t). All other features of Eq. 73 are elucidated by considering a slow pulsation, $AL/\bar{F} \ll \tau$ (i.e., n=0,q<<1 in Eq. 63). In that limit the last factor in Eq. 73 tends to unity, and what is left may be written in the form

$$\lim_{\tau \gg T} \bar{c}_0/c_0(\bar{F}) = 1 + \tfrac{1}{2}\,\varepsilon^2 \left(\frac{V_{max}}{\bar{F}K_m}\right)^2 \left[1 + \frac{c_0(\bar{F})}{K_m}\right]^{-3}, \tag{74}$$

where ε is the coefficient of variation of the temporal distribution of the flow rate:

$$\varepsilon^2 = \frac{1}{\tau} \int_t^{t+\tau} \frac{(F-\bar{F})^2}{\bar{F}^2}\, dt = \tfrac{1}{2}\left(\frac{F_1}{\bar{F}}\right)^2, \tag{75}$$

as is seen on inserting the F(t) given by Eq. 72. Eq. 74 coincides with a result derived in the next Section (Eq. 120) for the venous outflow from a liver comprising a set of parallel sinusoids which have a distribution of steady flow rates with a small coefficient of variation ε, the averages being calculated over the set of sinusoids to order ε^2. That means: when there are many transits in one pulsation period, $\bar{c}_0/c_0(\bar{F})$ is the same no matter whether the dispersion of F about its mean is sequential in one capillary, or simultaneous in a set of steadily perfused parallel capillaries differing only in perfusion rates. This may perhaps be regarded as a microvascular analogue of the ergodic hypothesis.

As a second application of uptake from unsteady flow, we reconsider published data determining the permeability to potassium ions of single capillaries in the frog mesentery (17). The rate of blood flow through a single capillary is so small that the injection of the requisite potassium-rich bolus causes appreciable unsteadiness in the flow at times when the data are recorded. A full and self-consistent calculation of the capillary permeability from such data requires therefore our extension of uptake calculations to the case of unsteady flow.

In the experiment (17), the intracapillary potassium concentration was monitored by two K^+-sensitive microelectrodes placed at a distance L from each other in a perfused single capillary. A potassium-rich bolus was injected upstream of both electrodes, and it generated the unsteadiness of concentrations shown schematically in Fig.3 as $c_i(t)$ at the upstream electrode, and $c_0(t)$ at the downstream electrode. The rate of escape of the extra potassium through the wall of the capillary is proportional to the local excess potassium concentration, which gives rise to first order uptake kinetics corresponding to the limit $c \ll K_m$ in irreversible metabolic wall uptake. In this mathematical isomorphism of the two kinds of uptake, which lasts until the onset of back-diffusion of potassium from extravascular spaces (cf. Introduction), V_{max}/K_m corresponds to the permeability-surface product PS for the capillary; it is PS which is to be determined

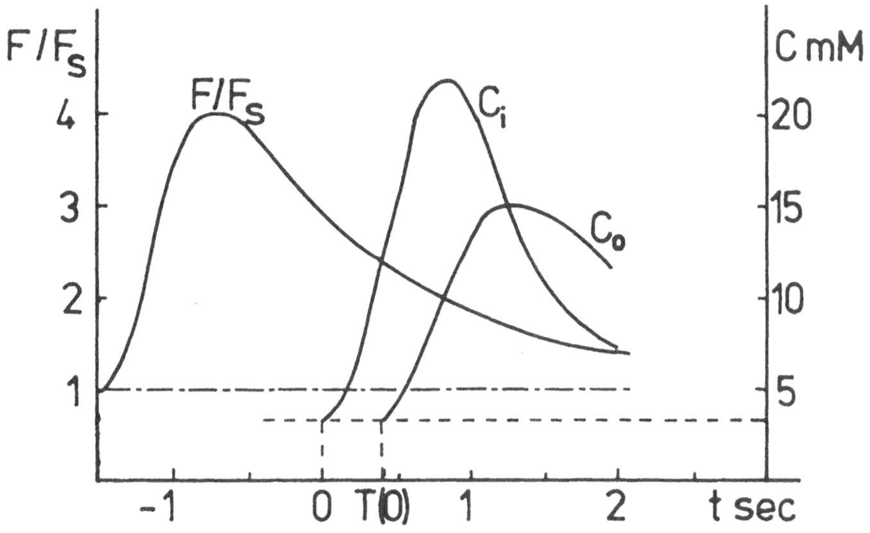

FIG.3

Three aspects of the passage of a potassium-rich bolus through a single capillary, drawn schematically on a common time-scale after (17). Flow rate F (left-hand scale: normalized to its steady pre- and post-bolus value F_s); potassium concentrations c_i and c_o at the upstream and downstream electrodes, respectively (right-hand scale), rising from the physiological background value at t=0 and t=T(0), respectively.

experimentally here. Accordingly, reduction of Eq. 59 to the limit of first-order kinetics (by dropping the non-logarithmic concentration terms), and replacement of V_{max}/K_m by PS, yields after rearrangement:

$$c_o(t) = c_i(t-T)e^{-\frac{PS}{AL}T} . \qquad (76)$$

We note that in the steady state Eq. 45 would hold, reducing Eq. 76 further to the familiar (13) counterpart of Eq. 5b.

In analyzing this experiment (19), we shall find it more convenient to use the time-variable t+T in place of t, so that we have in place of Eq. 76:

$$c_o(t+T) = c_i(t)e^{-\frac{PS}{AL}T} \qquad (76a)$$

where now T is defined by

$$AL = \int_t^{t+T} F(v)dv , \qquad (58a)$$

rather than by Eq. 58. As shown in Fig.3, we choose as t=0 the time of first appearance of the bolus at the upstream electrode, so that the time of first appearance at the downstream electrode is equal to T(0), i.e. to the initial value of the transit time as defined in Eq. 58a. The injection made the flow unsteady; by the times the bolus was passing the electrodes, the flow rate was falling monotonically back towards its steady base value, as shown schematically in Fig.3. Hence T(t) increased monotonically from its initial value T(0). In Eq. 76a the authors of (17) used T(0) as an approximation to all values of T from t=0 up to the time of the peak of c_i; they noted that this would result in an overestimate of the permeability, since in reality most of the indicator considered had remained longer than T(0) between the electrodes. We now quantify this qualitative assessment.

Since T(0) is the only directly measured value of T, we exploit it by developing T(t) in a series about t=0, confining ourselves to the linear term:

$$T(t) = T(0) + \dot{T}(0)t \; . \qquad (77)$$

To calculate $\dot{T}(0)$, we differentiate Eq. 58a through with respect to t, remembering that the limits of the integral depend on t explicitly as well as implicitly through T(t):

$$0 = F(t+T)(1+\dot{T}) - F(t) \; ,$$

or

$$\dot{T} = -\frac{F(t+T)-F(t)}{F(t+T)} \qquad (78)$$

without any approximations. Hence

$$\dot{T}(0) = -\frac{F[T(0)]-F(0)}{F[T(0)]} > 0 \qquad (79)$$

is exactly the relative change of the flow rate between the first appearance of the bolus at the electrodes. In what follows we shall use this dimensionless quantity as the measure of the unsteadiness of the flow. Measured values of F(0) and F[T(0)] are not available, but we shall be able to estimate $\dot{T}$(0) unambiguously from the available concentration data.

We substitute T(t) from Eq. 77 in Eq. 76a:

$$c_o[t+T(0)+\dot{T}(0)t] = c_i(t)e^{-\frac{PS}{AL}[T(0)+\dot{T}(0)t]} \; . \qquad (80)$$

Here PS/AL and $\dot{T}(0)$ are to be determined from the data. We do this by the method of least squares, seeking PS/AL and $\dot{T}(0)$ which minimize

$$Q(PS/AL,\dot{T}(0);t^*) = \int_0^{t^*} \left\{ c_o[t+T(0)+\dot{T}(0)t] - c_i e^{-\frac{PS}{AL}[T(0)+\dot{T}(0)t]} \right\}^2 dt, \qquad (81)$$

using data from t=0 up to a limiting time t*.

We study Q by digital computation using the observed $c_i(t)$ and $c_o(t)$ contained in Fig.4 of (17), which we converted carefully from graphical to digital form, and from which we subtracted the physiological background concentration shown in Fig.3. At least 80% of the rising limbs of c_i and c_o are linear, and we extrapolate these linear segments backward to the physiological background concentration to obtain an unambiguous initial transit time T(0). We thus obtain T(0)=0.31 sec, with a calculating error of less than 0.01 sec. All calculations that follow were made with T(0)=0.31 sec, and then repeated with T(0)=0.30 and 0.32 sec; the two latter sets of results do not differ substantially from those at 0.31 sec reported below.

We denote the time of the peak of c_i by t_p, and choose first $t^*=t_p$, in common with (17) and with other users of this "upslope method" of estimating PS (20). We display $Q(PS/AL,\dot{T}(0);t_p)$ as a function of the two parameters $PS/AL,\dot{T}(0)$ in Fig.4 by means of a family of contours of constant Q. The single minimum of this surface is so sharp that we draw the contours at values of Q each

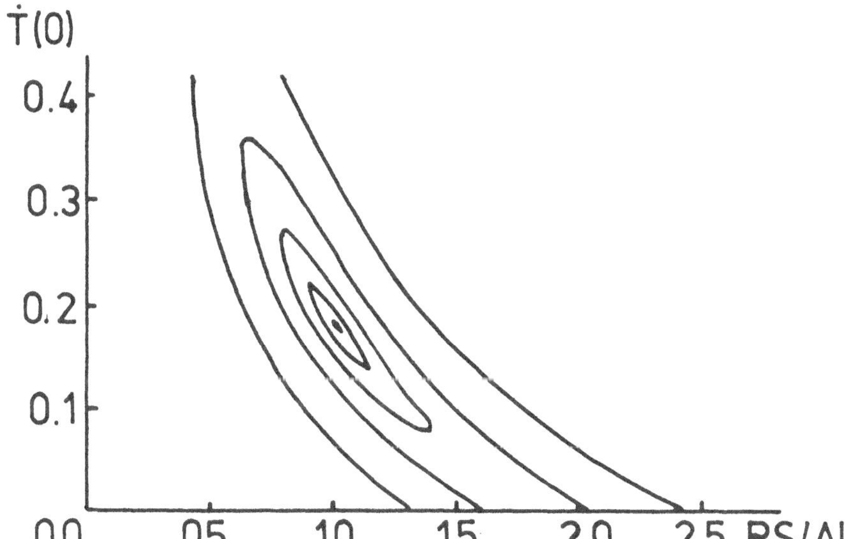

FIG.4

The sum-of-squares measure Q of the deviations of the theory from data in (17), evaluated throughout the rise of potassium concentrations (cf.Fig.3), and shown as a function of the normalized permeability PS/AL and of the measure $\dot{T}(0)$ of flow unsteadiness. Contours of constant Q are drawn (in the order of increasing size) at Q=0.2, 0.8, 3.2, 12.8, 51.2.

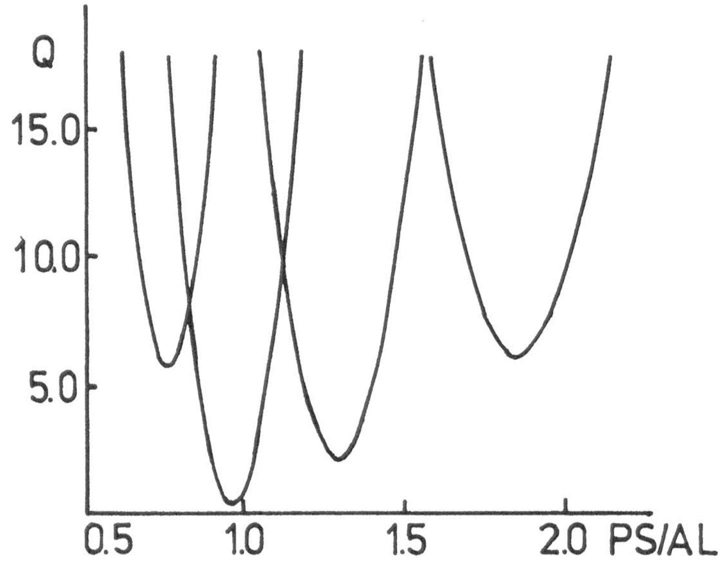

FIG.5

Intersections of the surface $Q(\dot{T}(0),PS/AL)$ of Fig.4, with planes $\dot{T}(0)$=const. From left to right: $\dot{T}(0)=0.3$, 0.2, 0.1, 0. Note the good fit of theory to data at $\dot{T}(0)=0.2$, PS/AL=0.96 (cf. Table 1).

of which is four times the preceding one (rather than at equal intervals of Q). The diagonal valley apparent in Fig.4 is detailed further in Fig.5, where four intersections of the surface with planes $\dot{T}(0)$=const. are drawn. A set of values of Q at the floor of the valley, denoted by $Q_{min}(t_p)$, is given in the second column of Table 1 (with corresponding values of $\dot{T}(0)$ in the first column, and of PS/AL in the third): the path through the valley leads through a deep minimum at $\dot{T}(0)=0.175$ and PS/AL=1.04, with a value of $Q_{min}(t_p)$ which is less than 1/20 of the values at $\dot{T}(0)=0$ and 0.3. The most probable reduction of the flow rate between the first appearances of the bolus at the two electrodes is thus estimated at 17.5%, and this value is associated with a substantially smaller permeability P than would be inferred by setting $\dot{T}(0)=0$: the reduction is by a factor of 1.04/1.84=0.565 from Table 1, since S/AL=2/r is fixed by the radius r of the capillary.

The time $t^*=t_p=0.85$ sec is only one of many choices of t^* small enough to exclude data influenced by back-diffusion of the indicator, and large enough to suppress the noise generated by the inaccuracy of the small increments of c_i and c_o at very early times (17). For all such times the minimum of Q should remain at the same values of PS/AL and of $\dot{T}(0)$ for any one capillary, since there is nothing in Eq. 80 to distinguish one choice of t^* from another. If this requirement of self-consistency of the theory

TABLE 1

Single Capillary Uptake from Unsteady Flow

$\dot{T}(0)$	$Q_{min}(t_p)$	$(PS/AL)_{t_p}$	$\overline{PS/AL}$	$Var(PS/AL)x10^2$
0.00	6.19	1.84	2.00	2.694
0.05	4.41	1.54	1.65	1.539
0.10	2.19	1.30	1.37	0.641
0.15	0.56	1.10	1.14	0.133
0.175	0.25	1.04	1.04	0.019
0.20	0.33	0.96	0.95	0.015
0.25	2.00	0.84	0.79	0.292
0.30	5.75	0.76	0.65	0.880

Note. Flow unsteadiness $\dot{T}(0)$; goodness of fit $Q_{min}(t_p)$ and normalized permeability $(PS/AL)_{t_p}$ at the time of concentration peak; the mean $\overline{PS/AL}$ and variance var(PS/AL) of PS/AL between 0.3 sec and 1 sec. Underlined numbers show how the best plateaux of PS/AL in time are associated with the best fits. Data from (17).

in the course of time was not satisfied, the distinctive minimum found at the single time $t^*=t_p$ would be of little avail. We emphasize that this additional test of the theory is obligatory only when data from single capillaries are available; in analogous studies on whole organs (capillary beds) extraction fractions from consecutive elements of the bolus may vary as a result of the heterogeneity of properties of the many capillaries acting in parallel (Section 6).

Fig.6 shows the values of PS/AL which minimize Q, plotted as a function of t^* at various fixed values of $\dot{T}(0)$. For example, at $t^*=t_p$ the ordinate of the highest curve in Fig.6 ($\dot{T}(0)=0$) is the abscissa of the minimum of the curve on the extreme right of Fig.5; since the curve in Fig.6 is falling monotonically, the minimum in Fig.5 would be further to the right at $t^*<t_p$ and further to the left at $t^*>t_p$. It is seen in all the curves in Fig.6 that the early noise subsides at about 0.3 sec, and that back-diffusion sets in at about 1 sec. In what follows we shall therefore consider t^* in the interval between 0.3 and 1.0 sec.

Now, consistency in the course of time requires that the curve in Fig.6 associated with the lowest Q's should also have the best plateau in the time-interval considered. We quantify the plateau by the variance of PS/AL in the interval between $t_1^*=$ 0.3 sec and $t_2^*=1$ sec:

$$\mathrm{var}(PS/AL) = \int_{t_1^*}^{t_2^*} (PS/AL - \overline{PS/AL})^2 dt/(t_2^*-t_1^*) \qquad (82)$$

which we tabulate in the last column of Table 1, next to the mean $\overline{PS/AL}$ taken over the same time-interval. Table 1 shows that as

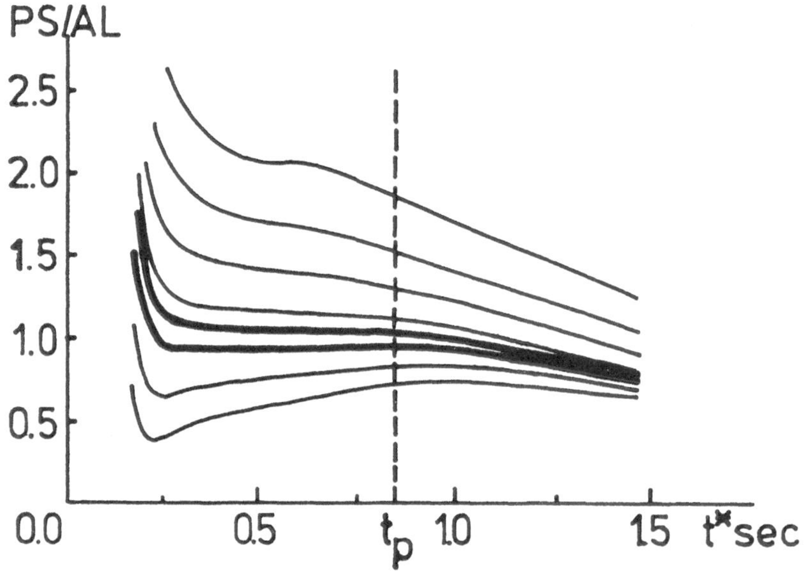

FIG.6

Best-fit values of the normalized permeability PS/AL, plotted as a function of the time t* up to which the fit is made, for different choices of the measure $\dot{T}(0)$ of flow unsteadiness. From the highest to the lowest curve: $\dot{T}(0)=0$ (steady flow), $\dot{T}(0)=0.05$, 0.10, 0.15, 0.175, 0.20, 0.25, 0.30. t_p is the value of t* to which Figs.4 and 5 refer. The best fits of the theory to the data (17) at each time between 0.3 sec and 1 sec generate the two curves with best plateaux (thick curves: $\dot{T}(0)=0.175$, 0.20).

$\dot{T}(0)$ is varied, var (PS/AL) goes through a sharp minimum at $\dot{T}(0)=0.20$, giving $\overline{PS/AL}=0.95$. On the other hand, $Q_{min}(t_p)$ was seen to have a sharp minimum at $\dot{T}(0)=0.175$, giving $(PS/AL)_{t_p}=1.04$; and we find by further calculation that Q_{min} as a function of $\dot{T}(0)$ remains minimal at $\dot{T}(0)=0.175$ or 0.20 also for t*=0.35, 0.40, 0.55, 0.70, 0.85 (=t_p) and 1.00 sec, the minimum becoming shallower towards earlier times. Thus the two independent minimization criteria give closely agreeing results; the relative differences in PS/AL and in $\dot{T}(0)$ so obtained are both about 10%, which could be regarded as an estimate of the accuracy of the determinations. By contrast, the hypothesis $\dot{T}(0)=0$ not only belongs to high values of Q, but also generates no plateau: its var(PS/AL) is rather more than 100 times larger than at $\dot{T}(0)=1.75$ and 0.20, confirming the visual impression gained from Fig.6. Therein lies the difficulty of the "matching of extraction and flow" (17), and its attainment at $\dot{T}(0)=0.175$ or 0.20. The halving of the estimated permeability of the capillary (cf. Table 1) demonstrates the practical importance of the matching. Moreover, this detailed application of the extended uptake theory to data which are free from the complicating effects of capillary heterogeneity occurring in whole organ studies (cf. Introduction, and Section 6), subjects this kind of "upslope" (13,20) method of determination of capillary permeability to quite severe testing. The validity of that determination is fully borne out by the analysis.

4. TRANSVERSE HETEROGENEITY OF ORGANS: STEADY-STATE ANALYSIS

Our next step towards physiological realism is to drop the assumption, characterizing the undistributed model of uptake (1), that all capillaries of an organ contribute equally to the extraction of a substrate or indicator infused through the inlet. We develop the resulting distributed model of organ uptake (6-8, 18) first for the case of irreversible metabolic uptake by the liver. From the undistributed model we retain the modeling of uptake by a single sinusoid, and the assumption that the Michaelis constant K_m is uniform throughout the organ for any particular enzyme-substrate interaction because it characterizes events at the molecular level. For Michaelis-Menten uptake, Eqs. 1-8 remain valid for each sinusoid, with sinusoidal v_{max} and f replacing their organ counterparts. The organ is now modeled as an ensemble of many sinusoids acting in parallel and having the common inlet concentration c_i of substrate. The values of c_o for individual sinusoids will no longer be the same when the values of v_{max}/f are not the same, as is apparent from Eq. 5.

The method of averaging over the ensemble is determined by the circumstance that venous samples are taken after the mixing of outflows from individual capillaries: the quantities which are additive in determining the venous concentration of the substrate are not the output concentrations c_o, but the outfluxes fc_o. The observed venous concentration is therefore the flow-weighted mean of the sinusoidal c_o's,

$$\bar{c}_o = \sum fc_o / \sum f , \tag{83}$$

where the summation is extended over the ensemble (organ). Thus

$$\sum f = F \tag{84}$$

is the organ rate of blood flow. Taking the flow-weighted mean on both sides of Eq. 1 written for one sinusoid, we obtain from Eqs. 83 and 84 the organ uptake rate V in the distributed model:

$$V = F(c_i - \bar{c}_o) . \tag{85}$$

What are now the predicted relations between the quantities c_i, $\bar{c}_o$, V and F observed on the ensemble (i.e., on the intact organ)? This question evidently cannot be answered without some knowledge of (or assumptions about) the distributions of v_{max} and f over the ensemble. Conversely, if we construct the relations theoretically, we can infer something about these distributions from the data.

In this we are greatly aided by a remarkable feature of all saturation kinetics (such as was exemplified by Eqs. 2 and 9 valid in the test-tube) when placed in the hepatic setting by the foregoing modeling. Consider an ensemble of N sinusoids perfused by blood at the total rate F given by Eq. 84, and having a total maximum (saturated) rate of uptake V_{max} as the high-concentration limit of V given by Eq. 85. We then have the mean values $\bar{f}=F/N$ and $\bar{v}_{max}=V_{max}/N$, about which sinusoidal values of f and v_{max} are distributed (dispersed). The remarkable feature is that <u>any</u> dispersion of f or v_{max} about the ensemble means $\bar{f}$, $\bar{v}_{max}$ must reduce the organ uptake rate V (except in saturation) or, equivalently, must increase the venous outflow concentration $\bar{c}_o$ as compared with an organ in which all sinusoids have the mean values $f=\bar{f}$, $v_{max}=\bar{v}_{max}$:

$$\bar{c}_o(c_i) \geq c_o(\bar{v}_{max},\bar{f}\,;c_i) \tag{86}$$

where c_i in the arguments indicates that the comparison is made at equal inlet concentrations. The equality sign refers to the limit of saturation, in which the architecture of the organ can be expected to have no effect on uptake. Before proving this result in general, we illustrate it by a simple example.

Consider two parallel sinusoids which have the same values of f but different values of v_{max}, namely $\bar{v}_{max}+\delta v_{max}$ and $\bar{v}_{max}-\delta v_{max}$; and let the common c_i be so small ($c_i \ll K_m$) that the limiting Eq. 5b holds for each sinusoid. The mean outflow concentration is then

$$\bar{c}_o = \tfrac{1}{2}c_i\left[\exp\left(-\frac{\bar{v}_{max}+\delta v_{max}}{fK_m}\right)+\exp\left(-\frac{\bar{v}_{max}-\delta v_{max}}{fK_m}\right)\right] \tag{87}$$

$$= c_o(\bar{v}_{max})\cosh(\delta v_{max}/fK_m) \tag{88}$$

using again Eq. 5b. For any $\delta v_{max}\neq 0$, the desired inequality follows. We note that the inequality is brought about by the convexity of the relation between c_o and v_{max}/f, rather than by the special exponential form used in this example.

We now turn to the more general problem arising when both f and v_{max} are distributed about the ensemble means. We generalize Eq. 3 for a single sinusoid by allowing for a wider choice of test-tube kinetics:

$$f\frac{dc}{dx} = -\rho(x)g(c) \tag{89}$$

where g(c) gives the concentration dependence of the uptake rate at each enzyme molecule, and

$$\int_0^L \rho(x)dx = v_{max}\ , \tag{90}$$

corresponding to Eq. 4. To the previously considered kinetics

$$g(c) = \frac{c^n}{c^n+K^n}, \quad n>0 \tag{91}$$

which includes Michaelis-Menten kinetics for n=1, we now add the simplest example of kinetics in which the rate is not a monotonically rising function of concentration:

$$g(c) = \frac{1+2(K_1/K_2)^{\frac{1}{2}}}{1+K_1/c+c/K_2} \tag{92}$$

which occurs in substrate inhibition (5). The maximum rate v_{max} is attained at large c according to Eq. 91, but at $c=(K_1K_2)^{\frac{1}{2}}$ according to Eq. 92. Separating Eq. 89 and integrating from inlet to outlet we obtain

$$\int_{c_i}^{c_o} \frac{dc}{g(c)} = -\frac{v_{max}}{f} \tag{93}$$

which expresses the dependence of c_o on c_i and on v_{max}/f in implicit form. For example, for Michaelis-Menten kinetics Eq. 93 reduces to Eq. 5 with V_{max}/F replaced by v_{max}/f. Note that c in Eq. 93 has become a dummy variable, and its dependence on x is immaterial to the input-output relation. K_1 and K_2 in Eq. 92 will be taken as uniform throughout the organ because, like K_m and K, they characterize events at the molecular level.

Because of the large number N of sinusoids in an intact liver (6), we shall use continuous probability densities for the dispersions of v_{max} and f. Because only the ratio v_{max}/f appears in Eq. 93, we prefer to work with distributions of f and of the ratio

$$w = v_{max}/f \; . \tag{94}$$

Let the probability of values in the intervals w, w+dw, and f, f+df in the ensemble be

$$\nu(w,f)dw\,df \; ,$$

defining the non-negative and normalized density function ν, from which all mean values over the ensemble are calculated. Since concentrations observed in the liver vein are flow-weighted mean values,

$$\bar{c}_o = \frac{1}{\bar{f}} \int_0^\infty \int_0^\infty f c_o \, \nu \, dw\, df \; , \tag{95}$$

where

$$\bar{f} = \int_0^\infty \int_0^\infty f \, \nu \, dw\, df = F/N \; . \tag{96}$$

The ratio v_{max}/f is the maximum arterial-venous concentration difference (cf. Eq. 5a) and accordingly its mean is also to be flow-weighted:

$$\bar{w} = \frac{1}{\bar{f}} \int_0^\infty \int_0^\infty f w \, \nu \, dw \, df = \frac{1}{\bar{f}} \int_0^\infty \int_0^\infty v_{max} \, \nu \, dw \, df = \frac{\bar{v}_{max}}{\bar{f}} . \qquad (97)$$

Hence we have the important result

$$\bar{w} = \overline{(v_{max}/f)} = (N\bar{v}_{max})/(N\bar{f}) = V_{max}/F . \qquad (98)$$

We now observe that because c_o depends on w but not on f according to Eq. 93, Eq. 95 can be simplified by defining (18) the flow-weighted density function:

$$\lambda(w) = \frac{1}{\bar{f}} \int_0^\infty f \, \nu \, (w,f) df . \qquad (99)$$

Since ν is normalized, λ is also normalized according to Eq. 96. The use of λ simplifies Eq. 95 to

$$\bar{c}_o(c_i) = \int_0^\infty c_o(c_i,w)\lambda(w)dw \qquad (100)$$

where $c_o(c_i,w)$ is given by Eq. 93. The function $\bar{c}_o(c_i)$ connects two observables and is available from experiments (3,7). If there is no dispersion about $\bar{w}$, λ is given by the Dirac impulse function $\delta(w-\bar{w})$ and Eq. 100 is reduced to the corresponding relation for the undistributed model: $\bar{c}_o(c_i)=c_o(c_i,\bar{w})$ (cf. Eq. 86).

We note that the function $\lambda(w)$ determines the relations between the observables in the context of uptake; uptake experiments cannot therefore determine the form of the density function $\nu(w,f)$. Indeed, there is an infinity of choices of ν consistent with a complete set of experimental results on uptake. For example, ν may be a product of a function of w and a function of f (each normalized), which describes the class of cases in which w and f are uncorrelated in the ensemble (6). If only v_{max} is dispersed but all f are equal to $\bar{f}$, as in our initial example, then

$$\nu(w,f) = \lambda(w)\delta(f-\bar{f}) . \qquad (101)$$

In the context of uptake, this non-uniqueness of the determination of ν is not a deficiency, since it is λ rather than ν which is the function governing the results of experiments considered hitherto. In forthcoming work we shall be able to throw further light on the structure of ν by bringing altogether new observables into play.

From the mathematical point of view, Eq. 100 is a Fredholm integral equation of the first kind in which the left-hand side is an empirically given function, $\lambda(w)$ is the unknown and

$c_o(c_i,w)$ is the kernel given by Eq. 93 for any choice of test-tube kinetics g(c). The mathematical problem of determining λ is particularly interesting and difficult because of the implicit definition of the kernel, and because the solution must be non-negative and normalized for positive values of its argument w.

For the case of Michaelis-Menten kinetics, Eq. 100 has been solved analytically (18), and numerically in relation to simulated data (34). The analytical solution proceeds through the transformation of Eq. 100 to convolution form, followed by the Fourier transform using certain convergence factors to ensure the existence of the transform, followed by solution in the transform space and by final inversion to $\lambda(w)$, which is expressed as an integral in the complex plane with a Fourier transform of the empirical relation $\bar{c}_o(c_i)$ involved in its integrand. It will come as no surprise to the reader that existing sets of data cannot support such a weight of mathematics (cf. last Section). While the mathematical structure of the problem has been greatly clarified by (18), practical application of the analytical solution must await much more numerous and accurate data, from a single preparation, than are available at present.

A much closer approach to practical applicability has been achieved by direct numerical analysis of Eq. 100 (34), using constrained least-square techniques in conjunction with a quadratic spline approximation to the unknown $\lambda(w)$. The data were produced by simulation in terms of the model, and included simulated random errors of the actual orders of magnitude (3). It was shown that if about 30 data pairs $\bar{c}_o,c_i$ were available from a single preparation and if they were distributed satisfactorily across the concentration range on both sides of K_m, the form of $\lambda(w)$ could be recovered to a good approximation. That is only three or four times more data pairs than have been available from existing experiments (cf. (3), and Fig.2), so that practical use of this method is almost within range of experimental work.

It is,however, a third approach (6,7,18) that has proved to be so fruitful in getting a grip on present-day data, that high levels of statistical significance were attained (7) in testing salient features of the distributed and undistributed uptake models. The exact as well as the approximate results of this approach are obtained from expanding the kernel c_o of Eq. 100 in a series about $\bar{w}$, whereby the integral is expressed in a series of central moments of $\lambda(w)$:

$$c_o(c_i,\bar{w}) = \sum_{n=0}^{\infty} \frac{1}{n!} c_o^{(n)}(c_i,\bar{w})(w-\bar{w})^n \qquad (102)$$

where $c_o^{(n)}$ denotes the n'th derivative of c_o with respect to w, evaluated from Eq. 93 and taken at $w=\bar{w}$. Substituting in Eq. 100 we get

$$\bar{c}_o(c_i) = \sum_{n=0}^{\infty} \frac{1}{n!} c_o^{(n)}(c_i,\bar{w})\mu_n \qquad (103)$$

where the moments of λ are given by

$$\mu_n = \int_0^\infty (w-\bar{w})^n \lambda(w)dw \ , \quad n = 0,1,2,3,\ldots \ . \tag{104}$$

In particular $\mu_0=1$, $\mu_1=0$, and $\mu_2=\sigma^2$ is the variance of $\lambda(w)$. The conditions for the existence of all μ_n, discussed in detail in (18), may be expected to hold in practice. But under what conditions are the expansions in Eqs. 102 and 103 justified? We can answer this question precisely by extending w and c_o into the complex domain and using the inverse function theorem (35). Differentiating $w=v_{max}/f$ with respect to c_o in Eq. 93, we obtain

$$dw/dc_o = -1/g(c_o) \ . \tag{105}$$

For definiteness we confine our attention to the Michaelis-Menten case in the discussion of convergence of the expansion. Then Eq. 93 gives the counterpart of Eq. 5 for the single sinusoid,

$$\frac{w}{K_m} = -\frac{c_o}{K_m} - \ln\frac{c_o}{K_m} + \frac{c_i}{K_m} + \ln\frac{c_i}{K_m} \ , \tag{106}$$

and the special case of Eq. 105:

$$dw/dc_o = -1 - \frac{K_m}{c_o} \ . \tag{107}$$

The derivative of the inverse function, dw/dc_o, vanishes at $c_o/K_m=-1$, where Eq. 106 gives

$$\frac{w}{K_m} = 1 + \frac{c_i}{K_m} + \ln\frac{c_i}{K_m} - \ln(-1) = 1 + \frac{c_i}{K_m} + \ln\frac{c_i}{K_m} - i\pi(1\pm 2m), \ m=0,1,2\ldots \tag{108}$$

and now w is complex, with v_{max}/f playing the role of the real part. This mapping of the complex c_o-plane on to the complex w-plane is discussed thoroughly in (18). Here we note only that the singularities (branch points) nearest to the expansion point $\bar{w}=v_{max}/f$ are those for m=0 and m=-1, as is seen in Fig.7. The radius of convergence R of the expansion, in Eq. 102, about $\bar{w}/K_m$ is therefore

$$R = \left[\left(1 + \frac{c_i}{K_m} + \ln\frac{c_i}{K_m} - \frac{V_{max}}{FK_m}\right)^2 + \pi^2\right]^{\frac{1}{2}} \ , \tag{109}$$

where we have introduced organ parameters by Eq. 98.

We thus see how the radius of convergence responds to changes in the physiological quantities. It has the minimum value π, so that if λ is zero outside the interval $\bar{w}-\pi K_m$, $\bar{w}+\pi K_m$, the series in Eq. 103 converges for all c_i and all F. It is apparent from Eq. 109 that R tends to infinity as c_i/K_m tends to zero or to infinity, so that the convergence in Eq. 103 is

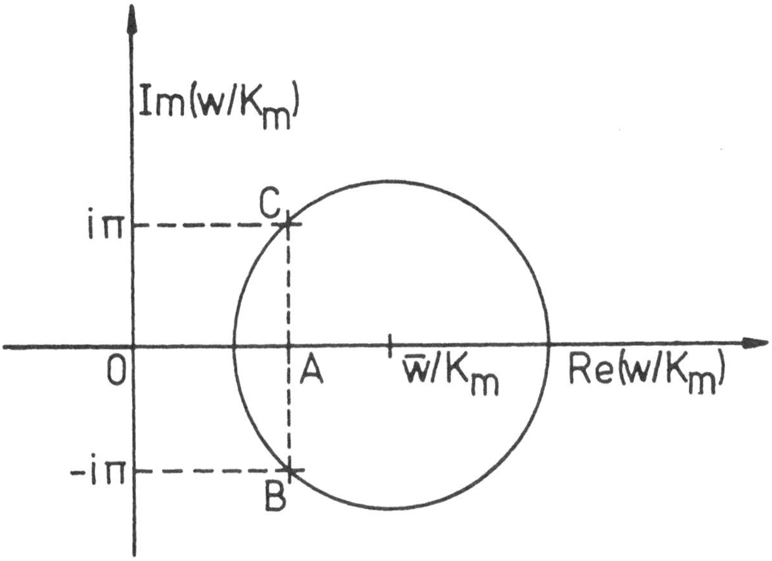

FIG.7

The circle of convergence for the expansion of the sinusoidal outlet concentration c_o in powers of $w-\bar{w} = v_{max}/f - V_{max}/F$. The radius of convergence is determined by the nearest singularities at B and C; A is at $1+c_i/K_m+\ln(c_i/K_m)$.

assured for first-order uptake, and also close to saturation, for all shapes of λ (which go to zero sufficiently rapidly as w tends to infinity: cf. (18)). In general, however, it may happen that the tails of $\lambda(w)$ will protrude out of the interval $\bar{w}-RK_m$, $\bar{w}+RK_m$, in which case the series in Eq. 103 will diverge, but will be asymptotic to $\bar{c}_o(c_i)$ (18,36).

Independently of the problem of convergence, exact results can be obtained by writing the series in finite terms with a remainder (7,18). Because of the importance of these results for data treatment and statistical hypothesis-testing (7) discussed in Section 7, we now return to Eq. 93 with its general kinetics g(c). We use Taylor's theorem with Lagrange's form of the remainder (35) in Eq. 102. Dropping the argument c_i for brevity, we obtain

$$c_o(w) = c_o(\bar{w}) + c_o'(\bar{w})(w-\bar{w}) + \tfrac{1}{2}c_o''(\bar{w}+\theta(w-\bar{w}))(w-\bar{w})^2, \quad 0 \leq \theta \leq 1 \qquad (110)$$

where θ may depend on w and $\bar{w}$. Substituting this in Eq. 100 and remembering that $\mu_0=1$ and $\mu_1=0$, we get the exact result

$$\bar{c}_o = c_o(\bar{w}) + \tfrac{1}{2}\int_0^\infty (w-\bar{w})^2 c_o''(\bar{w}+\theta(w-\bar{w}))\lambda(w)dw \ . \qquad (111)$$

To evaluate c_o'' from Eq. 93, we use Eq. 105 repeatedly:

$$\frac{d^2c_o}{dw^2} = -\frac{d}{dw}g(c_o) = -\frac{dg(c_o)}{dc_o}\frac{dc_o}{dw} = g(c_o)\frac{dg(c_o)}{dc_o}, \qquad (112)$$

so that c_o'' is expressed as a function of c_o rather than of $\bar{w}+\theta(w-\bar{w})$. However, since uptake must reduce c_i, all possible values of the argument of $g(c_o)$ are contained in the range

$$0 < c_o < c_i \ . \qquad (113)$$

If therefore dg/dc is positive throughout this interval, Eq. 112 implies that c_o'' is positive for all w when $g(c_o)$ is non-zero, and the last term in Eq. 111 is positive for <u>any</u> shape of $\lambda(w)$. Then Eq. 111 implies that $\bar{c}_o > c_o(\bar{w})$, as in relation 86, which we can now prove for the kinetics given by Eq. 91: the inequality holds for all finite c_o because g(c) rises monotonically with c, and the equality is attained asymptotically at high c_o (saturation) because g(c) tends to unity and so dg/dc_o tends to zero. Indeed it is now apparent that the important relation 86 holds for any saturation kinetics, if that class of kinetics is defined by a positive dg/dc which tends to zero as c tends to infinity. [By contrast, substrate inhibition kinetics defined by Eq. 92 must satisfy relation 86 only so long as $c_i<(K_1K_2)^{\frac{1}{2}}$; at higher c_i uptake may be reduced or increased by heterogeneity, depending on the detailed form of $\lambda(w)$.]

Thus $c_o(\bar{w})$ is a <u>lower bound</u> on $\bar{c}_o$; it is readily calculated from the undistributed model, or by considering that since Eq.106 holds for each sinusoidal w, it holds also for $\bar{w}$, which is equal to V_{max}/F according to Eq. 98. An <u>upper bound</u> on $\bar{c}_o$ is also available from Eq. 111 under the same conditions which make $c_o(\bar{w})$ a lower bound. If we replace c_o'' by its largest value in the interval 113, that is by the largest value of $g(dg/dc_o)$ according to Eq. 112, then the integral in Eq. 111 is increased to

$$\tfrac{1}{2}\sigma^2(g\ dg/dc_o)_{max} \geq \tfrac{1}{2}\int_0^\infty (w-\bar{w})^2 c_o''(\bar{w}+\theta(w-\bar{w}))\lambda(w)dw \qquad (114)$$

where $\sigma^2=\mu_2$ is the variance of $\lambda(w)$. Combining the upper and lower bounds we obtain

$$c_o(\bar{w}) < \bar{c}_o \leq c_o(\bar{w}) + \tfrac{1}{2}\sigma^2(g\ dg/dc_o)_{max} \qquad (115)$$

which holds for all c_o up to c_i when $dg/dc_o>0$. For example, for Michaelis-Menten kinetics it is easily shown by differentiation that

$$(g\ dg/dc_o)_{max} = 4/(27K_m) \qquad (116)$$

occurs at $c_o=K_m/2$. Defining the coefficient of variation of the distribution

$$\varepsilon = \sigma/\bar{w} = \sqrt{\mu_2}/\bar{w} \ , \tag{117}$$

and using Eq. 98, relations 115 become

$$c_o(V_{max}/F) < \bar{c}_o \leq c_o(V_{max}/F) + 2K_m\varepsilon^2(V_{max}/FK_m)^2/27 \ , \tag{118}$$

where $c_o(V_{max}/F)$ satisfies Eq. 5.

In experiments with c_i and $\bar{c}_o$ varied over a wide range (3), detection of transverse heterogeneity is greatly facilitated when its effects are known in advance to be insignificant in one limiting region of the concentration range: for then V_{max} and the chemical constants implicit in g(c) can be calibrated in that region for subsequent use at all concentrations. This is another example of a strategic range of concentration (cf. Section 2). A sufficient condition for finding such a calibrating concentration region is readily obtained from relations 115 by writing

$$\frac{\bar{c}_o - c_o(\bar{w})}{\bar{c}_o} \leq \tfrac{1}{2}\sigma^2(g\ dg/dc_o)_{max}/\bar{c}_o \ . \tag{119}$$

If the numerator on the right-hand side is independent of concentration (or, more generally, if it does not increase with concentration as fast as $\bar{c}_o$), then the difference between $\bar{c}_o$ and $c(\bar{w})$ can be made relatively insignificant by working at sufficiently high $\bar{c}_o$, and effects of heterogeneity on uptake disappear. For example, Michaelis-Menten kinetics gives a maximal difference $\bar{c}_o - c(\bar{w})$ which is independent of concentration according to relations 118, so that at sufficiently high $\bar{c}_o$ it becomes immaterial whether $\bar{c}_o$ or $c_o(\bar{w})$ is used in place of c_o of the undistributed model. This limiting situation has been called the homogeneous regime of uptake (6). Just how high a $\bar{c}_o$ is needed to attain this regime with some required accuracy depends also on ε, V_{max}/F and K_m according to relations 118. In practice this is considered in terms of the high-concentration segment of a suitable data plot, as we shall see below.

It is now easy to show that any saturation kinetics has the advantage of a homogeneous regime of uptake at high substrate concentrations. We have a positive dg/dc which tends to zero at large c, while g tends to a finite constant. Since evidently $g(0)=0$ and $g \geq 0$ for any kinetics, the product g dg/dc must have a maximum value at some finite concentration, determined by the chemical interaction constants implicit in g(c) (such as the value $4/(27K_m)$ in Michaelis-Menten kinetics). Then the numerator of the right-hand side in relation 119 is independent of concentration, and the conclusion follows as before.

An important example of g(c) for which no homogeneous regime exists is first-order kinetics, $g(c)=c$. Then $g(c_o)dg(c_o)/dc_o=c_o$, and this attains its greatest value in the interval 113 at $c_o=c_i$, so that $(g\ dg/dc_o)_{max}=c_i$. Then the upper bound on the relative difference in outflow concentrations, given by relation 119, is proportional to $c_i/\bar{c}_o$ which cannot be reduced at will by increasing concentration. Furthermore, first-order kinetics has the general property that nothing can be deduced about transverse heterogeneity of organs from steady-state experiments in which concentration is varied at constant organ flow. This is because $g(c)=c$ gives $c_0(c_i,w)=c_i\exp(-w)$ from Eqs. 93,94, so that the ratio $\bar{c}_0/c_i$ is independent of concentration according to Eq. 100. Experiments which do reveal heterogeneity under first-order kinetics involve changes in the organ flow rate, as we shall see in Sections 5 and 7.

We next wish to form an at least approximate picture of what happens between the precise bounds given by relations 115,118. The undistributed model gives a fair approximation to experimental data from at least some types of preparation (3,37). We therefore adopt the undistributed model as a lowest approximation, and perturb away from it in powers of a dimensionless parameter characterizing transverse heterogeneity. Relations 118 contain only one such parameter, namely the coefficient of variation ε of $\lambda(w)$ defined by Eq. 117; when $\varepsilon=0$, one recovers the undistributed model. The perturbation theory will therefore be developed by carrying the expansion in Eq. 103 to at least the μ_2-term on the assumption that w is distributed narrowly about $\bar{w}$, so that to successive moments of $\lambda(w)$ there correspond successively smaller contributions to the values of observable quantities. If for example $\lambda(w)$ is approximated by a narrow Gaussian distribution centred on $\bar{w}$ and having the variance $\sigma^2=\mu_2$, then $\mu_3=0$ by symmetry and the next non-vanishing term in Eq. 103 is proportional to ε^4. By using upper and lower bounds on the appropriate Taylor remainder (such as the remainder in Eq. 111, but taken after more terms), the sense in which the distribution of w should be narrow can be made precise (18,32). We shall now develop the perturbation theory to order ε^2 for Michaelis-Menten kinetics (6,18), aiming particularly at formulations that will make corrections to the undistributed model easily observable.

Calculating $c_0''(\bar{w})$ from Eq. 112 for $g=c/(c+K_m)$ and using the definition of ε in Eq. 117, we retain from the expansion in Eq. 103:

$$\bar{c}_0 = c_0(\bar{w})\left[1+\tfrac{1}{2}\varepsilon^2(V_{max}/FK_m)^2(1+c_0(\bar{w})/K_m)^{-3}\right] . \qquad (120)$$

We recall that $c_0(\bar{w})$ satisfies Eq. 106 for $w=\bar{w}$, so that we now have two equations from which we can eliminate $c_0(\bar{w})$ in favour of the observed venous concentration $\bar{c}_0$. Expanding the requisite terms in powers of ε^2 and working consistently to order ε^2, we thus find the correction to Eq. 5:

$$c_i-\bar{c}_0+K_m\ln(c_i/\bar{c}_0) = (V_{max}/F)\left[1-\tfrac{1}{2}\varepsilon^2(V_{max}/FK_m)\frac{K_m^2}{(\bar{c}_0+K_m)^2}\right] \qquad (121)$$

At high $\bar{c}_0$ we recover Eq. 5 as expected (homogeneous regime), but at low $\bar{c}_0$ we find something new: when $\bar{c}_0/K_m$ can be neglected against unity, Eq. 121 attains the same form as Eq. 5, but the constant on the right-hand side is reduced as if V_{max} was replaced with the smaller $\tilde{V}_{max}$ (say):

$$\tilde{V}_{max} = V_{max}\left[1 - \tfrac{1}{2}\varepsilon^2(V_{max}/FK_m)\right] < V_{max} . \qquad (122)$$

We can therefore expect that ε^2 will be revealed by first using high-concentration data to calibrate V_{max} and K_m, and then confronting these values with the prediction of the undistributed model that Eq. 5b should hold at very low concentrations. Alternatively, after the calibration of V_{max} and K_m at high concentrations, we can calculate $c_0(\bar{w})$ according to the undistributed model and then show that it is exceeded by $\bar{c}_0$-data according to Eq. 120 (7); see Section 7.

A particularly illuminating approach is to show how the perturbation by heterogeneity modifies Eqs. 6 and 7 which are valid for the undistributed model. The plot of Eq. 6 in inverse variables $1/V$, $1/\hat{c}_1$, known as the Lineweaver-Burk plot (5), is the straight line

$$1/V = 1/V_{max} + (K_m/V_{max})(1/\hat{c}_1) \qquad (123)$$

with the slope K_m/V_{max} and intercepts $1/V_{max}$, $-1/K_m$; these features of the undistributed model have been used (3) to estimate V_{max} and K_m of individual preparations from series of observed triplets (c_i, c_0, V), each of which gave the coordinates $(\hat{c}_1, V)$ of a point according to Eq. 7.

In the distributed model, the quantity c_0 in Eq. 7 has no unique meaning. It is natural to replace it by the observed venous concentration $\bar{c}_0$, so that now

$$\hat{c}_1 = \frac{c_i - \bar{c}_0}{\ln(c_i/\bar{c}_0)} \qquad (124)$$

in place of Eq. 7. Then Eq. 6 no longer holds, except at very high concentrations where heterogeneity has no effect (i.e., in the homogeneous regime of uptake). Since $\hat{c}_1$ is a mean of c_i and $\bar{c}_0$, high $\bar{c}_0$ implies high $\hat{c}_1$ and hence low $1/\hat{c}_1$: Eq. 123 continues to hold in the distributed model as the initial tangent to the modified Lineweaver-Burk plot (Fig.8). At the other extreme of very low concentrations, we have seen above that the distributed model (carried to order ε^2) is governed by equations of the same form as the undistributed model, provided that V_{max} is replaced by the smaller $\tilde{V}_{max}$ according to Eq. 122. Hence at very high $1/\hat{c}_1$ (low c_i implying low $\hat{c}_1$), Eq. 123 again holds in the distributed model, but with the larger slope $K_m/\tilde{V}_{max}$: it is the asymptote of the curved Lineweaver-Burk plot in Fig.8. The total change ΔS of the slope S of the curve, from the initial tangent to the asymptote, is readily calculated to order ε^2 using Eq.122:

$$\Delta S = \varepsilon^2/2F . \qquad (125)$$

Since the value of F is measured for each preparation, Eq. 125

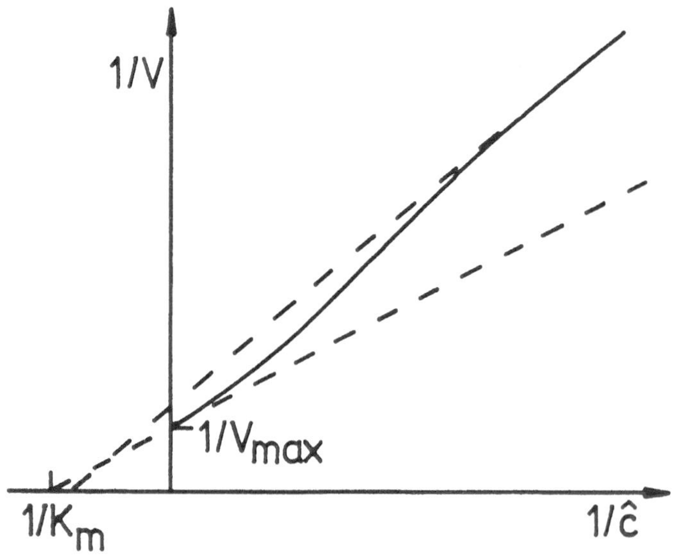

FIG.8

Inverse organ uptake rate plotted against the inverse logarithmic mean of the inlet and outlet concentrations of substrate. The solid curve is predicted by the distributed model, its initial tangent is the linear law predicted by the undistributed model for the same organ.

brings out the effect of ε^2 particularly clearly in a form well-suited for statistically significant analyses of data (7), discussed in Section 7.

For that purpose it is helpful to have a complete analysis of all possible relations between $1/V$ and $1/\hat{c}_1$ to order ε^2 (6,32). One can proceed as follows. The left-hand side of Eq. 121 can be written as $(V/F)(1+K_m/\hat{c}_1)$ using Eqs. 124 and 85. Next we express the $\bar{c}_0$ remaining in Eq. 121 in terms of V. Since that $\bar{c}_0$ occurs only in the coefficient of ε^2, we may estimate it from the undistributed model without introducing an error of order ε^2 in Eq. 121. Eliminating c_i from Eqs. 12 and 85 we get

$$\bar{c}_0 = (V/F)/(e^{(V_{max}-V)/FK_m}-1) + O(\varepsilon^2)\,, \qquad (126)$$

and use this to eliminate $\bar{c}_0$ from the right-hand side of Eq. 121. That equation is now written entirely in terms of V and $\hat{c}_1$ or, equivalently, in terms of their inverses. Its analysis classifies the curved Lineweaver-Burk plots into three types found in three ranges of the quantity V_{max}/FK_m. The intersection of the initial tangent and of the asymptote is particularly useful in data analysis (7); it occurs at

$$K_m/\hat{c}_1 = 2(V_{max}/FK_m)/(e^{V_{max}/FK_m}-1) - 1 , \qquad (127)$$

$$V_{max}/V = 2(V_{max}/FK_m)/(e^{V_{max}/FK_m}-1) , \qquad (128)$$

independently of ε^2.

In several of the following Sections we shall make practical use of the results of the perturbation theory to order ε^2. We note that some results of higher-order perturbations are available (32). These results require assumptions about more detailed features of $\lambda(w)$, and such assumptions are reflected in additional adjustable parameters in fitting data. As in the case of outright analytical and numerical solutions of the integral equation 100, convincing practical use of the higher-order results must await improvements in the number and accuracy of data available from single preparations.

5. WHEN IS THERE KINETIC EVIDENCE FOR RECRUITMENT OF CAPILLARIES?

In the foregoing Sections we have dealt with results of varying input concentrations c_i of substrates or indicators, at fixed rates F of blood flow through the extracting organ. Under such circumstances the number N of perfused capillaries in the ensemble comprising the organ can be expected to remain constant. However, when F is increased, hitherto unperfused capillaries may become perfused and contribute to organ extraction. Such an increase in N with increasing F is often seen in real capillary organs, and it is called recruitment of capillaries. Such recruitment is normally reversible (2), and the reduction in N with falling F can be regarded as negative recruitment. We shall see, however, that N may be constant over an appreciable range of values of F, in some organs at least.

The statistical mechanics of an organ in which N varies with F shall be developed in a forthcoming paper; the purpose of the present Section is more limited. The undistributed model for first-order uptake has been known for a long time, and it has been used for analyses of data from experiments in the steady (15) and unsteady (13) states. Analysis of such kinetic data in terms of the undistributed model (15) can point apparently unambiguously to recruitment of capillaries. We now show that when some of the same data are analysed in terms of the distributed model, they are consistent with effects of transverse heterogeneity of a fixed number N of capillaries. We shall apply these considerations to data (15) for which this alternative holds in just the range of flow rates in which the interpretation by recruitment is made doubtful by other experimental evidence (8,38).

At tracer concentrations of a substrate ($c_i \ll K_m$), the undistributed model predicts the steady-state input-output relation given by Eq. 5b. As shown in Section 3, we may re-interpret that relation for early uptake of diffusible indicators by replacing V_{max}/K_m with the permeability-surface area product PS (Eq. 76); but in view of the experiments to be discussed, we retain here the interpretation in terms of irreversible uptake of a substrate. We have shown in the preceding Section that when Eq. 5b is valid for the undistributed model, it can be adapted to hold for the narrowly distributed model by replacing c_o with $\bar{c}_o$, and V_{max} with $\tilde{V}_{max}$ given by Eq. 122. Taking logarithms on both sides of Eq. 5b so adapted, and changing sign, we obtain

$$\ln(c_i/\bar{c}_o) = V_{max}/FK_m - \tfrac{1}{2}\varepsilon^2(V_{max}/FK_m)^2 + R \ , \qquad (129)$$

where we have introduced, in addition, the remainder term R resulting from a more careful evaluation (8) of the perturbation of the undistributed model in powers of ε^2. R can be written in the form

$$R = e^{-p^2/2}/(2\pi)^{\frac{1}{2}}p \ , \quad p = 1/\varepsilon - \varepsilon V_{max}/FK_m \ . \qquad (130)$$

It is apparent that R goes to zero with ε much faster than ε^2. The perturbation theory to order ε^2 may be used so long as R is small as compared to the preceding term in Eq. 129.

Putting $\varepsilon^2=0$ in Eq. 129, we see that the undistributed model of first-order uptake predicts that $F\ln(c_i/\bar{c}_o)$ should be equal to V_{max}/K_m on any one preparation, and in the absence of recruitment this quantity should be independent of the choice of steady flow rate F. It has been noticed, for various perfused organs and various substrates (cf. references in (8)), that this prediction fails: at low flows, $F\ln(c_i/\bar{c}_o)$ in general increases with F, and it is natural to interpret this as an increase in organ V_{max} due to previously unused parts of the capillary bed coming into play. We shall concentrate our discussion on the results of the classic study (15) of uptake by the isolated perfused rat liver preparation.

Fig.9 summarizes the results of the measurements (15) of the steady uptake of labeled colloidal $CrPO_4$ by the Kupffer cells of isolated perfused rat livers, made at a series of different rates of flow F of full blood (solid curve). The first term on the right-hand side of Eq. 129 describes the initial straight line (extrapolated by the broken line), since $\ln(c_i/\bar{c}_o)$ is plotted against 1/F. Taking into consideration that uptake of the colloid is from plasma only, one finds the value V_{max}/K_m=1.03 ml/min.g liver (15,8) at these high values of F. As F is reduced from about 1/0.6=1.67 ml/min.g liver (i.e., as 1/F is increased), $\ln(c_i/\bar{c}_o)$ falls short increasingly of this straight line predicted by the undistributed model (ε^2=0). If this phenomenon is attributed to negative recruitment (V_{max} falling as F is reduced), one infers from Fig.9 that when F is reduced to 0.9 ml/min.g liver, V_{max} has been reduced by more than 25% from its value at high flow rates: Kupffer cells lining sinusoids which are no longer perfused, can no longer contribute to the extraction of the colloid.

Fourteen years later (38) the isolated perfused rat liver

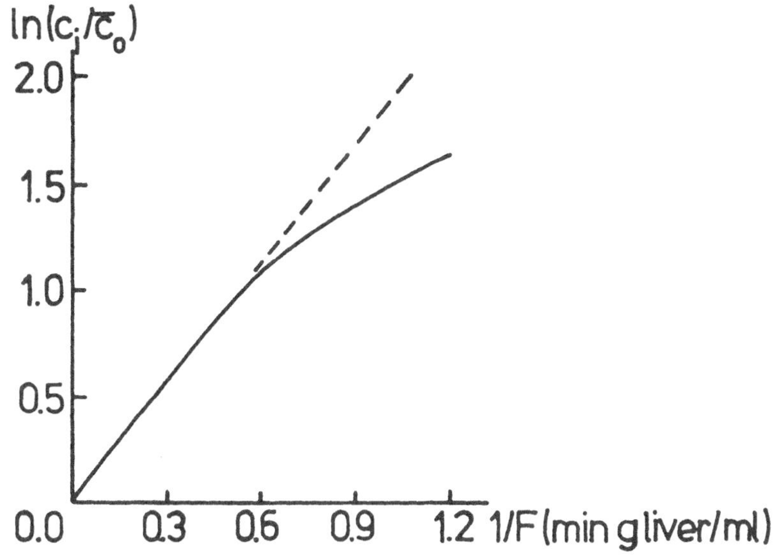

FIG.9

Effect of the rate F of perfusate flow on the steady extraction of labeled colloidal $CrPO_4$ by isolated perfused rat livers. Arterial radioactivity is c_i, venous radioactivity is $\bar{c}_o$. Schematically from data in (15).

preparation was used, in a different context, to examine the constancy of V_{max} for uptake of galactose (and the constancy of other physiological control variables) under variations of the flow rate F. Using the homogeneous regime of galactose uptake ($c \gg K_m$), that V_{max} was found to be independent of the value of F across the whole range of flow rates included in Fig.9, beginning to decline only when F was reduced below about 0.8 ml/min.g liver. It would seem likely that the liver should lose the services of hepatocytes (in which galactose is taken up), as well as of Kupffer cells in the unperfused parts of the capillary bed; but that argument is not conclusive in this simple form because galactose, in contrast to the $CrPO_4$ colloid, is not confined to blood. We shall therefore not assert here that the galactose V_{max} data refute the recruitment interpretation in the range of flow rates under consideration, but merely that the following alternative interpretation reconciles the two sets of data in an attractively simple way.

Returning to Eq. 129 in which V_{max}/K_m pertains to uptake of colloidal $CrPO_4$, we note that the second term on the right-hand side is negative, and is explicitly proportional to $(1/F)^2$. If ε^2 varies slowly with 1/F in comparison, that term can account for the concave deviation of the solid line in Fig.9 from the initial straight line. This is because the flow-dependence of

$\tilde{V}_{max}$, which replaces V_{max} in the presence of heterogeneity according to Eq. 122, simulates an effect of recruitment in the undistributed model. In more quantitative terms, the effect of an experimental change in F by some factor q can be modeled by supposing that all sinusoidal flow rates f in the ensemble will be changed by the same factor q, so long as q does not deviate too far from unity. Since the sinusoidal values of v_{max} will remain unchanged, all sinusoidal values of $w=v_{max}/f$ will change by the same factor 1/q, which will therefore cancel out when we form the coefficient of variation ε of the distribution of w over the ensemble. On this hypothesis, the data represented in Fig.9 were fitted (8) satisfactorily by the value $\varepsilon^2=0.137$. Using this value, and the value of V_{max}/K_m obtained above from high flow rates (initial straight line in Fig.9), the remainder term R in Eq. 129 turned out to be ten times smaller than the preceding term, as required.

Although the resulting estimate of ε^2 is consistent with estimates obtained by different methods from results of experiments of different design (cf. (7),(39), and below), all that we claim here for the foregoing application of Eq. 129 is that it creates a plausible alternative to the interpretation in terms of recruitment of capillaries. In particular, the foregoing argument for flow-independence of ε should be regarded as merely a provisional one. Since we know that at still lower flow rates (higher values of 1/F) some capillaries are in fact no longer perfused, our approach in forthcoming work will be to include both heterogeneity and recruitment of capillaries in modeling uptake at all flow rates for which data are available.

If ε^2 was independent of F, or if its dependence on F was known, we could use it to predict the transformation of the plot in Fig.8, on changing from one steady value of F to another. Since the initial tangent of the plot is independent of F, it would certainly stay in place, while the asymptote would move to give the new value of the total change of slope given by Eq. 125: it would swing around its intersection with the initial tangent (given by Eqs. 127,128) which is independent of ε. It is clear however, that in the present state of knowledge about the dependence of ε on F, estimates of ε^2 from variations of c_i at constant F ((7), and below) should be considered more reliable than estimates from effects of varying F.

6. TRANSVERSE HETEROGENEITY OF ORGANS: TRANSIENT ANALYSIS

Studies of the transient effects of injecting a concentrated pulse (bolus) of a substrate or indicator upstream of the organ of interest, are potentially more informative and certainly more convenient clinically than studies of steady states of uptake. The arterially injected bolus is fractionated by the vascular bed of the organ into elements which pass through the extracting capillaries and reunite in the vein, where the output concentration is seen with a time-dependence known as the dilution curve (20).

The instruments (sampling catheters), placed in blood vessels upstream and downstream of the organ of interest, are inevitably separated well from the extracting capillaries. The time T' (say) spent by an element of the bolus in travelling between the instruments is therefore longer than the time T during which extraction from the element occurs:

$$T' > T > 0 . \tag{131}$$

In fact, the major part of T' may be spent in traversing non-extracting arterioles and venules of the organ (40). This circumstance had only a trivial effect on time-dependent uptake by a single capillary in Section 3 (cf. Eqs. 54); but it has a major effect on the venous outflow $\bar{c}_0(t)$ from an organ because of the dispersion of the times T'. Consider two elements of the bolus taking different parallel paths between the instruments. Each will be subjected to extraction, but their effect on the form of $\bar{c}_0(t)$ will clearly depend also on whether they arrive at the mixing site in the vein at the same time (i.e. whether they have the same values of T'), or not. Thus the concentration $\bar{c}_0$ in any one venous sample is determined by two influences: the sample contains elements of the bolus that have been delivered after due extraction by capillaries, and it is diluted by blood from capillaries which have delivered their bolus fractions to earlier samples, or shall deliver them to later ones. In order to analyze the dilution curve $\bar{c}_0(t)$ from an organ, one needs therefore to know the distribution of the times T' which has no intrinsic connection with uptake, except for the constraint on the times T exerted by relation 131. By contrast, the times T spent under extraction do have an intimate connection with extraction, and their distribution can be modeled plausibly. Thus fT is the volume of distribution in one capillary (Section 3) in steady flow; if v_{max} was proportional to that volume with the same proportionality constant for each capillary of the organ, then the distribution of T over the ensemble would be the same (after normalization) as the distribution of v_{max}/f used in Section 4 because, on that hypothesis, $v_{max}/f=(v_{max}/fT)T=\text{const.}T$. Unfortunately the distribution of T is not observed, and further hypotheses are needed to connect it with the observed distribution of T' (14,41,42). These hypotheses are the Achilles' heel of the transient analysis of uptake. By contrast, the times T'-T spent in non-extracting regions have no observable effects in steady state analysis (cf. Section 4).

It is apparent that if one extended the work of Sections 3 and 4 to include effects of the dispersion of T', the resulting mathematical structure would surely lose its grip on data obtained from the extraction of a single substrate or indicator. Clearly a new experimental idea is needed at this stage: that is the idea of using <u>multiple indicators</u> (13,20). In developing this theme in the present Section, we shall keep to steady flow rates F=const., and we shall work in terms of the interpretation of capillary permeability to indicators (cf. Sections 1 and 3) taken up by first-order kinetics ($c \ll K_m$). In that limit we shall therefore replace v_{max}/K_m by the permeability - surface area product $\bar{p}s$ for each capillary, and V_{max}/K_m by the corresponding product

PS for the organ (see below). We recall that in this interpretation, our previous results hold strictly only until the onset of back-diffusion of the indicator from extravascular spaces; but we shall show how they can be used thereafter for the construction of certain bounds.

The indicator considered hitherto, which can leave the blood through pores or sites in the capillary wall, shall now be called diffusible indicator in order to contrast it with the newly introduced intravascular reference indicator confined to the blood, but chosen so as to match the diffusible indicator as closely as possible in all other relevant properties (20). The resulting method is often called the indicator diffusion (single injection) method (13). The main object is to deduce the organ value of PS for the diffusible indicator by comparing its venous outflow with that of the intravascular reference injected in the same bolus. A notable application of the method was to the quantitative demonstration and investigation of facilitated transfer of glucose across the blood-brain barrier (26). Instead of thus studying normal PS-values for various physiologically interesting diffusible indicators, one can use a suitable diffusible indicator(and reference) clinically to diagnose a pathological loss of active surface area of an organ (43).

If an element of the bolus enters a capillary with the concentration c_i, it leaves with the concentration

$$c_o = c_i e^{-\bar{p}s/f} \tag{132}$$

where $\bar{p}$ is the mean of the permeability p (weighted by wall surface area s) evaluated over the whole surface of the capillary:

$$\bar{p} = \frac{1}{s}\int pds \ .$$

This follows from the same reasoning as has led to Eq. 76 (with T/AL=1/F according to Eq. 45), but it is applied here to a single capillary from the point of view of an observer moving with the bolus fraction. Only the mean $\bar{p}$, not the longitudinal distribution of p along the capillary, matters in Eq. 132: this follows from the same reasoning as has shown the insensitivity of the input-output relations in steady flow to the longitudinal distribution of enzyme in Section 3 (Eqs. 42 and 38).

If the wall uptake of the diffusible indicator is by facilitated saturable transport (as for glucose entering the brain), the linearization of the uptake problem in Eq. 37 is applicable: $\bar{p}$ is replaced with $K\bar{p}_{max}/(K+c_M)$, where c_M is the local concentration of the mother substance of the labeled indicator, and K is the constant controlling the degree of saturation by c_M. The effect of the choice of c_M on organ uptake then permits an estimate of K and of the organ counterpart of $\bar{p}_{max}s$ (26).

Suppose now that an (infinitesimal) venous sample contains diffusible indicator contributed by only one capillary perfused by flow of rate f. Then the concentration $\bar{c}_o$ in the sample is given by mixing (flux conservation):

$$fc_i e^{-\bar{p}s/f} = fc_o = F\bar{c}_o \tag{133}$$

where F is again the sum of capillary f's over the ensemble, as in Eq. 84. We now make use of the intravascular reference indicator present in the same arterial bolus with the concentration C_i (say). Since that indicator is not extracted($\bar{p}$=0)but only diluted, the relations which correspond to Eqs. 133 are

$$fC_i = fC_o = F\bar{C}_o \ . \tag{134}$$

We can now eliminate the unobserved quantities c_o,C_o from Eqs. 133,134:

$$f/F = e^{\bar{p}s/f}\bar{c}_o/c_i = \bar{C}_o/C_i \ , \tag{135}$$

or, in correspondence with Eq. 132,

$$\frac{\bar{c}_o/c_i}{\bar{C}_o/C_i} = e^{-\bar{p}s/f} \ . \tag{136}$$

It is customary to define also the extraction fraction E, as in Eq. 13. From Eq. 132 we define it as

$$E = (c_i - c_o)/c_i = 1 - e^{-\bar{p}s/f} \ , \tag{137}$$

which is not in itself useful because c_o is not observed. However, the use of the intravascular reference permits expressing E in terms of the composition of venous samples by using Eq. 136:

$$E = 1 - \frac{\bar{c}_o/c_i}{\bar{C}_o/C_i} \ . \tag{138}$$

The time-courses of $\bar{c}_o(t)/c_i$ and $\bar{C}_o(t)/C_i$ contain all the data from which conclusions are drawn in the indicator diffusion method. A schematic example of such data is shown in Fig.10; a more realistic example follows in Fig.11.

Next the contributions $\bar{p}s$ of the individual capillaries must be summed over the organ in order to obtain the mean organ permeability P,

$$P = \sum\bar{p}s/\sum s \ , \quad \sum s = S \ , \tag{139}$$

where S is the total capillary wall area of the organ. We first illustrate the summation problem by obtaining the commonly used expression for PS (20) on the assumption, evidently implausible in a biological context, that all the capillaries of the organ are identical in their values of $\bar{p}$, s and f. We proceed in two steps (which we shall discard later).

(a) Instead of a single capillary, let a group of n identical capillaries acting in parallel contribute indicator and refer-

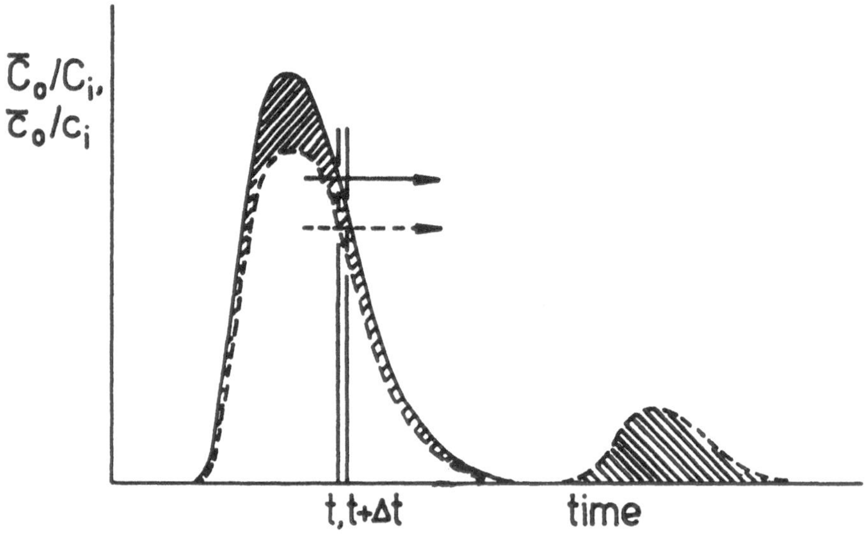

FIG.10

The ideal Crone case. The venous concentration of the indicator ($\bar{c}_o/c_i$, broken curve) and of the reference ($\bar{C}_o/C_i$, solid curve) normalized to the concentrations in the arterial bolus and drawn schematically as functions of time. In this idealized case, all indicator not recovered simultaneously with the reference is recovered after the reference bolus has passed, as shown by equal hatched areas. See text for the significance of the arrows.

ence to <u>one</u> (now finite) venous sample. Then the exponent in Eqs. 136 and 137 is $\bar{p}(ns)/(nf)=\bar{p}s/f$ independent of n, and so E in Eq. 138 is unchanged.

(b) Let all the capillaries contributing to <u>consecutive</u> venous samples be identical; then E given by Eqs. 136-138 is constant in time.

If the organ consists of N identical capillaries acting in parallel, then S=Ns, P=$\bar{p}$ and F=Nf. Then

$$PS = N\bar{p}s = F\bar{p}s/f = F \ln \frac{\bar{C}_o/C_i}{\bar{c}_o/c_i} \tag{140}$$

using Eq. 136. This is the familiar expression, in terms of observed quantities, for the permeability-surface product of an organ which has no heterogeneity of capillary extraction; it is often written in the form (13,20)

$$PS = -F \ln(1-E) , \tag{141}$$

where E is still given by Eq. 138. In reality the assumption of functional identity of all capillaries of an organ is contradicted by direct evidence from the study of single capillaries (17), by the evidence from steady-state uptake studies discussed in Sections 4,5 and 7, and most obviously by the observed time-dependence of E as given by Eq. 138 in many preparations, contrary to the prediction E=const. under (b), and to the meaning of PS/F in Eq. 141 in steady flow.

Before proceeding to a more realistic summation of $\bar{p}s$ over the organ in the presence of heterogeneities, it is important to distinguish between the two ways in which the assumption of functional identity of the capillaries can fail in the context of the indicator diffusion method. If step (a) fails because the capillaries involved do not extract equally, then the extraction fraction obtained from the <u>one</u> resulting venous sample is no longer given by Eq. 141. We have designated such capillary heterogeneity, which affects a venous sample taken at any one particular time, as organ heterogeneity of the <u>first kind</u> (14). It need not cause time-dependence of the extraction fraction E, since it may affect all consecutive samples equally. We shall show below that if heterogeneity of the first kind is present but disregarded, the calculated organ PS is always an underestimate of the true value.

By contrast, if step (b) fails because capillaries (or groups of capillaries) contributing indicator to <u>consecutive</u> samples do not extract equally, then the extraction fraction will be a function of time, E(t). We designate this kind of capillary heterogeneity as organ heterogeneity of the <u>second kind</u> (14). In this definition it is immaterial whether the time-varying E(t) is given at each time by Eq. 141 or by some other equation, such as may arise from heterogeneity of the first kind. Thus the two kinds of organ heterogeneity are not mutually exclusive.

Heterogeneity of the first kind is not readily recognized in data obtained by the indicator diffusion method (see below). By contrast, the presence of heterogeneity of the second kind is readily conjectured from time-dependence of the extraction fraction E calculated from data by using Eq. 138; in the literature of indicator diffusion, heterogeneity of the second kind is often referred to as "organ heterogeneity" without qualification.

However, heterogeneity of capillary extraction is not the only possible cause of a time-dependence of E in the indicator diffusion method, and additional causes (14) need to be allowed for in order to deduce organ PS-values from the data. The most important of these causes can operate even at the level of a single capillary: it is the aforementioned back-diffusion of previously extracted indicator back into the same (or into a neighbouring) capillary. The effect on the venous sample is to simulate reduced extraction and hence a reduced capillary permeability.

Next, for an organ <u>in situ</u>, re-circulated indicator and reference molecules making their second pass through the organ can mix in the vein with slower elements of the bolus making their first pass, thus obscuring the significance of the composition of venous samples (which now include twice-depleted elements of the indicator).

Such re-circulation effects can be reduced by the subtraction of the re-circulated contribution estimated conventionally by simple (semi-logarithmic) extrapolations of the dilution curves (20). Even better, recirculation can be removed completely in once-through perfusions, with the added advantage of a precise control and knowledge of the organ flow rate. Thus heterogeneity of capillary extraction, and back-diffusion remain as the two principal effects which must be dealt with theoretically in the calculation of organ PS from data. These two effects must lead to a modification or re-interpretation of Eqs. 140 and 141 whenever the extraction fraction E, as calculated from any actual set of indicator diffusion data, is found to depend on time.

If the first pass of the reference bolus through the organ was completed before the onset of appreciable back-diffusion of the indicator, the calculation of organ PS from data would be greatly facilitated. Since there is no intrinsic connection between the time-scales of these processes, one could in principle choose a diffusible indicator which would separate them completely. If furthermore the diffusion indicator had no metabolic sink in the organ, the fraction of its bolus not recovered simultaneously with the reference would be recovered completely at later times, as shown in Fig.10. Such temporal separation of the two parts of the outflow of the diffusible indicator would be in accord with the basic idea of the indicator diffusion method (13), and we therefore refer to this limiting case as the ideal Crone case (14). We first evaluate the organ PS for ideal Crone cases. The time-course of the venous appearance of the back-diffusing indicator, shown schematically in Fig.10, does not affect the calculation of PS.

Consider the values of $\bar{c}_o/c_i$, $\bar{C}_o/C_i$ observed in a short time-interval between t and t+Δt (Fig.10). If only one capillary had contributed indicator and reference to these concentrations, the resulting extraction and mixing would have been described already by Eqs. 134-138. Here we consider more generally a group of capillaries contributing tracer simultaneously to the venous outflow, and accordingly we replace f with the appropriate part ΔF of the total organ flow rate F, and $\bar{p}s$ with the corresponding part Δ(PS) of the organ PS. The remaining capillaries of the organ, perfused at the rate F-ΔF, are contributing tracer-free blood at this time. Then Eqs. 134, 136 and 138 give

$$\Delta F/F = \bar{C}_o/C_i \ , \tag{142}$$

$$\Delta(PS)/\Delta F = \ln\frac{\bar{C}_o/C_i}{\bar{c}_o/c_i} = -\ln(1-E) \tag{143}$$

on inverting Eq. 135. We note in passing that Eq. 142 can be a relation between infinitesimals, inasmuch as the actual arterial bolus approximates an ideal bolus ($C_i \rightarrow \infty$). We observe that Eqs. 142 and 143 would describe a steady state momentarily coincident with the actual state in the vein (cf. horizontal arrows in Fig.

10) if the capillaries now contributing tracer-free blood continued to do so, and if the capillaries now contributing the two tracers had been infused steadily with the concentrations C_i, c_i. For such an equivalent steady-state description of the venous outflow in an interval $t, t+\Delta t$, the organ divides itself into two notional suborgans with outputs mixed in the vein: a tracer-delivering suborgan perfused at the flow rate ΔF and containing the part $\Delta(PS)$ of the organ PS, and a complementary tracer-diluting suborgan perfused at the flow rate $F-\Delta F$. Proceeding thus by intervals Δt along the time-axis until all times are included at which there is a measurable venous concentration of the reference, the effect of the complete organ on the venous outflow is decomposed into sequential suborgan effects, each described by Eq. 143. The organ PS is then the sum of the contributions $\Delta(PS)$ of the tracer-delivering suborgans:

$$PS = \sum \Delta(PS) = \sum \Delta F \ \ln \frac{\bar{C}_o/C_i}{\bar{c}_o/c_i} \tag{144}$$

or, using Eq. 142,

$$PS = F \sum \frac{\bar{C}_o}{C_i} \ln \frac{\bar{C}_o/C_i}{\bar{c}_o/c_i} \ . \tag{145}$$

We shall perform the summation for a perfectly concentrated bolus, so that we can picture it without loss of generality as a rectangular pulse of duration Δt. Then, by conservation of the intravascular indicator,

$$FC_i \Delta t = F \int_0^\infty \bar{C}_o dt \ . \tag{146}$$

Using Eq. 146 to express C_i in the denominator of the first factor under the summation sign in Eq. 145, and proceeding to the limit $\Delta t \to 0$, we obtain

$$PS = F \frac{\int_0^\infty \bar{C}_o \ln \left(\frac{\bar{C}_o/C_i}{\bar{c}_o/c_i} \right) dt}{\int_0^\infty \bar{C}_o dt} \ . \tag{147}$$

We note that

$$\bar{C}_o / \int_0^\infty \bar{C}_o dt = h(t) \tag{148}$$

is the well-known frequency function of the transit times of the intravascular reference (20); using it, and the second of Eqs.143 in Eq. 147, we obtain (14)

$$PS = -F\int_0^{\infty} h(t)\ln[1-E(t)]dt \qquad (149)$$

as the generalization of Eq. 141 for the commonly encountered case when E, as calculated from data according to Eq. 138, turns out to be time-dependent even after allowing for recirculation and back-diffusion of the indicator.

We have thus taken into account heterogeneity of the second kind; what about the first kind? We return to the derivation of Eq. 143 and we note that it assumed that all capillaries within the tracer-delivering suborgan were extracting equally. In reality there will be some dispersion of extraction within any such suborgan belonging to an interval $t,t+\Delta t$, and we again characterize that dispersion by the coefficient of variation ε of the relevant distribution of $\bar{p}s/f$ (in place of v_{max}/fK_m) as in Section 4 (Eq. 117). However, now there is a coefficient of variation belonging to each time-interval, and we write therefore $\varepsilon(t)$. Using the perturbation theory of Section 4 to order ε^2 in the limit of first-order uptake, we need merely to translate Eq. 122 into the notation of the present interpretation: since ΔPS corresponds to V_{max}/K_m, the effect of heterogeneity on extraction by the suborgan is the same as if we replaced ΔPS by $\Delta\tilde{PS}$:

$$\Delta\tilde{PS} = \Delta PS\left[1 - \tfrac{1}{2}\varepsilon(t)^2(\Delta PS/\Delta F)\right] < \Delta PS \ , \qquad (150)$$

and it is this $\Delta\tilde{PS}$ that must be now inserted in the left-hand side of Eq. 143 in place of ΔPS. Solving Eq. 143 so modified for ΔPS to order $\varepsilon(t)^2$, we obtain

$$\Delta(PS)/\Delta F = -\ln(1-E) + \tfrac{1}{2}\varepsilon(t)^2[\ln(1-E)]^2 \ . \qquad (151)$$

Proceeding now through the same integration steps as from Eq. 144 to Eq. 149, we obtain the final expression for the organ PS in the ideal Crone case, accurate to order $\varepsilon(t)^2$:

$$PS = -F\int_0^{\infty} h(t)\ln(1-E)[1 - \tfrac{1}{2}\varepsilon(t)^2\ln(1-E)]dt \ . \qquad (152)$$

We note that if there is a non-zero $\varepsilon(t)$ at least at some time, the resulting correction term must increase the organ PS as compared with PS calculated from Eq. 149: neglect of an existing heterogeneity of the first kind leads therefore to an underestimate of organ PS. Thus Eq. 149 gives us a lower bound on organ PS in the ideal Crone case.

An upper bound is also available in this ideal case: we insert in Eq. 152 the value of ε^2 obtained for the organ by the steady-state methods of Section 4 (14). We need to show only that this ε is greater than $\varepsilon(t)$ of any tracer-delivering suborgan. If one envisaged suborgans formed from capillaries taken from the organ at random, the resulting ε's would be of the same order as the organ ε obtained in the steady state. However, in the indicator diffusion method the tracer-delivering suborgans form themselves from capillaries that deliver their bolus fractions at the same time, that is, from capillaries belonging to a common transit time T' between the instruments. If there was no dispersion of pre-capillary and post-capillary transit times, and if extraction by a single capillary was uniquely related to the capillary transit time T, then this self-organization of the suborgans would altogether remove heterogeneity of the first kind in the context of the indicator diffusion method: $\varepsilon(t)$ would vanish at all times. However, we can accept only that the transit times T and T' are correlated by the relation 131, so that capillaries in each suborgan will be more similar to each other than if they were taken from the organ at random. Therefore $\varepsilon(t)$ is always less than ε estimated on the same organ in the steady state, and the foregoing construction of the upper bound on PS follows. We note also that the relative smallness of $\varepsilon(t)$ makes our use of the perturbation theory more accurate in the present context than in steady state analysis.

It will now be apparent that extraction heterogeneity of the first kind, and its effect on the determination of organ PS through Eq. 152, cannot be analyzed further without modeling the connection between extraction and transit time T in each capillary, and then the connection between the distributions of T and T' for the organ. Deterministic (41,42) as well as probabilistic (14) models of these connections have been constructed, and the degrees of arbitrariness inherent at present in such modeling has been analyzed (14). Moreover, deterministic modeling of back-diffusion has been brought to bear on the analysis of indicator diffusion data (41). A very interesting extension of the indicator diffusion method for saturable wall uptake has been introduced (44): instead of linearizing tracer kinetics about a steady background of the mother substance, as discussed in the beginning of this Section in relation to Eq. 37 of Section 3, the mother substance is also confined to the bolus. This is particularly desirable clinically if some toxicity of the diffusible indicator is suspected (43). A fuller review of these developments is beyond the scope of this Section. Instead, we conclude it by showing how to apply the foregoing results in the presence of back-diffusion and recirculation of the indicators.

In a real venous outflow of indicator and reference (as distinct from the ideal Crone case), back-diffusing indicator appears before the reference bolus has passed (Fig.11a). The characteristic feature of the real case is the change from $\bar{c}_o/c_i < \bar{C}_o/C_i$ for $t < t_c$ to $\bar{c}_o/c_i > \bar{C}_o/C_i$ for $t > t_c$, where t_c is the time at which the two dilution curves cross while the magnitude of $\bar{C}_o/C_i$ is still appreciable. Some back-diffusion is likely at $t < t_c$, but without detailed modeling its presence is not certain until $t > t_c$, when the apparent extraction fraction given by Eq. 138 becomes negative. Similarly, it is likely that some extraction is still occurring at $t > t_c$, but without detailed modeling of back-diffusion we are certain of extraction only at $t < t_c$, when E

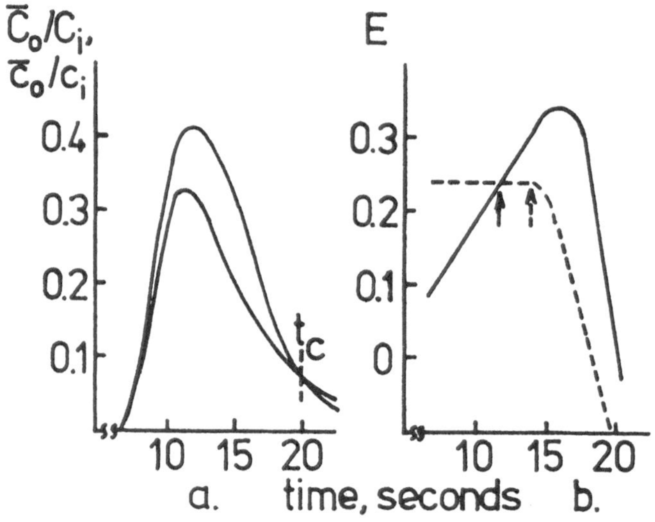

FIG.11

Examples of empirical indicator diffusion data (schematically after (41)). (a) As in Fig.10, but with a cross-over of the two dilution curves at the time $t=t_c$. (b) Extraction fractions as functions of time. The solid curve belongs to the case sketched in (a), the broken curve is from the same dog heart preparation in a different (vasodilated) state. Arrows indicate times of peak concentrations of the reference.

is positive (i.e., when there is a net diffusional outflux from the capillary).

We now calculate the best (highest) lower bound on organ PS that we can obtain without detailed modeling of back-diffusion and of recirculation. We proceed to simplify the calculation of PS in the real case, making sure that each simplifying step underestimates the true PS.

(a) We begin by neglecting all the possible extraction at $t > t_c$: in Eqs. 149 and 152 we integrate only up to $t=t_c$, leaving the denominator in Eq. 148 unchanged.

(b) Next we neglect all possible back-diffusion at $t < t_c$. If some of the observed $\bar{c}_o$ is in fact contributed by back-diffusion, this simplification underestimates extraction.

(c) If the preparation is perfused in a re-circulating system, we next perform the standard re-circulation correction (20) on the reference, but not on the diffusible indicator. It is the curve of $\bar{C}_o/C_i$ so corrected that is to be used in Eq. 148 and hence in Eqs. 149 and 152. The contribution of the re-circulated indicator (if any) then simulates lower extraction than is really the case.

(d) If we have no cogent prior estimate of the heterogeneity of the first kind, we set $\varepsilon(t)=0$ in Eq. 152, thus arriving at Eq. 149 as modified by the steps (a)-(c). We have shown above that this simplification must result in an underestimate of PS.

The outcome of the steps (a)-(d) is a secure lower bound on organ PS which is parsimonious (14) in the sense that no auxiliary parameters need to be determined, and no hypotheses associated with them need to be validated; the calculations proceed directly from the data provided by the indicator diffusion method at all times $t < t_C$. We note that a finite upper bound on organ PS cannot be obtained along similarly parsimonious lines. For without detailed modeling of back-diffusion we cannot exclude the possibility that some Δ(PS), making its effect in some time-interval $t, t+\Delta t$ at $t < t_C$, is arbitrarily large but that the observed $\bar{c}_0$ is provided by sufficiently fast back-diffusion.

These new methods of estimating organ PS have recently been applied (14) to a selection of data sets from the literature, including data from the intact human brain. Here we shall confine ourselves to data from a study of the extraction of ^{14}C-labeled sucrose by the myocardial capillaries of the functioning dog heart (41); these data are particularly interesting in that they contrast the vasoconstricted and vasodilated state of the same preparation. Fig.11a shows schematically the venous outflows of the indicator and of the ^{125}I-labeled albumin reference; there is a minor but noticeable deviation from the ideal Crone case visible from the time t_C onwards. Hence Eqs. 152 or 149 may be used as an approximation to organ PS, but only the foregoing lower bound on PS is valid strictly. The empirical time-courses of the extraction fractions E(t), which are used in Eqs. 149 or 152, are shown schematically in Fig.11b.

In order to see the quantitative importance of the foregoing considerations, it is interesting to compare the following practical results with older estimates of organ PS made by frequently used methods which first neglect all heterogeneity by using Eqs. 140, 141 and 138, and then attempt to correct that omission either by choosing E at a time when it might be particularly significant, or by making a weighted time-average of E(t). We shall consider four such estimates, referring to (20) and (14) for details and references. The initial extraction E_0 is obtained by extrapolating E(t) back to the time of first appearance of the indicators in the vein. The area-extraction E_A is constructed by using the fractional difference in the areas under the two dilution curves, taken as far as the time t_p of the peak $\bar{C}_0(t)$ (cf. Fig.11a). The extraction fraction $E(t_p)$ is E taken at the time t_p. The extraction E_{max} is the greatest extraction seen (as in Fig.11b) in the time-course of E(t). For the data pictured in Fig.11, we shall compare these four older estimates of PS with the lower bound (l.b. for short) calculated from Eq. 149 as modified by the steps (a)-(d). We calculate also the correction term proportional to $\varepsilon(t)^2$ in Eq. 152, assuming $\varepsilon(t)$=const. We thus obtain the results (14) set out in Table 2.

We observe that in the vasodilated state there is a clear plateau of E in time, which yields mutually consistent older estimates of PS/F which are higher by some 25% than the (uncorrected) lower bound. The vasoconstricted state of the same preparat-

TABLE 2

Estimates of organ PS

	E_o	E_A	$E(t_p)$	E_{max}	l.b.	ε^2-term
vasodilated:						
E	0.25	0.25	0.24	0.25		
PS/F	0.29	0.29	0.27	0.29	0.22	$0.028\ \varepsilon^2$
vasoconstricted:						
E	0.10	0.19	0.24	0.34		
PS/F	0.10	0.21	0.27	0.41	0.28	$0.046\ \varepsilon^2$

ion presents a remarkable contrast, which illustrates the demonstration (41) that heterogeneity of the second kind is greatly reduced by vasodilation of the myocardial capillaries. The plateau of E has disappeared, the four older estimates of PS/F are mutually at variance by factors of up to four, and both E_0 and E_A now give PS/F - estimates substantially below the lower bound. The dog heart study thus shows the four older estimates at their most consistent, and at their most ambiguous, in the same preparation.

We have seen in Section 5 that neglect of heterogeneity may lead to mistaken inferences about recruitment of capillaries from changes in organ PS (or V_{max}/K_m) with F. Similarly, Table 2 warns us against false conclusions that could arise from neglect of heterogeneity in inferring changes in organ PS per unit flow rate, PS/F, when the organ undergoes the important transition from the vasodilated to the vasoconstricted state. Vasoconstriction would seem to decrease PS/F according to E_0 and E_A, increase it according to E_{max}, and leave it unchanged according to $E(t_p)$, all from the same set of data. Actually, the lower bound of PS/F has been increased by the vasoconstriction. Since the data shown in Fig.11a are close to the ideal Crone case, the lower bounds will be close to the actual values of PS/F and so a real increase in PS/F by some 20-30% in vasoconstriction can be inferred from the data.

7.ANTIDOTE TO ADJUSTABLE PARAMETERS:NULL EXPERIMENTS

The data interpreted in this Chapter consist usually of discrete sets of concentration or radioactivity measurements, together with the corresponding values of time or some other parameter (flow rate, inlet concentration etc.). Confidence in an interpretation arises from a mixture of its simplicity, rationality and quantitative agreement with the data. The right mixture is hard to define, but a wrong one is easy to exemplify:

"Take, for example, the (licence) numbers of all the taxis that I have hired in the course of my life, and the times when I have hired them. We have here a finite set of integers and a finite number of corresponding times. If n is the number of the taxi that I hired at the time t, it is certainly possible, in an infinite number of ways, to find a function f such that the formula

$$n = f(t) \tag{153}$$

is true for all the values of n and t that have hitherto occurred. An infinite number of these formulae will fail for the next taxi I hire, but there will still be an infinite number that remain true." (45)

Since this was written, practical implementation of such procedures has become possible, at the touch of a few buttons, with the advent of high speed computers. Thus a sufficient number of adjustable parameters permits almost any theory to be brought into quantitative agreement with a finite set of data. In Section 2, for example, the subdivision of the two compartments into a sufficient number of communicating subcompartments would permit a quantitatively perfect (and physiologically uninformative) fit of all data in terms of the parameters of the subcompartments. It is clear that if the ill-defined concepts of simplicity and rationality of hypotheses were to become submerged in the fitting of data, using enough adjustable parameters and the powerful computational means now available, mathematical modeling could lose all its scientific value.

An important antidote to such indiscriminate use of adjustable parameters is to cast a model in such a form that a specified new experimental maneuver is predicted to produce no change in a specified combination of observables. Such null experiments (long important in physics) can be designed only for subject-matter that has reached a sufficient degree of theoretical development. We shall now discuss three such null experiments bearing on the foregoing work.

A snapshot of a liver sinusoid perfused with full blood would show parts of the sinusoidal wall occluded by red blood cells. Does this apparent occlusion reduce uptake of substrates confined to plasma? A theory of such a reduction would be very complicated in view of the motion of the blood cells, and their shapes in relation to the sinusoid: adjustable parameters would abound. However, a denial of such an effect provides our simplest example of a null experiment. In Section 5 we have discussed data (15) on the uptake of labeled $CrPO_4$ colloid by rat livers in terms of Eq. 129 and Fig.9. Whatever the interpretation of the concave part of the curve in Fig.9, it is clear that at sufficiently high values of the flow rate F, the quantity $F\ln(c_i/\bar{c}_o)$ must tend to V_{max}/K_m, which is the initial slope of the curve in Fig.9. If there is reduction of V_{max} by occlusion, it must depend on the proportion of the volume of the sinusoid taken up by blood cells, that is, on the haematocrit H of the perfusate. If there is no such reduction, then V_{max} is independent of H and we have the null prediction

$$\lim_{F\to\infty} \frac{\partial[(1-H)F\ \ln(c_i/\bar{c}_o)]}{\partial H} = 0 \tag{154}$$

where (1-H)F is the rate of flow of plasma. Here is a prediction which involves nothing but observed quantities. In fact, when H was varied from 0.0025 to 0.45, Eq. 154 was found to be satisfied with remarkable accuracy (15,8). It is clear that results of this fundamental null experiment would be basic also to studies of the kinetics of uptake from blood by other perfused organs.

For the undistributed model of Michaelis-Menten uptake, a powerful null experiment based on Eqs. 6 and 7 has been performed (46). Each of a set of ten isolated rat livers was perfused in a recirculating system in the steady state of galactose uptake determined by a constant infusion of galactose. Since V in Eq. 6 is equal to the constant rate of the infusion, and since V_{max} and K_m are constants for each preparation, Eq. 6 predicts that in such circumstances $\hat{c}_1$ must be independent of the choice of the steady rate of flow F of the perfusate:

$$\left(\frac{\partial \hat{c}_1}{\partial F}\right)_V = 0 \,, \tag{155}$$

where $\hat{c}_1$ is the logarithmic mean (Eq. 7) of c_i and c_o (each of which will depend on the choice of F). Again, Eq. 155 involves nothing but observable quantities when the definition of $\hat{c}_1$ by Eq. 7 is taken into consideration. One need not know the actual values of the constants V_{max} and K_m for each preparation, but the experimental rates of flow must be chosen within the range in which V_{max} and other physiological control variables are constant ((38),(46): cf. Section 5). The experiments were performed with the rates of flow 15 ml/min and 9 ml/min. No statistically significant change of $\hat{c}_1$ was found for the set of ten preparations $(P > 0.90)$. By contrast, c_o changed with F very significantly $(P < 0.01)$, incidentally refuting the venous equilibration model of liver uptake ((47), and references therein) sometimes used in pharmacokinetics.

When such a null experiment is viewed from the point of view of a more general theory, the predicted result may be no longer expressible in terms of directly observed quantities alone; but any additional hypothetical quantities (adjustable parameters) are likely to play a readily identifiable role in the observed or presumed deviations from the original prediction. We illustrate this by considering two different generalizations of the theory underlying Eq. 155.

(i) In the more general distributed model of uptake in Sections 4 and 5, c_o in Eq. 7 is replaced by $\bar{c}_o$ as in Eq. 124 while Eq. 6 is valid only in the limit of high concentrations, and the corresponding inverse (Lineweaver-Burk) plot is now curved as in Fig.8. To see qualitatively what deviation from Eq. 155 is predicted by the distributed model, we need only to continue the discussion of effects of changes in F at the end of Section 5. The slope of the initial tangent in Fig.8 is independent of F, the slope of the asymptote is greater by $\varepsilon^2/2F$. Consider a line V=const. (given by the galactose infusion into the recirculating system) and its intersection with the curve in Fig.8. If we reduce F, the asymptote swings further away from the initial tangent and the intersection with the line V=const. will move to smaller values of $1/\hat{c}_1$, that is, $\hat{c}_1$ will increase; the magnitude of the increase will be proportional to ε^2, and it will depend on the choice of V, and of the initial and final values of F. Thus the distributed model predicts a negative right-hand side of Eq. 155, proportional to ε^2. The failure to detect deviations from Eq. 155 in the experiment (46) means, from the point of view of the distributed model, that the actual value of ε^2 was too small to be detected within experimental errors on the set of ten perfused liver preparations. The null result thus imposes an upper bound on the admissible value of ε^2 at any chosen level of statistical significance. When these considerations were developed in detail (39), the reanalysis of the data (46) from the point of view of the distributed model yielded the upper bound $\varepsilon^2 < 0.18$ at the 0.05 level of statistical significance, in satisfactory relation to the outright estimate, ε^2=0.137, for the heterogeneity of uptake of colloidal $CrPO_4$ by Kupffer cells of the isolated perfused rat liver ((8); cf. Section 5).

(ii) Having thus seen that the results of this experiment (46) are rather insensitive to transverse heterogeneity of uptake, we can return to the undistributed model and generalize the theory in a different direction: we consider the class of cooperative saturation kinetics given by Eq. 9, which leads to Eqs. 10 and 11 for uptake by the intact organ. If the Hill constant n is different from unity, the same reasoning that has led us to Eq. 155 now leads to the same equation with $\hat{c}_1$ replaced with the $\hat{c}_n$ given by Eq. 11. For the true value of n, the combination $\hat{c}_n$ of the observed c_i and c_o should be independent of F: $\hat{c}_n$ should be a flow-invariant in the context of this experiment. In view of experimental errors, the stochastic counterpart of this statement for a set of perfused liver preparations (46) is that the changes in $\hat{c}_n$ resulting from a change in F should be distributed symmetrically about zero. By re-analyzing the statistics of the experimental results (46) afresh from this point of view for each of a range of values of n, we can construct a probability distribution for the true value of n (48). The distribution turns out to be peaked distinctly about the value n=1. That value was to be expected from our previous knowledge of galactose uptake by livers *in vitro* (31) and *in vivo* (3), but the good definition of the peak is good news: an effective method for estimating the Hill constant for hepatocellular enzymes *in vivo* can apparently be based on such a use of flow-invariants (48).

A conceptual counterpart to a real null experiment can be conducted by splitting a set of data into two subsets, and using one subset to formulate a null prediction for the other. It was by such a procedure that the most conclusive results about transverse heterogeneity in the steady state were deduced (7) from data obtained from a set of six isolated perfused pig livers eliminating galactose in the steady state (3). These data gave altogether 27 data triplets (V,c_i,c_o) and hence 27 points for plots of 1/V against $1/\hat{c}_1$ discussed in Section 4 (Fig.8). These were used first to examine the internal consistency of the undistributed model. Estimating V_{max} and K_m for each preparation from a least-square application of Eqs. 6 and 7 to the data, one can then pool all the data on a common Lineweaver-Burk plot of Eq. 123 (initial tangent in Fig.8) by using the normalized inverse variables V_{max}/V, $K_m/\hat{c}_1$. This gives an excellent straight line, which is not surprising considering that there are 12 adjustable parameters in this treatment of 27 points. Now for the antidote, inspired by our knowledge of the distributed model but administered to the undistributed model.

We split the data into a high concentration subset $\hat{c}_1 > K_m$ (17 points) and a low concentration subset $\hat{c}_1 < K_m$ (10 points), using the K_m obtained for each preparation in the previous step. We now estimate V_{max} and K_m again for each preparation as in the previous step, but using only the data in the high concentration subset. We use these new estimates of V_{max} and K_m to renormalize V_{max}/V and $K_m/\hat{c}_1$ for all 27 data points, and we reconstruct the pooled Lineweaver-Burk plot. For the 17 points of the high concentration subset, there is an excellent straight line (involving again the 12 adjustable parameters). By contrast, all but one of the 10 low concentration data points (which had not been used in the fitting) fall above that straight line. From the point of view of the undistributed model, the sample-splitting maneuver should result at most in an increased scatter of the low concentration points about the straight line obtained in our second step. However, the probability that the observed displacement of the group of 10 high concentration points occurs by chance was found to be less than 0.011 by the one-sided sign test, and less than 0.002 by Wilcoxon's one-sided signed rank test (7). This is convincing internal evidence against the undistributed model, despite the good fit in the initial step enforced by the use of adjustable parameters.

From the point of view of the distributed model, the foregoing results are immediately understandable (Fig.8): as we saw in Section 4, dispersion of v_{max}/f about its organ mean V_{max}/F reduces the uptake rate V, except in the limit of high concentrations. The high concentration points belong mainly to the initial tangent, the low concentration points mainly to the asymptote of the curved plot in Fig.8. When this was worked out quantitatively and Eqs. 125, 127 and 128 were used, the estimate $\varepsilon^2=0.196$ for the group of pig livers was arrived at (7). This satisfied the criteria of admissibility of the perturbation theory to order ε^2 as applied to the pig livers (as was the case with the very similar estimates for rat livers). Another analysis of the same data, but now involving also the measured values of F for each preparation, was based on relation 86 and Eq. 120. The same sample-splitting led to the same conclusions along this different route of analysis (7).

8. INTERCONVERTING SUBSTRATES: LONGITUDINAL HETEROGENEITY OF ORGANS

We have seen in Sections 1, 3 and 4 that for a single substrate or indicator, the relation between input concentration c_i and output concentration c_o is insensitive to the longitudinal distribution of uptake in the steady state, and in the unsteady state of concentrations in steady flow. This insensitivity disappears when a precursor substrate is converted by liver cells into a metabolite which in turn is eliminated (conjugated) in liver cells. This can be expected intuitively, since it must matter to the venous outflows of the metabolite and its conjugate whether, for example, the metabolizing machinery of the liver is located upstream of the conjugating machinery, or vice versa. We shall develop the mathematics of this new chapter of steady-state tracer kinetics (10,12,49) with particular reference to a set of data from an ingenious experiment devised in a different context (16).

Each liver cell (hepatocyte) may possess some capability to convert the precursor into the metabolite, as well as some capability to eliminate (conjugate) the metabolite. The metabolite is used with two labels: one label is shared with the precursor, the other labels metabolite which is introduced into the liver preformed. The precursor and the preformed metabolite infused into the liver with the blood through the inlet enter the hepatocytes, where the metabolite (either preformed or formed there from the precursor) may be eliminated by the formation of its conjugate. The precursor, the metabolite and its conjugate are exchanged steadily between each hepatocyte and the ambient blood, which sweeps all these species towards the hepatic vein.

We develop the theory of this interconversion process in terms of the undistributed model of uptake, and recall that it will apply to a single sinusoid by a minor reinterpretation (Section 1). In place of a single steady-state concentration profile $c(x)$ on the interval $0 \leq x \leq L$, we shall have five: $P(x)$ for the precursor, $M(x)$ for its metabolite, $\tilde{M}(x)$ for its conjugate; $M^*(x)$ for the preformed metabolite, and $\tilde{M}^*(x)$ for its conjugate.

We begin with the simpler kinetics of the preformed metabolite. We use Eqs. 3 and 4 for its elimination by conjugation, with the following slight modifications. We consider first-order uptake of the tracers ($c \ll K_m$), and we denote the dimensionless quantity V_{max}/FK_m by m. Moreover, in place of the density function $\rho(x)$, we use the density function $g(x)=\rho(x)/V_{max}$, so that $g(x)$ is now normalized to unity on the interval from 0 to L. We thus obtain in place of Eqs. 3 and 4 :

$$\frac{dM^*}{dx} = -mg(x)M^* , \tag{156}$$

$$\int_0^L g(x)dx = 1 , \tag{157}$$

where $g(x)$ is non-negative. The input and output concentrations (radioactivities), M_i^* and M_o^*, are observed. The equation for the conjugate is $d\tilde{M}^*/dx=mg(x)M^*$.

The equations for the depletion of the precursor by conversion into metabolite are formally quite analogous to Eqs. 156,157. In place of the effective rate constant m we write p, and in place of the density distribution $g(x)$ we write $f(x)$, since the enzymes for metabolism may be distributed along the sinusoids differently from those for conjugation:

$$\frac{dP}{dx} = -pf(x)P \ , \tag{158}$$

$$\int_0^L f(x)dx = 1 \ , \tag{159}$$

where again f(x) is non-negative but otherwise unspecified. The loss of the precursor is the source of the metabolite, which is in turn depleted by conjugation by enzymes already introduced in Eqs. 156, 157:

$$\frac{dM}{dx} = pf(x)P - mg(x)M \ . \tag{160}$$

The conjugate is again governed by the equation $d\tilde{M}/dx=mg(x)M$; but in what follows we shall not consider the conjugates any further (see however (16), (49)). We note that if the tracers are superposed on chemical quantities of their mother substances which are subject to kinetics other than first order, then we can modify the tracer rate constants m,p to depend on the concentrations of the mother substances as in Section 3.

The role of the preformed metabolite satisfying Eq. 156 is limited but important; separating Eq. 156, integrating from inlet to outlet and using Eq. 157, we obtain

$$m = \ln(M_i^*/M_o^*) \tag{161}$$

so that in any one experimental preparation, m is calibrated for the use in Eq. 160: m is no longer an adjustable parameter. From Eqs. 158 and 159, we obtain similarly

$$p = \ln(P_i/P_o) \tag{162}$$

where P_i and P_o are observed at the inlet and outlet. Thus only the two longitudinal distribution functions f(x), g(x) remain to be investigated by studying the interconversion of the tracers described by Eq. 160. The metabolite with the label of the precursor, described by M(x), is produced entirely in the liver from the precursor:

$$M_i = 0 \ , \tag{163}$$

while M_o is observed.

We now calculate the observable ratio M_o/P_i in terms of the functions f(x), g(x). Separating Eq. 158 and integrating from the inlet to a general position x yields

$$P(x) = P_i \exp[-p\int_0^x f(x')dx'] \tag{164}$$

where x' denotes a dummy variable. This P(x) is now substituted in Eq. 160. Multiplying the latter through with the integrating factor

$$\exp[m\int_0^x g(x')dx'] ,$$

rearranging, integrating from inlet to outlet and using Eqs. 157 and 159 yields

$$M_o/P_i = pe^{-m}\int_0^L f(x'')\exp[-p\int_0^{x''} f(x')dx']\exp[m\int_0^{x''} g(x')dx']dx'' , \quad (165)$$

where both x' and x" are dummies. Thus M_o/P_i depends on f(x) and g(x) as a functional (in the sense of the calculus of variations: see Section 9). There are however three important special cases independent of the form of these functions.

When $f(x)\neq 0$ upstream of $g(x)\neq 0$ and there is no overlap, the exponent of the third factor in the integrand is zero for any x" for which the first factor is non-zero; hence the third factor can be replaced by unity. Then M_o/P_i becomes independent of the form of f(x"), since the substitution

$$u(x'') = p\int_0^{x''} f(x')dx' \quad (166)$$

transforms Eq. 165 into

$$M_o/P_i = e^{-m}\int_0^p e^{-u}du = e^{-m}(1-e^{-p}) . \quad (167)$$

Next, if the non-zero parts of f(x), g(x) are interchanged (with respect to the direction of blood flow), it follows by similar reasoning that

$$M_o/P_i = 1-e^{-p} . \quad (168)$$

Next, when f(x)=g(x) (i.e., when all hepatocytes function equally) and the second and third factors in the integrand of Eq. 165 are combined, it is apparent that the substitution given by Eq. 166 can again be used, provided that p is replaced with p-m. Then Eq. 165 yields, again independently of the form of f(x"),

$$M_o/P_i = p(e^{-m}-e^{-p})/(p-m) . \quad (169)$$

Since Eqs. 167,168,169 involve only the parameters p,m calibrated experimentally on each preparation, the underlying hypotheses can be tested against data without the intervention of adjustable parameters (cf. Section 7). Eq. 167 represents the hypothesis that all metabolism takes place upstream of conjugation, and Eq. 168 represents the reversed situation. Eq. 169

represents the classical view of the hepatocyte (11), according to which all hepatocytes are functionally the same.

Table 3 gives an analysis (12) of data obtained from perfused in situ rat livers eliminating the metabolite acetaminophen (paracetamol), both preformed and formed in the livers from the precursor phenacetin, in a series of eight once-through preparations in the steady state (16).

It is apparent from Table 3 that Eq. 169 fails: all the predicted M_o/P_i are greater than the observed ones, so that the sign test alone refutes the hypothesis of functional identity of hepatocytes at the significance level $P=2^{-8} < 0.004$. Eq. 168 fails likewise, since its predictions are necessarily even higher than those of Eq. 169. By contrast, Eq. 167 does remarkably well, with differences between predictions and observations distributed fairly symmetrically about zero. Thus, $P > 0.94$ from the(two-sided) Wilcoxon signed rank test (49). These contrasting results indicate that the foregoing developments lead to a non-destructive kinetic method for examining, for any precursor-metabolite pair, the zonal structure of liver function which has been long postulated but has only recently begun to be detected by enzymological and histochemical methods (see (11) and (49) for references). In the case of phenacetin and acetaminophen, the success of Eq. 167 implies that almost all the metabolism takes place in a zone located upstream of a zone in which conjugation takes place.

It is helpful to view these input-output relations in terms of extraction fractions. For the preformed metabolite with the input concentration M_i^*, the extraction fraction is defined as in Eq. 13:

$$E^* = 1-M_o^*/M_i^* = 1-e^{-m} , \tag{170}$$

using also Eq. 161. By contrast, "input" of the metabolite made in the liver from the precursor ($M_i=0$, as in Eq. 163) occurs inside the hepatocytes, the total input being equal to P_i-P_o which is missing from the precursor. The appropriate extraction fraction of this metabolite is therefore

$$E = 1-M_o/(P_i-P_o) = 1-(M_o/P_i)/(1-e^{-p}) \tag{171}$$

TABLE 3

Kinetics of phenacetin and acetaminophen in rat liver

From	M_o/P_i for liver no. 1	2	3	4	5	6	7	8	Mean
Equation 169	0.487	0.359	0.336	0.531	0.484	0.429	0.407	0.462	0.437
Equation 167	0.346	0.220	0.217	0.410	0.339	0.297	0.251	0.318	0.2997
Observed M_o,P_i	0.338	0.276	0.309	0.415	0.284	0.253	0.250	0.279	0.3005

using also Eq. 162. The factor M_o/P_i has been calculated in Eq. 165.

If we assume the validity of Eq. 167 and substitute for M_o/P_i in Eq. 171, we get E=E* (cf. Eq. 170): since all metabolite is made from the precursor upstream of the zone of conjugation, the metabolite is as good as "preformed" as far as conjugation is concerned. Using the data (16) which have been used to construct Table 3, one finds the mean values for the eight preparations (49):

$$\bar{E}^* = 0.670 \pm 0.025 \text{ S.E.M.}, \quad \bar{E} = 0.673 \pm 0.019 \text{ S.E.M. } (N=8). \quad (172)$$

This close agreement is an aspect of the success of Eq. 167 in Table 3. If on the other hand we assume the validity of Eq. 168 and substitute for M_o/P_i in Eq. 171, we get the null prediction E=0 (falsified by Eq. 172): all the metabolite has missed the zone of conjugation because it has been created downstream of it from the precursor. If we use M_o/P_i from Eq. 169, we obtain a prediction which fails by being systematically too low: metabolite is being created from the precursor downstream of some part of the conjugating machinery.

A satisfactory aspect of the close agreement between $\bar{E}$ and $\bar{E}^*$ in Eq. 172 is that it confirms the rapidity of equilibration of the metabolite across the hepatocyte membrane: if there was an appreciable delay, the metabolite created from the precursor inside the hepatocyte would in general have a better chance of conjugation than when it is presented from the blood, so that E would be greater than E*.

How much overlap of the distributions f(x) and g(x) would be consistent with the data leading to Eqs. 172? This was investigated carefully by two statistical methods (distribution free, and Bayesian) for overlaps of rectangular f(x) and g(x). The most probable overlap was zero, the median overlap was 17%, and the odds against an overlap greater than 50% were 40 to 1 (49).

If the direction of blood flow through a given preparation could be reversed without change of the microvascular pathways, would Eq. 168 hold in place of Eq. 167? The answer would be in the affirmative if the longitudinal distributions f(x), g(x) of the effective rate constants p,m depended only on densities of enzymes which are confined to the interior of hepatocytes and do not redistribute themselves in response to changes in the rate of blood flow. However, the rate of conversion of the precursor phenacetin to the metabolite acetaminophen depends also on ambient oxygen concentration, and the rate of conjugation of the metabolite acetaminophen depends on the presence of the conjugating sulfates and glucuronides. Oxygen, sulfates and glucuronides are mobile co-reactants with longitudinal distributions influenced by the rate and direction of blood flow, so that the effective first-order rate constants p,m have an implicit dependence on F in addition to their explicit proportionality to 1/F (10). The experimentally difficult subject of flow reversal effects is at present under investigation in several laboratories.

The mobile co-reactants are responsible for the distinction between enzyme densities and enzyme activities, which is particularly important in the context of the intact perfused organ (10). Enzymological studies (cf. references in (11),(16),(49)) have found enrichment of metabolizing enzymes downstream of an enrichment of conjugating enzymes; if enzyme densities made the decisive contributions to the forms of f(x) and g(x), then Eq.168 should hold more closely than Eq. 167, and E should be substantially smaller than E*. However, the foregoing kinetic analysis detects distributions of enzyme activities rather than densities. The gradients of the mobile co-reactants favour the hypothesis underlying Eq. 167 (10), and it seems from Eqs. 172 and from Table 3 that they have much greater influence on the form of f(x) and g(x) than existing distributions of enzyme densities. If this interpretation is correct, then we would not expect Eq. 167 to be replaced by Eq. 168 on reversing the direction of blood flow.

Whereas the foregoing kinetic analysis yields information about locations of functional zones relative to the direction of blood flow (upstream-downstream relations), it reveals nothing about the actual physical sizes of these zones in the organ. That gap can be filled from a quite different point of view. Having noted in Section 3 that the indifference of input-output relations of a single substrate to a longitudinal organization of uptake is removed when the flow is unsteady, we now sketch an experimental method for estimating the spatial domain in which uptake takes place. To complement the results obtained above, the substrates to be investigated could be phenacetin, and preformed acetaminophen. For simplicity we continue to use mainly the undistributed model of uptake, and we shall assume rectangular longitudinal distributions f(x), g(x), as for $\rho(x)/V_{max}$ in Eqs. 54 in Section 3.

We return to the calculations of uptake from blood pulsating with the period τ about a mean flow rate $\bar{F}$ (Section 3, Eqs. 60-74). Extraction was seen to be detectably higher at short τ than at long τ: the essential point is that here τ is "short" and "long" as compared with $T=AL/\bar{F}$, where AL is the actual volume in which uptake takes place in the organ. Now, if τ is varied experimentally by a suitable control of the pump perfusing a preparation, so that the change in extraction is detected at some $\tau=\tau^*\approx T$, then $AL\cong\bar{F}\tau^*$ can be inferred. While the discussion (i)-(iii) following Eq. 66 holds for any shape and amplitude of the periodic pulsation, the essentials of the change of uptake with τ are brought out explicitly in Eqs. 72-75. At very long τ we have from Eq. 73 the effect of heterogeneity on uptake according to Eq. 74, which is familiar from Section 4 except that here we generate our own temporal heterogeneity by the control of the perfusion pump. The non-negative second term on the right-hand side of Eq. 73 gives the extra venous outflow of the substrate (in excess of $\bar{c}_o=c(\bar{F})$) due to the temporal heterogeneity, for all values of τ. We see that as we reduce τ experimentally from the high values for which Eq. 74 is valid, the first zero of the heterogeneity term is encountered when $AL/\bar{F}\tau^*=1$, where $\bar{F}$ and $\tau=\tau^*$ are observed. Subsequent zeros of the heterogeneity term at $AL/\bar{F}\tau=2,3,4...$ are less distinct because the magnitude of the heterogeneity term varies with the inverse square of $AL/\bar{F}\tau$.

Thus the volume AL may be estimated for each of several substrates of interest in the same preparation. If in addition the mean transit times $\bar{T}'$ of the substrates between instruments are estimated by standard methods (20), then we can estimate for each substrate the fraction $T/\bar{T}'=AL/\overline{FT}'$ of the time spent in the relevant uptake zone, which is approximately equal to the fractional path length through that zone. We note that the actual transverse heterogeneity of uptake (Section 4) will replace the zeros of the second term in Eq. 73 by non-zero minima, since the sinusoidal counterparts of $AL/\bar{F}$ cannot be expected to be identical for all pathways through the relevant uptake zone. The importance of this complication remains to be seen in actual experimental effects. Here we note only that it may be helpful to study the area under $\bar{c}_0/c(\bar{F})-1$ plotted as a function of τ: Eq. 74 gives the maximum value of the ordinate, while the predicted area can be calculated exactly from Eq. 73 because the integral of $\sin^2 x/x^2$ (with $x=\pi AL/\bar{F}\tau$) along all of the positive real axis is $\pi/2$.

To show the practicality of the proposed experiment, we recall that the volume of a human or pig liver is of the order of 1 l, and the physiological rate of blood flow is of the order of 1 l/min; for the rat liver both these quantities are reduced by a factor of about 10^{-2}. About a quarter of each volume is filled with blood, and about a half with hepatocytes. The transit time of an intravascular substance is thus of the order 0.25 min = 15 sec, while a substance equilibrated between blood and hepatocytes has transit time of the order of 45 sec. If the microcirculatory pathways through each of three consecutive functional zones (11) were about equally long, zone-specific substrates would be taken up for some 15 sec in a single pass. Thus the proposed experimental scanning of pulsation periods τ from longer to shorter than any of the aforementioned transit times would impose no impracticable demands on the control of a perfusion pump, or on the durability of an isolated perfused preparation used over many pulsation periods. Moreover, the equilibration of the relevant substrates across the hepatocyte membrane (25) could keep pace readily with the periodic changes in flow rates at the requisite frequencies.

9. OPTIMAL CONTROL OF HEPATIC DETOXIFICATION?

In comparing the predictions of the ratio M_0/P_i for three special arrangements of f(x) and g(x) with data from phenacetin and acetaminophen in Section 8, we had noted that the two unsuccessful Eqs. 168 and 169 predicted systematically larger values of M_0/P_i than the successful Eq. 167. We now show that Eq. 167 predicts the smallest M_0/P_i that can be obtained by <u>any</u> choice of functions f(x), g(x) which are non-negative and normalized on the interval $0 \le x \le L$. We shall see that the solution of the problem of minimizing the functional M_0/P_i given by Eq. 165 is highly non-unique, but that all the minimizing pairs f,g yield the same minimum given by Eq. 167. After proving this result, we shall generalize the problem to other uptake kinetics, and discuss its possible physiological significance.

Since we expect (and shall find) the minimizing f(x) and g(x) to be zero on parts of the interval, the classical Euler-Lagrange variational approach is inadmissible because it would violate the non-negative character of f and g. We proceed as follows. We define the non-decreasing functions

$$\phi(x) = \int_0^x f(u)du \ , \quad \phi(0) = 0 \ , \quad \phi(L) = 1 \tag{173}$$

$$\psi(x) = \int_0^x g(u)du \ , \quad \psi(0) = 0 \ , \quad \psi(L) = 1 \ , \tag{174}$$

and furthermore

$$X(x) = e^{-p\phi} \ , \quad X(0) = 1 \ , \quad X(L) = e^{-p} \tag{175}$$

$$Y(x) = e^{m\psi} \ , \quad Y(0) = 1 \ , \quad Y(L) = e^{m} \ . \tag{176}$$

Then, from Eq. 165,

$$I = e^m M_o/P_i = p\int_0^L \phi' e^{-p\phi+m\psi}dx = \int_{e^{-p}}^1 YdX \ ; \tag{177}$$

here and below, prime denotes a derivative with respect to x. Using X and Y as rectangular Cartesians in Fig.12, we need to connect the points (1,1) and (e^{-p},e^m) by a curve which minimizes the area I under it. That curve, represented parametrically in term of x, is constrained by the conditions

$$X' = -pe^{-p\phi}\phi' \leqq 0 \ , \quad Y' = me^{m\psi}\psi' \geqq 0 \tag{178}$$

which follow from Eqs. 173-177 because f and g are non-negative: hence dY/dX must not be positive. The minimum area is obtained by first proceeding from (e^{-p},e^m) parallel to the Y-axis to $(e^{-p},1)$, and then parallel to the X-axis to (1,1). The x-dependence of ϕ and ψ is thus immaterial as long as the change in ϕ from 0 to 1 is completed before the change in ψ commences; that is, as long as f(x) and g(x) do not overlap, and $f(x)\neq 0$ at smaller x than $g(x)\neq 0$. Hence, from Fig.12,

$$M_o/P_i = e^{-m}I_{min} = e^{-m}(1-e^{-p}) \ , \tag{179}$$

as in Eq. 167. Similarly, the maximum of M_o/P_i is, from Fig. 12,

$$M_o/P_i = e^{-m}I_{max} = 1-e^{-p} \ , \tag{180}$$

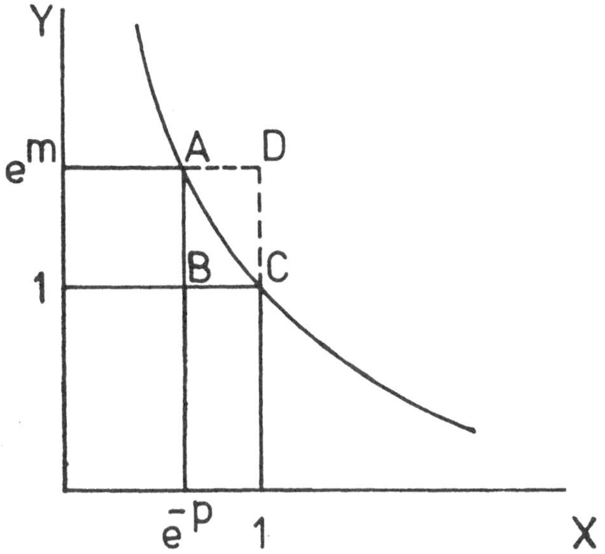

FIG.12

The two unknown functions of x can be transformed to X(x), Y(x) so that the path ABC minimizes, and ADC maximizes, the integral of interest. The hyperbolic path AC expresses a classical view of liver cells.

as in Eq. 168: here the positions of the non-overlapping f(x) and g(x) are interchanged. These results seem to be intuitively transparent from the kinetic point of view. The outflux of M is minimized if all metabolite is created from the precursor upstream of the conjugating enzymes, so that none misses any opportunity of being conjugated. On the other hand, if all creation of the metabolite from the precursor takes place downstream of the conjugating enzymes, then there is no conjugation, and M_o/P_i is maximal. By contrast, the classical hypothesis of the functional homogeneity of liver cells (11) implies f(x)=g(x) ($\phi=\psi$), so that

$$Y = X^{-m/p} \tag{181}$$

from Eqs. 175 and 176; this is the hyperbola drawn in Fig.12. In that case

$$M_o/P_i = e^{-m}I = \frac{p}{p-m}(e^{-m}-e^{-p}) , \tag{182}$$

as in Eq. 169.

We note that the minimization and maximization results are the same in the undistributed and distributed models: P_i is the same for all sinusoids because of their common inlet, so that if M_o/P_i is minimized (maximized) for each sinusoid, it is minimized (maximized) for the whole liver.

A much more difficult minimization problem for M_o/P_i arises when the first-order kinetics of tracers in Eqs. 156, 158 and 160 is replaced by Michaelis-Menten or other non-linear kinetics, such as that in Eqs. 91 or 92. Then the functional M_o/P_i can no longer be calculated explicitly as in Eq. 165, but it remains implicit in the differential equations and their boundary conditions. We shall deal with this novel mathematical problem elsewhere. Here we remark only that the foregoing choices of f and g which minimized M_o/P_i for linear kinetics, cannot be expected to solve the general problem. Suppose for example that the kinetics of metabolization is again first-order, but that conjugation is subject to substrate inhibition as in Eq. 92. If $f(x)\neq 0$ was wholly upstream of $g(x)\neq 0$, inhibition of conjugation could be increased at will by choosing a sufficiently large P_i. However, if some of the metabolization was transferred to a location downstream of the conjugation, some metabolite would lose its chance of conjugation, but that effect might be more than balanced by the effect of reducing the inhibition of conjugation.

It is tempting to speculate (10)about the possible advantages (in the sense of natural selection) of a zonal arrangement of liver functions. The variety of substances which can be synthesized and modified by the liver would be greatly restricted if no by-products toxic to the brain and other organs (9) were to occur. This obstacle to evolution would be removed by placing all potentially deleterious hepatic production in a zone located upstream of a detoxifying zone. If we regard acetaminophen produced in the liver from phenacetin as the model of an endogeneously produced toxic substance, then the actual minimization of its output concentration M_o (at any given level of P_i), demonstrated in Section 8 from data (16), exemplifies optimal control of detoxification brought about by the zonal structure of liver function.

10.CONCLUDING REMARKS

The reader will have noted our efforts, throughout this Chapter, to bring theory and experiment (mathematical modeling and clinical practice) to bear on each other. In addition to the obligation imposed on us by the subtitle of the present volume, we have philosophical reasons for this attitude.

The author of the thoughtful article (50) entitled "The unreasonable effectiveness of mathematics in the natural sciences" was concerned with physics and chemistry. After attempting to revive our astonishment (blunted by familiarity) at that effectiveness, he concluded that there is an unresolved and perhaps unresolvable mystery about it.

Is there a corresponding effectiveness of mathematics in the biological sciences? We think that the question is still unanswered, and that it can be answered only by careful attention to data. Since we do not know the reason for the effectiveness of mathematics in physics and chemistry (50), we can make no prediction for biology. In particular, we cannot assume that the most elegant a priori mathematical constructions are most likely to be true in biology. We cannot improve on the classic formulation of our basic concerns (51):

"Everyone is agreed that figures have the right of entry into Natural Science, but when it becomes a matter of reasoning about these figures, or of dealing mathematically with them, there is encountered a resistance, a repugnance. Why is this? It must be admitted that this resistance does not always come from narrowmindedness or from conservatism. Reasoning in general does not frighten a naturalist, but mathematical reasoning startles him, because he is in the habit of verifying each step by experiment. In reasoning, experimental results are subjected to a series of logical operations. The accuracy of the ultimate result depends on that of the initial data, and also on the number and nature of the logical operations carried out between the premise and the conclusion. In ordinary reasoning, this number is not very great, and successive stages are always verifiable. In mathematical reasoning, the steps are taken too quickly, and a result is reached which may appear to be, and very often is, arbitrary or untrue. The reason for this is that in establishing a biological equation, the problem is simplified by sacrificing a number of factors or a number of details, and these sacrifices distort the results that emerge from the logical method. Inexact yet acceptable initial hypotheses are transformed into gross errors by a few turns of the crank of the logical apparatus. Simplification gives rise to paradox. This is a fact that cannot be denied, and one that is common to all experimental sciences. In purely mathematical problems, the mathematician is certain of his premise and the number and nature of the operations is of interest only from the aesthetic point of view; but in dealing with applications of mathematics, the position is quite different. A long period of development has been necessary to secure unquestioning acceptance of the agreement between reasoning and experiment in mechanics, physics and astronomy. Perhaps in biology this development will be more rapid by virtue of an acquired impetus. In any case, long and continuous collaboration between mathematicians and biologists is necessary before reaching the same assurance as in the physical sciences."

Developments in the half century since this was written have, if anything, underlined the need for caution. In Section 7 we have touched upon the risks inherent in the power of high speed computers to enforce quantitative agreement between theories and data. At the other extreme, mathematical analyses of qualitative features of families of possible biological equations (52) are unlikely to generate amongst biologists confidence in the effectiveness of mathematics, until refutability in some quantitative, statistically significant sense is brought about by a closer relation to real data.

If the work of this Chapter has shown some biological effectiveness of non-trivial mathematics, it is because principles of biological function entail simplifications that lend leverage to mathematically simple concepts. For example, optimal blood-tissue interaction is attained in perfused organs by manifolding the organ blood flow through capillaries just wide enough to permit passage of blood cells. The resulting motion of thin plugs of plasma (delimited by blood cells) through the capillaries brings about the simplifications in the description of flow and uptake, which were exploited above. If this was not so, substrate diffusion in the blood would enforce overall modeling by partial differential equations of the second order (e.g., (53)) rather than of first order (e.g., (25),(27-30)). The resulting difficulty would not be in solving the mathematical problem of uptake (by digital computer), but in formulating it: the requisite boundary conditions would now require the specification of the precise geometry of all capillaries or (in practice) their replacement by copies of some representative capillary. The weakness of this last proposal "is, however, obvious to all who have looked at functioning capillaries under a microscope" (33). Modeling by first order partial differential equations can thus be regarded as more robust than by second order equations, because in the former case the results are insensitive to architectural details of capillary shapes which Nature would surely not reproduce precisely in millions of copies in any one organ.

Another example of the influence of functional design on mathematical structure is the good first approximation furnished by the undistributed model of liver uptake, which permits the perturbation by heterogeneity to be introduced as a higher approximation (Section 4). The liver is so positioned in the circulation that substances from the intestines, toxic substances in particular, must first pass through it before reaching other organs. If the distribution of $w=v_{max}/f$ in Section 4 (and hence the extractive properties of the sinusoids) was too widely dispersed about the ensemble average $\bar{w}=V_{max}/F$, the detoxifying function of the first-pass arrangement would be lost, as in pathological states such as liver cirrhosis. Another, rather more speculative example of a functional design resulting in a mathematically simple concept was developed in Section 9.

We emphasize that the influence of such biological design principles on the success or failure of mathematical models and techniques can be recognised only *a posteriori*, expecially in relation to analyses of data.

FOOTNOTE

*Now at the Department of Nuclear Physics, Weizmann Institute of Science, Rehovot, Israel.

ACKNOWLEDGMENTS

The hitherto unpublished material in Section 2 owes much to discussions with Dr. K. Winkler and Prof. N. Tygstrup; that in Section 3, to additional information from Prof. C. Crone on the experiment in (17), and to the computational skills of Mr. J. Zornig. Our gratitude to many colleagues is recorded in papers quoted below, and so is our appreciation of financial support from Australian and Danish granting bodies.

REFERENCES

1. Bass L, Keiding S, Winkler K, Tygstrup N: Enzymatic elimination of substances flowing through the intact liver. J theor Biol 61:393-409, 1976

2. Brauer RW: Liver circulation and function. Physiol Rev 43: 115-213, 1963

3. Keiding S, Johansen S, Winkler K, Tønnesen K, Tygstrup N: Michaelis-Menten kinetics of galactose elimination by the isolated perfused pig liver. Amer J Physiol 230: 1302-1313, 1976

4. Johansen S, Keiding S: A family of models for the elimination of substrate in the liver. J theor Biol 89: 549-556,1981

5. Dixon M, Webb EC: Enzymes. 3rd edition. London, Longman, 1979

6. Bass L, Robinson PJ, Bracken AJ: Hepatic elimination of flowing substrates: the distributed model. J theor Biol 72: 161-184, 1978

7. Bass L, Robinson PJ: Effects of capillary heterogeneity on rates of steady uptake by the intact liver. Microvasc Res 22: 43-57, 1981

8. Bass L: Flow-dependence of first-order uptake of substances by heterogeneous perfused organs. J theor Biol 86: 365-376, 1980

9. Mitchell JR, Jollows DJ: Metabolic activation of drugs to toxic substances. Gastroenterology 68: 392-410, 1975

10. Bass L: Functional zones in the liver. Gastroenterology 81: 976-977, 1981

11. Gumucio JJ, Miller DL: Functional implications of liver cell heterogeneity. Gastroenterology 80: 393-403, 1981

12. Bass L: On the location of cellular functions in perfused organs. J theor Biol 82: 347-351, 1980

13. Crone C: The permeability of capillaries in various organs as determined by use of indicator diffusion method. Acta Physiol Scand 58: 292-305, 1963

14. Bass L, Robinson PJ: Capillary permeability of heterogeneous organs: a parsimonious interpretation of indicator diffusion

data. Clin Exp Pharmacol Physiol 9: 363-388, 1982.

15. Brauer RW, Leong GF, McElroy RF, Holloway RJ: Circulatory pathways in the rat liver as revealed by P^{32} chromic phosphate colloid uptake in the isolated perfused liver preparation. Amer J Physiol 184: 593-598, 1956

16. Pang KS, Gillette JR: Kinetics of metabolite formation and elimination in the perfused rat liver preparation: differences between the elimination of preformed acetaminophen and acetaminophen formed from phenacetin. J Pharmacol Exp Ther 207: 178-194, 1978

17. Crone C, Frøkjaer-Jensen J, Friedman JJ, Christensen O: The permeability of single capillaries to potassium ions. J General Physiol 71: 198-220, 1978

18. Bracken AJ, Bass L: Statistical mechanics of hepatic elimination. Math Biosci 44: 97-120, 1979

19. Tygstrup N: Determination of hepatic galactose elimination capacity after a single intravenous injection in man. Acta Physiol Scand 58: 162-172, 1963

20. Lassen NA, Perl W: Tracer kinetic methods in medical physiology. New York, Raven Press, 1979

21. Crick FHC: Thinking about the brain. Sci American 241: 181-188, 1979

22. Tygstrup N, Winkler K: Kinetics of galactose·elimination. Acta Physiol Scand 32: 354-362, 1954

23. Vink CLJ: The half-life concept in the determination of the functional capacity of the liver. Clin chim Acta 4: 583-590, 1959

24. Burgen ASV: A theoretical treatment of glucose reabsorbtion in the kidney. J Biochem Physiol 34: 466-474, 1956

25. Bass L, Bracken AJ: Time-dependent elimination of substrates flowing through the liver or kidney. J theor Biol 67: 637-652, 1977

26. Crone C: Facilitated transfer of glucose from blood into brain tissue. J Physiol 181: 103-113, 1965

27. Sangren WC, Sheppard CW: Mathematical derivation of the exchange of a labeled substance between a liquid flowing in a vessel and an external compartment. Bull Math Biophys 15: 387-394, 1953

28. Goresky CA, Ziegler WH, Bach GG: Capillary exchange modeling. Circul Res 27: 739-764, 1970

29. Goresky CA, Bach GG, Nadeau BE: On the uptake of materials by the intact liver. The transport and net removal of galactose. J clin Invest 52: 991-998, 1973

30. Goresky CA: The interstitial space in the liver: its partitioning effects. Capillary Permeability (C Crone and NA Lassen, Eds), pp 415-430, Copenhagen, Munksgaard, 1970

31. Ballard FJ: Purification and properties of galactokinase from pig liver. Biochem J 98: 347-352, 1966

32. Robinson PJ: Aspects of mathematical liver kinetics. Ph.D. Thesis, University of Queensland, 1979. Univ.Microfilms Int., Ann Arbor, Mich.

33. Crone C: Capillary permeability - techniques and problems. Capillary Permeability (C Crone and NA Lassen, Eds), pp 15-31, Copenhagen, Munksgaard, 1970

34. Holt JN, Bracken AJ: First-kind Fredholm equation of liver kinetics: numerical solution by constrained least squares. Math Biosci 51: 11-24, 1980

35. Jeffreys H, Jeffreys BS: Methods of Mathematical Physics. 2nd edition. London, Cambridge University Press, 1950

36. Copson ET: Asymptotic Expansions. London, Cambridge University Press, 1950

37. Keiding S, Johansen S, Midtboll I, Rabøl A, Christiansen L: Ethanol elimination kinetics in human and pig liver in vivo. Amer J Physiol 237(4): 316-324, 1979

38. Keiding S, Vilstrup H, Hansen L: Importance of flow and haematocrit for metabolic function of perfused rat liver. Scand J clin Lab Invest 40: 355-359, 1980

39. Bass L, Robinson PJ: How small is the functional variability of liver sinusoids? J theor Biol 81: 761-769, 1979

40. Crone C, Christensen O: Transcapillary transport of small solutes and water. International Review of Physiology,18 (AC Guyton and DB Young, Eds), pp 149-212, Baltimore, University Park Press 1979

41. Rose CP, Goresky CA: Vasomotor control of capillary transit time heterogeneity in the canine coronary circulation. Circul Res 39: 541-554, 1976

42. Bronikowski TA, Linehan JH, Dawson CA: A mathematical analysis of the influence of perfusion heterogeneity on indicator extraction. Math Biosci 52: 27-51, 1980

43. Gillis CN, Cronan LH, Mandel S, Hammond GL: Indicator dilution measurement of 5-hydroxytryptamine clearance by human lung. J Appl Physiol 46: 1178-1183, 1979

44. Bronikowski TA, Dawson CA, Linehan JH, Rickaby DA: A mathematical model of indicator extraction by the pulmonary endothelium via saturation kinetics. Math Biosci 61: 237-266, 1982

45. Russell B: Human Knowledge : Its Scope and Limits. London, Allen and Unwin, 1948, pp 329-330

46. Keiding S, Chiarantini E: Effects of sinusoidal perfusion on galactose elimination in perfused rat liver. J Pharmacol Exp Ther 205: 465-470, 1978

47. Bass L: Current models of hepatic elimination. Gastroenterology 76: 1504-1505, 1979

48. Bass L: Estimates and implications of co-operativity for enzyme kinetics in the intact liver: method of flow invariants. J theor Biol 100:113-121

49. Bass L: Functional zones in rat liver: the degree of overlap. J theor Biol 89: 303-319, 1981

50. Wigner EP: The unreasonable effectiveness of mathematics in the natural sciences. Symmetries and Reflections. Bloomington & London, Indiana University Press, 1967, pp 222-237

51. Kostitzin VA: Mathematical Biology. London, G. Harrap, 1939, pp 16-17

52. Thom R: Stabilité Structurelle et Morphogénèse. New York, Benjamin, 1972

53. Bassingthwaighte JB, Knopp TJ, Hazelrig JB: A concurrent flow model for capillary-tissue exchanges. Capillary Permeability (C Crone and NA Lassen, Eds), pp 60-80, Copenhagen, Munksgaard, 1970

APPENDIX I

The case of capillary uptake rate and cross-section varying along the flow

In this general case Eq. 36 is

$$A(x)\frac{\partial c}{\partial t} + F(t)\frac{\partial c}{\partial x} = -\rho(x)\frac{c}{c+K_m} , \qquad (I.1)$$

and we seek solutions $c(x,t)$ in $0 \leq x \leq L$, given some $A(x)$, $\rho(x)$,

F(t), and the input concentration $c_i(t)=c(0,t)$ at all times. In particular, we seek the output concentration $c_o(t)=c(L,t)$. Again, Eq.38 transforms Eq. (I.1) into

$$A\frac{\partial u}{\partial t} + F\frac{\partial u}{\partial x} = -\rho \; . \tag{I.2}$$

The equations of characteristics belonging to Eq. (I.2) are

$$dx/F(t) = dt/A(x) = -du/\rho(x) \; . \tag{I.3}$$

The first of these equations determines the motion of any element of the indicator or substrate from inlet to outlet. If the element enters the capillary at time t and leaves it at time t', that equation gives by integration

$$\int_0^{x(t')} A(\xi)d\xi = \int_t^{t'} F(v)dv \; , \tag{I.4}$$

where ξ and v are dummy variables; the time variable t' is in the interval $t \leq t' \leq t+T$. T is defined here (as in Eq.58a) by the complete transit starting at time t and sweeping out the volume of the capillary:

$$\int_0^{L} A(\xi)d\xi = \int_t^{t+T} F(v)dv \; . \tag{I.5}$$

Eq. (I.4) specifies x(t') implicitly, without involving T. If A is constant along the capillary, Eq. (I.4) gives x(t') explicitly, since the left-hand side becomes Ax(t').

We thus know x(t') for any element that has entered the capillary at time t, so that the second of Eqs. (I.3) can be written

$$-du = \frac{\rho[x(t')]}{A[x(t')]}dt' \; , \tag{I.6}$$

where the right-hand side is a function of t' through the x given by Eq. (I.4). Integrating from the inlet x=0 which is passed at t'=t, to the outlet x=L passed at t'=t+T, we obtain

$$u(L,t+T) - u(0,t) = -\int_t^{t+T} \frac{\rho[x(t')]}{A[x(t')]}dt' \; . \tag{I.7}$$

Reverting to the original variable through Eq. 38 we obtain:

$$c_o(t+T) + K_m \ln c_o(t+T) = c_i(t) + K_m \ln c_i(t) - \int_t^{t+T} \frac{\rho[x(t')]}{A[x(t')]}dt' \; , \tag{I.8}$$

where $x(t')$ is given by Eq. (I.4), and T by Eq. (I.5).

Changing the time variable from t to t-T in Eqs. (I.5) and (I.8), we obtain the desired generalization of Eq. 59. When F and A are constants, Eq. (I.4) gives

$$Ax(t') = F(t'-t) \ , \quad Adx(t') = Fdt' \ . \tag{I.9}$$

Using this, and AL=FT from Eq. (I.5), to change the variable from t' to x(t'), the integral in Eq. (I.8) becomes V_{max}/F according to Eq. 4.

APPENDIX II

Uptake from flow pulsating with a small amplitude

We consider the periodic flow rate given by Eq. 72, in the form

$$F = \bar{F}[(1+F_1/F)\cos\omega t] \ , \tag{II.1}$$

where $F_1/\bar{F}$ is small, and

$$\omega = 2\pi/\tau \ . \tag{II.2}$$

We show that Eq. 75 is valid to order $(F_1/\bar{F})^2$. Since the input concentration c_i is independent of time, Eq. 59 becomes

$$c_o(t) + K_m \ln c_o(t) = c_i + K_m \ln c_i - V_{max}T/(AL) \ , \tag{II.3}$$

where the transit time T is defined by Eq. 58.

We first calculate T explicitly to order $(F_1/\bar{F})^2$. Substituting Eq. (II.1) in Eq. 58 we obtain a transcendental equation for T:

$$T = AL/\bar{F} + (F_1/\omega\bar{F})[\sin\omega(t-T) - \sin\omega t] \ . \tag{II.4}$$

Iterating twice and expanding in powers of $(F_1/\bar{F})$ gives

$$T = AL/\bar{F}+(F_1/\omega\bar{F})[\sin\omega(t-AL/\bar{F})-\sin\omega t][1-(F_1/\bar{F})\cos\omega(t-AL/\bar{F})], \tag{II.5}$$

neglecting terms of order $(F_1/\bar{F})^3$ and higher.

Next we calculate $c_o(t)$ to order $(F_1/\bar{F})^2$. According to Eq. (II.3), c_o depends on t only through T, which differs little from $AL/\bar{F}$ according to Eq. (II.5). We therefore expand c_o about $T=AL/\bar{F}$:

$$c_o(t)=c_o[T(t)]=c_o(AL/\bar{F})+(dc_o/dT)(T-AL/\bar{F})+\tfrac{1}{2}(d^2c_o/dT^2)(T-AL/\bar{F})^2+\ldots \tag{II.6}$$

where the derivatives of c_o with respect to T are evaluated at $T=AL/\bar{F}$, and the dots indicate terms of order $(F_1/\bar{F})^3$ and higher. We evaluate dc_o/dT and d^2c_o/dT^2 from Eq. (II.3):

$$dc_o/dT = -(V_{max}/AL)c_o/(c_o+K_m) \ ,$$

$$d^2c_o/dT^2 = \left[\frac{d}{dc_o}\left(\frac{dc_o}{dT}\right)\right]\frac{dc_o}{dT} = (V_{max}/AL)^2 K_m c_o/(c_o+K_m)^3 \ .$$

Noting that when $T=AL/\bar{F}$, c_o is the solution $c_o(\bar{F})$ of the problem of steady flow with rate $\bar{F}$, we have from Eq. (II.6):

$$c_o(t)=c_o(\bar{F})-\left(\frac{V_{max}}{AL}\right)\frac{c_o(\bar{F})}{c_o(\bar{F})+K_m}(T-AL/\bar{F})+\tfrac{1}{2}\left(\frac{V_{max}}{AL}\right)^2\frac{K_m c_o(\bar{F})}{(c_o(\bar{F})+K_m)^3}(T-AL/\bar{F})^2. \tag{II.7}$$

To calculate the time-averaged outflux $\overline{Fc_o}$, we multiply Eq. (II.7) through with the F(t) given by Eq. (II.1), substitute for $T-AL/\bar{F}$ from Eq. (II.5), and integrate over a full cycle with respect to t (and divide with $\tau = 2\pi/\omega$). A lengthy but straightforward calculation shows that all terms vanish or cancel out except

$$\overline{Fc_o}=\bar{F}c_o(\bar{F})+\tfrac{1}{2}\bar{F}\left(\frac{V_{max}}{AL}\right)^2\frac{K_m c_o(\bar{F})}{(c_o(\bar{F})+K_m)^3}\left(\frac{F_1}{\omega\bar{F}}\right)^2\overline{[\sin\omega(t-AL/\bar{F})-\sin\omega t]^2} \ ,$$

and the last factor is $2\sin^2(\omega AL/2\bar{F})$. Using Eq. (II.2), the definition of $\bar{c}_o = \overline{Fc_o}/\bar{F}$ by Eq. 61, and some rearrangement, we arrive at Eq. 73.

BASIC PRINCIPLES UNDERLYING RADIOISOTOPIC METHODS FOR ASSAY OF BIOCHEMICAL PROCESSES *IN VIVO*

Louis Sokoloff and Carolyn B. Smith

Laboratory of Cerebral Metabolism,
National Institute of Mental Health, Bethesda, MD

INTRODUCTION

Radioisotopes are frequently used to facilitate the assay of biochemical reactions. Usually they are used to study chemical reactions *in vitro*, and the procedure is to label one of the reactants and to measure the rate of accumulation of a labeled product (see General Equation in Fig.1B). From assay or knowledge of the specific activity of the reactant molecule, the rate of the overall reaction rate can be calculated from the rate of radioactive product formation. The application of this approach generally necessitates, however, specialized biochemical procedures to isolate and identify the labeled product and to limit the measurement of the radioactivity to the chemical product of the reaction.

Quantitative autoradiography makes it possible to measure the concentrations of isotopes in tissues of animals labeled *in vivo*. In a few cases, the administration of a judiciously selected labeled chemical compound and the design of an appropriate procedure has made it possible to use this capability to measure the rate of a chemical process in animals *in vivo*. Emission tomography, and particularly positron-emission tomography, provides a means to extend this capability to man and to assay the rates of biochemical processes in human tissues *in vivo*. It does not, however, obviate the need to adhere to established principles of chemical and enzyme kinetics and tracer theory.

A chemical reaction is the conversion of one species of molecule to another. The rate of this reaction can be measured by determining the rate of disappearance of one or more of the reactants or the formation of one or more of the products. The addition of a radioactive label to one of the reactants in molecular concentrations too negligible to alter the kinetics of the reaction facilitates the measurement of either the reactants or the products, but it does not solve all the problems. The rate of chemical transformation of the labeled species can easily be measured, but this is not the rate of the reaction of interest. To derive the rate of the total reaction from measurement of the reaction rate of the labeled species, it is necessary to know the integrated specific activity (i.e., the ratio of labeled to total molecules) of the precursor pool. Occasionally the labeled species exhibits a kinetic difference from the natural compound, the so-called isotope effect; this isotope effect can be evaluated and appropriate correction made for it. In assays of biochemical reactions in vivo it is generally impossible to measure the integrated specific activity of the precursor pool directly. This would require the measurement of the complete time courses of the concentrations of the labeled and unlabeled precursor molecules in the tissue at the enzyme site. It is, therefore, necessary to determine the precursor pool specific activity indirectly from measurements in the blood supplied to the tissue. The specific activity in the arterial blood or plasma can be readily measured directly, and the precursor-specific activity calculated from it by correcting for the lag in the equilibration of the precursor pool in the tissue with that of the plasma. To apply this correction it is necessary to know the kinetics of the equilibration process between the precursor pools in the tissue and plasma.

The rate of a chemical reaction can be determined by measurement of precursor disappearance or product accumulation; generally the errors are smaller with the latter measurement because the percent increase in amount of product is much greater than the percent loss in amount of precursor. Autoradiography and emission tomography, which measure only the total concentration of the radioactive molecules, cannot distinguish among the various chemical species which may be labeled, neither the precursor nor any of the possible labeled products. Strategies must, therefore, be developed that ensure that the radioactivity is contained exclusively in the precursor and/or in one or more of the products specific to the chemical reaction to be assayed. The labeled precursor should be so selected that its chemical transformations are limited only to the pathway under study.

These general principles have been more or less successfully applied in two currently operational methods for the measurement of energy metabolism in the nervous system of animals and man. One method is the steady-state O_2 consumption technique which is based on the measurement of substrate disappearance (1). Cerebral blood flow is measured by positron-emission tomography with $C^{15}O_2$ and, when multiplied by arterial O_2 content, provides the steady state delivery of O_2 to the tissues. Local cerebral O_2 extraction from the blood is measured by positron-emission tomography with $^{15}O_2$. The product of local oxygen extraction, blood flow, and arterial O_2 content provides the values for local O_2 consumption. The other method is the radioactive deoxyglucose technique for the measurement of local cerebral glucose utilization. It has been used extensively in animals with autoradiography (2,3), but it has been adapted to man by the use of $[^{18}F]$fluorodeoxyglucose and positron-emission tomography. The deoxyglucose technique is based on the measurement of product accumulation. Because it encompasses almost all the principles to be considered in the measurement of biochemical processes _in vivo_, it will serve as an informative example of their application. A comparable method, but one designed to measure local rates of cerebral protein synthesis, is currently under development (4), and it serves to illustrate additional problems in the assay of biochemical processes _in vivo_.

THE DEOXYGLUCOSE METHOD

Theoretical Basis

The deoxyglucose method was developed to measure the rates of glucose utilization simultaneously in all structural and/or functional components of the central nervous system in conscious animals (2). It was developed first for use with [^{14}C]deoxyglucose and was designed specifically to take advantage of the localization made possible by quantitative autoradiography although its principles are equally applicable with any type of emission tomography as well. Although the purpose was to measure the local rates of glucose utilization, the analogue of glucose, 2-deoxy-D-glucose, rather than glucose itself, was selected as the labeled precursor because its biochemical properties make it easier to adhere to the essential biochemical principles for the measurement of a biochemical process *in vivo* by autoradiography or other emission tomographic techniques. If radioactive glucose is used as the precursor, some of the labeled products of glucose metabolism, particularly CO_2 or water, are lost too rapidly from the tissue, and many other labeled products dependent on additional chemical reactions other than glucose metabolism are retained. With radioactive deoxyglucose as precursor, the label is retained in the tissues in either of two chemical species, the unmetabolized precursor molecule or the immediate product of its metabolism. As will become clear subsequently, the use of deoxyglucose serves to isolate the chemical process under study to a well-defined reaction, the hexokinase-catalyzed phosphorylation of the hexose, the first step in the biochemical pathway of glucose metabolism.

The method was derived by analysis of a model based on the biochemical properties of 2-deoxyglucose and glucose in brain (Fig.1A) (2). 2-Deoxyglucose (DG) is transported bi-directionally between blood and brain by the same carrier that transports glucose across the blood-brain barrier. In the cerebral tissues it is phosphorylated, like glucose, by hexokinase to produce 2-deoxyglucose-6-phosphate (DG-6-P). Deoxyglucose and glucose are, therefore, competitive substrates for both blood-brain transport and hexokinase-catalyzed phosphorylation. Unlike glucose-6-phosphate, however, which is metabolized further eventually to CO_2 and water, DG-6-P cannot be converted to fructose-6-phosphate, and it is also a poor substrate for glucose-6-phosphate dehydrogenase. There is relatively little glucose-6-phosphatase activity in brain and even less deoxyglucose-6-phosphatase activity. Deoxyglucose-6-phosphate, once formed, remains, therefore, essentially trapped in the cerebral tissues, at least for 45 minutes (5).

If the interval of time is kept short enough, for example, 45 minutes, to allow the assumption of negligible loss of $[^{14}C]$DG-6-P from the tissues, then the quantity of $[^{14}C]$DG-6-P accumulated in any cerebral tissue at any given time following the introduction of $[^{14}C]$DG into the circulation is equal to the integral of the rate of $[^{14}C]$DG phosphorylation by hexokinase in that tissue during that interval of time. This integral is in turn related to the amount of glucose that has been phosphorylated over the same interval, depending on the time courses of the relative concentrations of $[^{14}C]$DG and glucose in the precursor pools and the Michaelis-Menten kinetic constants for hexokinase with respect to both $[^{14}C]$DG and glucose. With cerebral glucose consumption in a steady state, the amount of glucose phosphorylated during the interval of time equals the steady state flux of glucose through the hexokinase-catalyzed step times the duration of the interval, and the net rate of flux of glucose through this step equals the rate of glucose utilization.

These relationships can be rigorously combined into a model (Fig.1A) which can be mathematically analyzed to derive an operational equation (Fig.1B), provided that the following assumptions are made: 1) steady state for glucose (i.e., constant plasma glucose concentration and constant rate of glucose consumption) throughout the experimental period; 2) homogeneous tissue compartment within which the concentrations of $[^{14}C]$DG and glucose are uniform and exchange directly with the plasma; and 3) concentrations of $[^{14}C]$DG (i.e., molecular concentrations of free $[^{14}C]$DG essentially equal to zero). The operational equation

A

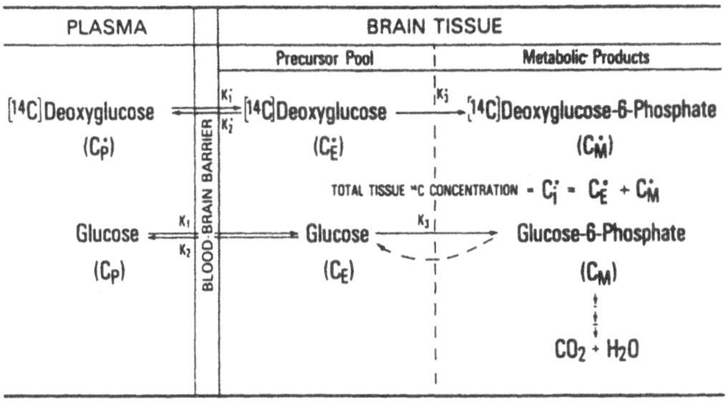

B

Functional Anatomy of the Operational Equation of the [14C] Deoxyglucose Method

General Equation for Measurement of Reaction Rates with Tracers:

$$\text{Rate of Reaction} = \frac{\text{Labeled Product Formed in Interval of Time, 0 to T}}{\begin{bmatrix}\text{Isotope Effect}\\ \text{Correction Factor}\end{bmatrix}\begin{bmatrix}\text{Integrated Specific Activity}\\ \text{of Precursor}\end{bmatrix}}$$

Operational Equation of [14C]Deoxyglucose Method:

$$R_i = \frac{\overbrace{\underbrace{C_i^*(T)}_{\substack{\text{Total }^{14}\text{C in Tissue}\\ \text{at Time, T}}} - \underbrace{k_1^* e^{-(k_2^*+k_3^*)T}\int_0^T C_p^* e^{(k_2^*+k_3^*)t}\,dt}_{^{14}\text{C in Precursor Remaining in Tissue at Time, T}}}^{\text{Labeled Product Formed in Interval of Time, 0 to T}}}{\underbrace{\left[\frac{\lambda \cdot V_m^* \cdot K_m}{\Phi \cdot V_m \cdot K_m^*}\right]}_{\substack{\text{Isotope Effect}\\ \text{Correction}\\ \text{Factor}}}\underbrace{\left[\underbrace{\int_0^T \left(\frac{C_p^*}{C_p}\right) dt}_{\substack{\text{Integrated Plasma}\\ \text{Specific Activity}}} - \underbrace{e^{-(k_2^*+k_3^*)T}\int_0^T \left(\frac{C_p^*}{C_p}\right) e^{(k_2^*+k_3^*)t}\,dt}_{\substack{\text{Correction for Lag in Tissue}\\ \text{Equilibration with Plasma}}}\right]}_{\text{Integrated Precursor Specific Activity in Tissue}}}$$

FIG. 1

Theoretical basis of radioactive deoxyglucose method for measurement of local cerebral glucose utilization (2). A. Diagrammatic representation of the theoretical model. C_i^* represents the total ^{14}C concentration in a single homogeneous tissue of the brain. C_P^* and C_P represent the concentrations of [^{14}C]deoxyglucose and glucose in the arterial plasma, respectively; C_E^* and C_E represent their respective concentrations in the tissue pools that serve as substrates for hexokinase. C_M^* represents the concentration of [^{14}C]deoxyglucose-6-phosphate in the tissue. The constants k_1^*, k_2^*, and k_3^* represent the rate constants for carrier-mediated transport of [^{14}C]deoxyglucose from plasma to tissue, for carrier-mediated transport back from tissue to plasma, and for phosphorylation by hexokinase, respectively; the constants k_1, k_2, and k_3 are the equivalent rate constants for glucose. [^{14}C]Deoxyglucose and glucose share and compete for the carrier that transports both between plasma and tissue and for hexokinase which phosphorylates them to their respective hexose-6-phosphates. The dashed arrow represents the possibility of glucose-6-phosphate hydrolysis by glucose-6-phosphatase activity, if any. B. Operational equation of the radioactive deoxyglucose method and its functional anatomy. T represents the time of termination of the experimental period; λ equals the ratio of the distribution space of deoxyglucose in the tissue to that of glucose; Φ equals the fraction of glucose which once phosphorylated continues down the glycolytic pathway; and K_m^* and V_m^* and K_m and V_m represent the familiar Michaelis-Menten kinetic constants of hexokinase for deoxyglucose and glucose, respectively. The other symbols are the same as those defined in A.

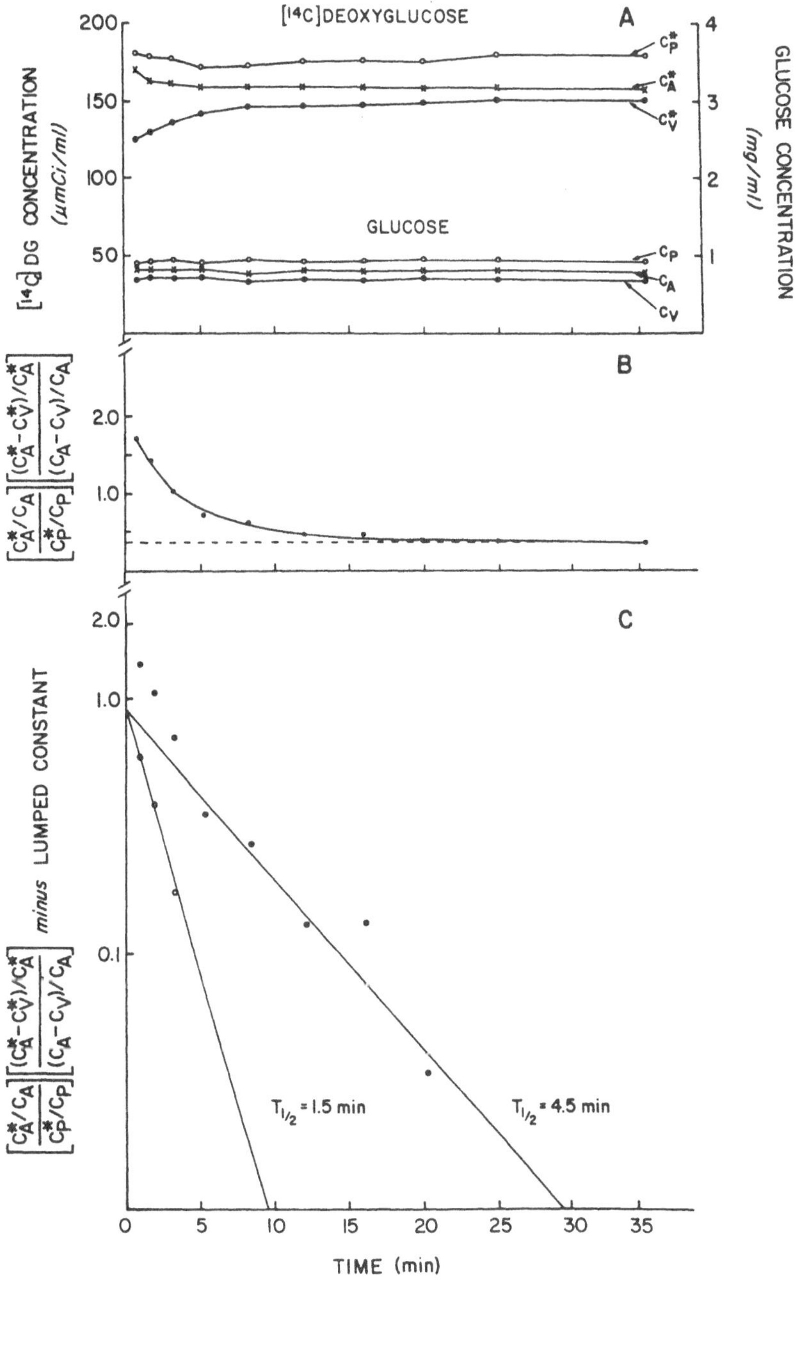

[14C]DEOXYGLUCOSE
A
B
C
GLUCOSE
[14C] DG CONCENTRATION (μmCi/ml)
GLUCOSE CONCENTRATION (mg/ml)
C_P^*
C_A^*
C_V^*
C_P
C_A
C_V
200
150
100
50
4
3
2
1
2.0
1.0
0.1
$\left[\frac{C_A^*/C_A}{C_P^*/C_P}\right]\left[\frac{(C_A^*-C_V^*)/C_A^*}{(C_A-C_V)/C_A}\right]$
minus LUMPED CONSTANT
$T_{1/2}$ = 1.5 min
$T_{1/2}$ = 4.5 min
0
5
10
15
20
25
30
35
TIME (min)

FIG. 2

Data obtained and their use in determination of the lumped constant and the combination of rate constants, $(k_2^* + k_3^*)$, in a representative experiment. (A) Time courses of arterial blood and plasma concentrations of [^{14}C]DG and glucose and cerebral venous blood concentrations of [^{14}C]DG and glucose during programmed intravenous infusion of [^{14}C]DG. (B) Arithmetic plot of the function derived from the variables in A and combined as indicated in the formula on the ordinate against time. This function declines exponentially, with a rate constant equal to $(k_2^* + k_3^*)$, until it reaches an asymptotic value equal to the lumped constant, 0.35, in this experiment (dashed line). (C) Semilogarithmic plot of the curve in B less the lumped constant, i.e., its asymptotic value. Solid circles represent actual values. This curve is analyzed into two components by a standard curve-peeling technique to yield the two straight lines representing the separate components. Open circles are points for the fast component, obtained by subtracting the values for the slow component from the solid circles. The rate constants for these two components represent the values of $(k_2^* + k_3^*)$ for two compartments; the fast and slow compartments are assumed to represent gray and white matter, respectively. In this experiment the values for $(k_2^* + k_3^*)$ were found to equal 0.462 (half-time = 1.5 min) and 0.154 (half-time = 4.5 min) in gray and white matter, respectively (6).

which defines R_i, the rate of glucose utilization per unit mass of tissue, i, in terms of measurable variables is presented in Fig.1B.

The rate constants, k_1^*, k_2^*, and k_3^*, are determined in a separate group of animals by a non-linear, iterative process which provides the least squares best-fit of an equation which defines the time course of tissue ^{14}C concentration in terms of the time, the history of the plasma [^{14}C]DG concentration and the rate constants to the experimentally determined time courses of tissue and plasma concentrations of ^{14}C (2). The λ, Φ, and the enzyme kinetic constants are grouped together to constitute a single, lumped constant (see equation in Fig.1B). It can be shown mathematically that this lumped constant is equal to the asymptotic value of the product of the ratio of the cerebral extraction ratios of [^{14}C]DG and glucose and the ratio of the arterial blood to plasma specific activities when the arterial plasma [^{14}C]DG concentration is maintained constant (2). The lumped constant is also determined in a separate group of animals from arterial and cerebral venous blood samples drawn during a programmed intravenous infusion which produces and maintains a constant arterial plasma [^{14}C]DG concentration (Fig.2) (2,6).

Despite its complex appearance, the operational equation is really nothing more than a general statement of the standard relationship by which rates of enzyme-catalyzed reactions are determined from measurements made with radioactive tracers (Fig.1B). The numerator of the equation represents the amount of radioactive product formed in a given interval of time; it is equal to C_i^*, the combined concentrations of [^{14}C]DG and [^{14}C]DG-6-P in the tissue at time, T, measured by the quantitative autoradiographic technique or emission tomography, less a term that represents the free unmetabolized [^{14}C]DG still remaining in the tissue. The denominator represents the integrated specific activity of the precursor pool times a factor, the lumped constant, which is equivalent to a correction factor for an isotope effect. The term with the exponential factor in the denominator takes into account the lag in the equilibration of the tissue precursor pool with that of the plasma.

By the use of labeled 2-deoxyglucose as a probe, a single biochemical reaction, the first step in the pathway of glucose metabolism has been isolated (Fig.3). This is the hexokinase-catalyzed phosphorylation of glucose. The total amount of radioactive product formed and the integrated specific activity of the precursor at the enzyme site can be determined. From these data and the use of a correction factor, the "lumped constant", for the difference in the kinetic behavior of deoxyglucose and glucose, the net rate of glucose phosphorylation can be calculated by the operational equation. In a steady state the net rate through any step in a pathway equals the net rate through the overall pathway. The deoxyglucose method, therefore, measures *in vivo* the net rate of glucose phosphorylation and in a steady state the net rate of the entire glycolytic pathway.

Applications of Biochemical Principles to Design of Procedure

The operational equation dictates the variables to be measured to determine the local rates of cerebral glucose utilization. The specific procedure employed is designed to evaluate these variables and to minimize potential errors that might occur in the actual application of the method. If the rate constants, k_1^*, k_2^*, and k_3^*, are precisely known, then the equation is generally applicable with any mode of administration of $[^{14}C]$DG and for a wide range of time intervals. At the present time the rate constants have been fully determined for $[^{14}C]$DG only in the conscious rat (2) (Table 1). Partial determination of the rate constants indicates that they are similar in the monkey (6). These rate constants can be expected to vary with the condition of the animal, however, and for most accurate results should be re-determined for each condition studied. The structure of the operational equation suggests a more practical alternative. All the terms in the equation that contain the rate constants approach zero with increasing time if the $[^{14}C]$DG is so administered that the plasma $[^{14}C]$DG concentration also approaches zero. From the values of the rate constants determined in normal animals and the usual time course of the clearance of $[^{14}C]$DG from the arterial

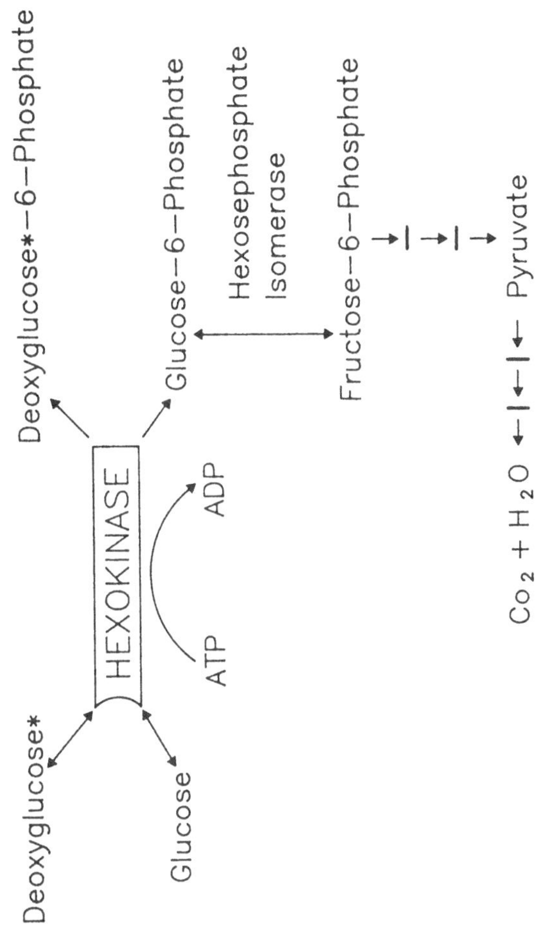
Deoxyglucose*
Glucose
HEXOKINASE
ATP
ADP
Deoxyglucose*–6–Phosphate
Glucose–6–Phosphate
Hexosephosphate
Isomerase
Fructose–6–Phosphate
Pyruvate
Co2 + H2O

FIG. 3

Schema illustrating the fundamental principle of the radioactive deoxyglucose method for the measurement of local cerebral glucose utilization. Glucose utilization commences with the hexokinase-catalyzed phosphorylation of glucose by ATP, but the product of this reaction, glucose-6-phosphate, is not retained in the tissues. Instead, it is metabolized further to products, like CO_2 and H_2O, that leave the tissue. Deoxyglucose, an analogue and competitive substrate with glucose in the hexokinase reaction, leads to a product, deoxyglucose-6-phosphate, that does accumulate in the tissue quantitatively for a reasonable length of time. By putting a label on the deoxyglucose, it is possible to measure the rate of labeled deoxyglucose-6-phosphate formation. From a knowledge of the time course of the relative concentrations of labeled deoxyglucose and glucose in the tissue at the enzyme site and the relative Michaelis-Menten constants of hexokinase for the two substrates, it is possible to calculate how much glucose must have also been phosphorylated during the production of the measured amount of deoxyglucose-6-phosphate. The integrated relative concentrations of labeled deoxyglucose and glucose in the tissue are calculated from the measured time courses of the two compounds in the arterial plasma by subtracting from the integrated plasma specific activity a term that corrects for the lag of the tissue behind the plasma.

TABLE 1. VALUES OF RATE CONSTANTS IN THE NORMAL CONSCIOUS ALBINO RAT

Structure	Rate Constants (min^{-1}) k_1^*	k_2^*	k_3^*	Distribution Volume (ml/g) $k_1^*/(k_2^*+k_3^*)$	Half-Life of Precursor Pool (min) $Log_e 2/(k_2^*+k_3^*)$
		Gray Matter			
Visual Cortex	0.189 ± 0.048	0.279 ± 0.176	0.063 ± 0.040	0.553	2.03
Auditory Cortex	0.226 ± 0.068	0.241 ± 0.198	0.067 ± 0.057	0.734	2.25
Parietal Cortex	0.194 ± 0.051	0.257 ± 0.175	0.062 ± 0.045	0.608	2.17
Sensory-Motor Cortex	0.193 ± 0.037	0.208 ± 0.112	0.049 ± 0.035	0.751	2.70
Thalamus	0.188 ± 0.045	0.218 ± 0.144	0.053 ± 0.043	0.694	2.56
Medial Geniculate Body	0.219 ± 0.055	0.259 ± 0.164	0.055 ± 0.040	0.697	2.21
Lateral Geniculate Body	0.172 ± 0.038	0.220 ± 0.134	0.055 ± 0.040	0.625	2.52
Hypothalamus	0.158 ± 0.032	0.226 ± 0.119	0.043 ± 0.032	0.587	2.58
Hippocampus	0.169 ± 0.043	0.260 ± 0.166	0.056 ± 0.040	0.535	2.19
Amygdala	0.149 ± 0.028	0.235 ± 0.109	0.032 ± 0.026	0.558	2.60
Caudate-Putamen	0.176 ± 0.041	0.200 ± 0.140	0.061 ± 0.050	0.674	2.66
Superior Colliculus	0.138 ± 0.054	0.240 ± 0.166	0.046 ± 0.042	0.692	2.42
Pontine Gray Matter	0.170 ± 0.040	0.246 ± 0.142	0.037 ± 0.033	0.601	2.45
Cerebellar Cortex	0.225 ± 0.066	0.392 ± 0.229	0.059 ± 0.031	0.499	1.54
Cerebellar Nucleus	0.207 ± 0.042	0.194 ± 0.111	0.038 ± 0.035	0.892	2.99
Mean S.E.M.	0.189 ± 0.012	0.245 ± 0.040	0.052 ± 0.010	0.647 ± 0.073	2.39 ± 0.40
		White Matter			
Corpus Callosum	0.085 ± 0.015	0.135 ± 0.075	0.019 ± 0.033	0.552	4.50
Genu of Corpus Callosum	0.076 ± 0.013	0.131 ± 0.075	0.019 ± 0.034	0.507	4.62
Internal Capsule	0.077 ± 0.015	0.134 ± 0.085	0.023 ± 0.039	0.490	4.41
Mean S.E.M.	0.079 ± 0.008	0.133 ± 0.046	0.020 ± 0.020	0.516 ± 0.171	4.51 ± 0.90

From Sokoloff et al., (2).

plasma following a single intravenous pulse at zero time, it has been determined that an interval of 30-45 minutes after a pulse is adequate for these terms to become sufficiently small that considerable latitude in inaccuracies of the rate constants is permissible without appreciable error in the estimates of local glucose consumption (2). An additional advantage derived from the use of a single pulse of [^{14}C]DG followed by a relatively long interval before killing the animal for measurement of local tissue ^{14}C concentration is that by then most of the free [^{14}C]DG in the tissues has been either converted to [^{14}C]DG-6-P or transported back to the plasma; the radioactivity in the tissues and the optical densities in the autoradiographs then represent mainly the concentrations of the product, [^{14}C]DG-6-P, and, therefore, reflect directly the relative rates of glucose utilization in the various cerebral tissues.

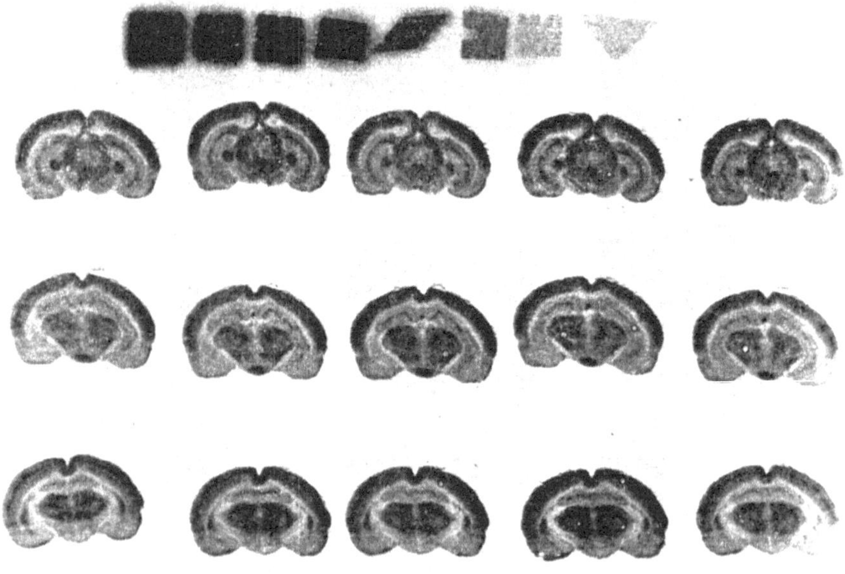

FIG. 4

[^{14}C]Deoxyglucose autoradiographs of sections of conscious rat brain and of calibrated [^{14}C]methylmethacrylate standards used to quantify ^{14}C concentration in tissues by quantitative densitometry (2).

The experimental procedure (2) is to inject a pulse of $[^{14}C]$DG intravenously at zero time and to decapitate the animal and freeze the brain at a measured time, T, 30-45 minutes later; in the interval timed arterial samples are taken for the measurement of plasma $[^{14}C]$DG and glucose concentrations. To ensure that tracer conditions are maintained, the dose of $[^{14}C]$DG should not exceed 2.5 μmoles of deoxyglucose per kg of body weight. Tissue ^{14}C concentrations, C_i^*, are measured at time, T, by quantitative autoradiography of 20 μm frozen dried sections prepared serially from the entire brain and calibrated radioactive standards (Fig.4) (2). Local cerebral glucose utilization is then calculated by the operational equation.

Theoretical and Practical Considerations

The design of the deoxyglucose method is based on an operational equation, derived by the mathematical analysis of a model of the biochemical behavior of $[^{14}C]$deoxyglucose and glucose in brain (Fig.1). Although the model and its mathematical analysis are as rigorous and comprehensive as reasonably possible, it must be recognized that models almost always represent idealized situations and cannot possibly take into account every single known, let alone unknown, property of a complex biological system. There remained, therefore, the possibility that extensive experience with the $[^{14}C]$deoxyglucose method might uncover weaknesses, limitations, or flaws serious enough to limit its usefulness or even to invalidate it. Several years have now passed since its introduction, and numerous applications of it have been made. The results of this experience generally establish the validity and worth of the method. There still remain, however, some potential problems in specialized situations, and several theoretical and practical issues need further clarification.

The main potential sources of error are the rate constants and the lumped constant. The problem with them is that they are not determined in the same animals and at the same time when local cerebral glucose utilization is being measured. They are measured in separate groups of comparable animals and then used subsequently in other animals in which glucose utilization is being measured. The part played by these constants in the method is defined by their role in the operational equation of the method (Fig.1B).

Rate Constants: The rate constants, k_1^*, k_2^*, and k_3^*, for deoxyglucose have thus far been fully determined for various cerebral tissues only in the normal conscious albino rat (2) (Table 1). Partial determination of the rate constants in the normal conscious Rhesus monkey indicates that they are quite similar to those in the rat. All the rate constants vary from tissue to tissue, but the variation among gray structures and among white structures is considerably less than the differences between the two types of tissues (Table 1). The rate constants, k_2^* and k_3^*, appear in the equation only as their sum, and $(k_2^* + k_3^*)$ is equal to the rate constant for the turnover of the free [^{14}C]deoxyglucose pool in the tissue. The half-life of the free [^{14}C]deoxyglucose pool can then be calculated by dividing $(k_2^* + k_3^*)$ into the natural logarithm of 2 and has been found to average 2.4 minutes in gray matter and 4.5 minutes in white matter in the normal conscious rat (Table 1).

The rate constants vary not only from structure to structure but can be expected to vary with the condition. For example, k_1^* and k_2^* are influenced by both blood flow and transport of [^{14}C]deoxyglucose across the blood-brain barrier, and because of the competition for the transport carrier, the glucose concentrations in the plasma and tissue affect the transport of [^{14}C]deoxyglucose and, therefore, also k_1^* and k_2^*. The constant, k_3^*, is related to phosphorylation of [^{14}C]deoxyglucose and will certainly change when glucose utilization is altered. To minimize potential errors due to inaccuracies in the values of the rate constants used, it was decided to sacrifice time resolution for accuracy. If the [^{14}C]deoxyglucose is given as an intravenous pulse and sufficient time is allowed for the plasma to be cleared of the tracer, then the influence of the rate constants, and the functions that they represent, on the final result diminishes with increasing time until ultimately it becomes zero. This relationship is implicit in the structure of the operational equation (Fig.1B); as C_p^* approaches zero, then the terms containing the rate constants also

OPERATIONAL EQUATION:

$$R_i = \frac{C_i^*(T) - k_1^* e^{-(k_2^* + k_3^*)T} \int_0^T C_p^* e^{(k_2^* + k_3^*)t} \, dt}{\left(\frac{\lambda V_m^* K_m}{\Phi V_m K_m^*}\right)\left[\int_0^T (C_p^*/C_p)\, dt - e^{-(k_2^* + k_3^*)T} \int_0^T (C_p^*/C_p)\, e^{(k_2^* + k_3^*)t} \, dt\right]}$$

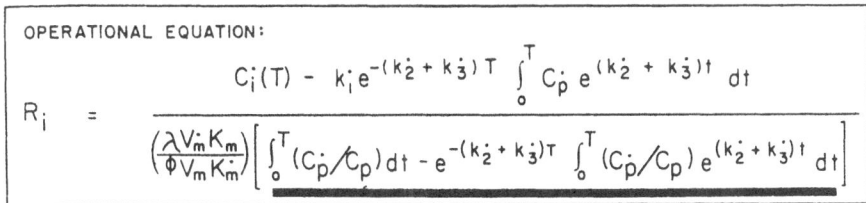

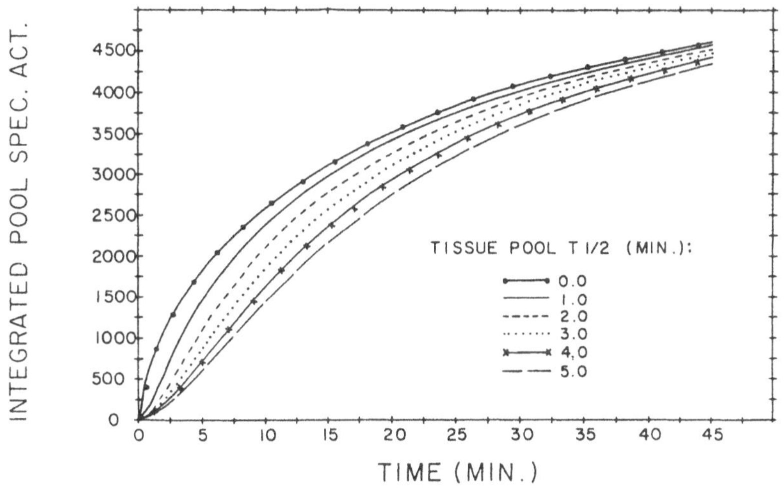

FIG. 5

Influence of time and rate constants, $(k_2^* + k_3^*)$, on integrated precursor pool specific activity in a normal conscious rat given an intravenous pulse of 50 μCi of [^{14}C]deoxyglucose at zero time. The time courses of the arterial plasma [^{14}C]deoxyglucose and glucose concentrations were measured following the pulse. The portion of the equation underlined, corresponding to integrated pool specific activity, was computed as a function of time with different values of $(k_2^* + k_3^*)$, as indicated by their equivalent half-lives, calculated according to T 1/2 = 0.693/$(k_2^* + k_3^*)$ (24).

approach zero with increasing time. The significance of this relationship is graphically illustrated in Fig.5. From typical arterial plasma [^{14}C]deoxyglucose and glucose concentration curves obtained in a normal conscious rat, the portion of the denominator of the operational equation underlined by the heavy bar was computed with a wide range of values for ($k_2^* + k_3^*$) as a function of time. The values for ($k_2^* + k_3^*$) are presented as their equivalent half-lives calculated as described above. The values of ($k_2^* + k_3^*$) vary from infinite (i.e., T 1/2 = 0 min) to 0.14 per min (i.e., T 1/2 = 5 min) and more than cover the range of values to be expected under physiological conditions. The portion of the equation underlined and computed represents the integral of the precursor pool specific activity in the tissue. The curves represent the time course of this function, one each for every value of ($k_2^* + k_3^*$) examined. It can be seen that these curves are widely different at early times but converge with increasing time until at 45 minutes the differences over the entire range of ($k_2^* + k_3^*$) equal only a small fraction of the value of the integral. These curves demonstrate that at short times enormous errors can occur if the values of the rate constants are not precisely known, but only negligible errors occur at 45 minutes, even over a wide range of rate constants of several fold. In fact, it was precisely for this reason that [^{14}C]deoxyglucose rather than [^{14}C]glucose was selected as the tracer for glucose metabolism. The relationships are similar for glucose. Because the products of [^{14}C]glucose metabolism are so rapidly lost from the tissues, it is necessary to limit the experimental period to short times when enormous errors can occur if the rate constants are not precisely known. [^{14}C]Deoxyglucose permits the prolongation of the experimental period to times when inaccuracies in rate constants have little effect on the final result.

It should be noted, however, that in pathological conditions, such as severe ischemia or hyperglycemia, the rate constants may fall far below the range examined in Fig.5. There is evidence, for example, that this occurs with hyperglycemia and ischemia (7).

In such abnormal conditions it may be necessary to redetermine the rate constants for the particular condition under study.

Lumped Constant: The lumped constant is composed of six separate constants. One of these, Φ, is a measure of the steady-state hydrolysis of glucose-6-phosphate to free glucose and phosphate. Because in normal brain tissue there is little such phosphohydrolase activity (8), Φ is normally approximately equal to unity. The other components are arranged in three ratios: λ, which is the ratio of distribution spaces in the tissue for deoxyglucose and glucose; V_m^*/V_m; and K_m/K_m^*. Although each individual constant may vary from structure to structure and condition to condition, it is likely that the ratios tend to remain the same under normal conditions. For reasons described in detail previously (2), it is reasonable to believe that the lumped constant is the same throughout the brain and is characteristic of the species of animal, but only in normal tissue. Although reasonable, it is not certain, and there are theoretical possibilities that it may not be so. Empirical experience thus far indicates that it is. The greatest experience has been accumulated in the albino rat. In this species the lumped constant for the brain as a whole has been determined under a variety of conditions (2). In the normal conscious rat local cerebral glucose utilization, determined by the [^{14}C]deoxyglucose method with the single value of the lumped constant for the brain as a whole, correlates almost perfectly ($r = 0.96$) with local cerebral blood flow, measured by the [^{14}C]-iodoantipyrine method, an entirely independent method (9). It is generally recognized that local blood flow is adjusted to local metabolic rate, but if the single value of the lumped constant did not apply to the individual structures studied, then errors in local glucose utilization would occur that might be expected to obscure the correlation. Also, the lumped constant has been directly determined in the albino rat in the normal conscious state, under barbiturate anesthesia, and during the inhalation of 5% CO_2; no significant differences were observed (Table 2). The lumped constant does vary with the species of animal. It has now

TABLE 2

VALUES OF THE LUMPED CONSTANT IN THE ALBINO RAT, RHESUS MONKEY, CAT AND DOG

Animal	No. of Animals	Mean ± S.D.	S.E.M.
Albino Rat:			
Conscious	15	0.464 ± 0.099*	± 0.026
Anesthetized	9	0.512 ± 0.118*	± 0.039
Conscious (5% CO_2)	2	0.463 ± 0.122*	± 0.086
Combined	26	0.481 ± 0.119	± 0.023
Rhesus Monkey:			
Conscious	7	0.344 ± 0.095	± 0.036
Cat:			
Anesthetized	6	0.411 ± 0.013	± 0.005
Dog (Beagle Puppy):			
Conscious	7	0.558 ± 0.082	± 0.031

* No statistically significant difference between normal conscious and anesthetized rats ($0.3 < p < 0.4$) and conscious rats breathing 5% CO_2 ($p > 0.9$).

Note: The values were obtained as follows: rat (2); monkey (6); cat (M. Miyaoka, J. Magnes, C. Kennedy, M. Shinohara, and L. Sokoloff, unpublished data); dog (10).

also been determined in the Rhesus monkey (6), cat (M. Miyaoka, J. Magnes, C. Kennedy, M. Shinohara, and L. Sokoloff, unpublished data), and Beagle puppy (10), and each species has a different value (Table 2). The values for local rates of glucose utilization determined with these lumped constants in these species are very close to what might be expected from measurement of energy metabolism in the brain as a whole by other methods (Table 3).

TABLE 3. REPRESENTATIVE VALUES FOR LOCAL CEREBRAL GLUCOSE UTILIZATION IN THE NORMAL CONSCIOUS ALBINO RAT AND MONKEY (μmoles/100g/min)

Structure	Albino Rat* (10)	Monkey† (7)
	Gray Matter	
Visual Cortex	107 ± 6	59 ± 2
Auditory Cortex	162 ± 5	79 ± 4
Parietal Cortex	112 ± 5	47 ± 4
Sensory-Motor Cortex	120 ± 5	44 ± 3
Thalamus: Lateral Nucleus	116 ± 5	54 ± 2
Thalamus: Ventral Nucleus	109 ± 5	43 ± 2
Medial Geniculate Body	131 ± 5	65 ± 3
Lateral Geniculate Body	96 ± 5	39 ± 1
Hypothalamus	54 ± 2	25 ± 1
Mamillary Body	121 ± 5	57 ± 3
Hippocampus	79 ± 3	39 ± 2
Amygdala	52 ± 2	25 ± 2
Caudate-Putamen	110 ± 4	52 ± 3
Nucleus Accumbens	82 ± 3	36 ± 2
Globus-Pallidus	58 ± 2	26 ± 2
Substantia Nigra	58 ± 3	29 ± 2
Vestibular Nucleus	128 ± 5	66 ± 3
Cochlear Nucleus	113 ± 7	51 ± 3
Superior Olivary Nucleus	133 ± 7	63 ± 4
Inferior Colliculus	197 ±10	103 ± 6
Superior Colliculus	95 ± 5	55 ± 4
Pontine Gray Matter	62 ± 3	28 ± 1
Cerebellar Cortex	57 ± 2	31 ± 2
Cerebellar Nuclei	100 ± 4	45 ± 2
	White Matter	
Corpus Callosum	40 ± 2	11 ± 1
Internal Capsule	33 ± 2	13 ± 1
Cerebellar White Matter	37 ± 2	12 ± 1

Note: The values are the means ± standard errors from measurements made in the number of animals indicated in parentheses.

* From Sokoloff et al. (2).

† From Kennedy et al. (6).

Although there is yet no experimental evidence to indicate that the lumped constants change under physiological conditions, they may change in pathological states. In severe hypoglycemia there is a marked increase in the lumped constant (11), and in severe hyperglycemia there is a moderate decrease (12). Tissue damage may also disrupt the normal cellular compartmentation, and there is no assurance that λ, the ratio of the distribution spaces for $[^{14}C]$deoxyglucose and glucose, is the same in damaged tissue as in normal tissue. In pathological states there may be release of lysosomal acid hydrolases that may hydrolyze glucose-6-phosphate and thus alter the value of Φ. It is advisable, therefore, to re-evaluate the lumped constant in pathological states.

Glucose-6-Phosphatase: Although relatively low the activity of glucose-6-phosphatase in brain is not zero (5). This enzyme is capable of hydrolyzing the product, $[^{14}C]$deoxyglucose-6-phosphate, back to free $[^{14}C]$deoxyglucose and thus cause loss of product. Fortunately, the product and enzyme are in separate cellular compartments, at least for a time. The $[^{14}C]$DG-6-P is formed in the cytosol and must be transported into the cisterns of the endoplasmic reticulum where the glucose-6-phosphatase resides, before the hydrolysis can occur. This compartmentalization provides a period of time before the effects of glucose-6-phosphatase become significant. If the experimental period is kept within 45 minutes, then the influence of glucose-6-phosphatase is negligible and can be ignored (2,5). If, however, it is necessary to extend the experimental period to longer intervals, as, for example, in studies in man with positron emission tomography (13), then it is necessary to account for the effects of glucose-6-phosphatase activity. This has been done by modifying slightly the original model to include a k_4^*, the rate constant for $[^{14}C]$DG-6-P hydrolysis by glucose-6-phosphatase, and deriving a modified operational equation that incorporates it (5,14).

Computerized Image-Processing

The regional localization obtained with the deoxyglucose method is achieved by the use of quantitative autoradiography. The autoradiographs contain an immense amount of information that cannot be practically recovered by manual densitometry or adequately represented by tabular presentation of the data. A computerized image-processing system has, therefore, been developed to analyze and transform the autoradiographs into color-coded pictorial maps of the rates of local glucose utilization throughout the CNS (15). The autoradiographs are scanned automatically by a computer-controlled scanning microdensitometer. The optical density of each spot on the autoradiograph, from 25 to 100 μm as selected, is stored in a computer, converted to ^{14}C concentration on the basis of the optical densities of the calibrated ^{14}C plastic standards, and then converted to local rate of glucose utilization by solution of the operational equation. Colors are assigned to narrow ranges of the rates of glucose utilization, and the autoradiographs are then displayed on a monitor in color along with a calibrated color scale for identifying the rate of glucose utilization in each spot of the autoradiograph from its color. The display is similar to that used by Lassen, Ingvar, and associates (16) for regional cortical blood flow, but it represents the rates of glucose utilization in all parts of the brain down to a resolution of at least 200 μm. This image-processing system has been adapted for use with positron-emission tomographic data obtained in man, but then, of course, the resolution is much less and limited by that of the tomography.

THE [^{18}F]FLUORODEOXYGLUCOSE TECHNIQUE

The deoxyglucose method was originally designed for use in animals with quantitative autoradiography and the radioactive isotopes most suitable for film autoradiography, ^{14}C or ^{3}H. Its basic physiological and biochemical principles apply, however, to man as well, and it is applicable to man provided the local tissue concentrations of isotope can be measured in the brain. Film autoradiography is a type of emission tomography that for obvious reasons cannot be used in man, but recent developments in computerized tomography have made it possible to determine local concentrations of γ-emitting isotopes in the cerebral tissues. The only possible γ-emitting isotopes that could be incorporated into 2-deoxyglucose are ^{11}C or ^{15}O, but the short half-lives of these isotopes present problems in the synthesis of the compounds. Alternatively, an analogue of 2-deoxyglucose with another γ-emitting isotope but with similar biochemical properties could be used. It is a common experience that the substitution of the very small atom, F, in place of a hydrogen at a judicious site in the molecule often does not alter the basic biochemical behavior of metabolic substrates. 2-[^{18}F]Fluoro-2-deoxy-D-glucose has been synthesized, found to retain the biochemical properties of 2-deoxyglucose, and used to measure cerebral glucose utilization in man by means of single photon emission tomography (17). ^{18}F is actually a positron-emitter, and the absorption of positrons in the tissues gives rise to two coincident annihilation γ-rays of equal energy traveling at almost 180° to each other. Positron emission tomography takes advantage of these coincident annihilation γ-rays and, therefore, is inherently capable of better spatial resolution than single photon tomography. The [^{18}F]fluorodeoxyglucose method is, therefore, now generally used with positron emission tomography (13). Positron emission tomography with [^{18}F]fluorodeoxyglucose is still relatively slow, and it may take up to two hours to obtain sufficient counts for accurate measurements of local ^{18}F concentrations in all parts of the brain. Although low in brain, glucose-6-phosphatase activity is not zero, and its effect becomes significant after the first 45 minutes after the pulse of tracer (5). It has, therefore, been necessary to modify the model to include a rate constant for the hydrolysis of the phosphorylated product by the glucose-6-phosphatase and to derive a new operational equation that takes this activity into account (5,13,14). The [^{18}F]fluorodeoxyglucose technique for the measurement of local cerebral glucose utilization in man is now operational and in use for studies of the human brain in health and disease in a number of laboratories throughout the world.

LOCAL CEREBRAL PROTEIN SYNTHESIS

The basic biochemical principles for the measurement of metabolic rates *in vivo*, which were so effectively applied in the deoxyglucose technique, also apply to other metabolic processes. A metabolic activity of broad interest is protein synthesis. This biochemical activity is not likely to reflect directly functional activity, at least not acutely, but it may well be involved in slower more gradual processes in the nervous system, such as growth and development, plasticity, regeneration and repair, response to drugs and hormones, and possibly learning and memory. Protein synthesis may also be altered in pathological states, such as brain tumors, mental retardation due to metabolic errors, aging and senility, Alzheimer's disease, Huntington's disease, endocrine diseases, etc.

A method for the measurement of local rates of protein synthesis in the nervous system is under development (4). Like the deoxyglucose method it is designed to achieve localization by quantitative autoradiography although eventually it should be adaptable to positron-emission tomography. Also like the deoxyglucose methods it is based on the same biochemical principles described above, but their application to the measurement of local cerebral protein synthesis may be far more complex because of still undefined properties and kinetics of the equilibration of the precursor amino acid pool in the tissue with the circulating amino acid pool in the plasma.

The two essential variables which must be determined in any quantitative radioactive assay of the rate of a reaction are the amount of product formed and the integrated precursor specific activity over a measured interval of time. Because autoradiographic or emission tomographic techniques measure the concentration only of the radioisotope and not that of the radioactive product itself, it is essential that the method be so designed that the label in the tissue is confined only to the product molecule itself or, at least, in well-defined chemical species which can be quantified separately. This problem is mitigated by the use of carboxyl-labeled L-leucine, an essential amino acid which is prevalent in most proteins and which if not incorporated into protein follows a single simple pathway of metabolic degradation. In the pathway of degradation, the amino acid is first transaminated and then rapidly decarboxylated; the label is then lost as radioactive CO_2, which because of dilution by the large pool of unlabeled CO_2 constantly generated by carbohydrate metabolism, the relatively slow rate of CO_2 fixation, and the rapid removal of CO_2 from brain tissue by the blood flow, is removed from the tissues. The label is then retained only in the product of the reaction, labeled protein, and in the residual unincorporated amino acid. The concentration of free labeled amino acid can be calculated from the history of the plasma concentration and the kinetic constants for the equilibration of the tissue free amino acid pools and the plasma. The concentration of free labeled amino acid in the tissue at the time of killing can be minimized by its intravenous administration as a pulse at zero time followed by the allowance of a sufficiently long time for its clearance from the plasma and tissue. One hour after the pulse the fraction of total radioactivity in the tissue that is in the free amino acid pool is small (about 10%) in the rat. In adult monkey and probably in man, however, it is large (30-50%) because of the relatively slow rates of protein synthesis and of clearance of the free amino acid pools. The error in subtracting a poorly defined free amino acid pool concentration from a total concentration that is not a great deal larger may, of course, be enormous.

An even more difficult problem is the determination of the integrated precursor pool specific activity in the tissue from measurements in the plasma. To accomplish this, it is necessary to know the kinetics of the equilibration of the precursor pool in the cells with that of the plasma. What makes this problem particularly perplexing is that there is evidence that amino acids in the cells are compartmentalized with only a fraction of the total intracellular amino acid content representative of the pool that serves as precursor for protein synthesis. Therefore, although it is relatively simple to measure the rate constants for the equilibration of the total amino acid pool with that of the plasma, there is little assurance that this pool reflects the kinetic behavior of the fraction of it that is the precursor for protein synthesis. A further complication is the possibility of significant dilution of the intracellular precursor amino acid pool by unlabeled amino acid derived from the slow but continuous turnover of the protein components of the cell. The magnitude of this potential dilution is even more difficult to evaluate. Nevertheless, studies are currently in progress in our laboratory that are designed to resolve these problems. If successful, they will not only determine the rate constants for the turnover of the true precursor pool but also the degree of admixture of unlabeled amino acids derived from protein breakdown with the labeled amino acids in the precursor pool.

Although the method is not yet fully developed, experiments with our first and most primitive model already indicate the potential usefulness for a technique that measures local cerebral protein synthesis. Model I is essentially the same as that for the deoxyglucose method; it assumes a single tissue pool of free amino acid, all of which equilibrates uniformly with the plasma and serves as the precursor pool for protein synthesis with no dilution by unlabeled amino acids derived from protein degradation (4). Although the quantitative values obtained with this version of the method are probably not accurate and may be underestimates of the true rates of L-leucine incorporation into protein, the results demonstrate that the rates of protein synthesis do change in specific regions of the brain in response to altered function. For example, in the rat section of one hypoglossal nerve is followed by increased protein synthesis in the ipsilateral hypoglossal nucleus after a lag of close to four days (18). The increase reaches a maximum between 20-30%, and protein synthesis does not return to normal until regeneration and restoration of functional activity in the hypoglossal nerve are complete (C.B. Smith, unpublished observations).

The method has also been used to study plasticity in the binocular visual system of the newborn Rhesus monkey (19). The outputs from the retinae of the two eyes are crossed approximately 50 percent, and the optic tracts terminate in the lateral geniculate nuclei in six discrete laminae, 1, 4, and 6, the sites of termination of the pathways from the contralateral retina and 2, 3, and 5, the laminae supplied by the ipsilateral eye. The cells in these laminae project via the geniculocalcarine tracts to the ipsilateral striate cortex in such a way that the two retinal outputs for each point in the visual field converge to two adjacent cortical columns, one for each eye, for the same spot in the visual field. These are the ocular dominance columns, first described by Hubel and Wiesel (20), and demonstrated autoradiographically by the [^{14}C]deoxyglucose method (21). The visual system of the newborn monkey exhibits plasticity. Chronic occlusion of one eye in a newborn monkey leads to widening of the ocular dominance columns for the functioning eye at the expense of the columns for the deprived eye until eventually the columns disappear, and the entire striate cortex is taken over to subserve the function of the undeprived eye (22,23). Presumably the axonal terminals of the geniculocalcarine pathway for the functioning eye grow into, and take over, the synaptic connections in the adjacent column normally reserved for the deprived eye. If so, changes in protein synthesis required for axonal growth and sprouting could be involved, and the protein synthesis used for this process occurs in the cell bodies of origin of the pathway, i.e., in the lateral geniculate nuclei. Illustrated in Fig.6 are the results of application of the local protein synthesis technique to this question. The laminae in the geniculate bodies are clearly visible and relatively uniform in the autoradiographs of the 25 day-old normal monkey. Acute monocular deprivation for 3 hours does not alter the rates of protein synthesis in any of the laminae, including those for the deprived eye. Chronic monocular deprivation from 2 days to 25 days of age results in marked reductions in protein synthesis in the laminae served by the deprived eye. Apparently chronic reduction in functional activity, in contrast to the acute state, results in a lowering of protein synthesis in the affected pathway. These results suggest that the loss of ocular dominance columns in the striate cortex for the chronically deprived eye is the result of depressed protein synthesis and deficient axonal growth in the geniculocalcarine pathways for the deprived eye.

It is hoped that measurement of local rates of protein synthesis in the nervous system may be useful to study normal and

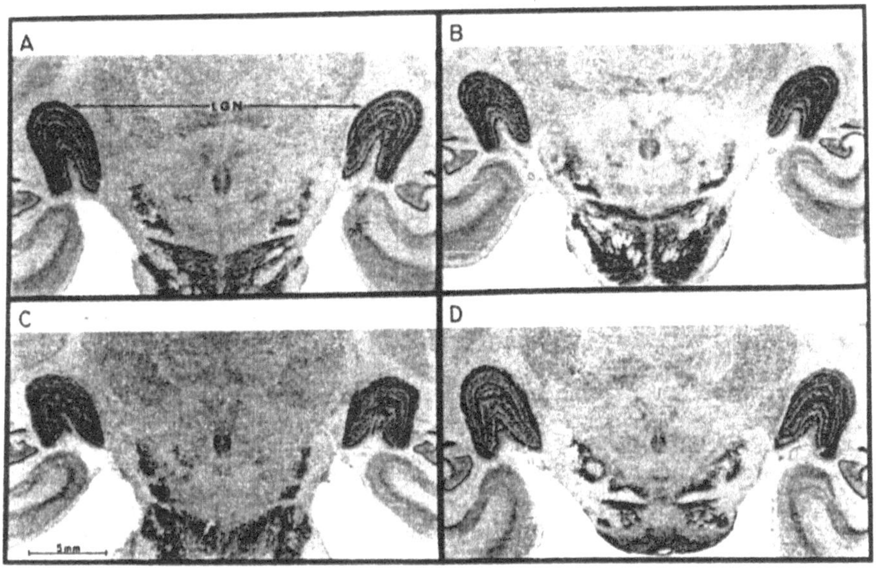

FIG. 6

Autoradiographs of coronal sections of monkey lateral geniculate nuclei (LGN) obtained with the [^{14}C]leucine method. The left side of the brain is on the left side of the autoradiographs. (A) Twenty-five-day-old monkey with intact binocular vision. (B) Twenty-five-day-old monkey with acute occlusion of the left eye. (C) Twenty-five-day-old monkey with chronic occlusion of right eye initiated on second day of life. (D) Twenty-five-day-old monkey with chronic occlusion of left eye initiated on second day of life. Note the decreased labeling and, therefore, rate of protein synthesis in the laminae 1, 4, and 6 of the lateral geniculate ganglion contralateral to the deprived eye and in laminae 2, 3, and 5 of the ganglion ipsilateral to the deprived eye (19).

abnormal processes that may not be accessible to other autoradiographic and tomographic procedures, processes such as growth, maturation, plasticity, actions of hormones. The full potential of this approach must, however, await the development of an accurate and reliable method.

REFERENCES

1. Frackowiak RSJ, Lenzi G-L, Jones T, Heather JD: Quantitative measurement of regional cerebral blood flow and oxygen metabolism in man using ^{15}O and positron emission tomography. J Computer-Assisted Tomography 4:727-736, 1980

2. Sokoloff L, Reivich M, Kennedy C, Des Rosiers MH, Patlak CS, Pettigrew KD, Sakurada O, Shinohara M: The [^{14}C]deoxyglucose method for the measurement of local cerebral glucose utilization: theory, procedure, and normal values in the conscious and anesthetized albino rat. J Neurochem 28:897-916 1977

3. Sokoloff L: Localization of functional activity in the central nervous system by measurement of glucose utilization with radioactive deoxyglucose. J Cereb Blood Flow Metab 1:7-36, 1981

4. Smith CB, Davidsen L, Deibler G, Patlak C, Pettigrew K, Sokoloff L: A method for the determination of local rates of protein synthesis in brain. Trans Amer Soc Neurochem 11:94, 1980

5. Sokoloff L: The radioactive deoxyglucose method. Theory, procedure, and applications for the measurement of local glucose utilization in the central nervous system. In Agranoff BW and Aprison MH, Eds. Advances in Neurochemistry, Vol. 4. New York, Plenum Publishing Corp, 1982, pp 1-82

6. Kennedy C, Sakurada O, Shinohara M, Jehle J, Sokoloff L: Local cerebral glucose utilization in the normal conscious Macaque monkey. Ann Neurol 4:293-301, 1978

7. Hawkins R, Phelps M, Huang SC, Kuhl D: Effect of ischemia upon quantification of local cerebral metabolic rates for glucose with 2-(F-18)fluoro-deoxyglucose (FDG). J Cereb Blood Flow Metab 1(Suppl 1):S9-S10, 1981

8. Hers HG: Le Métabolisme du Fructose. Bruxelles, Editions Arscia, 1957, p 102

9. Sokoloff L: Local cerebral energy metabolism: its relationships to local functional activity and blood flow. In Purves MJ and Elliott K, Eds. Cerebral Vascular Smooth Muscle and Its Control, Ciba Foundation Symposium 56. Amsterdam, Elsevier/Excerpta Medica/North-Holland, 1978, pp 171-197

10. Duffy TE, Cavazzuti M, Cruz NF, Sokoloff L: Local cerebral glucose metabolism in newborn dogs: effects of hypoxia and halothane anesthesia. Ann Neurol 11:233-246, 1982.

11. Suda S, Shinohara M, Miyaoka M, Kennedy C, Sokoloff L: Local cerebral glucose utilization in hypoglycemia. J Cereb Blood Flow Metab 1(Suppl 1):S62, 1981

12. Schuier F, Orzi F, Suda S, Kennedy C, Sokoloff L: The lumped constant for the [^{14}C]deoxyglucose method in hyperglycemic rats. J Cereb Blood Flow Metab 1(Suppl 1):S63, 1981

13. Phelps ME, Huang SC, Hoffman EJ, Selin C, Sokoloff L, Kuhl DE: Tomographic measurement of local cerebral glucose metabolic rate in humans with (F-18)2-fluoro-2-deoxy-d-glucose: validation of method. Ann Neurol 6:371-388, 1979

14. Huang SC, Phelps ME, Hoffman EJ, Sideris K, Selin CJ, Kuhl DE: Noninvasive determination of local cerebral metabolic rate of glucose in man. Am J Physiol 238:E69-E82, 1980

15. Goochee C, Rasband W, Sokoloff L: Computerized densitometry and color coding of [^{14}C]deoxyglucose autoradiographs. Ann Neurol 7:359-370, 1980

16. Lassen NA, Ingvar DH, Skinhøj E: Brain function and blood flow. Sci Amer 239:62-71, 1978

17. Reivich M, Kuhl D, Wolf A, Greenberg J, Phelps M, Ido T, Casella V, Fowler J, Hoffman E, Alavi A, Som P, Sokoloff L: The [^{18}F]fluoro-deoxyglucose method for the measurement of local cerebral glucose utilization in man. Circ Res 44:127-137, 1979

18. Agranoff BW, Smith CB, Sokoloff L: Regional protein synthesis in rat brain after hypoglossal axotomy. Trans Amer Soc Neurochem 11:95, 1980

19. Kennedy C, Suda S, Smith CB, Miyaoka M, Ito M, Sokoloff L: Changes in protein synthesis underlying functional plasticity in immature monkey visual system. Proc Natl Acad Sci USA 78:3950-3953, 1981

20. Hubel DH, Wiesel TN: Receptive fields and functional architecture of monkey striate cortex. J Physiol 195:215-243, 1968

21. Kennedy C, Des Rosiers MH, Sakurada O, Shinohara M, Reivich M, Jehle JW, Sokoloff L: Metabolic mapping of the primary visual system of the monkey by means of the autoradiographic [^{14}C]deoxyglucose technique. Proc Natl Acad Sci USA 73:4230-4234, 1976

22. Hubel DH, Wiesel TN, LeVay S: Plasticity of ocular dominance columns in monkey striate cortex. Phil Trans R Soc Lond B278:377-409, 1977

23. Des Rosiers MH, Sakurada O, Jehle J, Shinohara M, Kennedy C, Sokoloff L: Functional plasticity in the immature striate cortex of the monkey shown by the [^{14}C]deoxyglucose method. Science 200:447-449, 1978

24. Sokoloff L: The [^{14}C]deoxyglucose method: four years later. Acta Neurol Scand (Suppl 70) 60:640-649, 1979

TRACER STUDIES OF PERIPHERAL CIRCULATION

Niels A. Lassen and Ole Henriksen

Bispebjerg Hospital, Copenhagen, Denmark

INTRODUCTION

Studying the blood flow of the various tissues by tracers (also called indicators) one assumes steady state conditions for the system. It means, that the relevant parameters of the system are taken to be constant, the flow, oxygen uptake, etc. Systemic steady state is elementary for deriving the basic equations. It must persist during the time needed for making the measurement. This does not mean, however, that some degree of variability of the systemic parameter in question cannot be allowed. Consider for example the determination of cardiac output by injection of below-body-temperature saline in the right side of the heart with downstream temperature measurement in the pulmonary artery ("heat" clearance). In this case the flow rate of the blood in the system measured oscillates enormously. Yet, because the duration of the period of oscillation is fairly short relative to the duration of the heat clearance curve itself, one can get a good estimate of the average blood flow. In contrast to the systemic parameters, the tracer parameters, as for example the blood concentration, often vary as a function of time, i.e. for the tracer the steady state condition does not (in many cases) pertain.

We can only comment briefly on the many different tracers used for measuring peripheral circulation. Practical considerations regarding accurate measurement of their amount or concentration are important. The tracer must be inert in the amount used, i.e. it must cause only a minimal perturbation of the system. As long as systemic steady state is maintained, the system is stationary (two identical tracer applications, one delayed relative to the other, give, after the delay, the same response). In most instances linearity of tracer response must also be assumed (double dose gives double response): This property is inherent in the tracer concept of using an "infinitely small amount" that does not alter the system. Stationarity and linearity of tracer response are necessary for deriving the convolution principle, one of the basic concepts in tracer methods.

To trace blood flow the substance must mix with the blood. Mixing at the inlet to the organ must pertain in many cases. This means that the tracer concentration is at any time the same everywhere in a cross-section of the inlet. In other words the tracer enters the system in precisely the same way as the substance to be traced (the "mother substance", in this case the blood). In other words, inlet mixing of tracer and mother substance means that the two substances have equivalent entry.

For most tracers we assume that no fraction of the molecules is permanently retained: as the blood itself we assume, that what goes in must also sooner or later come out. In this sense the system is conservative or "non-active" relative to the tracer. This underlies the mass-balance concept used extensively, consisting of a quantitative bookkeeping, that accounts for all indicator molecules, a concept termed the Law of Conservation of Matter, also in circulation physiology called the Fick Principle or simply Mass Balance.

The Constant Infusion Method (Stewart principle)

Consider a fluid flowing through a tube at the constant rate F ml/min and with a site of cross-stream mixing anywhere inside the system or at its inlet or outlet. For example consider the right side of the heart where the passage of the blood through the ventricular cavity gives a fairly good mixing. Upstream of, or at the mixing site, we infuse tracer at the constant influx rate of j_{in} mg/min in form of a concentrated standard solution of concentration C_{st} mg/ml being infused at a slow inflow rate F_{st} ml/min. Thus

$$j_{in} = F_{st} \cdot C_{st} \quad \text{mg/min} \tag{1}$$

Downstream of the mixing site one blood sample is collected at a time when this concentration has reached its constant maximum, steady state, value $C_{out}(\infty)$. The steady state outflux, $j_{out}(\infty)$ equals $(F + F_{st})C_{out}(\infty)$. This must balance the influx, as the amount inside the system is constant in the steady state. Hence

$$F_{st} \cdot C_{st} = (F + F_{st})C_{out}(\infty) \quad \text{ml/min} \tag{2}$$

As the rate of tracer solution infusion F_{st} can be kept very small relative to the system's flow rate F, it follows that $(F + F_{st}) \simeq F$. Therefore equation 2 can be solved for F simply by writing

$$F \simeq \frac{F_{st} \cdot C_{st}}{C_{out}(\infty)} \quad \text{ml/min} \tag{3}$$

In other words, for sufficiently small tracer-solution infusion rates F_{st}, the flow is as many times greater than the tracer solution infusion flow, as the dilution factor $C_{st}/C_{out}(\infty)$. As shown in Fig. 1, even if the system has multiple outlets, the method is valid as in the steady state all outlets have the same concentration. This classical tracer dilution method was first applied by Stewart in 1897 (1) for blood flow measurement using NaCl as indicator and conductivity as a measure of concentration. It was the first practical application of tracers to flow measurements in biological systems.

Note that the general flux equation is not given by equation 1 as it only contains a term for convective (flow related) flux omitting diffusive fluxes of the form-DS dc/dx in the axial (inflow) direction (with D being diffusion coefficient, S cross-sectional area and dc/dx the concentration gradient). This is correct as during the steady state of infusion equation 2 correctly states the influx through the infusion catheter and the outflux as there can be no diffusion gradients at the outlet in the steady state.

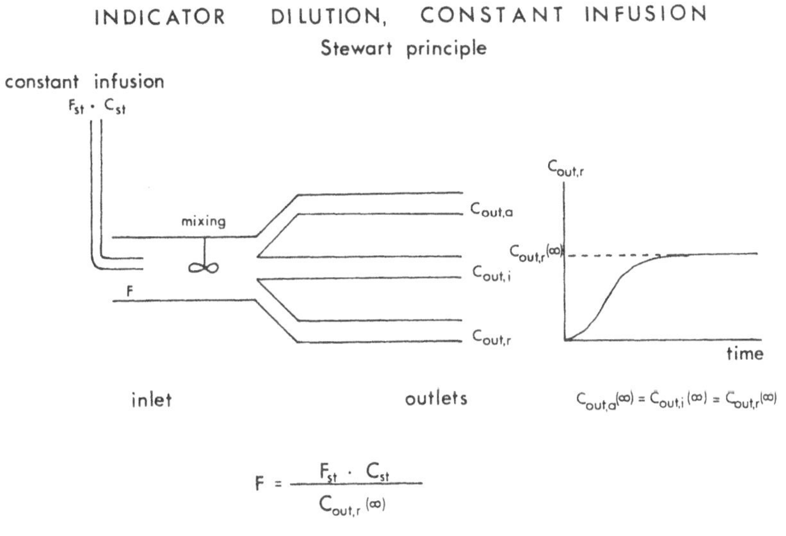

FIG. 1

Diagram illustrating constant infusion, outlet sampling experiment (Stewart principle).

Recirculation of tracer is often a problem: before tracer steady-state has been reached, in many situations, blood containing tracer has made a complete circuit and is adding to the flux of indicator passing the outlet. A constant maximal concentration is therefore not observed. Instead a continuously rising curve is seen. A method of correcting for recirculation exists if biraterally symmetrical organs such as kidneys or forearms are studied. Then sampling also from the outlet of the non-injected side gives the concentration to be subtracted from that of the injected side. This difference's constant maximal value as measured after the initial transient should be used in equation 3.

Other means of correcting for recirculation exist, notably by using the convolution theorem and knowing the recirculation at the inflow (usually the arterial) site (see below). However, one should always strive to minimize the effect of recirculation. This can be done by 1) infusing the tracer as close as possible upstream to the mixing site and sampling close downstream of the site; 2) using an indicator that recirculates minimally or not at all (heat/cold is the only indicator for which recirculation can be ignored; inert gases show little recirculation, as they leave the circulation at the tissues and at the lungs).

The Constant Infusion Method in the Case of Constant Recirculation (Fick Principle)

In his classical note of 1870 A Fick (2) proposed to measure cardiac output with oxygen as the tracer for blood flow. The system studied is the lung having a blood flow of F ml/min. The indicator influx j mMol/min is the uptake of oxygen in the lung, the metabolic rate of the lungs being considered negligible. Oxygen recirculates at a constant rate from the body as it is carried back by the venous return flowing at essentially the same flow rate F with a constant concentration C_{in} being the oxygen concentration of mixed venous blood $C_{\bar{v}}$. Mass balance means that the combined influx equals the outflux, that is

$$j + F \cdot C_{in} = F \cdot C_{out} \tag{4}$$

Solving for F yields the well known relation

$$F = \frac{j}{C_{out}(\infty) - C_{in}(\infty)} = \frac{\text{oxygen uptake rate}}{\text{outlet minus inlet conc.}} \tag{5}$$

where $C_{out} - C_{in}$ is $C_a - C_{\bar{v}}$ for oxygen.

The oxygen concentration of mixed venous blood $C_{\bar{v}}$ may be obtained by sampling from the pulmonary artery. An often used (but less accurate) means of getting it, is to calculate it as the average of the oxygen content of two blood samples, one collected from the superior vena cava and one from the inferior vena cava.

The system studied is not quite the same as for the constant infusion method discussed in the first section of this chapter. Because, with the Fick method we must have two cross-stream mixing sites, one upstream of the inlet sampling site and one upstream of the outlet sampling site. This requirement frequently poses serious problems. Consider for example the use of Fick's method for calculating hepatic blood flow with constant intravenous indocyanine infusion ("Cardiac green"). Here the constant i.v. infusion is taken to represent the steady state uptake in the liver, because the non-hepatic clearance is negligible. The mass balance consideration yields equation 5 with C_{in} and C_{out} being reversed, because the liver is not the site of tracer addition but the site of its removal, i.e. $F = j/(C_{in} - C_{out})$. In this case no physical means of mixing exists at inlet (v. portae and a. hepatica) or at outlet (the hepatic veins). It is therefore important to check, that the concentration is the same at the various inlets and outlets.

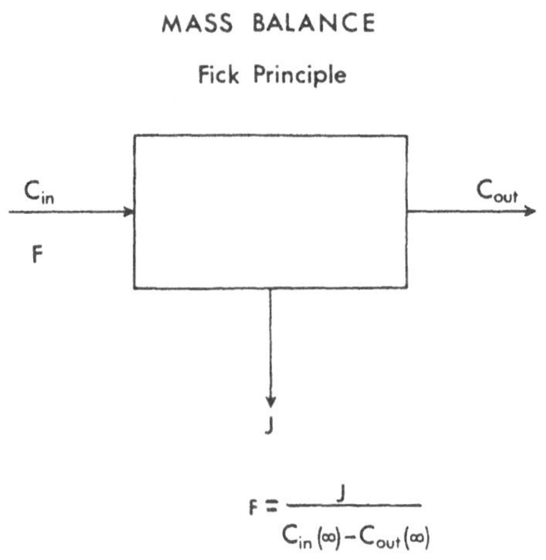

FIG. 2

Diagram illustrating the mass balance concept (Fick principle).

EXTRACTION AND CLEARANCE

The extraction of the tracer, E, is defined as the fraction of the inflowing amount, that is taken (removed from) the blood in a single passage through the system. Thus E is uptake divided by delivery

$$E = \frac{F(C_{in} - C_{out})}{F \cdot C_{in}}$$

$$= \frac{C_{in} - C_{out}}{C_{in}} \qquad (6)$$

The complement of E leaving the system by the effluent blood is termed the transmitted fraction, T, i.e. E + T = 1.

Another important concept for describing the uptake within the system is clearance, Cl, defined as the flow of reference fluid carrying the amount of tracer taken up per unit time, i.e.

$$Cl = \frac{F(C_{in} - C_{out})}{C_{ref}} \qquad (7)$$

where C_{ref} is the concentration in the reference fluid.If C_{in} is used as the reference fluid, then equation 6 and 7 can be combined to

$$Cl = E \cdot F \qquad (8)$$

It should be emphasized that Cl has only a physical meaning in special circumstances, e.g. when the substance is completely extracted from the reference fluid (E = 1). Another example is the inulin clearance in the glomeruli. Since no exchange of inulin occurs across the tubular membrane the urinary excretion of inulin equals the amount ultrafiltered from arterial plasma water. Thus using plasma water as reference fluid inulin clearance equals the glomerular water filtration rate, GFR. Using equation 8 it is apparent, that the extraction fraction of inulin equals the glomerular filtration fraction FF, i.e. GFR divided by the renal plasma water flow, viz. plasma flow multiplied by the fractional content of water in plasma, that normally is appr. 0.93. Generally clearance must be regarded as a non-existing equivalent flow. The linearity of the system's response to the tracer means that the tracer obeys first order kinetics, i.e. the uptake increases in direct proportion to the tracer concentration and hence the fractional uptake, E, is constant.

The choice of reference fluid is arbitrary, but may be of importance for interpreting Cl. Consider, for example, the case of a substance cleared from the blood by diffusion across a membrane offering the main barrier to exchange (capillary membrane) and assume that the outside concentration remains essentially zero. Then the capillary concentration decreases mono-exponentially along the capillary as shown by Crone (3) and Renkin (4) giving

$$C_{out} = C_{in} \cdot e^{-\frac{PS}{F}} \qquad (9)$$

where PS is the permeability-surface area product defined as the membrane's tracer flux per unit concentration gradient.

Solving equation 9 for PS gives

$$PS = F(\ln C_{in} - \ln C_{out}) \qquad (10)$$

Multiplying both sides of equation 10 with $(C_{in} - C_{out})$ and rearranging gives

$$PS = \frac{F(C_{in} - C_{out})}{(C_{in} - C_{out})/(\ln C_{in} - \ln C_{out})} \qquad (11)$$

The denominator defines the socalled logarithmic averate concentration, $\hat{C}$, a concentration lying between C_{in} and C_{out}.

Using $\hat{C}$ as concentration in the reference fluid it is seen, that

$$PS = \frac{F(C_{in} - C_{out})}{\hat{C}} = Cl \qquad (12)$$

Thus, this example demonstrates that with a simple first order kinetic uptake, and assuming no back-diffusion, the clearance calculated using $\hat{C}$ equals the capillary diffusion capacity, PS, which may be conceived as a virtual volume of fluid crossing (being totally cleared at) the capillary membrane.

Bolus Injection Method (Henriques-Hamilton-Bergner Principle)

The amount, m_0, of a tracer is injected into the system with a well-mixed outlet, where the flow of carrier fluid is F. The outlet concentration at time t is $C_{out}(t)$. Assuming that the tracer does not change F and the volume injected is insignificant compared to the flow rate, the amount of tracer leaving the system in a short time interval dt from time t to time t + dt is

$$dm(t) = F \cdot dt \cdot C_{out}(t)$$

since $C_{out}(t)$ can be considered constant throughout the short time interval dt.

INDICATOR DILUTION, BOLUS INJECTION

Henriques – Hamilton principle

$$F = \frac{m_o}{\int_o^\infty C_{out}(t)\,dt}$$

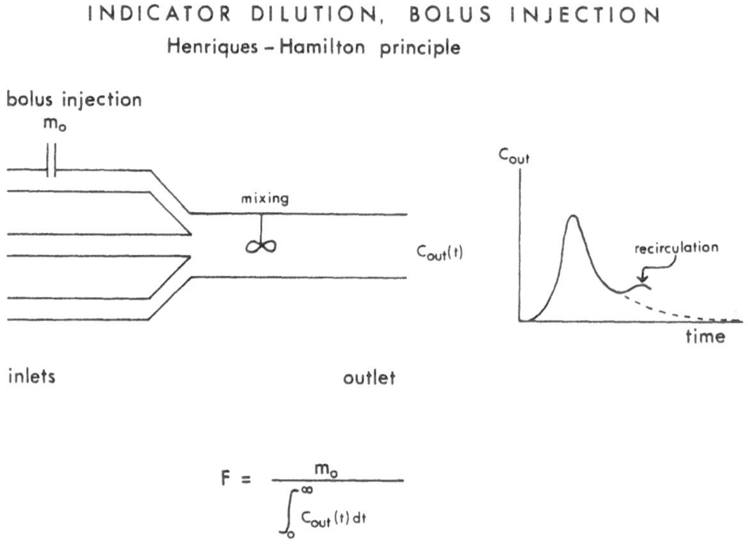

FIG. 3

Diagram illustrating the bolus injection out-flow sampling method in a multiple-inlet single-outlet system (Henriques-Hamilton principle).

When all tracer molecules have left the system and provided no recirculation occurs, then the total amount entering, the dose m_0, equals the sum of all amounts leaving

$$m_0 = F\int_0^\infty C_{out}(t)dt \tag{13}$$

or

$$F = \frac{m_0}{\int_0^\infty C_{out}(t)dt} = \frac{\int_0^\infty j_{in}(t)dt}{\int_0^\infty C_{out}(t)dt} \tag{14}$$

where the sign ∞ (infinity) denotes any time after T, the longest transit time, i.e. the time at which the tracer has left the system completely. m_0 equals the product of the volume of injectate (standard) V_{st} and its concentration C_{st}. It is also the integral of the instantaneous influx, $j_{in}(t)$. Note that the area in the denominator of equation 14 can be obtained by a single cumulative sampling from time zero to time T, provided that the entire amount of injected tracer has passed the sampling site before time T. If so, then $\int_0^\infty C_{out}(t)dt = \int_0^T C_{out}(t)dt = \bar{C}_{out} \cdot T$, where $\bar{C}_{out}$ is the average concentration in the cumulative sample.

Thus equation 14 states that $F \cdot T$, the cumulative volume flowing out from the start of sampling to time T is as many times greater than the injected standard volume, V_{st}, as the measured dilution factor $C_{st}/\bar{C}_{out}$ (5, 6, 7).

The derivation of equation 14 depends on the mass balance concept as applied to a single well-mixed outlet. In this context it should be mentioned, that even a single tube with laminar flow constitutes a multiple outlet system. It can, however, be shown that the cross-stream mixing site can be located anywhere in the system, even at its inlet. As will be shown below, the area under a C(t) curve obtained at any of a multitude of outlets downstream a cross-stream mixing site equals the area that would be observed by mixing all outlets, i.e. by artificially creating a single well-mixed outlet.

The proof is afforded by the stimulus-response theorem (8), which states that in any arbitrary system, which is stationary and linear, any arbitrary tracer parameter being regarded as the stimulus s and any other parameter as the resulting response r, then the ratio, R of stimulus and response is the same in the constant infusion (steady-state) experiment ss, as the ratio of the corresponding time integrals to time infinity in the bolus experiment b, i.e.

$$R = \left[\frac{s(\infty)}{r(\infty)}\right]_{ss} = \left[\frac{\int_0^\infty s(t)dt}{\int_0^\infty r(t)dt}\right]_b \qquad (15)$$

Note that if we combine equation 3 and equation 14 we get

$$F = \frac{j_{in}(\infty)}{C_{out}(\infty)} = \frac{\int_0^\infty j_{in}(t)dt}{\int_0^\infty C_{out}(t)dt} \qquad (16)$$

Thus the two indicator-dilution methods sofar described actually express the stimulus-response theorem. But, then it also follows that in any system where the constant-infusion equation is valid, the bolus equation is valid too.

Now consider a single inlet - multiple outlet system where the indicator is applied by constant infusion. After a sufficient long time has elapsed, the concentration of all n outlets has reached the same maximum value, viz that at the inlet. In this situation F equals $j_{in}(\infty)/C_{out,r}(\infty)$, r denoting any one of the n outlets. Using the stimulus-response theorem according to which j_{in} corresponds to $\int_0^\infty j_{in}(t)dt$ and $C_{out,r}(\infty)$ to $\int_0^\infty C_{out,r}(t)dt$, we get

$$F = \frac{j_{in}(\infty)}{C_{out,r}(\infty)} = \frac{\int_0^\infty j_{in}(t)dt}{\int_0^\infty C_{out,r}(t)dt} = \frac{m_0}{\int_0^\infty C_{out,r}(t)dt} \qquad (17)$$

It is thus seen that even in the bolus-experiment sampling from outlet r can be used for calculating flow.

Therefore it is possible to use any of the n outlets. Even an artificially extra outlet can be used, e.g. in form of sampling inside the system downstream of the mixing site. This must be correct, as all outlets have the same area. This constitutes the important "equal area rule" which is valid in a single-phase system down-stream from a mixing site (9). In circulation physiology Bergner's proof is valuable. It relaxes the sampling requirement in a very important way, because, as one cannot in actual fact readily sample at a mixing site as assumed when deriving the equation from the mass balance consideration. Note, however, that one cannot "jump" from one outlet r to another u during the sampling, as we cannot be sure that $\int_0^T C_r(t)dt = \int_0^{t_1} C_r(t)dt + \int_{t_1}^T C_u(t)dt$. This "jump" is possible in the steady state (Constant infusion) experiment as clearly $C_r(\infty) = C_u(\infty)$.

The indicator dilution methods described above have been widely used. In particular the bolus injection method has been used for determination of cardiac output injection at the right side of the heart and following the concentration of the tracer as a function of time in a systemic artery (the rth outlet). The main difficulty with this method is correcting for recirculation. Often mono-exponential extrapolation to time infinity is used, i.e. the curve to be expected if complete mixing of indicator in the vascular volume between the injection and sampling site pertained. Actually this extrapolation procedure slightly underestimates the area under the outflow curve and hence cardiac output correspondingly is a little overestimated. Correction for recirculation may be improved by sampling of the recirculating blood from the inlet as this renders possible to calculate the first part of the contribution of recirculation by convolution as described later.

Another approach has been to fit the outflow curve before recirculation becomes significant to a γ-variate function (10). Using heat as flow indicator problems due to recirculation are avoided (11).

The indicator dilution method with bolus injection can also be used for determination of the clearance of a substance.

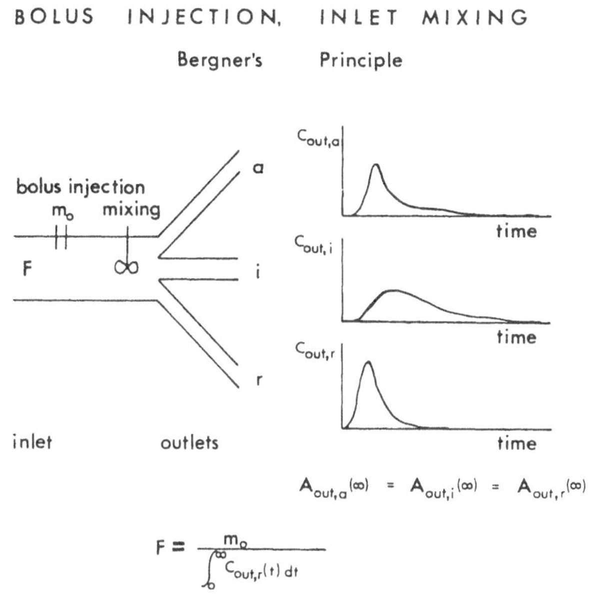

FIG. 4

Diagram illustrating the "equal area rule" of Bergner (9) when sampling from any of the multiple outlets including artificial ones downstream to a cross mixing site.

Recalling that in the steady-state $Cl = j/C_{ref}(\infty)$ the stimulus-response theorem can be used to obtain the bolus injection equation

$$Cl = \frac{j}{C_{ref}(\infty)} = \frac{\int_0^\infty j(t)dt}{\int_0^\infty C_{ref}(t)dt} = \frac{m_0}{\int_0^\infty C_{ref}(t)dt} \qquad (18)$$

The bolus technique has been applied for determining renal clearance of ^{51}Cr-EDTA. Since this substance essentially is excreted by glomerular filtration, the dose over plasma-curve area (equation 18) practically equals GFR (12, 13).

Bolus Fractionation Principle

Consider a situation where an amount, m_0, of an indicator is injected as a bolus. Assuming complete mixing between the indicator and blood at the inlet then the fraction of the dose m_{tissue}/m_0 reaching a given area equals the fraction F_{tissue}/F_0 of the labeled blood flow F_0 that goes to the tissue in question

$$\frac{F_{tissue}}{F_0} = \frac{m_{tissue}}{m_0} \tag{19}$$

It is necessary that total retention at the indicator in the tissues is attained. Sapirstein (14) developed the principle using radioactive potassium. A better degree of tissue retention is obtained by using radioactively labeled inert particles of uniformly small size, microspheres. They are usually injected into the left atrium to label the entire cardiac output (F_0 in equation 19) uniformly. The method can be calibrated simply by taking a single arterial blood sample.

Rearrangement of equation 19 gives

$$\frac{m_{tissue}}{F_{tissue}} = \frac{m_{blood\ sample}}{F_{blood\ sample}} = \frac{m_0}{F_0}$$

Thus

$$F_{tissue} = m_{tissue} \cdot \frac{F_{blood\ sample}}{m_{blood\ sample}} \tag{20}$$

m_{tissue} is the amount of tracer retained in the tissue and $m_{blood\ sample}$ is the amount in the blood sample collected at the rate $F_{blood\ sample}$ ml/min.

The bolus injection - tissue sampling method of Sapirstein is a variant of the bolus injection - venous sampling method of Henriques, Hamilton and Bergner as equation 20 can be shown to equal the dose/area ratio: the tracer dose to the tissue in question is the amount of tracer in that tissue m_{tissue}, and the F/m ratio of the sample equals 1/area as $m_{sample} = \bar{C}a\ F_{sample}T = F_{sample} \int_0^\infty C_a(t)dt$. Because of inlet mixing all areas are equal and thus, had we been able to inject the dose selectively into the inflow to the tissue volume in question, then the area both on the arterial and venous side (if no retention had occurred) is the one measured.

The bolus distribution technique can be used in all organs or tissues provided the areas of interest are not so small that the number of retained indicator particles is too small for statistical evaluation.

Axial accumulation may give a maldistribution of the microspheres which depends of the size used. These problems may be significant in the kidney and in the myocardium where the method has been extensively used. The assumption of mixing at the inlet can be checked by taking blood samples at different sites downstream of the injection site. According to the equal area concept of Bergner (9) (Eq. 17) the area under the concentration curves should be the same. Otherwise complete mixing with the inflowing blood has not been achieved.

The microspheres are not readily applicable to studies of peripheral circulation in man, because they require intracardiac injection and measurement of the tracer concentration in the tissue. The principle has, however, been extensively used in man for determination of blood flow distribution in the lungs using Technetium-99m labeled macroaggregated albumin, a method which has great clinical importance.

Complete mixing with the inflowing blood is more readily accomplished using highly diffusible lipophilic indicators, C^{14} labeled butanol or C^{14} labeled iodo-antipyrine, with an initial extraction of more than 90 per cent. This variant of the microsphere is the local blood flow method of Kety as used for very short experimental periods, as will be discussed below. Recently a tracer with high initial extraction and prolonged retention in the brain and in other tissues as well, has been described by Winchell (15). This molecule, isopropyl-iodo-amphetamine, labeled with Iodine-123 constitutes a "chemical microsphere" that can be injected intravenously. The prolonged retention allows time for external detection with SPECT (Single Photon Emission Computerized Tomography) as used for measurement of regional cerebral blood flow in man.

Highly diffusible tracers with a short physical half-time compared to the shortest transit times in the system studied (e.g. $Krypton^{81m}$ with $t_{\frac{1}{2}}$ 13 sec) constitutes another related approach. With such tracers the steady-state distribution of the indicator in the organ studied during constant infusion, equals practically, that after a bolus injection of microspheres. This approach has been used for determination of blood flow distribution in lungs (16) and brain (17). The distribution of activity is usually recorded by a γ-camera. The advantage is that the recorded activity can be summed up over a long period of time reducing the statistical scatter of the measurement and improving the spatial resolution or allowing a tomographic recording to be made. It should be noted, that blood flow in areas with high flow rates tends to be underestimated, because significant wash-out by effluent blood occurs despite the short physical half-time of the indicator. This non-linearity of the concentration/flow relationship can be corrected for.

THE MEAN TRANSIT TIME METHODS, I

Non-compartmental Analysis ("Black Box" Analysis)

Determination of the mean transit time, $\bar{t}$, of an indicator in a given organ or tissue gives possibility for calculating the flow, F, if the volume of distribution, V_D, is known

$$F = V_D/\bar{t} \tag{21}$$

This formula was proved for intravascular indicators by Meier and Zierler (18). A proof including freely diffusible indicators will be given in a later section (see the section: The volume of distribution-flow ratio, V_D/F).

The mean transit time is the weighted average of all transit times in the system, each time being weighted by the fraction of transits having that transit time (the frequency of that particular transit time).

The concept of a single mean transit time presupposes a single inlet and a single outlet. However, using external recording of a radio-active tracer (residue-detection) converts a system with many outlets to an equivalent single-outlet system.

The volume of distribution of a tracer in a given system is defined as the amount of tracer in the system during tracer steady-state $m(\infty)$ divided by the blood concentration $C_{blood}(\infty)$, i.e.

$$V_D = \frac{m(\infty)}{C_{blood}(\infty)} \tag{22}$$

According to this definition V_D is obtained after constant infusion in such a way that full saturation (tracer steady-state) is achieved.

Another important parameter in this context is the tissue to blood partition coefficient, λ, defined as

$$\lambda = \frac{C_T(\infty)}{C_B(\infty)} \tag{23}$$

It is seen that λ equals the ratio of concentrations in tissue and blood during steady-state. Since the amount of tracer in the tissue at time infinity, $m(\infty)$, equals the weight of tissue W_T times $C_T(\infty)$ equation 22 can be written as $V_D = W_T \cdot C_T(\infty)/C_B(\infty)$ or $C_T(\infty)/C_B(\infty) = V_D/W_T$ giving according to equation 23

$$\lambda = \frac{V_D}{W_T} \tag{24}$$

Thus λ expresses the volume of distribution pr. gram of tissue. If λ is known it is possible to measure blood flow pr. gram of tissue by determination of $\bar{t}$: Dividing equation 21 on both sides with the tissue weight, W_T, we get, $F/W_T = (V_D/W_T)/\bar{t}$

$$f = \frac{\lambda}{\bar{t}} \tag{25}$$

where f is the perfusion coefficient often expressed in $ml \cdot min^{-1} \cdot (100g)^{-1}$, i.e. as $100 \cdot \lambda/\bar{t}$.

Expressing λ in the units ml/g we have used the definition originally given by Kety and Schmidt (19). It is important to stress that in this context V_D, W and λ all refer to the tissue including the blood located in the tissue.

Normally the tissue in a system or organ is not homogeneous, but may be regarded as a sum of homogeneous tissues (e.g. muscle, fat, collagen fibrils etc.). In this case it is necessary to calculate an average partition coefficient, $\bar{\lambda}$ taking into account all the different tissue components of the organ. As the concentration during indicator steady state in the ith tissue component equals V_{Di}/W_i we have according to equation 24 that $V_{Di} = \lambda_i \cdot W_i$. Summing up for all tissue components yields the total volume of distribution

$$V_D = \Sigma V_{Di} = \Sigma \lambda_i \cdot W_i \tag{26}$$

Dividing equation 26 by the total weight, W_T gives

$$\frac{V_D}{W_T} = \frac{\Sigma \lambda_i \cdot W_i}{W_T} \tag{27}$$

Since $\bar{\lambda}$ equals V_D/W_T we get

$$\bar{\lambda} = \Sigma \lambda_i \cdot \frac{W_i}{W_T} \tag{28}$$

It is seen that $\bar{\lambda}$ is the weighted average of all the λ_i in the organ, the weighting factor being the fractional weight of each tissue component.

The λ-concept plays an important role in all inert gas indicator methods, because for these freely diffusible tracers λ is practically independent of the functional state of the tissue, which may include changes in blood volume.

During indicator steady state the gas tension of an inert gas is the same throughout the system. The volume of gas dissolved per unit mass of tissue, $C_T(\infty)$ equals $\alpha_T \cdot P$, where α_T is the solubility coefficient of the gas in the tissue at a given temperature with the dimension ml gas (STPD) $\cdot g^{-1} \cdot atm^{-1}$. P is the partial pressure with the dimension of atm^{-1}. Similarly $C_B(\infty)$ equals $\zeta_B \cdot \alpha_B \cdot P$, with ζ_B being the specific gravity of the blood in $g \cdot ml^{-1}$, yielding

$$\lambda = \frac{C_T(\infty)}{C_B(\infty)} = \frac{\alpha_T}{\zeta_B \; \alpha_B} \; ml \cdot g^{-1} \tag{29}$$

Since α_T for an inert gas in an inhomogeneous system equals the weighted sum of the solubility coefficient of the single tissue components $\alpha_{T,i}$ we have

$$\alpha_T = \Sigma \, \alpha_{T,i} \cdot \frac{W_{T,i}}{W_T} \tag{30}$$

This means that the total amount of gas dissolved in a whole system per unit pressure equals the sum of gas amounts dissolved in each tissue component per unit pressure. As the same equation can be written for gas dissolved in the blood, we get

$$\frac{\alpha_T}{\alpha_B} = \frac{\zeta_B \; V_B}{W_T} \cdot \frac{\Sigma \, \alpha_{T,i} \cdot W_{T,i}}{\Sigma \, \alpha_{B,i} \cdot \zeta_{B,i} \; V_{B,i}} \tag{31}$$

where V_B is the total blood volume in the system. Substituting α_T/α_B in equation 29 yields

$$\bar{\lambda} = \frac{V_B \, \Sigma \, \alpha_{T,i} \cdot W_{T,i}}{W_T \, \Sigma \, \alpha_{B,i} \cdot \zeta_{B,i} \; V_{B,i}} \tag{32}$$

Thus it is possible to calculate $\bar{\lambda}$ for an inert gas in a whole system if the composition of the system is known. Since an inert gas as Xe is more soluble in hemoglobin than in plasma, the hematocrit in the blood becomes an important variable. $\bar{\lambda}$ is independent of the functional state of the tissue, as the inert gas solubility at a given temperature depends practically only upon the concentration of water, lipid and protein in the tissue. Based on equation 32 Yeh and Peterson (20) calculated $\bar{\lambda}$ for Xe in various tissues.

As stated above, a great advantage of using freely diffusible tracers compared to intravascular tracers is, that λ is practically independent of changes in blood volume in the tissue. As an example the change in $\bar{\lambda}$ due to venous stasis will be estimated. If we take muscle tissue and assume that normal blood volume is 5g/100g, the water content 60g/100g, the lipid content 1g/100g, and the protein content is 34g/100g, we have from equation 28 and using Yeh and Peterson's values:

$$\bar{\lambda} = \frac{1}{100} \cdot (5 \cdot 1.00 + 60 \cdot 0.45 + 34 \cdot 0.82 + 1 \cdot 10.2)$$

$$= 0.70 \text{ ml} \cdot g^{-1}$$

for a hematocrit of 0.45.

Assuming that venous stasis causes a 2-fold increase in blood volume $\bar{\lambda}$ becomes

$$\bar{\lambda} = \frac{1}{100} \cdot (10 \cdot 1.00 + 57 \cdot 0.45 + 32 \cdot 0.82 + 0.95 \cdot 10.2)$$

$$= 0.72 \text{ ml} \cdot g^{-1}$$

Thus doubling the blood volume only changed $\bar{\lambda}$ by about 3 per cent. In tissues with higher $\bar{\lambda}$ values as subcutaneous tissue, the influence of blood volume changes would be even less. On the other hand using intravascular tracers a doubling of the blood volume would cause an 100 per cent increase in $\bar{\lambda}$.

This is the reason why for example the ^{133}Xe washout method is suitable for measurement of blood flow in cases with distended veins, where venous occlusion plethysmography cannot be used.

Another important issue is that $\bar{\lambda}$ for inert gases with high solubility in lipid is very sensitive to changes in the lipid content of the tissue in question. Using the example from skeletal muscle and assuming that the fat content has increased from 1 to 3 per cent, $\bar{\lambda}$ becomes 0.9 ml/g, a change of about 33 per cent. This is especially important in lean tissues as muscle and cutis. Great variations of the lipid content in the liver constitutes also a major draw back for the use of inert gas indicators for measurement of blood flow in this organ.

Development of edema is another important functional change in a tissue. In lean tissues as muscle and cutis edema formation for example correcponding to 50 per cent of the tissue weight causes a decrease in $\bar{\lambda}$ for Xe from 0.70 ml $\cdot$ g^{-1} to 0.60. With unchanged flow rate $f = k \cdot \lambda$ per gram tissue, the decrease in $\bar{\lambda}$ tends to increase the washout rate constant of Xe by about 14 per cent. However, the decrease in capillary density of about 33 per cent influence the washout rate in the opposite direction, the net result being a reduction in the washout rate constant of about 22 per cent (assuming constant flow in each capillary). In tissues with high $\bar{\lambda}$ values as subcutaneous adipose tissue, the washout rate of Xe at a given capillary flow rate is less influenced by edema formation because changes due to decrease in $\bar{\lambda}$ are almost exactly counterbalanced by the concomitant decrease in capillary density. As example take abdominal subcutaneous tissue with a $\bar{\lambda}$ value of 10 ml · g^{-1}. Edema corresponding to 50 per cent of the tissue weight will cause a decrease in $\bar{\lambda}$ to 6.9 ml · g^{-1}. This taken together with the decrease in capillary density of 33 per cent means that the washout rate of Xe will be reduced by only 2-3 per cent.

Frequency Function of Transit Time, h(t)

Consider a single-inlet - single-outlet system where the amount m_0 of a tracer is injected at the inlet as an ideally brief bolus (impulse). h(t) is defined as the fractional rate at which the tracer leaves the system at time t. It has the dimension of t^{-1}, i.e. by definition

$$h(t) = \frac{FC(t)}{F\int_0^\infty C(t)dt} = \frac{C(t)}{\int_0^\infty C(t)dt} \quad \text{min}^{-1} \tag{33}$$

h(t) is thus the normalized (normalized to unit area) outflow concentration curve for the idealized impulse type of bolus injection.

Since h(t) remains practically constant in a very short time interval dt, we have that h(t) · dt is the fraction of the bolus leaving the system between time t and time t + dt. Thus h(t) · dt is the frequency of transit times in the time interval from time t to time t + dt, which shall be used to weight the transit time t in calculating $\bar{t}$.

According to the definition of $\bar{t}$ we therefore have

$$\bar{t} = \int_0^\infty t\, h(t)dt \tag{34}$$

or, as $h(t) = C(t)/\int_0^\infty C(t)dt$,

$$\bar{t} = \frac{\int_0^\infty t \cdot C(t)dt}{\int_0^\infty C(t)dt} \tag{35}$$

where C(t) is the outlet's concentration curve for an impulse input.

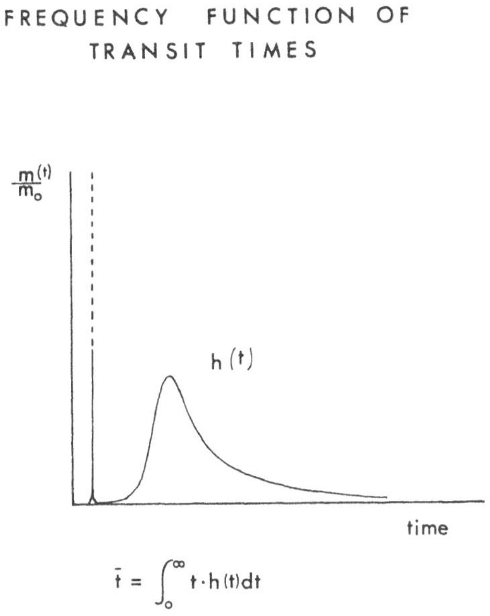

FIG. 5

h(t) function defined as fractional washout rate of tracer as a function of time.

Cumulative Outflux and Residue

The cumulative fraction of the dose which has left the system at time t is H(t) and can be written as

$$\text{Fractional Cumulative Outflux} = H(t) = \int_0^t h(t)dt \qquad (36)$$

The fraction remaining in the system at time t is the complement of the cumulative outflux giving

$$\text{Fractional Residue} = 1 - H(t) = 1 - \int_0^t h(t)dt \qquad (37)$$

Convolution Principle

Generally the input is not an ideally brief bolus, but if the system is stationary and linear, the impulse response, $h(\tau)$, can be used to calculate the response for any arbitrary input.If for example the bolus lasts a finite time during which the inlet concentration $C_{in}(t)$ differs from zero, the influx per unit dose $h_{in}(\tau)$ is spread out in time, so that in the interval τ, $\tau + d\tau$, the fraction $h_{in}(\tau)d\tau$ enters. The convolution principle consists in calculating the response by considering the input as a series

RESIDUE DETECTION

CUMULATIVE OUTFLOW SAMPLING

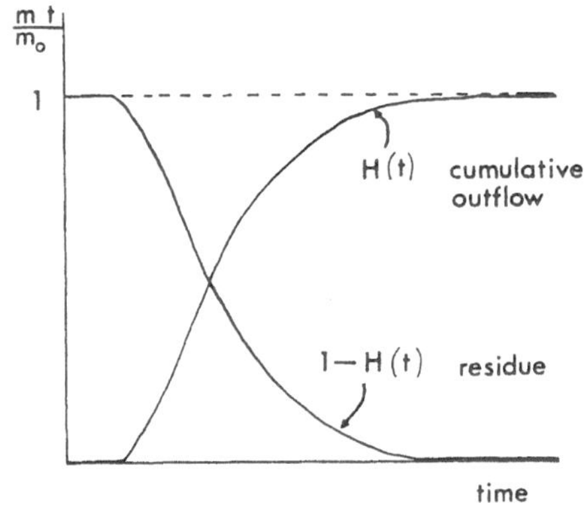

$$\bar{t} = \int_0^\infty [1 - H(t)]\,dt$$

FIG. 6

Residue curve, (1-H(t)) and cumulative outflow curve, (H(t)) after injection of the tracer as an ideally brief bolus, (impulse).

of ideally brief bolus inputs each of the amount $h_{in}(\tau) \cdot d\tau$. For each of these, the response is obtained by using $h(\tau)$ adjusted to take into account the time of entrance τ of $h(\tau)d\tau$. The contribution at the outlet of the system at time t of the bolus $h_{in}(\tau)d\tau$ entering at time τ is the product of the amount entering at time τ and the response per unit of bolus entering at time τ, $h(t-\tau)d\tau$. Adding all the contributions gives the fractional output at time t

$$h_{out}(t) = \int_0^t h_{in}(\tau) \cdot h(t-\tau)d\tau \qquad (38)$$

τ is an integration variable with the dimension of time and going from zero to t.

The convolution principle thus consists of integrating the product of the two functions where the one, $h_{in}(\tau)$ goes from zero to t, while the other function, $h(t-\tau)$ goes from t to zero, or vice versa.

This is expressed by writing equation 38

$$h_{out}(t) = h_{in}(t) * h(t) \tag{39}$$

with the asterisk denoting the convolution procedure described above in equation 38.

Based on this formalism it is possible to calculate the concentration of the outlet at time t after any injection of indicator, simply by scaling with m_0, because the influx is $F \cdot C_{in}(t) = m_0 \cdot h_{in}(t)$ and the outflux is $F \cdot C_{out}(t) = m_0 \cdot h_{out}(t)$. Thus multiplying equation 39 with m_0/F gives

$$C_{out}(t) = C_{in}(t) * h(t) \tag{40}$$

For this reason h(t) may be regarded as the elementary response of the system, a transfer function that in a precisely known way transfers or transforms any known input curve to the curve at the outlet.

MEAN TRANSIT TIME DETERMINED BY CONSTANT INFUSION AND INLET-OUTLET SAMPLING

Saturation experiment (Kety & Schmidt (19))

Consider the situation where the indicators are supplied by constant infusion at the inlet. Sampling is performed at the inlet $C_{in}(t)$ and at the outlet $C_{out}(t)$. The mass balance concept gives that the indicator uptake in the system in the time interval t, t+dt, dm(t) can be written as

$$dm(t) = F(C_{in}(t) - C_{out}(t))dt$$

Hence the total uptake at time infinity is obtained by integrating on both sides

$$m(\infty) = F\int_0^{\infty}(C_{in}(t) - C_{out}(t))dt \tag{41}$$

Since $m(\infty)$ equals the tissue weight W_T times the average indicator concentration for $t = \infty$, $C_T(\infty)$ and the latter equals $\lambda \cdot C_{blood}(\infty)$ (Eq. 23) we therefore get $m(\infty) = W_T C_T(\infty) = W_T \lambda C_{blood}(\infty)$, which inserted into equation 41 yields

$$\frac{F}{W_T} = f = \frac{\lambda \cdot C_{blood}(\infty)}{\int_0^\infty C_{in}(t)dt - \int_0^\infty C_{out}(t)dt} \qquad (42)$$

$C_{blood}(\infty)$ is the indicator concentration at the time infinity, when indicator steady-state is obtained, i.e. $C_{out}(\infty) = C_{in}(\infty) = C_{blood}(\infty)$.

CONSTANT INFUSION, INLET-OUTLET SAMPLING

Kety – Schmidt Principle

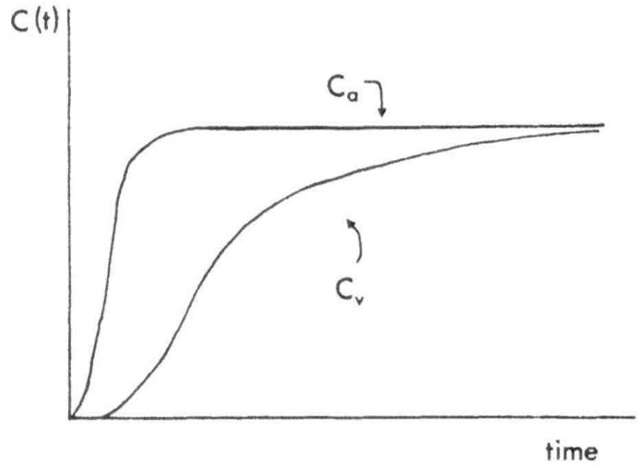

$$f = \frac{\lambda \cdot C_{blood}(\infty)}{\int_0^\infty C_a(t)dt - \int_0^\infty C_v(t)dt}$$

FIG. 7

Diagram illustrating the constant infusion experiment with inlet-outlet sampling, (Kety-Schmidt experiment).

Since f equals $\lambda/\bar{t}$ (Eq. 25) it is seen that the area between the curves divided by their height at equilibrium is the mean transit time of the system

$$\bar{t} = \frac{\int_0^\infty C_{in}(t)dt - \int_0^\infty C_{out}(t)dt}{C_{blood}(\infty)} \qquad (43)$$

As will be shown in the following, a proof for this relationship can also be obtained by using the convolution theorem, Eq. 40. For simplicity we assume that $C_{in}(t)$ reaches the equilibrium level in an instantaneous step and remains constant, i.e. $C_{in}(t) = C_{in}$. According to equation 40 we have

$$C_{out}(t) = C_{in} * h(t) = \int_0^{\tau} C_{in}(t-\tau)h(\tau)d\tau$$

or, as C_{in} is a constant

$$C_{out}(t) = C_{in} \cdot \int_0^t h(t)dt = C_{in} \cdot H(t) \tag{44}$$

Substituting $C_{out}(t)$ in equation 43 with equation 44 and using $C_{blood}(\infty) = C_{in}$ the right hand side in equation 43 becomes

$$\frac{\int_0^{\infty} (C_{in}(\infty) - C_{in}(\infty) \cdot H(t))dt}{C_{in}(\infty)}$$

or

$$\int_0^{\infty} (1 - H(t))dt$$

Integrating by parts and recalling that $\bar{t} = \int_0^{\infty} t \cdot h(t)dt$ yields

$$\int_0^{\infty} 1 \cdot (1 - H(t))dt = t(1 - Ht))\Big|_0^{\infty} + \int_0^{\infty} t\, h(t)dt$$

$$= t(1 - H(t))\Big|_0^{\infty} + \bar{t}$$

i.e.

$$\bar{t} = \int_0^{\infty} (1 - H(t))dt \tag{45}$$

because the first term on the right hand side is zero in both time limits (for $t \to \infty (1 - Ht))$ goes to zero, because $h(t)$ has the area of unity, i.e. $H(t) = \int_0^t h(t) \to 1$ as $t \to \infty$). Thus the correctness of equation 43 has been proven by the convolution theorem.

The constant infusion experiment with inlet-outlet sampling was introduced by Kety and Schmidt in 1945 (19) using inert gas saturation for quantitative determination of the perfusion coefficient f in the brain. The method gives an average value of the brain perfusion pr. gram of tissue calculated according to equation 42.

Air containing N_2O with a constant concentration (30% or less) is inhaled over a period of about 10-12 min. The concentration is measured in blood sampled from an artery and from the internal jugular vein. Using as Kety and Schmidt an equilibration time of only 10 min the area between the arterial and venous concentration curves is underestimated. However, using the concentration in venous blood at 10 min as the height, this is also underestimated and that reduces the error. Lassen and Munck (21) employing ^{85}Kr as indicator emphasized that the indicator uptake theoretically should be followed to time infinity. Monoexponential extrapolation was applied in calculating the total area between the curves to time infinity.

A similar approach has been used for determination of the perfusion coefficient in the human kidney (22). As in the case of the brain too short time was used for complete saturation of the tissues especially the regions of the kidney with low perfusion (medulla). For that reason the calculated perfusion coefficient is dominated by the perfusion in the cortex.

The method has also been applied for determination of myocardial blood flow (23), venous blood from the myocardium was sampled from the coronary sinus. Like in the case of brain and kidney this has the advantage of allowing simultaneous determination of the myocardial arterio-venous difference of oxygen and various metabolites, i.e. the metabolic rate can be calculated. Again, the area between the arterial and venous concentration curves can be measured accurately only for a few minutes (usually 5 min) a time too short for full equilibration and the area is underestimated. Thus, saturation of the tissue components with slow perfusion relative to solubility are not fully taken into account and the calculated perfusion coefficient is therefore dominated by tissue components with high perfusion. This approach is therefore similar to that of using the initial wash-out rate (initial slope) of externally recorded γ-emitting inert gases following a close intra-arterial injection as a brief bolus (see later).

Note that the Kety-Schmidt method gives no information of regional distribution of blood flow inside the tissue studied.

Desaturation Experiment

In a saturation experiment described above it is seen from equation 44 that the outlet concentration per unit step input $C_{out}(t)/C_{in}$ equals the cumulative outflow following a brief bolus injection, H(t). In the desaturation experiment the infusion starts at time minus infinity and full saturation being achieved, at time zero, the infusion is stopped and the inlet concentration is assumed to drop instantaneously from its constant value C_{in} to zero. Thus $C_{in}(t) = C_{in}$ for $t \leqslant 0$ and $C_{in}(t) = 0$ for $t > 0$.

$$C_{out}(t) = \int_{-\infty}^{t} C_{in}(\tau) \cdot h(t-\tau)d\tau$$

Splitting the integral into two parts by integrating from $(-\infty)$

to time zero and from zero to t yields with $t-\tau = u$

$$C_{out}(t) = C_{in} \int_{-\infty}^{0} h(t-\tau)d\tau = C_{in} \int_{t}^{\infty} h(u)du$$

$$= C_{in}(\int_{0}^{\infty} h(u)du - \int_{0}^{t} h(u)du)$$

$$= C_{in}(1 - H(t))$$

or

$$\frac{C_{out}(t)}{C_{in}} = 1 - H(t) \tag{46}$$

Thus the outlet concentration curve during desaturation for a unit step input equals the residue curve following a brief bolus injection (see below).

Thus, as $C_{in} = 0$, the area/height ratio during desaturation becomes $\int_0^\infty(1-H(t))dt = \bar{t}$ just as in the saturation experiment described above.

The desaturation experiment is often more accurate than the saturation experiment as the arterial curve descends very smoothly (leaks at the mask are not important during desaturation). On the other hand it presupposes a prolonged preceeding saturation period (20 to 30 min in the case of the brain).

MEAN TRANSIT TIME DETERMINED BY CONSTANT INFUSION AND RESIDUE DETECTION

Desaturation

In this case the amount in the tissue, also called the _residue_ of the tracer in the tissue, is recorded as a function of time m(t). The tracer is infused into the local artery in such a way, that it is possible to obtain an abrupt transition from the constant arterial concentration, C_{in} to zero.

The amount of tracer in the tissue after full saturation to equilibrium between tissue and blood $m(\infty)$ is calculated as the unit bolus residue function $(1-H(t))$ convoluted by the constant input $F \cdot C_{in}$:

$$m(\infty) = F \cdot C_{in} * (1 - H(t))$$

$$= F \cdot C_{in} \cdot \int_{0}^{\infty}(1 - H(t))dt$$

$$= F \cdot C_{in} \cdot \bar{t}$$

or

$$\bar{t} = \frac{m(\infty)}{F \cdot C_{in}} \tag{47}$$

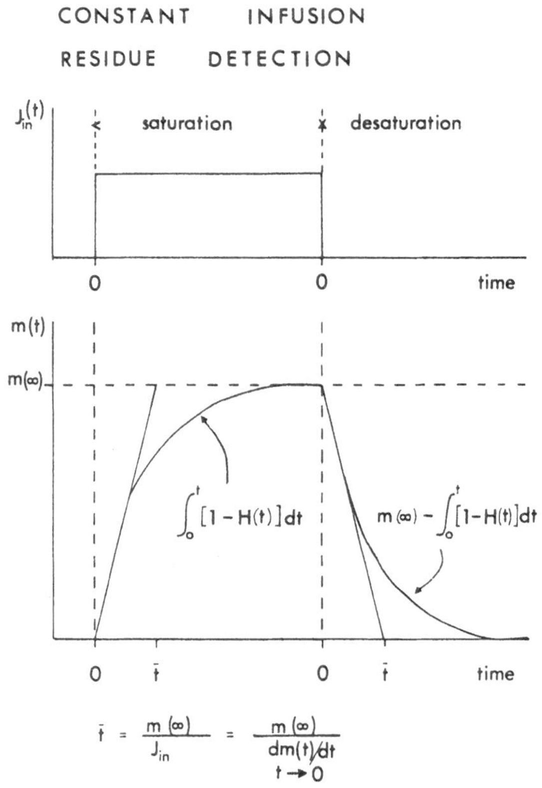

FIG. 8

Diagram illustrating the constant infusion, residue detection experiment.

At time zero the infusion is stopped and C_{in} drops instantaneously to zero. Since the initial washout rate -dm/dt, $t \to 0$ equals the outflux during equilibrium $F \cdot C_{out}(\infty)$ and $C_{out}(\infty) = C_{in}(\infty)$, we get

$$\bar{t} = \frac{m(\infty)}{-dm/dt_{\,t \to 0+}} = \frac{\text{equilibrium height}}{\text{initial slope}} \tag{48}$$

Inserting $\bar{t} = \frac{\lambda}{f}$ and solving for f yields

$$f = \lambda \frac{-dm/dt}{m(\infty)}_{t \to 0+} = \lambda \frac{|\text{slope at } t \to 0|}{\text{height at equilibrium}} \qquad (49)$$

Saturation

In this case the infusion starts at time zero i.e. C_{in} increases instantaneously from zero to its constant value C_{in}. The initial increase in amount of tracer in the system dm/dt within a time period corresponding to the shortest transit times in the system equals $F \cdot C_{in}$ (no outflow). Recalling that the amount at equilibrium $m(\infty) = F \cdot C_{in} \cdot \bar{t}$ we have

$$\bar{t} = \frac{m(\infty)}{dm/dt}_{t \to 0+} \qquad (50)$$

Comments on the Residue Detection During Desaturation or Saturation (the Initial Slope Method) with Special Regard to the Use of Freely Diffusible Indicators

As only the ratio of the residue $m(\infty)$ and its initial slope, dm(t)/dt for $t \to 0+$, must be measured it follows, that the absolute residual amount need not to be determined. When using external counting of a radioactive indicator we therefore do not have to know the counting efficiency (the counting "geometry") as long as it remains constant. The rate of tracer infusion is also immaterial.

The major difficulty of the initial slope method consists in the possibility (or even the likelyhood) that only a very short time may exist during which the influx has truly changed stepwise, while yet the outflux remains at its previous steady state value. Consider for example that we were studying by external counting the initial rate of decrease of Iodine-131-labeled serum albumin after stopping an intra-arterial constant infusion abruptly. Even if one stops the infusion pump abruptly, the influx of tracer does not drop to zero instantaneously, because the tracer concentration in the blood at the inlet cannot change truly stepwise. Perhaps it will take 1 or 2 seconds for it to reach a negligible level. Following this delay there may be a brief period, perhaps 3 to 5 seconds, during which the outflux can be assumed still to continue at the same (maximum) rate as during the infusion. It is during this brief period, say from the 2nd to the 5th or 7th second that the initial slope must be recorded. Clearly, this slope cannot be recorded accurately in so short a time, especially if the slope is relatively shallow.

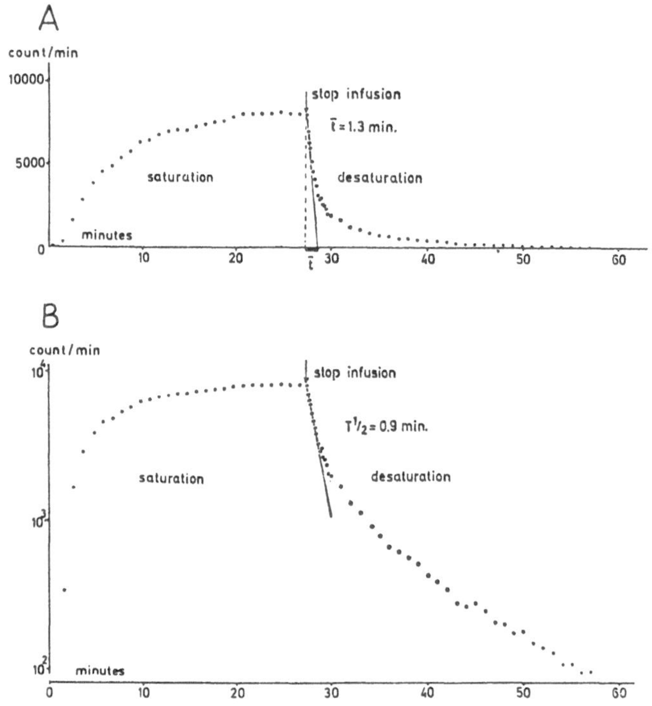

FIG. 9

Linear plot (upper curve) and semilogarithmic plot (lower curve) of ^{133}Xe washout from isolated cat gastrocnemius muscle following close intra-arterial constant infusion.(Sejrsen & Tønnesen (25)).

This discussion demonstrates, that although the residue detection method is quite analogous to the inlet-outlet detection method (the Kety-Schmidt method), in practice the two methods are quite different. The difficulties involved in determining the initial linear slope dm(t)/dt for $t \to 0+$ are of such a magnitude that to our knowledge the method has never been used (and should not be used either!). It is the initial or, more precisely, the steepest semilogarithmic slope one employs.

The justification for making a semilogarithmic plot is that, with freely diffusible indicators many tissues will initially during desaturation behave like a single well-mixed system, a "compartment" as discussed below. We shall here just mention, that its residue desaturation curve is monoexponential, i.e.

$$m(t) = m(\infty)e^{-k\,t}$$

$$\text{with } k = 1/\bar{t} = f/\lambda \qquad (51)$$

For this curve the relative slope $\dot{m}/m$ has the constant numerical value of

$$-\dot{m}(t)/m(t) = k = 1/\bar{t}$$

Hence it follows that with the use of a freely diffusible indicator in a given system and under certain circumstances, where the curve decreases monoexponentially for a substantial fraction of the residue (until $t = t_1$), we have

$$k = -\dot{m}(0)/m(0) \simeq -\dot{m}(t)/m(t) = d \ln m(t)/dt \quad (\text{for } t < t_1) \qquad (52)$$

Thus the parameter on the left hand side, that we want to measure, $k = -\dot{m}(0)/m(0)$ can be calculated from the right hand side, viz. from the observed slope of the semilogarithmic plot, where the slope is a straight line for a much longer time than on the linear plot, Fig. 9.

The use of the initial semilogarithmic slope for a freely diffusible tracer $k = -d \ln m(t)/dt$ can also be explained by reference to a multicompartmental system all subelements assumed to obey equation 51 and assumed to be arranged in parallel. For this system the residue curve is

$$m(t) = \Sigma W_i C_{in}(\infty) \lambda_i \exp.(-f_i/\lambda_i)t \qquad (53)$$

The logarithmic slope is thus for short times

$$-d \ln m/dt \simeq -\dot{m}/m = \frac{\Sigma W_i C_{in}(\infty) \lambda_i \cdot f_i/\lambda_i}{\Sigma W_i C_{in}(\infty) \lambda_i} - \frac{f}{\lambda} = k \qquad (54)$$

This way of deriving equation 52 is more rigorous. It explains that the initial maximal semilog slope of a multiexponential curve can be used to estimate the average blood flow $\bar{f}$ if one experimentally has observed that a quasi-semilogarithmic initial segment exists (this in its turn is the same as to state that a sizable part of the system represents the highest flow compartments).

In summary, instead of the correct but impractical linear slope one can for freely diffusible tracers with good approximation use a semilogarithmic slope. This approximation was proposed by Lassen and Ingvar (24) for measurement of blood flow in the cerebral cortex and verified experimentally by Sejrsen and Tønnesen (25) using ^{133}Xe as tracer for blood flow in skeletal muscle and comparing the result to the directly metered outflow, Fig. 10.

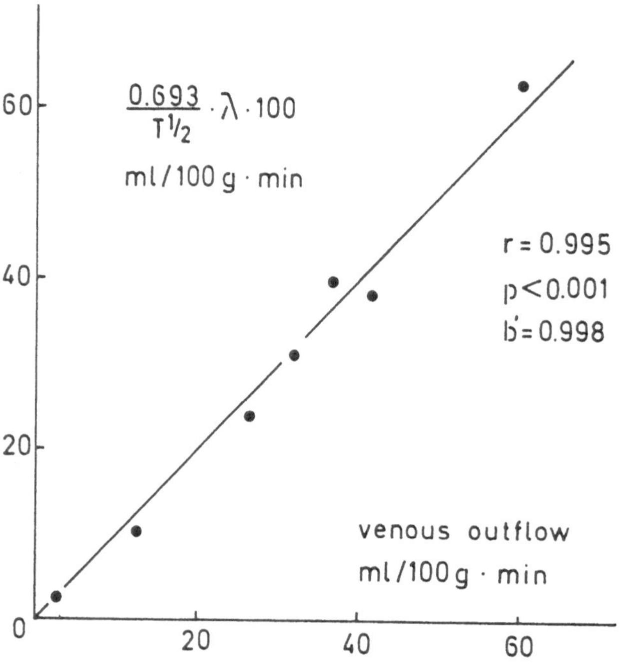

FIG. 10

Comparison between directly measured blood flow as venous outflow rate and blood flow calculated from the initial slope in a semilogarithmic plot (Eq. 52) of the ^{133}Xe desaturation curves in the isolated cat gastrocnemius muscle following intraarterially step input.
From Sejrsen and Tønnesen (25) by permission of the American Heart Association, Inc.

In the above description the tracer was introduced by constant infusion into the inflowing blood. Another approach using freely diffusible tracers (e.g. inert gases) is to label the tissue directly by letting the tracer diffuse into the tissue from the surface or by injecting the tracer into the tissue and externally recording the washout of the tracer (residue). In this situation all the tissue components are equally labeled and due to the high diffusibility of the tracers in question, diffusion equilibrium between the tissue and the effluent blood is maintained (26). As the argument leading to the semilogarithmic slope is based on the concept of well-mixed compartments organized in parallel, these methods will be discussed in a following section. All that was aimed at in the above paragraph was to stress the very close relationship between the "black box" result (linear initial slope) and the "multicompartmental" result (semilogarithmic initial slope).

MEAN TRANSIT TIME BY BOLUS INJECTION AND RESIDUE DETECTION: The Height over Area Equation of Zierler (27).

In this experiment a radioactive tracer is injected by close intra-arterial injection at the single inlet as a brief bolus. The washout from the organ or tissue is followed by an external detector. The initial part of the curve shows the abrupt arrival of the tracer followed by a brief plateau of constant maximum actively denoting that the entire dose, m_0 remains inside the system until the shortest transit time is exceeded. Thereafter a steady washout is seen.

Assuming no recirculation we have, according to equation 37, that the amount of tracer per unit dose remaining in the system at time t, $m(t)/m_0$ equals $1 - H(t)$ or

$$m(t) = m_0 (1 - H(t)) \tag{55}$$

In the actual experiment the total dose is seldom measured because the detection efficiency is included. However, the recorded initial maximum height, A_{max} is a relative measure of the dose, m_0 as measured with the same efficiency as the entire recorded washout function.

Thus, since $m_0 = \varepsilon \cdot A_{max}$, where ε denotes the detection efficiency we can rewrite equation 55

$$\varepsilon A(t) = \varepsilon A_{max}(1 - H(t))$$

or

$$A(t) = A_{max}(1 - H(t)) \tag{56}$$

The area under the recorded residue curve to time infinity is

$$\int_0^\infty A(t)dt = A_{max}\int_0^\infty (1 - H(t))dt = A_{max} \cdot \bar{t}$$

since $\bar{t} = (1 - H(t))dt$ (Eq. 45).

Thus

$$\bar{t} = \frac{\int_0^\infty A(t)dt}{A_{max}} = \frac{\text{Area under residue curve}}{\text{Height}} \tag{57}$$

Since $f = \lambda/\bar{t}$ the perfusion coefficient in $ml \cdot min^{-1}$ equals

$$f = \lambda \cdot \frac{A_{max}}{\int_0^\infty A(t)dt} = \lambda \cdot \frac{\text{Height}}{\text{Area}}\ ml \cdot g^{-1} \cdot min \tag{58}$$

From equation 56 it is seen that it is essential that the total dose and the washout function if measured with the same efficiency. Furthermore it is necessary, that the obtained washout function is representative for the whole system studied. It is also important, that the bolus is so brief, that the total dose has entered the system within a time interval shorter than the shortest transit times in the system.

It is seen that Zierler's final equation (Eq. 58) is precisely the same as that used in the Kety-Schmidt experiment (Eq. 42) and the two methods are basically identical. An advantage of performing residue detection using a number of external detectors is, that is is possible to record the delivery from discrete regions of an organ and thus obtaining regional distribution of blood flow as measured in the human brain by Lassen and Ingvar (24, see also 28).

Tønnesen and Sejrsen (29) has used ^{133}Xe and the bolus injection residue detection method for determination of blood flow in the isolated autoperfused gastrocnemius muscle. The results agreed well with directly measured flow.

The bolus injection-residue detection method has also been applied for determination of blood flow in the myocardium (30,31) and kidney (32). For both organs the washout of ^{133}Xe after close intra-arterial injection followed a multiexponential course. Using the "area/height" formula, equation 57 and a λ value of 0.7 $ml \cdot g^{-1}$ too low blood flow values were obtained. The explanation is, that ^{133}Xe is accumulating in pericardial fat tissue in the heart and perirenal fat tissue in the kidney. This means that the true average λ for the whole organ is larger than the values used.

Since the fat content may vary considerably, it is virtually impossible to obtain the correct λ in the individual case. The best method of analyzing the ^{133}Xe washout curves is to use the <u>initial slope</u> in a semilogarithmic plot. This slope is dominated by the washout of tracer from the fast flow component, i.e. the practically homogeneously perfused myocardium in heart and cortex in kidney.

The initial slope, k may be calculated as ln 2 divided by the half time $T_{\frac{1}{2}}$ of the initial monoexponential part of the wash-out curve. Since $\bar{t}$ equals 1/k (see under compartmental analysis) we have that the perfusion coefficient in the fast flow component is approximated as

$$f_1 \simeq \lambda_1 \cdot \frac{\ln 2}{T_{\frac{1}{2}} \text{ initial}} \tag{59}$$

where λ_1 is the tissue to blood partition coefficient for the fast flow component.

In the brain the washout curves of ^{133}Xe are biexponential following bolus injection in the internal carotid artery. Again the initial mono-exponential part of the washout curve is dominated by washout of tracer from the fast flow component, i.e. grey matter of the brain (33).

To emphasize this point it should be mentioned that in the bolus experiment the initial slope in a semilogarithmic plot is basically quite different from the corresponding slope in the saturation-desaturation experiment. The difference may be expressed by using the multicompartmental approach on both experiments. As already shown in equation 53 during desaturation each tissue element i contributes to $-\dot{m}/m(t\to0)$ in proportion to its volume of distribution ($W_i\ \lambda_i$), while in the bolus experiment the contribution is proportional to the total flow through that tissue $W_i\ f_i$. This is a direct consequence of the bolus' distribution, i.e. each tissue, i getting tracer amounts in proportion to $F_i = W_i\ f_i$.

Thus, desaturation experiment (Eq. 54):

$$-\dot{m}/m_{\,t\to0} = \Sigma\, W_i\ \lambda_i\ k_i / \Sigma\, W_i\ \lambda_i$$

bolus experiment:

$$-\dot{m}/m_{\,t\to0} = \Sigma\, W_i\ f_i\ k_i / \Sigma\, W_i\ f_i \tag{60}$$

MEAN TRANSIT TIME BY BOLUS INJECTION AND INLET-OUTLET SAMPLING

Often the bolus input is not an ideal impulse. The actual shape of the input curve may be regarded as the outflow from an imaginary input system located in front and in series with the actual system studied. The imaginary input system is characterized by a frequency function of transit times, $h_{in}(t)$ and its input is the ideal brief impulse.

According to equations 34 and 35 the mean transit time for the input system t_{in} equals

$$\bar{t}_{in} = \int_0^\infty t\, h_{in}(t)dt = \frac{\int_0^\infty t\, C_{in}(t)dt}{\int_0^\infty C_{in}(t)dt} \qquad (61)$$

The outflow curve normalized to unit area is the frequency function of transit times, $h_{out}(t)$ in the combined system, i.e. the imaginary input system and the actually system studied thus

$$\bar{t}_{out} = \int_0^\infty t\, h_{out}(t)dt = \frac{\int_0^\infty t\, C_{out}(t)dt}{\int_0^\infty C_{out}(t)dt} \qquad (62)$$

BOLUS INJECTION, INLET - OUTLET SAMPLING

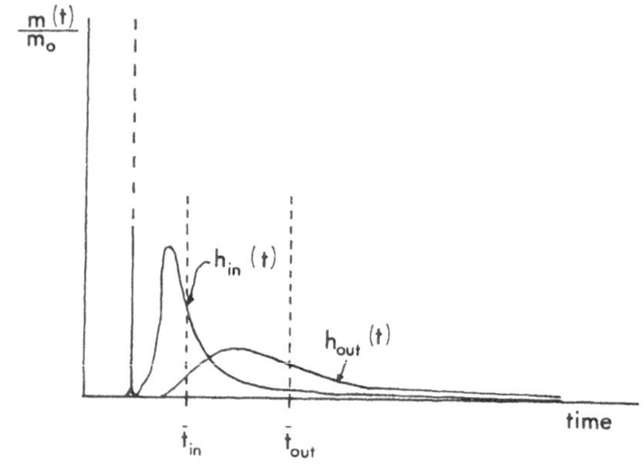

$$\bar{t}_{system} = \bar{t}_{out} - \bar{t}_{in} = \int_0^\infty t \cdot h_{out}(t)dt - \int_0^\infty t \cdot h_{in}(t)dt$$

FIG. 11

Bolus experiment, inlet-outlet sampling

The mean transit times in systems coupled in series are additive. Consider two systems coupled in series with the volumes of distribution of V_{D1} and V_{D2} respectively and the flow, F

Since $V_{D1}/F + V_{D2}/F = (V_{D1} + V_{D2})/F$

and $\bar{t} = V_D/F$, we have

$$\bar{t}_1 + \bar{t}_2 = \bar{t}_{1+2} \tag{63}$$

That is, the sum of the mean transit times of the two systems in series gives the mean transit time of the total system.

Based on this we have, that the mean transit time of the system actually studied, $\bar{t}_{system}$ equals $\bar{t}_{out} - \bar{t}_{in}$ or

$$\bar{t}_{system} = \int_0^\infty t \cdot h_{out}(t)dt - \int_0^\infty t \cdot h_{in}(t)dt$$

$$= \frac{\int_0^\infty t \cdot C_{out}(t)dt}{\int_0^\infty C_{out}(t)dt} - \frac{\int_0^\infty t \cdot C_{in}(t)dt}{\int_0^\infty C_{in}(t)dt} \tag{64}$$

Although the actual experiment is the same as the indicator dilution method discussed previously for measuring blood flow (dose over area) the analysis of the mean transit time is based on a completely different set of assumptions, i.e. a single inlet - single outlet system,i.e. cross stream mixing occurs at the inlet as well as at the outlet.

Another important implication of equation 63 is, that it is possible to correct errors in calculation of $\bar{t}$ based on outflow measurements, where the obtained $\bar{t}$ value may include the mean transit time of the tracer in the collecting catheter, $\bar{t}_{cath}$, since $\bar{t}_{total} = \bar{t}_{system} + \bar{t}_{cath}$ according to equation 63 and as $\bar{t}_{cath}$ equals the volume of the catheter, V_{cath} divided with the sampling rate F_{cath}, we have

$$\bar{t}_{total} = \bar{t}_{system + cath} - V_{cath}/F_{cath} \tag{65}$$

VOLUME OF DISTRIBUTION - FLOW RATIO, V_D/F

The methods for measurement of blood flow of the tracer, by determining the mean transit time in the system are based on the fundamental equation, $\bar{t} = V_D/F$.

It has been rigorously shown, that $\bar{t}$ can be obtained from the outflow either in a constant infusion experiment (as the normalized area) or in bolus-experiment (as the weighted normalized area). Here we shall offer a simple and yet rigorous proof of the mean transit time theorem $\bar{t} = V_D/F$. The constant infusion experiment offers a particular easy way of proving that this theorem is correct for any tracer, including the freely diffusible tracers. Consider the constant infusion experiment, where the concentration in the inflowing blood is the constant C_{in} starting at time $t = 0$ to time $t = \infty$. During indicator steady state, where full saturation of the system is obtained, we have according to equation 47 that the amount of indicator in the system is

$$m(\infty) = F \cdot C_{in} \cdot \bar{t} \tag{66}$$

As shown earlier (Eq. 22) the residue can also be expressed as

$$m(\infty) = V_D \cdot C_{in} \tag{67}$$

yielding

$$\bar{t} = V_D/F \tag{68}$$

According to the stimulus response theorem (8), see equations 15 and 16, the ratio of stimulus and response is the same in the constant infusion (steady state) experiment as the corresponding time integrals to $t = \infty$ in the bolus experiment.

The same relationship holds true for the mean transit time analyzed above, hence

$$\bar{t} = \underset{\text{steady state}}{\frac{m(\infty)}{F \cdot C_{in}(\infty)}} = \underset{\text{bolus}}{\frac{\int_0^\infty m(t)dt}{F\int_0^\infty C_{in}(t)dt}} = \underset{\text{bolus}}{\frac{\int_0^\infty m(t)dt}{m_{max}}} = V_D/F \tag{69}$$

These important equations state that $\bar{t}$, which can be obtained from constant infusion experiments as well as bolus experiments, equals V_D/F. It is consequently not necessary to assume that the tracer remains inside the plasma (cf. the proof by Meier and Zierler(18)). The relationship holds also true for freely diffusible indicators passing through the capillary membrane.

SUMMARY OF BLACK-BOX ANALYSIS FOR MEASURING $\bar{t}$ AND HENCE FLOW BY $f = \lambda/\bar{t}$.

Bolus Injection

Residue Detection: This curve represents if scaled to unit height the fraction of the bolus remaining (residing) in the tissue as a function of time, i.e. $(1 - H(t))$. Hence its area is $\bar{t}$ as $\int_0^\infty (1 - H(t)dt = \int_0^\infty t\, h(t)dt = \bar{t}$. If normalization to unit height is omitted, it is necessary to scale afterwards by dividing the area by the height. If one cannot make so brief an injection, that the height represents the total amount of tracer, then the $\bar{t}$ = area/height is invalid.

Using freely diffusible tracer and bolus injection the initial slope in a semilogarithmic system may descend quasi-monoexponentially for a substantial fraction of the residue (e.g. until 50% of the residue has been washed out). This signifies that the fastest flow component is a fairly large component of the tissue. The slope of this semilogarithmic curve (for $t < t_1$) is an approximate measure (a slight underestimate) of the time constant of that dominant fast flow tissue, i.e. $d \ln m(t)/dt$ (for $t < t_1$) $\simeq k_i = 1/\bar{t}_i = f_i/\lambda_i$. By convolution it can be shown that even if the bolus is not very brief so, that the height underestimates the total bolus, the initial steepest slope still can be used essentially without added error.

Outlet Sampling: Injecting an ideally brief bolus the curve recorded at the outlet is, after scaling to unit area $h(t)$. Thus in this experiment, that cannot be carried out in practice, $\bar{t} = \int_0^\infty t \cdot C(t)dt / \int_0^\infty C(t)dt$. Under realistic experimental conditions the mean time of bolus entrance $\bar{t}_{in}$ must be subtracted as must also the delay incurred by the sampling. In both cases the volume/flow ratio may be used for the correction. In order to emphasize that the inlet's $\bar{t}_{in}$ must be known, the method was in the above text termed the inlet-outlet sampling method, without implying, however, that one need to take blood samples at the inlet!

Constant Infusion

Residue Detection: Saturating the tissue by an abruptly starting constant infusion (step function) $\bar{t}$ is the full saturation residue divided by the initial slope. In the mirror-image experiment stopping the infusion abruptly after full saturation, (i.e. the desaturation experiment), $\bar{t}$ is the full saturation residue divided by the numerical value of the initial slope.

These two initial slope calculations are based on recording the initial slope in a linear plot of the curve. This initial slope cannot be recorded accurately and that invalidates the approach. Instead the initial slope in a semilogarithmic plot can be often used with freely diffusible indicators as the early part of the curve decreases (respectively increases towards saturation) in a quasi-monoexponential manner with a time constant k being the reciprocal of the mean transit time for the entire system, $k = 1/\bar{t}$.

Outlet Sampling: Saturating a tissue by constant infusion of ideal step-function shape the outlet curve rises towards its final value $C(\infty)$ with the function $C(t) = C(\infty)\ H(t)$. Hence $\bar{t}$ is the area between this final plateau value and the outlet curve divided by the plateau value $\bar{t} = \int_0^\infty (C(\infty) - C(\infty)\ H(t))dt$.

Abrupt desaturation results in a curve descending from the constant saturation value $C(\infty)$ with the function $C(\infty)\ (1 - H(t))$, i.e. the area underneath gives after dividing by the height the mean transit time $\bar{t}$.

In practice we must correct for the fact that the ideal step function cannot be achieved, this is done by recording the inlet curve and calculating $\bar{t}$ as the area between inlet and outlet curves divided by their height (Kety-Schmidt approach).

Recirculation

As already stressed, in the mean transit time methods inert gases are widely used. This tends to reduce the recirculation problem to a negligible level. For example when using ^{133}Xe and bolus injection in one carotid artery in man and external detection over the brain, the recirculation only increases the area by 1 - 2%, an error that can easily be estimated by injecting the same dose intravenously. The low level of recirculation is mainly due to the very effective elimination of ^{133}Xe in the lungs.

Extrapolation: The Achilles heel of the flow methods so far discussed, viz. the mass balance methods and the non-compartmental mean transit time methods lies in the requirement of knowing the entire fate of the bolus respective of its integral. Consider for example the Stewart constant-infusion method first mentioned. In this case it is necessary to wait for the maximal (the steady-state) outlet concentration. Theoretically an extrapolation procedure might be needed in order to take into account the "final" increase of $C_{out}(t)$ towards its asymptotic value $C_{out}(\infty)$, that only can be truly reached when the longest transit time has been exceeded. Precisely the same holds for the bolus injection method for measuring flow or clearance (Henriques, Hamilton, Bergner). And in the mean transit time methods the problem of extrapolation is even worse, as the "tail" of h(t) is weighted heavily (by t) to calculate $\bar{t}$.

Conventionally a mono-exponential extrapolation procedure is used throughout. The rationale for this approach is discussed in the final section of this chapter.

Comment on the Initial Slope Techniques: In the above text we introduced the logarithmic initial slope approach. Both the one after full saturation that (under certain conditions) may give an estimate of $\bar{t}$, the mean transit time of the entire system, and the one after bolus injection that (under practically the same conditions) may yield a slightly underestimated value for $\bar{t}_i$, the mean transit time of the fastest "compartment".

This analysis is clearly not a true black-box approach, as precise assumptions are made as to the nature of the tracer (freely diffusible) and of the system (the fastest flow component behaving as a single compartment and being of sufficient size to dominate the initial curve segment). Yet, the analysis is not compartmental in the sense of requiring the resolution of the curve in a series of exponentials. In the desaturation experiment the approach is rather a hybrid one as shown by transition at time zero, where $-m/\dot{m}$ reaches the "black box value" $(-m/\dot{m})_0 = \bar{t}$.

Of the two initial slopes mentioned the one after bolus injection is clearly the less precise one: how can one be sure, that this initial slope will underestimate k_i to the same extent in all situations? The answer is clearly that one cannot be sure. However, if under certain conditions blood flow changes proportionally in all the compartments (that are also assumed to remain of constant relative size), then it follows from equation 60 that the initial slope will bear a constant relationship to k_i (e.g. $-\dot{m}/m = 0.82\ k_i$). This aspect has been termed "curve transformation" meaning, that all that changes (is transformed) is the time axis, the shape of the curve remains constant (33). It also follows from equation 60 that if blood flow only changes in the fast component, then the initial slope correctly indicates the direction of the flow change and the order of magnitude of this change.

In discussing the initial slope after bolus injection it should be recalled that (as mentioned in the text) the Kety-Schmidt saturation/desaturation experiment essentially is of the same "initial" nature if only carried out to a finite time (5 or 10 min). This approach will overlook tissue component with very low flow, a critique long ago expressed in the classic paper by Sapirstein and Ogden (34), who tried to use the method for blood flow determination in the legs. Kety's response to this critique has been to assert that the method should simply not be used for this purpose. Yet, the critique is basically correct even for other applications performing short term experiment. In disease states areas with very low flow may well exist in brain, myocardium or kidney, areas that will not be fully included in the average flow calculated in short term experiments. Theoretically this does not mean that the Kety-Schmidt method is incorrect, because extending the time for introducing the tracer (hours) these poorly perfused areas will be fully saturated and thus contribute to the tracer washout proportional to their size. In practice, however, it may be quite impossible to perform such long term experiments.

Comment on Terminology (Why not to Use the Term "Stochastic")

The non-compartmental (black-box) analysis is sometimes called the "stochastic" analysis. Stochastic means statistical or probabilistic. The word may therefore be said to convey an element of uncertainty. That is incorrect and truly not what is implied when using the word. The basis for using the word "stochastic analysis" is namely the formal identity between the probability density function for one single tracer molecule's traversal of a system and the frequency function of transit times h(t). In principle the bolus consists of infinitely many tracer molecules, so that h(t) can (theoretically) be determined with any desired accuracy. Thus h(t) is actually deterministic (= uniquely and precisely determined by the tracer, the system and its state) and not stochastic (= subject to random variations governed by the statistical laws of probability). For this reason we prefer not to use the word "stochastic" that, moreover, conveys little meaning to readers unfamiliar with the statistical formalism mentioned.

MEAN TRANSIT TIME METHODS, II

Compartmental Analysis ("Exponential Analysis")

A compartment is a system that is well mixed or behaves as if it were well mixed. Mixing means that a constant fraction of the residue k leaves the system per unit time, with k being the flow/volume ratio, i.e. $1/\bar{t}$. This may be illustrated by reference to a tissue assumed to consist of one single capillary and its surrounding cylinder of cells and interstitial fluid. Mixing means that the steady state relationship $C_{tissue}(\infty)C_{blood}(\infty) = \lambda$ is valid at all times, i.e.

$$\text{(mixing)} \qquad C_{tissue}(t)/C_{blood}(t) = \lambda \qquad (70)$$

From this it follows, that the amount leaving the system per unit time and per gram of tissue is

$$\text{(outflux)} \qquad f\ C_{blood}(t) = f/\lambda\ C_{tissue}(t) \qquad (71)$$

As the residue per gram of tissue is $C_{tissue}(t)$ it follows that the outflux/residue ratio is indeed constant at f/λ for all times with this constant being $f/\lambda = k = 1/\bar{t}$, the time constant. Assuming that we are in a simple washout situation with no influx, then the rate of change of C_{tissue} is solely due to the outflux, i.e.

$$-d\ C_{tissue}(t)/dt = f/\lambda\ C_{tissue}(t) \qquad (72)$$

or

$$\frac{-d\,C_{tissue}(t)}{C_{tissue}(t)} = f/\lambda\ dt \qquad (72a)$$

$$-d\ \ln C_{tissue}(t) = f/\lambda\ dt \qquad (72b)$$

Assuming f and λ are constant integration yields

$$-\ln C_{tissue}(t)\Big|_o^t = f/\lambda \cdot t\Big|_o^t$$

$$\ln C_{tissue}(t) - \ln C_{tissue}(0) = -f/\lambda \cdot t$$

$$C_{tissue}(t)/C_{tissue}(0) = e^{-f/\lambda\ \cdot\ t} \qquad (73)$$

or, multiplying by the tissues weight W the residue curve $m(t) = W \cdot C(t)$ is

$$m_{tissue}(t)/m_{tissue}(0) = e^{-f/\lambda\ \cdot\ t} \qquad (73a)$$

With n identical capillaries and tissue cylinders arranged in parallel the basic equation (eq. 70) implies that

$$1/n\ (C_{tissue,1}(t) + C_{tissue,2}(t) + \ldots\ldots C_{tissue,n}(t)) =$$
$$1/n\ \lambda(C_{blood,1}(t) + C_{blood,2}(t) + \ldots\ldots\ldots C_{blood,n(t)}) \qquad (74)$$

$$\underline{\bar{C}_{tissue}(t) = \lambda\ \bar{C}_{blood}(t)} \qquad (75)$$

Accordingly also equations 71, 72, and 73 are valid. Thus it follows that even if there is no physical means of mixing, then such a homogeneous tissue behaves as if it were mixed. Note, that it was not assumed in deriving the average concentration, that the individual concentrations are the same in all tissue cylinders. This implies that diffusion processes inside a homogeneous (isotropic) tissue do not change the tissue's monoexponential washout curve: By reference to equation 74 it follows that even if diffusion, e.g. between tissue cylinder 1 and 2, takes place it only means, that for these two subelements the curve deviates from monoexponentiality, but the curve for the combined tissue (1+2) is monoexponential throughout, as equation 75 and hence 73 both remain valid. Local injection of a freely diffusible indicator give rise to such gradients, that consequently can be ignored.

In deriving equation 73 it was assumed, at the integration step, that $k = 1/\bar{t} = f/\lambda$ remained constant. It is interesting, however, to consider the case when the partition coefficient λ remains constant, but f varies as a function of time, f(t). In this case equation 72a becomes, after multiplying by the tissue weight W,

$$f(t) = \lambda\ (-d\ m(t)/dt) \cdot (1/m(t))$$

$$= \lambda\ (-d\ \ln m(t)/dt) \qquad (76)$$

Thus plotting m(t) in a semilogarithmic plot, f(t) is λ times the slope of this curve. Accordingly, by the severe restraint of assuming mixing one "gains" the advantage of being able to measure f as a function of time. Accurate values for the slope as a function of time cannot easily be obtained. I may be advantageous to calculate an average value of f(t) over a time interval for example from l_1 to t_2: by integrating equation 76

$$\bar{f}_{1\to 2} = \frac{\int_{t_1}^{t_2} f(t)dt}{t_2 - t_1} = \lambda \frac{\ln m(t_1) - \ln m(t_2)}{t_2 - t_1} \qquad (77)$$

This approach has been used for determination of subcutaneous blood flow during 24 h in patients with occlusive arterial disease in the legs (35).

Single Compartment with Arbitrary Input: This experimental procedure has been used extensively for determination of regional blood flow first described by Kety in 1948 (36), see also (37). Using the convolution principle the residue per gram of tissue to time t, C(t) with the arbitrary input function Ca(t) can be written

$$C(t) = f \cdot \int_0^t Ca(\tau) \cdot e^{-(t-\tau)/\bar{t}}\ dt \qquad (78)$$

τ is an integration variable with the dimension of time varying between zero and t. Using $k = 1/\bar{t}$ yields

$$C(t) = f \cdot e^{-kt} \cdot \int_0^t Ca(\tau) \cdot e^{k\cdot\tau} d\tau \qquad (79)$$

If the tracer is retained in the tissue, then the unit bolus residue is 1 and equation 62 becomes simply

$$C(t) = f\int_0^t Ca(\tau)d\tau \qquad (80)$$

This equation slightly rewritten is the same as equation 20, the bolus fractionation method.

Compartmental Analysis based on mono-exponential washout curves of inert gases has been extensively used for determination of blood flow in various tissues.

Theoretically the washout of the tracer is monoexponential and the perfusion coefficient is based on equation 73a, i.e.

$$f = \lambda \cdot k \cdot 100\ ml \cdot min^{-1}\ (100g)^{-1} \qquad (81)$$

where λ is the tissue to blood partition coefficient in ml/g and k the washout rate constant in min^{-1} (37).

Adipose Tissue: Larsen et al. (38) observed that the washout of ^{133}Xe injected subcutaneously after an initial phase of about 30 min follow a monoexponential course. The ratio of washout rates of ^{133}Xe and ^{85}Kr equals the ratio of λ suggesting that diffusion equilibrium is achieved at any time during the washout.

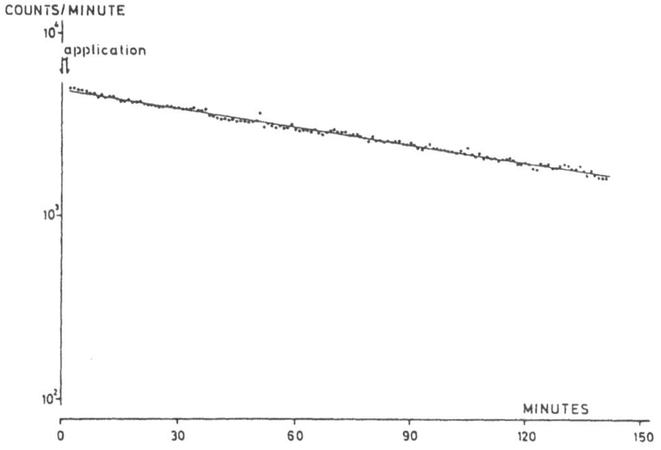

FIG. 12

^{133}Xe washout curve from the ingvinal fat pad in cat following atraumatic labeling. Note that the washout function is strictly monoexponential. From Sejrsen, 1969 (39).

The initial faster washout rate was assumed to be caused by the injection trauma including local hyperemia. This interpretation is supported by the finding, that the washout of ^{133}Xe from the ingvinal fat pad is strictly monoexponential following atraumatic labeling (39) (fig. 12) and there is a good agreement between blood flow calculated from the ^{133}Xe washout curves and directly recorded venous outflow (40) (fig. 13). In the same preparation Levin Nielsen (41) found that following injection the tracer blood flow calculated from the monoexponential washout curve obtained after the injection-trauma has become insignificant (more than 30 min) agreed with the directly recorded venous outflow rate.

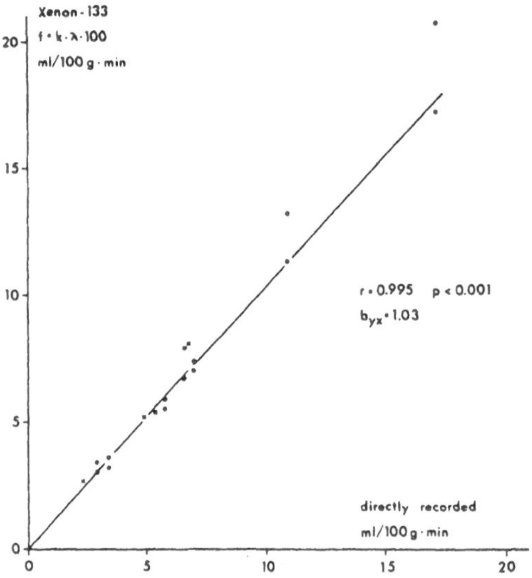

FIG. 13

Comparison between blood flow in rabbit ingvinal fat pad calculated from ^{133}Xe washout curves following atraumatic labeling and directly recorded venous outflow rate. From Nielsen (74).

These findings suggest that the assumptions underlying the derivation of equation 58 are valid in adipose tissue. A source of error is the injection trauma induced local hyperemia, which subsides to become insignificant within 30 min. In the above mentioned studies λ was determined in each case by analysis of the tissue content of water, lipid and protein. Values ranging between 9 and 12 ml/g was found. Usually a λ value of 10 ml/g is used (42). However, the λ value is very sensitive to the lipid content of subcutaneous adipose tissue. This lipic concentration may vary considerably in different locations. This may be especially when patients are studied. The variation in the ^{133}Xe washout rate due to variations in λ in subcutaneous tissue can be considerably reduced by using a double isotope washout technique. Bjerre-Jepsen et al. (43) measured simultaneously the washout of ^{131}I-Antipyrine and ^{133}Xe.

Since f is the same for the two tracers, we have

$$\frac{\lambda_{^{133}Xe}}{\lambda_{Antipyrine}} = \frac{k_{Antipyrine}}{k_{^{133}Xe}}$$

or

$$\lambda_{^{133}Xe} = \lambda_{Antipyrine} \frac{k_{Antipyrine}}{k_{^{133}Xe}} \qquad (82)$$

$\lambda_{Antipyrine}$ in oil/water ranges between 1 - 1.5 ml/g (44). There is no reliable measurement of $\lambda_{Antipyrine}$ in adipose tissue. Bjerre-Jepsen et al. (43) used 1 ml/g in calf and foot. This may give an underestimation especially in abdominal subcutaneous tissue with a high lipid content.

In situations where $\lambda_{^{133}Xe}$ is unknown it is still possible to measure relative blood flow accurately during different experimental conditions, where λ remains constant.

$$\frac{f_{test}}{f_{control}} = \frac{\lambda \cdot k_{test}}{\lambda \cdot k_{control}} = \frac{k_{test}}{k_{control}} \qquad (83)$$

This technique has been used by Henriksen (45) in a series of studies at local control of human subcutaneous blood flow.

Changes in detection-geometry due to movements is a major source of error. The area must be carefully immobilized for example by using a vacuum-fixation pillow. Correction for changes in detection-geometry caused by movements for example in exercise studies can be performed by simultaneously recording the activity from a fixed radioactive source placed on the surface of the skin just above the area under study (45).

Skeletal muscle: It is essential to mention the pioneer study of Kety (36), which first described the theory of the local washout method. He used ^{24}Na but diffusion equilibrium between tissue and effluent blood may not be achieved at high blood flow rates, where ^{133}Xe maintains equilibrium much better(47) and currently ^{133}Xe introduced by Lassen et al. (48) is now used almost exclusively.

Even following non-traumatic labeling the washout of ^{133}Xe in resting skeletal muscle follows a multiexponential course(25).

The slope of the initial monoexponential part of the washout curve corresponds to directly recorded venous outflow. However, after some minutes during which about 30-40% of the depot has been washed out, the slope gradually declines to reach a level corresponding to only approximately 50% of the directly recorded venous outflow rate (range 40-80%). In these studies all visible fat was carefully removed and the underestimation of blood flow from the slow part of the washout curve can probably be ascribed by reentering of tracer into the tissue due to venoarterial shunting by diffusion of ^{133}Xe (49), a phenomenon demonstrated in the brain too (50). The recruitment phenomenon implying a very large effective radius of the tissue cylinder in resting skeletal muscle may also be implied.

Following intra-muscular injection the initial part of the washout curve is influenced by the injection trauma induced local hyperemia, and consequently the initial slope of the washout curve gives too high values for the average perfusion coefficient in the muscle tissue (51) (fig. 14). Since the late part of the curve gives an underestimation of the blood flow with great variation, it is obviously impossible to obtain reliable values for blood flow in resting skeletal muscle.

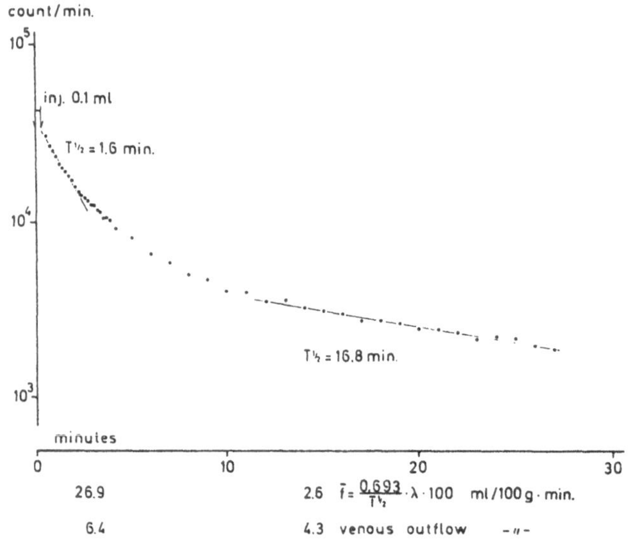

FIG. 14

^{133}Xe washout curve from isolated cat gastrocnemius muscle following intra-muscular injection. From Tønnesen and Sejrsen (51).

During muscle exercise initiated about 10 minutes after the local injection, blood flow calculated from the ^{133}Xe washout resembled that of directly measured venous outflow (second slope technique) (see fig. 15 & 16). During these circumstances the contribution of veno-arterial shunting by diffusion and recruitment reduces the effective radius of the tissue cylinder.

In these calculations a λ value of 0.7 ml/g has been used. However, in human studies accumulation of ^{133}Xe in fat tissue lining the vessels and separating the muscle bands may delay the washout rate and lead to underestimation of muscle blood flow. In humans the anterior tibial muscle is typically lean containing a low percentage of fat, whereas other muscles like the gastrocnemius and the soleus contains more fat.

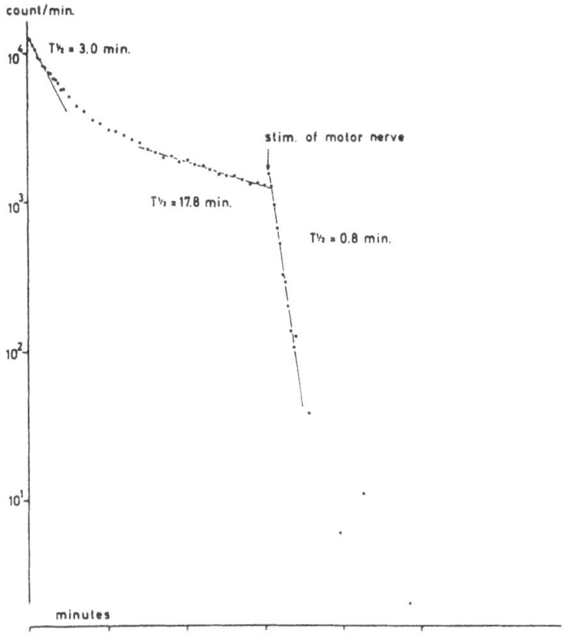

FIG. 15

Diagram showing the "second slope technique" for determination of muscle blood flow in isolated cat gastrocnemius muscle by the local ^{133}Xe washout technique following i.m. injection. After the effects of the injection trauma has become insignificant, muscle exercise is initiated and a steep monoexponential washout of the tracer is seen. The washout rate during these circumstances agrees with average muscle blood flow recorded as venous outflow rate, see fig. 16. Tønnesen and Sejrsen (51).

Thus, in humans the second slope technique may give reasonable values for blood flow in exercising muscles. However, as mentioned before, it is not possible to obtain reliable values for blood flow in resting skeletal muscle. Nevertheless, relative changes in resting blood flow may still be assessed correctly by observing variations in the slope of the washout curve after the injection trauma has become insignificant (52) appr. 10 min after injection.

Even after this time the washout curve may not be strictly monoexponential. Hence it is important to perform a control measurement just before and after the test situation in order to take the spontaneous change of the washout curve into account.

From equation 83 we have

$$f_{test}/f_{control} = k_{test}/1/2(k_{control_1} + k_{control_2}) \qquad (84)$$

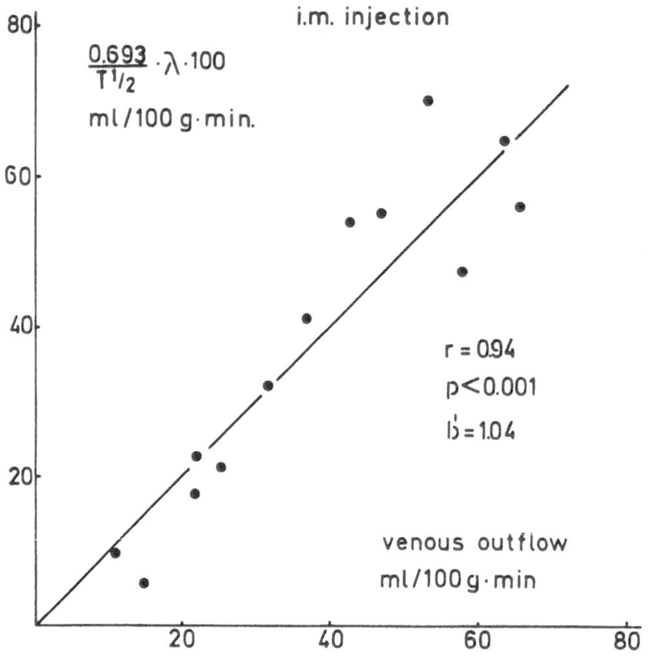

FIG. 16

Comparison of blood flow in isolated cat gastrocnemius muscle calculated from the ^{133}Xe washout curves, using the "second slope technique" and directly recorded venous outflow rate. Tønnesen and Sejrsen (51).

Myocardium: Haunsø et al. (53) showed in dogs that the washout of ^{133}Xe applied atraumatically to the exposed myocardium and detected with narrow collimation follows a monoexponential course. Thus errors due to veno-arterial shunting by diffusion and accumulation of indicator in fat tissue discussed in the section on muscle blood flow above, are insignificant in the myocardium in the described "detection set up". Furthermore the injection trauma seems also to be of no importance in myocardium, since no difference in the washout was seen following local injection and atraumatic labelling (53), see fig. 16.

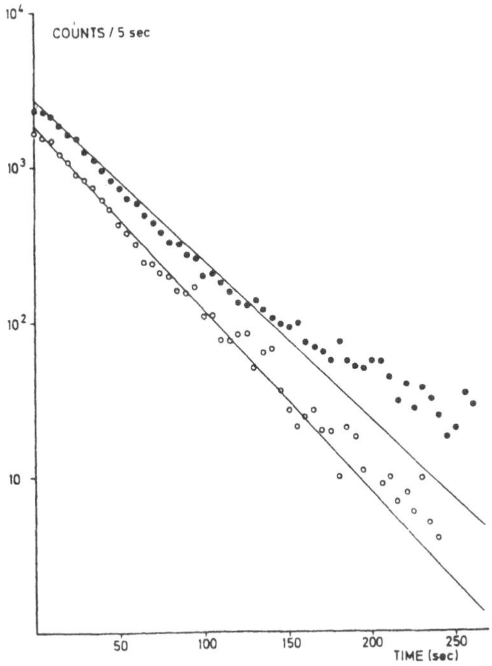

FIG. 17

^{133}Xe washout from canine myocardial tissue. Upper curve recorded with broad collimation, lower recorded with narrow collimation. Note in the latter situation the curve is almost monoexponential. From Haunsø et al. (53).

Thus, the washout of locally deposited freely diffusible tracers from the myocardium, corresponds to the washout from a single compartment and consequently $f = \lambda \cdot k \cdot 100\ ml \cdot min^{-1}\ (100g)^{-1}$.

This technique may give interesting information peroperatively of regional myocardial blood flow before and after coronary by-pass operation.

Compartmental Analysis Based on Biexponential Washout of Inert Gases

Human Cutaneous Tissue: Measurement of blood flow in cutaneous tissue is complicated by the underlying subcutaneous tissue. The washout of ^{133}Xe from human skin following atraumatic labelling follows a biexponential course. Sejrsen (39) proposed a 2 compartment model, where a part of the ^{133}Xe removed from cutaneous tissue is accumulating in the underlying subcutaneous tissue, which functions as a sink for the tracer because of the high solubility of ^{133}Xe in the fat containing subcutaneous tissue. The tracer reaches the subcutaneous tissue mainly by diffusion through the walls of the veins draining the overlying cutaneous tissue.

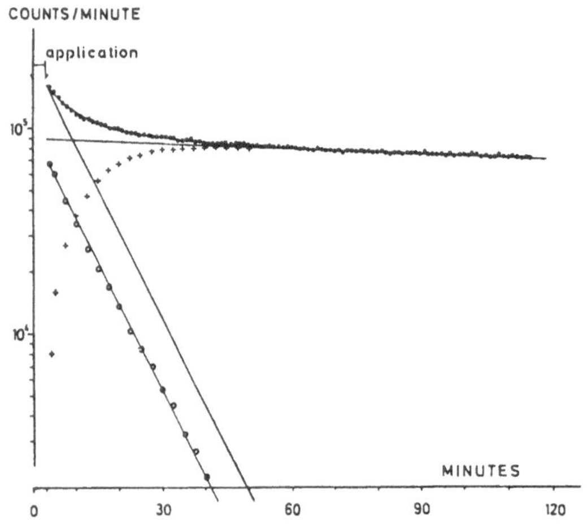

FIG. 18

^{133}Xe washout curve from human cutaneous tissue following atraumatic epicutaneous labeling. Note the curve is biexponential with the fast component reflecting the washout from cutaneous tissue and the slow component reflecting the washout from subcutaneous adipose tissue. The crosses indicate the initial uptake of ^{133}Xe in subcutaneous tissue. From Sejrsen (39).

A crucial point is, that ^{133}Xe does not reenter the cutaneous tissue from subcutaneous tissue due to the great difference in solubility of ^{133}Xe in the two tissue components.

Thus resolution of the biexponential washout curves into the two monoexponential components gives the washout from cutaneous tissue (fast component) and from subcutaneous tissue (slow component). Experimental evidence supporting the washout model proposed by Sejrsen (39) is the observation of a monoexponential washout function from cutaneous (see fig. 19) as well as subcutaneous tissue (see fig. 12) when studied separately (39). Thus blood flow in cutaneous tissue is calculated as

$$f_c = \lambda_c \cdot k_c \cdot 100 \ \text{ml} \cdot \text{min}^{-1} \ (100\text{g})^{-1}$$

where k_c is the washout rate constant of the fast monoexponential component and λ_c is the cutaneous tissue to blood partition coefficient (0.7 ml/g).

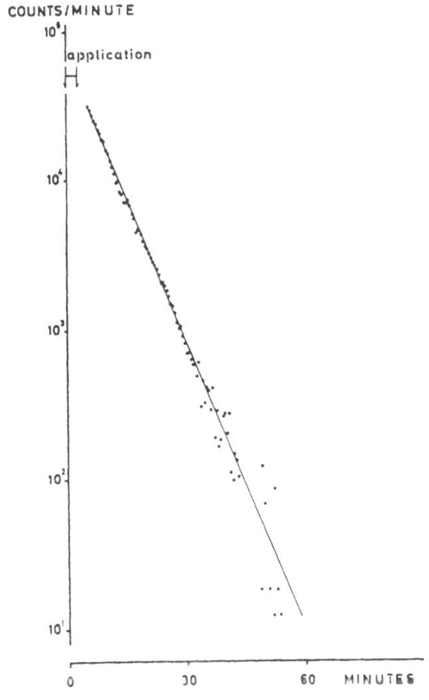

FIG. 19

^{133}Xe washout from cutaneous tissue of the skinfold between the 1st. and 2nd. finger following atraumatic labeling. Note that the curve is strictly monoexponential down to background values. From Sejrsen (39).

Intracutaneous injection of ^{133}Xe dissolved in isotonic saline induces an initial hyperemic reaction (injection trauma) lasting about 15 min. This reaction is seen as an initial slope of the washout curve, which subsequently levels off to equal that seen after epicutaneous atraumatic labeling (39). Thus, resting cutaneous blood flow can be determined after intra-cutaneous injection of ^{133}Xe, provided one waits until the influence of the injection has become insignificant.

It is often necessary to record the ^{133}Xe washout curve for 1½ to 2 h to perform a reliable curve resolution. This may be difficult in clinical studies. It is, however, possible to estimate relative changes in cutaneous blood flow by varying the experimental conditions within the time interval of the initial almost monoexponential part of the washout curve following atraumatic labeling. This part of the curve, lasting about 10-15 min, is particularly at high cutaneous flow rates, dominated by the cutaeous washout component (54).

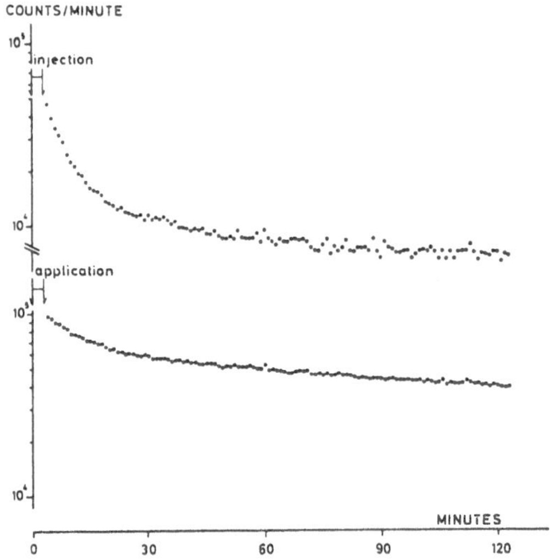

FIG. 20

^{133}Xe washout curves from the skin on the anterolateral side of crus on both sides. Upper curve shows the washout after intra-cutaneous injection and lower curve shows the washout after atraumatic epicutaneous labeling. Note that after about 15 min hyperemia due to the injection trauma has ceased to become insignificant and the shape of the curves is hereafter virtually identical. From Sejrsen (39).

A source of error is elimination of ^{133}Xe by sweating. In intact non-sweating skin loss of ^{133}Xe through the skin surface is less than 1% of the washout by the blood flow. In profusely sweating skin 10-20% of the ^{133}Xe is lost via the sweat. The magnitude can be estimated on the extremities by inducing circulatory arrest with a tourniquet as the loss by sweating continues (55). Loss of ^{133}Xe through the skin can be substantial in patients with dermatological diseases with damage of the epidermal diffusion barrier. However, the relatively gastight normal epidermal membrane can be imitated by a Myelar membrane (20 µmm thick) placed on the surface of the skin with a drop of water interposed.

Injection of ^{85}Kr dissolved in saline has been proposed for measuring cutaneous blood flow with recording of the β-radiation. This approach, however, is invalidated by the injection artefact and diffusion processes altering the detection efficiency (56).

Brain: The residue-washout curves of ^{133}Xe in the brain following a bolus injection into the internal carotid artery follows a biexponential course. Using a two-compartment in-parallel model (no interchange between the two compartments) the residue function m(t) is the weighted average of the washout from the two tissue compartments of the brain.

$$m(t) = I_g \cdot e^{-t/\bar{t}_g} + I_w \cdot e^{-t/\bar{t}_w}$$

where I_g and I_w are the initial amounts of tracer in the grey and white matter of the brain respectively. $\bar{t}_g$ and $\bar{t}_w$ are the mean transit time in grey and white matter respectively, which equals the λ/f ratios.

The relative weights of grey and white matter W_g/W_w can be deduced using the bolus fractionation principle

$$I_g = m_o \cdot F_g/(F_g + F_w) = m_o \cdot f_g \cdot W_g/(F_g + F_w) \qquad (85)$$

$$I_w = m_o \cdot F_w/(F_g + F_w) = m_o \cdot f_w \cdot W_w/(F_g + F_w) \qquad (86)$$

F_g and F_w are the total blood flow in grey and white matter respectively, and m_o is the total dose injected.

Dividing equation 81 by equation 82 and solving for W_g/W_w yields

$$\frac{W_g}{W_w} = \frac{I_g}{I_w} \cdot \frac{f_w}{f_g} \qquad (87)$$

The ratio W_g/W_w is based on anatomical studies about 60/40 and in blood flow studies about 50/50 (57), indicating that the described two-compartments in parallel model is almost correct at least for the normal brain. This may be different in different disease states, which may alter the washout conditions in the brain. If, for example the blood flow in the grey matter is severely reduced, the difference in washout rate constants in grey and white matter may be too small to allow a reliable curve resolution. Furthermore there may at low flow rates be a significant intercompartmental exchange of tracer by diffusion or by combined diffusion and convection changing the washout model.

The initial slope is dominated by the blood flow in the grey matter at normal and high flow rates and may be useful in clinical studies using a multidetector equipment. The number of regions recorded from one hemisphere has increased from 8 to 256 (58). In these studies the initial slope of the ^{133}Xe washout curves has been used for estimating regional distribution of blood flow in the grey matter, because it is possible to perform a fast computation of the initial slope of the numerous regional washout curves (59).

Comments on the Interpretation of a Biexponential Washout Function and on Multicompartmental Analysis

The washout models proposed for the biexponential washout functions in skin and brain are based on experimentally obtained knowledge of the washout functions of the subsystems involved. Many other washout models including in parallel models with or without intercompartmental exchange, in-series models, combined in series in parallel models, and mamillary models, which all may give a truly biexponential washout curve. The rate constants of the two monoexponential components obtained from graphical resolution of the curve are, except for the pure in parallel model, not identical to the relevant rate constants of the biological exchange processes.

From these considerations it is obvious that possible compartment models explaining a multiple exponential washout function are numerous and such models should be taken with great reservation. For example the three compartment in parallel models proposed for the multiexponential washout function of close intraarterially injected inert gases in the kidney must be regarded as speculative. Because of the complex vasculature in this organ with vessels transversing the different regions interchange of tracer between the different regions is moreover very likely to occur.

The tracer mass balance relationships in n-compartmental systems can with matrix notation be written in symmetrical and compact form. The n-compartmental form with n being an arbitrarily large number cannot be solved to yield explicit analytical expressions for the masses and fluxes of the individual compartment. However, by using the matrix notation it is possible to derive all the general properties of the system as first shown by Nosslin (60) and Bergner (9). A detailed discussion of deriving the stimulus-response theorem (equations 15 and 16) based on the matrix notation is given by Lassen and Perl (61). It is important to stress that solving the series of first order differential equations underlying the multicompartmental approach leads to single integral equations expressing the described results of the non-compartmental (black-box) analysis yet using a more complicated formalism. The two modes of analysis are thus basically identical .

Compartmental Analysis for Monoexponential Extrapolation to Time Infinity

In the nom-compartmental analysis extrapolation to time infinity is often necessary to calculate the area, $\int_0^\infty c(t)dt$ or the time-weighted area, $\int_0^\infty t\,C(t)dt$. Multicompartmental analysis with a high number of compartments predicts that after a sufficiently long time has elapsed the washout curve is practically monoexponential. This means that after this time the contribution to the washout curve from the faster components are negligible compared to the slowest one (final slope). Thus the compartmental approach is essential for the monoexponential extrapolation procedure in non-compartmental analysis for determination of $\bar{t}$.

A simple probabilistic argument supports the monoexponential approach. Suppose that after a long time has elapsed after an intra-arterial bolus injection a small residue, 1%, 0.1% or even less of the injected dose is distributed in locations with the worst probability of washout because all other favorable sites has been washed down to very low concentrations. At this time the remainder of the washout function must be practically monoexponential. This must be true because after a further time T has elapsed, this small worst residue has been reduced to for example one-half its value; then this remaining half is distributed in precisely the same manner as the shole residue T min before. Because the distribution is unchanged - it cannot be worse than worst - the probability of washout is constant and hence the fractional change in tissue concentration with time is constant. Consequently the washout curve is monoexponential.

The final slope concept presented here is very important and the procedure of extrapolation to obtain the area to time infinity can be expressed as

$$\int_0^\infty C(t)dt = \int_0^\tau C(t)dt + \int_\tau^\infty C(\tau)e^{-k(t-\tau)}d\tau \qquad (88)$$

This is equal to the measured area from 0 to $\tau + C(\tau) \cdot \bar{t}_{final}$, where $\bar{t}_{final} = 1/k_{final} \simeq t_{\frac{1}{2}final}/0.693$ and τ is the time when the washout of the tracer becomes monoexponential. Similarly

$$\int_0^\infty t\,C(t)dt = \int_0^\tau t \cdot C(t)dt + \int_\tau^\infty t \cdot C(\tau) \cdot e^{-k(t-\tau)}dt \qquad (89)$$

This equals the measured time-weighted area from 0 to $\tau + C(\tau) \cdot \bar{t}_{final} \cdot (\bar{t}_{final} + \tau)$.

Experimental evidence that the final slope has been reached may be very difficult to obtain, since the concept itself is an approximation. This is inherent in the multicompartmental formulation, which implies that one must wait until the faster components have died out, when they in fact never really die out; they just become increasingly insignificant. Strong experimental evidence that the final slope in fact has been reached, i.e. $t > \tau$ in the above notation, can be obtained if simultaneous observations of residue and outflow can be made for long transit times without influence of recirculation.

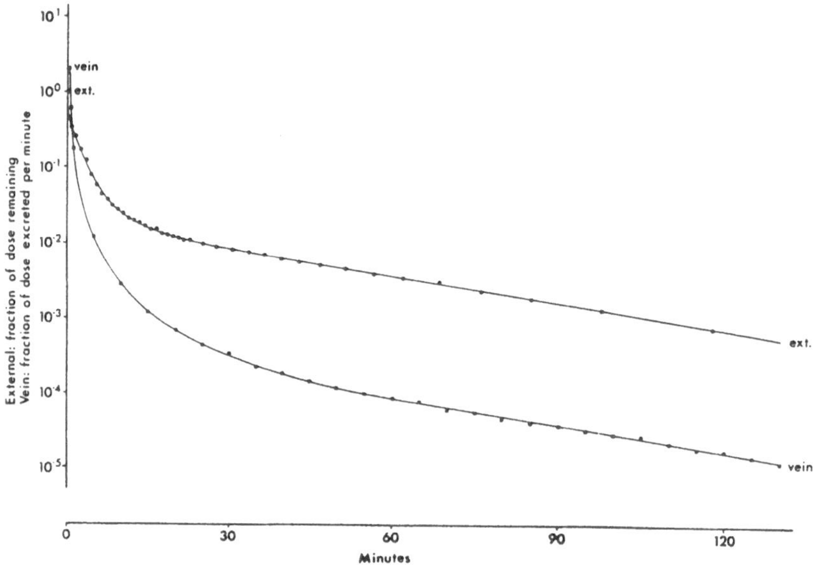

FIG. 21

Semilogarithmic plot of simultaneously recorded fractional residue, upper curve and fractional outflow rate, lower curve of ^{51}Cr-EDTA in isolated cat gastrocnemius muscle following a close intra-arterial bolus injection. Note that after some time the curves become straight and parallel indicating that at this time the "final slope" has been reached. Lassen and Sejrsen (62).

In this situation the residue can be expressed as

$$m(t) = m(\tau) \cdot e^{-k(t-\tau)}, \quad t \geq \tau$$

The outflow curve ($F \cdot C_{out}(t)$) equals the time derivative of m(t) and $C_{out}(t)$ are plotted in a semilogarithmic diagram, they must be straight and parallel lines, when the final slope has been reached, i.e. $t \geq \tau$, see fig. 21 (62).

CORRECTION FOR RECIRCULATION

Inlet Sampling: For the constant infusion experiment a correction for recirculation is achieved by inlet sampling. This is the Fick principle, where correction for recirculation consists of subtracting the inlet concentrations from the outlet concentrations during indicator steady-state. In the bolus experiment with inflow and outflow detection correction for recirculation can be performed using the elementary convolution theory if the response to a brief delta input (impulse) h(t) is known. Assuming cross-stream mixing at the inlet, the response of the system in any input, at time t, $j_{in}(t) = F \cdot C_{in}(t)$ can be calculated from equation 38. Multiplying equation 38 on both sides by m_o/F yields

$$C_{out}(t) = \int_0^t C_{in}(\tau) \cdot h(t-\tau)d\tau$$

Often h(t) is not a priori known, but this approach may still be used. Consider the situation where a brief bolus had been injected into the inlet of the system and that after a lag time of about for example 30 s recirculation sets in at the inlet. If the shortest transit time measured at the outlet after a bolus (appearance time) is 5 s, the appearance of the recirculation at the outlet can be expected 30 s + 5 s after the bolus injection. Thus the outflow curve in the time interval from 0 to 35 s has the form of h(t). This gives the possibility to calculate the contribution of recirculation to the outlet concentration in the time interval 35 s to 70 s, and thereby correct the error due to recirculation. This approach gives a more accurate correction for recirculation than that obtained by the classic simple monoexponential extrapolation of the outflow curve. In fact correction for recirculation using the convolution integral often reveals a non-monoexponential downslope.

Simultaneous, Symmetrical Sampling: Experimental correction for recirculation can be achieved by simultaneously sampling from the outlet of the system studied and from a symmetrical system (organ, region) in the circulation, if available. The correct first passage curve can be calculated by subtracting the curve of the symmetrical organ from the system studied.

Similar approach can be used when residue detection is performed. In this situation it is essential, that the detection efficiency is equal for the two systems studied.

Additional bolus injection at the outlet; residue detection: If it is not possible to record the recirculatory function simultaneously from a symmetrical organ (region), correction for recirculation in calculating $\bar{t}$ can be obtained by performing an extra bolus injection at the outlet of the system studied and recording the recirculatory function by residue detection as proposed by Larson and Snyder (63). Since this approach is difficult to perform in man a detailed discussion is beyond the scope of this article. A detailed presentation of this method is given in the original article of Larson and Snyder (63) and by Lassen and Perl (61).

REFERENCES

1. Stewart GN: Researches on the circulation time and on the influences which affect it. IV. The output of the heart. J Physiol London 15:159-183, 1897.

2. Fick A: Uber die Messung des Blutquantums in den Hertzventrikeln. Verhl Phys Med Ges Würzburg 2: 16, 1870.

3. Crone C: The permeability of capillaries in various organs as determined by use of the "indicator diffusion" method. Acta Physiol Scand 58:292-305, 1963.

4. Renkin EM: Transport of potassium-42 from blood to tissue in isolated mammalian skeletal muscles. Am J Physiol 197:1205-1210, 1959.

5. Henriques V: Uber die Verteilung des Blutes vom linken Herzen zwischen dem Herzen und dem übrigen Organismus. Biochem Z 56:230-248, 1913.

6. Hamilton WF, Moore JW, Kinsman JM and Spurling RG: Simultaneous determination of the pulmonary and systemic circulation times in man and of a figure related to the cardiac output. Am J Physiol 84:338-344, 1928.

6a. Hamilton WF, Moore JW, Kinsman JM and Spurling RG: Simultaneous determination of the greater and lesser circulation times, of the mean velocity of blood flow through the heart and lungs, of the cardiac output and an approximation of the amount of blood actively circulating in the heart and lungs. Am J Physiol 85:377-378, 1928.

7. Hamilton WF, Moore JW, Kinsman JM and Spurling RG: Studies on the circulation. IV. Further analysis of the injection method, and of changes in hemodynamics under physiological and pathological conditions. Am J Physiol 99:534-551, 1932.

8. Perl W: Heat and matter distribution in body tissues and the determination of tissue blood flow by local clearance methods. J Theoret Biol 2:201-235, 1963.

9. Bergner P-EE: Tracer dynamics and the determination of pool-sizes and turnover factors in metabolic systems. J Theoret Biol 6:137-158, 1964.

10. Thompson HK, Starmer CF, Whalen RE and McIntosh HD: Indicator transit time considered as a gamma variate. Circ Res 14:502-515, 1964.

11. Hosie KF: Thermal dilution techniques. Circ Res 10: 491-504, 1962.

12. Nosslin B: Determination of clearance and distribution volume with the single injection technique. Acta Med Scand Suppl. 442, 1965.

13. Bröchner-Mortensen J and Rödbro P: Selection of routine method for determination of glomerular filtration rate in adult patients. Scand J clin Lab Invest 36: 35-43, 1976.

14. Sapirstein LA: Fractionation of the cardiac output of rats with isotopic potassium. Circ Res 4:689-692, 1956.

15. Winchell HS, Horst WD, Braun L et al.: N-isopropyl-(^{123}I)p-iodoamphetamine: Single-pass brain uptake and washout; binding to brain synaptosomes; and localization in dog and monkey brain. J Nucl Med 21:947-952, 1980.

16. Ciofetta G, Pratt TA and Hughes MB: Comparison of krypton 81m and technetium 99m-human serum albumin for measurement of pulmonary perfusion distribution. Br J Radiol Spec Rep 15:38-43, 1978.

17. Fazio F and Giuntini C: Determination of extravascular lung water by dilution method. II Technique and results in dog and man. J Nucl Med All Sci 23:97-107, 1979.

18. Meier P and Zierler KL: On the theory of the indicator-dilution method for measurement of blood flow and volume. J Appl Physiol 6:731-744, 1954.

19. Kety SS and Schmidt CF: The determination of cerebral blood flow in man by the use of nitrous oxide in low concentrations. Am J Physiol 143:53-66, 1945.

20. Yeh SY and Peterson RE: Solubility of krypton and xenon in blood, protein solutions, and tissue homogenates. J Appl Physiol 20:1041-1047, 1965.

21. Lassen NA and Munck O: The cerebral blood flow in man determined by the use of radioactive krypton. Acta Physiol Scand 33:30-49, 1955.

22. Conn HL, Wood YC and Schmidt CF: A comparison of renal blood flow results obtained in the intact animal by nitrous oxide (derived Fick) and by para-aminohippurate (direct Fick) method. J Clin Invest 32:1180, 1953.

23. Eckenhoff JE, Hafkenschiel JH, Harmel MH et al.: Measurement of coronary blood flow by the nitrous oxide method. Am J Physiol 152:356-364, 1948.

24. Lassen NA and Ingvar DH: The blood flow of the cerebral cortex determined by radioactive krypton-85. Experientia 17: 42-45, 1961.

25. Sejrsen P and Tønnesen KH: The inert gas diffusion method for measurement of blood flow using saturation techniques: comparison with directly measured blood flow in the isolated gastrocnemius muscle of the cat. Circ Res 22:679-693, 1968.

26. Lassen NA: On the theory of the local clearance method for measurement of blood flow including a discussion of its application to various tissues. Acta Med Scand Suppl. 472:136-145, 1967.

27. Zierler KL: Equations for measuring blood flow by external monitoring of radioisotopes. Circ Res 16: 309-321, 1965.

28. Ingvar DH and Lassen NA: Regional blood flow of the cerebral cortex determined by Krypton-85. Acta Physiol Scand 54:325-338, 1962.

29. Tønnesen KH and Sejrsen P: Inert gas diffusion method for measurement of blood flow. Comparison of bolus injection to directly measured blood flow in isolated gastrocnemius muscle. Circ Res 20:552-564, 1967.

30. Ross RS, Ueda K, Lichtlen PR et al.: Measurement of myocardiac blood flow in animals and man by selective injection of radioactive inert gas into the coronary arteries. Circ Res 15: 28-41, 1964.

31. Bassingthwaighte JB, Strandell T and Donald DE: Estimation of coronary blood flow by washout of diffusible indicators. Circ Res 23:259-278, 1968.

32. Kemp E, Høedt-Rasmussen K, Bjerrum JK et al.: A new method for determination of divided renal blood flow in man. Lancet 1:1402-1403, 1963.

33. Olesen J, Paulson OB and Lassen NA: Regional cerebral blood flow in man determined by the initial slope of the clearance of intra-arterially injected ^{133}Xe. Stroke 2:519-540, 1971.

34 Sapirstein LA and Ogden E: Theoretic limitations of the nitrous oxide method for the measurement of regional blood flow. Circ Res 4:245-257, 1956.

35. Bjerre-Jepsen K, Faris I, Henriksen, O and Lassen NA: Subcutaneous blood flow over 24-hour periods in patients with severe leg ischaemia. Clin Physiol 2:357-362, 1982.

36. Kety SS: Quantitative measurement of regional circulation by the clearance of radioactive sodium. Am J Med Sci 215:352-353, 1948.

37. Kety SS: Theory and applications of the exchange of inert gas at the lungs and tissues. Pharmacol Rev 3: 1-41, 1951.

38. Larsen OA, Lassen NA and Quaade F: Blood flow through human adipose tissue determined with radioactive xenon. Acta Physiol Scand 66:337-345, 1966.

39. Sejrsen P: Blood flow in cutaneous tissue in man studied by washout of radioactive Xenon. Circ Res 24:215-229, 1969.

40. Nielsen SL: Measurement of blood flow in adipose tissue from the washout of Xenon-133 after atraumatic labelling. Acta Physiol Scand 86:187-196, 1972.

41. Nielsen SL: Adipose tissue blood flow determined by the washout of locally injected ^{133}Xe. Scand J clin Lab Invest 29:31-36, 1972.

42. Sejrsen P: Measurements of cutaneous blood flow by freely diffusible radioactive isotopes. Thesis, Copenhagen 1971. Dan Med Bull Suppl 18:9-38, 1971.

43. Bjerre-Jepsen K, Faris I, Henriksen O and Tønnesen KH: Determination of the subcutaneous tissue to blood partition coefficient in patients with severe leg ischaemia by a double isotope washout technique. Clin Physiol 2:479-484, 1982.

44. Epstein RM: Non uniform distribution of 4-iodo-antipyrine in body water. Fed Proc 17:366-374, 1958.

45. Henriksen O: Local sympathetic reflex mechanism in regulation of blood flow in human subcutaneous adipose tissue. Acta Physiol Scand Suppl 450:7-48, 1977.

46. Bülow J and Madsen J: Compensation for geometric changes during monitoring of ^{133}Xe washout from subcutaneous adipose tissue. Scand J clin Lab Invest 35:641-644, 1975.

47. Lassen NA: Muscle blood flow in normal man and in patients with intermittent claudication evaluated by simultaneous Xe^{133} and Na^{24} clearances. J Clin Invest 43:1805-1812, 1964.

48. Lassen NA, Lindbjerg IF and Munck O: Measurement of blood flow through skeletal muscle by intramuscular injection of Xenon-133. Lancet 1:686-689, 1964.

49. Sejrsen P and Tønnesen KH: Shunting by diffusion of inert gas in skeletal muscle. Acta Physiol Scand 86: 82-91, 1972.

50. Brodersen P, Sejrsen P and Lassen NA: Diffusion bypass of Xenon in brain circulation. Circ Res 32:363-369, 1973.

51. Tønnesen KH and Sejrsen P: Washout of ^{133}Xenon after intramuscular injection and direct measurement of blood flow in skeletal muscle. Scand J clin Lab Invest 25:71-81, 1970.

52. Henriksen O and Sejrsen P: Local reflex in microcirculation in human skeletal muscle. Acta Physiol Scand 99:19-26, 1977.

53. Haunsø S, Amtorp O and Larsen B: Regional blood flow in canine myocardium as determined by local washout of a freely diffusible radioactive indicator. Acta Physiol Scand 106:115-121, 1979.

54. Kristensen JK and Henriksen O: Local regulation of blood flow in cutaneous tissue in generalized scleroderma. J invest Derm 70:260-262, 1978.

55. Sejrsen P: Epidermal diffusion barrier to ^{133}Xe in man and studies of clearance of ^{133}Xe by sweat. J Appl Physiol 24:211-216, 1968.

56. Sejrsen P: Diffusion processes invalidating the intra-arterial krypton-85 beta particle clearance method for measurement of skin blood flow in man. Circ Res 21: 281-295, 1967.

57. Sveinsdottir E, Torlöf P, Risberg J et al.: Monitoring regional cerebral blood flow in normal man with a computer-controlled 32-detector system. In Fieschi C, Ed. Cerebral Blood Flow and Intracranial Pressure, Basel, S Karger, AG, 1972, pp 228-233.

58. Sveinsdottir E, Larsen B, Rommer P and Lassen NA: A multidetector scintillation camera with 254 channels. J Nucl Med 18:168-174, 1977.

59. Caprani O, Sveinsdottir E and Lassen NA: SHAM, a method for biexponential curve resolution using initial slope height, area and moment of the experimental decay type curve. J Theoret Biol 52:299-315, 1975.

60. Nosslin B (1962). In: Metabolism of Human Gamma Globulin. Andersen SB (Thesis), Blackwell, Oxford, 1964, pp. 115-119.

61. Lassen NA and Perl W: Tracer Kinetic Methods in Medical Physiology, Raven Press, New York, 1979.

62. Lassen NA and Sejrsen P: Monoexponential extrapolation of tracer clearance curves in kinetic analysis. Circ Res 19:76-87, 1971.

63. Larson KB and Snyder DL: Measurement of relative blood flow, transit-time distributions and transport-model parameters by residue detection when radiotracer recirculates. J Theoret Biol 37:503-529, 1972.

TRACER KINETIC MODELING IN POSITRON COMPUTED TOMOGRAPHY

Sung-Cheng Huang, Richard E. Carson, Michael E. Phelps

UCLA Medical School, Los Angeles, CA

INTRODUCTION

The tracer technique uses a measurable substance to trace a dynamic process, such as flow, transport, or chemical reactions. The technique is neither new nor rarely used. For example, it has been used in our daily lives to estimate intuitively the flow speed in a river by observing the drifting of floats in the river. The application of the technique to physiological systems in the 19th century by injecting dye in the circulatory system to measure cardiac output(1,2). The success of this application has led to many biomedical tracer techniques, including the measurement of cerebral blood flow in man(3). After the development of radioisotope tracer techniques(4) and external detection capabilities, tracer techniques have become widely used in many applications(5-9). With the recent development of positron emission computed tomography, i.e., positron CT(10), tracer techniques became an essential, integral part of this new technique for measuring many physiologic or biochemical parameters in man(11,12). Studies dealing with the principles and treatment of tracer techniques developed in parallel and have become more rigorous (13-17). As a result, the fundamental basis of tracer kinetics has been expanded and they have been applied to complicated systems(18-23). This chapter reviews the principles of the tracer kinetic technique, particularly for its application to positron CT, and examples illustrate the essential points.

The technique requires the introduction of an appropriate tracer which resembles the natural substance that it will trace. The degree of resemblance required depends on the application. For example, in biochemical applications, radioisotope tracers which have the same or very similar chemical and physical properties as their natural counterparts, except for a small difference in mass, are considered to be ideal tracers. However, in applications where molecular diffusion is a limiting process, effects due to the small difference in mass may have to be considered.

The tracer introduced is assumed to be in a small enough quantity that the process to be measured is not perturbed by the tracer introduced (i.e., the tracer exerts no mass effects). Otherwise, the results obtained could reflect the effects of the tracer and not the original process that one wants to measure.

If the amount of tracer introduced is a two orders of magnitude smaller than the natural substance in the system, the disturbance caused by the tracer is generally considered to be insignificant. For any particular experiment, this needs to be verified.

Usually, the dynamic process to be traced is implicitly assumed to be in a steady state. That is, the rate of transport or reaction is not changing with time, and the amount of substance in any pool is constant during the measurement time. Rigorously, for biological systems that change all the time to adapt to the environment, there is no steady state. However, the steady state condition is generally considered to be satisfied if the amount of change is negligible within the time of measurement.

In tracer kinetic experiments, measurements are taken after tracers have been introduced. Inference about the system or process is then made, based on the measurements. In some cases, the rate of increase/decrease of the measured tracer activity or the time integral of the tracer concentration would provide directly the information required(8). For example, the measure of the mean transit time (τ) of a tracer through a system is equal to the ratio of the distribution volume(V) of the tracer to the convective flow(F) through the system(14,16).

$$\tau = V/F \tag{1}$$

This relationship, usually called the central volume principle, holds regardless of the configuration of the system, as long as the tracer is not involved in chemical reactions. However, the amount of information that can be obtained from these general characteristics is quite limited. As the system/process studied becomes more complicated and the amount of information expected increases, more extensive modeling is required. Modeling is a general mathematical method of incorporating some known a priori information to help the interpretation of observations. In tracer kinetics, linear compartmental models are traditionally used to describe physiologic processes(5-9).

Compartmental Modeling and Linearity of Response

A compartment is usually a space, in which the tracer is assumed to be distributed uniformly. The amount of tracer exiting from the compartment is proportional to the amount in the compartment. The proportionality constant between the amount of exiting tracer to the amount in the compartment is called the rate constant(k). The rate constant has the units of inverse time and is the fraction of tracer leaving the compartment per unit time (i.e., k=0.2/min means that 20 per cent of the tracer in the compartment is transported per minute). The inverse of the sum of all the rate constants of a compartment is called the turnover time of the compartment. The turnover time divided by 0.693 is the half time and is equal to the time for the tracer in the compartment to drop to one half of its original value, if no more tracer is brought into the compartment. Based on these compartments, the tracer kinetics of the system can be described in terms of first order, constant coefficient, linear ordinary differential equations. (Although there are nonlinear or time-variant compartmental models, the linear, time-invariant ones are the most frequently used and are the most successful.) The solutions to such differential equations consist of sums of exponential terms, if the input function is an impulse. In other words, if the tracer is introduced to the system of interest as an impulse-like bolus(i.e., the duration of the bolus is shorter than the minumum transit time through the organ or region of the organ examined), the measured tracer activity as a function of time will be a sum of exponential components. This sum of exponentials is usually called the impulse response function or simply the response function of the system. Furthermore, the number of exponential components in the response function is equal to the number of compartments in the model(24).

When the input function is not an impulse, the measured tracer quantities will be the convolution of the input function with the response function of the system. This is a direct result of the linearity of the compartmental models. Strictly speaking, not very many physiologic processes are linear systems. However, because the amount of tracer introduced is always very small as compared to the natural substance, the transport or chemical transfer of tracer usually can be considered as linear (or first order)(6,25). Measurement of the input function allows it to be deconvolved from the tissue tracer curve to yield the impulse response of the tissue. The impulse response reflects the kinetic process in the tissue without interference from effects in the rest of the body.

Measurement Techniques and Tracer Kinetic Models

The kind of system/process that can be modeled to provide useful information is very much related to the measurement techniques available. For a long time the amount of tracer in blood or in urine was the only quantity that could be measured non-invasively in man. Thus, the models developed for this kind of measurements invariably consider the blood pool in the circulatory system as a single compartment that communicates with other body organs, which also are usually treated as single compartments(26). In these models, the gross approximation of considering a whole organ or a group of organs as a uniform pool has to be made, and the amount of information and the accuracy attainable from the use of these models are very limited. After the development of radioisotope tracers and external detection techniques (e.g. scintillation probes and Anger cameras, measurement of tracer in an organ or part of an organ became possible, and models were formulated to describe the detailed transport of tracers in organs(27,28,29). In these models, functionally different tissue spaces or different chemical forms of tracers can be modeled as separate compartments. However, because of the non-uniformity of the detection efficiency in depth and the overlap of many tissues, the measurements are limited in quantitation and the spatial hetereogeneity in an organ cannot be differentiated from functionally different pools.

Recently, with the development of positron CT, the amount of radioactivity in small local regions of body can be quantitatively and non-invasively measured. This new capability has a big influence on the kind of models that can be employed to obtain useful physiologic or biochemical information. Models can now focus on the description of tracers within a small and more homogeneous tissue element. As far as the tracer is concerned, the only connection between the small tissue element and other parts of the organ/body is the tracer delivery and clearance in the tissue element through the blood flow, of which the tracer concentration can be measured from peripheral blood samples. This change in modeling allows one to look more in detail at the various processes a tracer goes through in tissue and thus provides more detailed information about the tissue. However, to maximally utilize this new capability provided by positron CT, one needs to understand fully the charateristics of positron CT, including its advantages and its limitations.

Development and Characteristics of Positron CT

Like other CT techniques, positron CT basically uses the same mathematical reconstruction technique, which generates the two-dimensional tomographic distribution from its line integrals measured at many angles and transverse positions(30). In positron CT, the distribution is the concentration of positron emitters in the body and the line integrals are measured by coincidence detection of positrons, which generate a pair of photons at opposite directions when annihillated(10,31). Because the coincidence detection is obtained by detectors positioned outside the body, the measurement procedure is completely non-invasive. Modern positron CT scanners can provide a spatial resolution of under one centimeter(32-38) and newer techniques allow resolutions on the order of 3 to 5 mm (39). A complete set of positron CT images of human brain is shown in Figure 1. These images were obtained by NeuroECAT(Ortec Corp., OakRidge, Tenn.) with a spatial resolution of 8.4 mm. The convolutions of the cortical ribbon and many subcortical structures are clearly delineated in these images. Quantitation accuracy on the order of 2 to 3 percent is attainable, although this depends very much on the care in carrying out the actual measurement procedures (such as attenuation correction, calibration, and external measurements of chemical and activity concentrations).

Due to the inherent noise enhancement property of the mathematical reconstruction of CT techniques, positron CT is also very sensitive to random noise(37,38,39). In other words, a sufficiently large number of coincidence counts is usually required to provide a clear and detailed distribution of the positron emitters in the body. This usually means a longer collection time. This limits the temporal sampling frequency of positron CT measurements to less than 10 to 20 samples per minute, although this limitation depends very much on the particular scanner and tracer used. This limitation thus normally excludes positron CT from measurements of compartments or dynamic processes

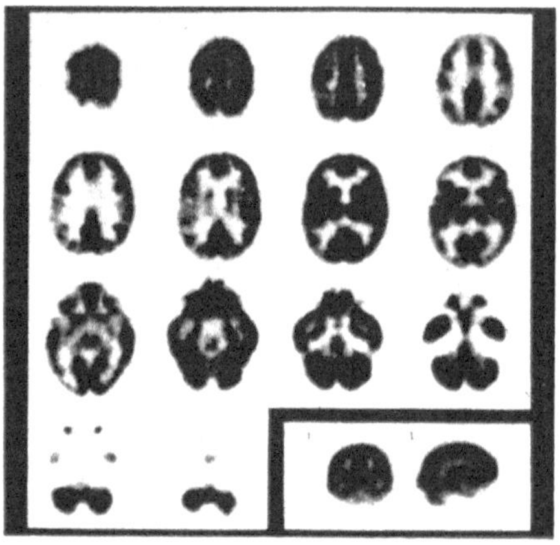

FIG. 1

Positron CT images of normal human brain from the top to the base at 8 mm intervals parallel to the orbito-meatal plane. The two images at lower right are rectilinear images that can be used to help positioning the subject for positron CT imaging. The images were obtained by NeuroECAT system with an 8.4 mm resolution. The tracer was FDG, which is used to determine the cerebral utilization rate of glucose. The convolutions of the cortical ribbon and many subcortical structures(inclucing the thalamus, caudate and the putamen-globus pallidus complex) are clearly delineated in these positron CT images.

that have turnover times on the order of 10 seconds or shorter.

Since positron CT scanners only detect the annihilation of positrons, tracers need to be labelled with positron emitting isotopes to be measured. Most essential atoms in organic compounds have positron emitting isotopes (e.g., ^{11}C, ^{15}O, ^{13}N) which can be incorporated in the compound to form tracers to follow certain processes. There is no positron emitting isotope for hydrogen. The fluorine isotope ^{18}F is often substituted because of its atomic dimensions and the strong C-F bond. Other positron emitters like ^{68}Ga, ^{82}Rb, ^{77}Kr, are also used for various tracers. However, positron emitters have short half lifes, usually ranging from a couple of minutes (^{15}O) to a couple of hours (^{18}F). If the turnover times of the compartment/process is longer than the half life of the positron emitter, the measurements could have too high a noise level to be useful before the end of the measurement period, which is generally required to be at least a few turnover times of the process. Therefore, the positron CT technique is restricted to measurements of processes with turnover times not longer than a couple of hours.

In positron CT scanners, the concentrations of positron emitters in all resolution elements in the imaged sections are measured simultaneously. Because of the high resolution of the new scanners, the amount of data that is obtained and needs to be processed is very large, especially as compared to the amount collected in traditional measurement techniques. In order to handle this large amount of data, efficient data processing algorithms are needed even with the availability of fast digital computers. This data processing consideration becomes increasingly important, as the spatial and the temporal resolution of positron CT scanners are being improved.

Requirements of Tracer Kinetic Modeling in Positron CT

Generally, models are used to describe the response of a system and to estimate the physiologic and biochemical parameters from the observations. This is the same for tracer kinetic models in positron CT, except that the requirements are more stringent. Due to the quantitative nature of positron CT, more accurate and reliable estimates of the processes are expected. Plus, more complex physical and biochemical processes are involved. This requires that models in positron CT describe as accurately as possible the physical and chemical processes and that measurements and parameter estimation be optimized. Also because of the non-invasiveness of the technique, tracer kinetic models in positron CT are expected to be used in clinical environments. That is, they need to describe the processes in question over a wide range of physiologic and biochemical conditions. And, for each subject/patient studied, an accurate and reliable estimate of the process is expected, so that meaningful clinical information can be obtained. In other words, models in positron CT not only are used to obtain the physiological and biochemical information for a certain population, but are also required to provide reliable information for each subject/patient studied. Because of these requirements, the modeling process in positron CT needs to be involved with the study procedures to obtain the optimal estimates while keeping the study convenient to use, i.e., minimum patient dose, study time, and discomfort.

TRACER SELECTION

For one physiological process, there are many possible tracers that one can use. Even the same chemical compound can usually be labeled at different molecular positions or with different positron emitters. Since tracer kinetic models are to provide a priori information about the transport process of tracers, the choice of tracer can affect the structure of the model and its complexity. This will eventually determine the success and usefulness of the model and the tracer for use in positron CT.

General Criteria for Selecting Appropriate Tracers

The proper tracer to use in positron CT depends critically on the process to be measured. It also depends on the kind of tracers available. The right tracer to use needs to be examined individually for each case. However, there are some general guidelines to follow in selecting the appropriate tracers. First, the tracer must be related to the process of concern, and the turnover time of the tracer is within the time window of the positron CT technique and the radioactive decay time as discussed above. Secondly, it is preferrable that the tracer not be related to other processes, so the tracer kinetics will reflect only the process of concern. This is not always possible. For example, all tracers must be related to blood flow for their transport to the tissue, even though blood flow may not be the principle process of interest. However, this dependence can be reduced by selecting tracers that have low extraction fractions across the capillary wall, so the uptake of a tracer is not critically dependent on the blood flow. Other desirable features of tracers that can minimize the dependence on other processes include (a) the trapping of tracer product in a slow turnover pool after the tracer has gone through the process of primary interest so the kinetics will not be related to the tracer clearance, (b) the elimimation of other possible branch processes by using tracers labeled in a specific position or analogs that are specific to only one pathway, (c) small pool size (rapid turnover rate) for the precursor pool, (d) fast clearance of tracer from blood to a low plasma concentration, and (e) the blood activity remain primarily in the form of the label tracer originally administered during the course of the study. These desirable features can reduce the background influence and result in a measured signal of high information content for the process of primary interest. Furthermore, the kinetics of a tracer having these features are likely to be easily describable with a model of simple structure that can give good estimates of the process. Other practical considerations for tracer selection in positron CT will be discussed later.

Various Choices of Tracers and Their Tradeoffs

For each process of interest, there are usually many choices of tracers in terms of their chemical forms, labelling position, and the half life of the labelling isotope . As discussed above, the proper choice depends on the process and needs to be evaluated individually. In the following, the general tradeoffs between various possible choices will be discussed and illustrated with some practical tracer examples.

Natural Substrates Versus Analogs: Various chemical analogs that have similar chemical structures and functional properties as the natural substrate have been synthesized and used in biochemistry for isolating and studying specific biochemical reactions(12,40,41). These analogs, when labelled with positron emitters, can be used in positron CT to trace the specific reaction which reflects the rate of utilization of the corresponding natural substrate. The advantage in the use of analogs is that some desirable features for tracers as outlined above can be more easily achieved. The disadvantage, however, is that the relationship between the analog and its natural substrate needs to be verified and understood over a wide range of physiological conditions.

Labelled natural substrates will be identical to their tracees (other than some small mass effects due to the radioisotopes), so they do not have the same problem as analogs. However, for labelled natural substrates, one is more restrictive in terms of incorporating the desirable characteristics into the tracer. In other words, even by the selection of the isotope and the molecular position for labelling, one may not be able to achieve the above mentioned features to minimize the background signals for the tracer.

The most frequently used tracer for measuring glucose utilization with positron CT is (^{18}F)-fluorodeoxyglucose (FDG)(20,21,42). The chemical structure of FDG is identical to glucose, except that the hydroxyl group in the second carbon position is replaced by a fluoride-18 atom(43). It represents an example of fluorine substitution for hydrogen in that the hydrogen in the 2 position of deoxyglucose is replaced by fluorine. This alteration of natural glucose results in FDG only tracing the glycolytic pathway through transport and phosphorylation to the end product of FDG-6-PO_4(20,21,44). Furthermore, FDG-6-PO_4 is not a substrate for glycogen synthesis or the pentose shunt and does not leave the cell except through slow hydrolysis back to free FDG, which can then be transported to plasma or rephosphorylated. Figure 2 illustrates the transport and reaction pathways of FDG as compared to glucose in cerebral tissue. FDG only follows glucose in its transport from plasma to tissue and in its phosphorylation, the rate of which, under a steady state and with appropriate correction for dephosphorylation of glucose, is equal to the utilization rate of exogenous glucose(20,21). Therefore, the tracer FDG has the desirable features a,b,e discussed above. The desirable feature d is only partially satisfied by FDG. Although FDG in blood is excreted by the kidneys, it usually takes more than 40 minutes before its concentration in blood and the tissue precursor pool drop to a small level(20,21). The relationship between FDG and glucose in their membrane transport and phosphorylation is characterized by a parameter called the lumped constant, which is based upon the principles of competitive substrate kinetics(19-21). The value of the lumped constant in cerebral and myocardial tissues under various conditions has been extensively studied (19-21, 45, 46), so the utilization rate of glucose is predictable from the kinetics of FDG.

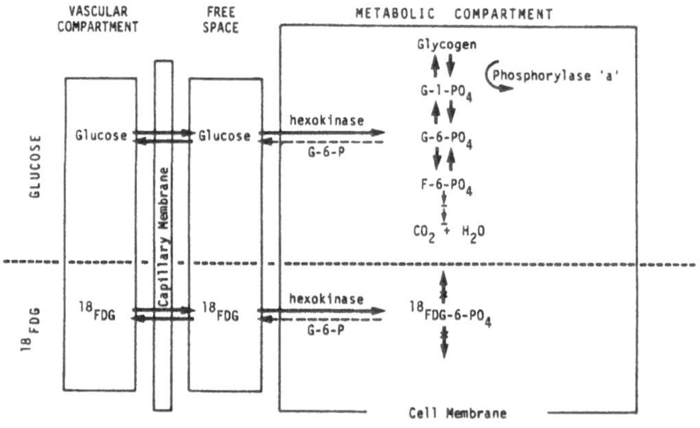

FIG. 2

Diagram illustrating the transport and reaction pathways of FDG in cerebral tissue. Similar to glucose, FDG can cross the blood brain barrier and be phosphorylated to FDG-6-PO_4. However, the phosphorylated FDG is not a substrate for further glycolytic reactions or for conversion to glycogen. Also, FDG-6-PO_4 can not cross the cell membrane and leave the tissue except through a slow dephosphorylation back to free FDG. These properties make FDG a desirable tracer for estimating utilization rate of exogenous glucose in cerebral tissues.

Another glucose analog that has been synthesized for positron CT is ^{11}C deoxyglucose (DG)(47). DG has similar characteristics as FDG except the value of the lumped constant for DG is expected to be somewhat different, and the half life of ^{11}C is shorter than ^{18}F (20 min vs. 110 min). The shorter half life of ^{11}C is less desirable because the tracer concentration in blood and precursor pools needs more than 40 minutes to reach a low level. Commercial positron CT scanners do not permit scanning the whole organ at one time (i.e., different sections of an organ are scanned in sequence at different times). The 20 minutes half life of ^{11}C DG poses an additional restriction on the length of time that the tracer study can be carried out. On the other hand, the shorter half life of ^{11}C allows repeated studies during the day, permitting a subject to serve as his own control(88).

For measurement of glucose utilization, labelled natural

glucose (^{11}C labelled) are also available for positron CT use(29). The compound can be either uniformly labelled or labelled at a specific carbon position. However, regardless of how the compound is labelled, the label ^{11}C goes through a substantial number of reaction steps in the glycolytic pathway before it is cleaved away as CO_2 or labeled products that are removed by the venous flow. Also, some ^{11}C labelled metabolic intermediates generated throughout the body will appear in the blood shortly after the introduction of the tracer. In other words, ^{11}C glucose has few of the desirable features and the kinetic measurements of the tracer are expected to contain information about many kinetic processes that are not directly related to the utilization of glucose by tissue. These unrelated processes will make the estimation of glucose utilization from the ^{11}C glucose kinetic data more difficult and less reliable, although, with the natural substrate, there is no need for the correction embodied in the lumped constant used with FDG.

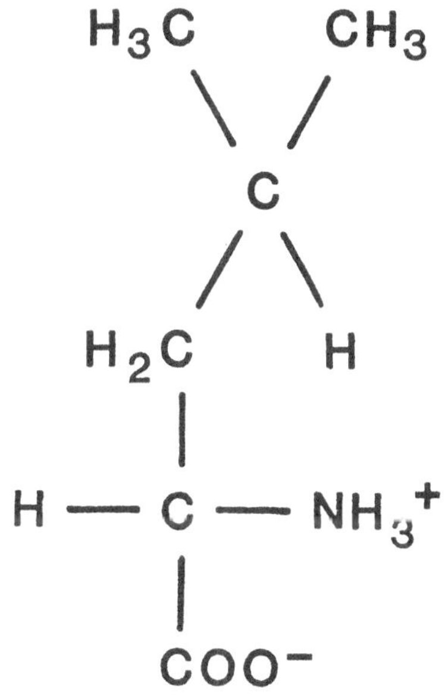

FIG. 3

Diagram showing the chemical structure of leucine. This amino acid can be labelled with ^{13}N in the amine group or with ^{11}C in any of the carbon positions.

The use of different labelling isotopes or labelling positions on the same compound could reflect completely different processes. This large effect on the kinetics of a tracer due to the labelling is best shown by the labelling of leucine for protein synthesis in cerebral tissues(22,23). Leucine is chosen over other amino acids primarily because of its higher extraction across the blood brain barrier(48) and the rapid turnover rate of the tissue precursor pool. Leucine can be labelled with ^{13}N in the amine group or with ^{11}C at any of the carbon positions as shown in Figure 3. Through blood flow, leucine is transported and extracted into tissue. Some fraction of the leucine will be incorporated into protein and some will be transported back to the blood pool, but the rest will go through the metabolic pathway as shown in Figure 4. Different functional groups or atoms of the molecule would go through different routes and end up in different metabolic products. For example, if the molecule is labelled with ^{13}N, the label will end up in glutamate, which has a slow turnover rate because of its large pool size in tissue(49). Within one to two hours, the label in glutamate is kinetically similar to that incorporated into protein, which, like glutamate, has a very slow turnover rate. In other words, the information that can be obtained from the kinetic data will be the combined rate of protein synthesis and leucine metabolism. Also, the labelled glutamate or its products in tissue could be washed out to blood, thus adding different labelled amino acids to the blood pool and making the problem more complicated. However, if the molecule is labelled with ^{11}C at the first carbon position, the label ends up in CO_2 after the second step in the metabolic pathway(i.e., decarboxylation) and the labelled CO_2 will be cleared from tissue by the venous blood flow at a fast rate. Therefore, only labelled leucine that is incorporated into protein will have a slow turnover rate, and protein synthesis can be more clearly isolated from other processes in the kinetic measurements. If ^{11}C label is at other carbon positions, it will be involved in more reaction steps and there will be more variability in the kinetic measurements that is unrelated to protein synthesis. Thus, labelling at other carbon positions is not as desirable as at the first carbon.

Similar strategy was adopted (87) for use of 2-^{11}C-palmitate (CPA) for the study of oxidation of free fatty acids in myocardium. The label ^{11}C is transferred to CO_2 at the beginning step of oxidation. In addition to oxidation, CPA can also be transported back to the blood pool or be converted to triglycerides or phospholipids that have slow turnover rates(50). Therefore, the transport and reactions of CPA in tissue are very similar to those of ^{11}C-leucine, except that the process of main interest for CPA is the oxidation step, while for leucine it is the incorporation into the slow turnover pool of protein.

Other Considerations

As illustrated above, tracer kinetics allow the identification and separation of only pathways or compartments that are kinetically separable--the greater the separation, the higher the accuracy and reliability. A desirable tracer should

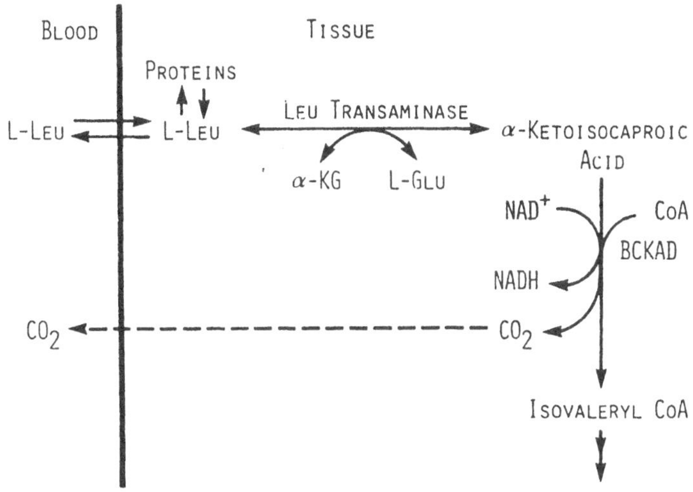

FIG. 4

Diagram illustrating the biochemical pathways of L-leucine in tissue. In addition to its incorporation into protein, leucine can be metabolized in tissue. In the metabolic route, the amine group is transferred to glutamate in the transamination reaction. So, if the compound is labelled with ^{13}N, the label would be in the tissue glutamate pool that has a slow turnover rate. If the compound is labelled with ^{11}C at the first carbon position, the label would come off as $^{11}CO_2$ and be rapidly cleared from tissue by the venous blood flow. Thus, the majority of the ^{11}C label in tissue is incorporated in protein.

have its kinetics primarily related to the process of interest, thus practically isolating the process for study. With such a tracer, the modeling is simplified and the estimates of the rates of the process by the use of the model will be reliable. However, there are other practical considerations that need to be evaluated and could determine the final selection of the tracer to use for a particular study. Among these, the half life of the labelling isotope has already been discussed. Usually a critical problem is the synthesis of the compound. A compound that has all the desirable features but cannot be synthesized quickly or have a high yield is useless for positron CT studies. In other words, the tracer to be selected is restricted to those that can be synthesized conveniently. The criteria for desirable tracers discussed above can be used to point to the research direction for synthesis developments of new tracers.

In order to obtain good counting statistics without violating the criterion of minimal mass effect for tracer kinetic studies, the specific activity of the tracer sometimes can be a problem. This is especially crucial when the concentration of the natural substrate of concern is low. For example, the concentration of neuroreceptors in brain is rather low (in the pmole/gm range)(51). To study the concentration of these receptors, the labelled tracers should not occupy more than 1 to 5 percent of the receptor sites, which usually corresponds to a fraction of a pmole/gm. With a detection efficiency of 40,000 counts/sec/μCi/cc/image plane for a positron CT scanner, it requires a specific activity of at least 50 Ci/mmole to give an image of 500,000 counts in a 10 min scan. For most other processes, the requirement is not so demanding. However, the higher the specific activity, the smaller amount (in cold mass) of tracer is needed, and the less the tracer will disturb the process to be measured.

Consideration of radiation dose to the subject will also influence the selection of tracers. Radiation dose is related to the physical half life of the isotope, the biological clearance and distribution of the tracer. As far as radiation dose is concerned, an ideal tracer should be taken up only by the target organ and have a half life that is long enough to give good quality measurements but will quickly decay away so little radiation is left in body after the measurements. In reality, there are few such ideal tracers, and compromises and tradeoffs between different considerations have to be made in selecting a proper tracer to use for a particular study.

MODEL CONFIGURATIONS

As discussed earlier, tracer kinetic models are basically used to incorporate a priori information in the interpretation of tracer kinetic measurements. Incorrect a priori information could lead to wrong interpretations. Therefore, models should be structured as faithfully as possible to the transport and subsequent reactions of tracers in tissue. On the other hand, too complicated a model is difficult, if not impossible, to use. Compartmental models generally provide a compromise between the fidelity requirements and the mathematical tractibility. Compartmental models offer many attractive mathematical properties and at the same time can describe tracer kinetic data very well. In such models, compartments can represent either physically separated spaces or different chemical forms of tracer in the same physical space. However, the question of what space should be included or be considered as separate compartments is related to the tracer and the process being studied. Usually, a comprehensive model that identifies the different spaces and their interconnections needs to be first formulated. The comprehensive model is then reduced to form a practical model.

Also, a model needs to be validated before it is used for interpreting data. It is a fair statement that tracer kinetic data alone can rarely be used to structure a model, but with the appropriate model they can provide accurate estimates of the process under study. Biochemical studies or knowledge is necessary to structure models. These steps in developing a tracer kinetic model are discussed in detail in the following sections. Examples are used to show the procedure in each step.

Formulation of Comprehensive Models

For a given tracer kinetic measurement, there are many compartmental models that can adequately describe the measurements(18,52). However, not all of these models can be used to help extract useful information. To ensure that the model is physiologically or biochemically meaningful, the physiological and biochemical information about the tracer needs to be incorporated into the model. If, in building the initial model, a preliminary compartment is included for each physical space or chemical form of the tracer and the assignments of connections among these compartments are guided by the physiologic and biochemical information, the model parameters can be easily associated with physiologically meaningful information.

In general, tracers are transported to tissue through the capillary blood flow and extracted into cells across the capillary and cellular membrane. After entering the cells, the tracer could participate in various reactions depending on the characteristics of the tracer. The exact configuration of a comprehensive model would depend on the tracer used. Figure 5 shows an example of a comprehensive model for the tracer FDG. There are separate compartments for the vascular space, the interstitial space, the cellular space and for various labelled chemical compounds. Transport between the compartments is also shown. The magnitude and properties of these transport rates could determine the final model configuration. The general characteristics of each of these transports are discussed below.

Delivery, Extraction and Clearance: Tracers are usually introduced in the body through intravenous injection or through inhalation. Through either method, tracers are well mixed in blood when going through the heart chambers, so all arterial blood should have the same concentration. Because of this condition, tracer concentration delivered to the tissue capillaries can be obtained from any peripheral artery (like the radial artery), and the amount of tracer delivered to tissue is proportional to the blood flow.

Once in the capillaries, some portion of the tracer (except for vascular tracers) will be extracted into tissue across the capillary wall, while the unextracted portion will be rapidly washed away from tissue by the venous blood flow. The size of the fraction that is extracted across capillary wall depends on the surface area(S) of the capillary wall, the permeability (P) of the capillary wall for the tracer, and the capillary blood flow. The surface area and the permeability directly affect the extraction of tracer across the capillary and the venous flow clears the

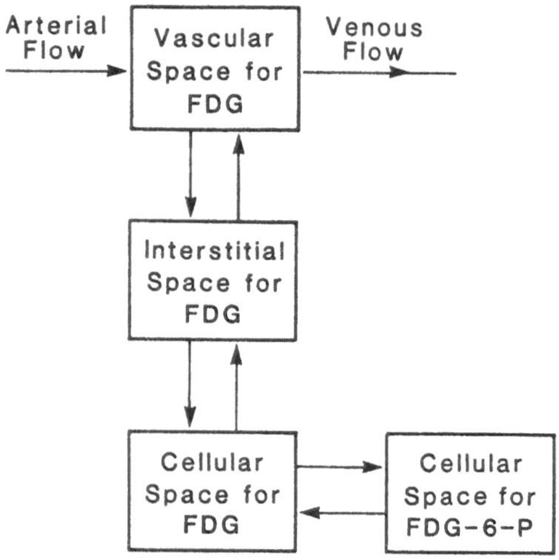

FIG. 5

Diagram showing a comprehensive model of FDG in cerebral tissue. Every tissue space of FDG is represented by a separate compartment. The arrows indicate transport or chemical conversions among compartments.

tracer from the capillaries in competition with the extraction process. This competition for the tracer has been modelled by Kety(13), Renkin(53) and Crone(54) by a rigid cylindrical tube model (usually referred to as the Renkin-Crone model). According to this model, the fraction of tracer that is extracted across the capillary wall when the tracer goes through the capillaries can be expresed as

$$E=1-\exp(-PS/F) \qquad (2)$$

where P, in units of cm/min, denotes the permeability of tracer across the capillary, S, in unit of cm^2/gm, is the surface area of the capillaries in a gram of tissue, and F is the blood flow(ml/min/gm). PS is usually called the permeability-surface product. The higher the value of PS, the larger the amount of tracer extracted in tissue. But the relationship is not linear. As a function of the blood flow, the extraction fraction drops as flow increases. However, assuming the same arterial tracer concentration, the amount of tracer delivered to capillaries increases linearly with the blood flow. This increase more than compensates for the decrease in the extraction fraction and results in a net increase in the total amount of tracer extracted across the capillary wall (equal to E*F). The relative amount of tracer extracted as a function of blood flow is show in Figure 6 for various PS values.

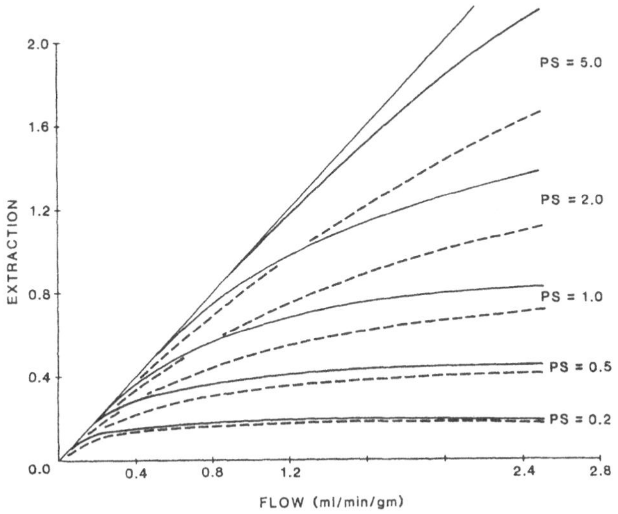

FIG. 6

Graph showing the extraction of substrate across the capillary wall as a function of blood flow for various capillary PS values. The solid curves are according to the Renkin-Crone model. The dashed lines are based on the compartmental model shown in Figure 7. Both models show nonlinearity as a function of flow. At low PS values, the relationships due to the two models are shown to be similar.

A simple compartmental model can also be used to describe the relationship between blood flow and extraction and is shown in Figure 7. According to this model, the extraction fraction E is related to F and PS as

$$E=PS/(PS+F) \tag{3}$$

In this model, the capillary space is assumed to be a compartment of uniform concentration. The extraction and venous flow compete through the pool for the tracers. According to this model, the relative amount of tracer extracted in tissue as a function of blood flow is also shown in Figure 6 for comparison to the Renkin-Crone model.

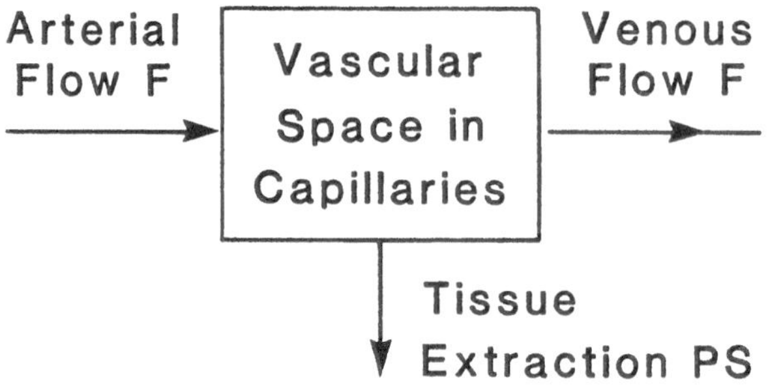

FIG. 7

A compartmental model for the vascular space in tissue that can be used to indicate the relationship between the extraction of substrates into tissue and the clearance by the venous flow. The amount of extraction as a function of flow for various PS values are shown in Figure 6 as dashed lines.

In the relationships shown in Figure 6, the PS values are assumed to be constant (independent of flow). However, the PS values are generally expected to be larger as the blood flow is increased(55,56). This dependence of PS on flow, if known for a particular organ, can be incorporated in the above two models easily .

Transport Mechanisms: In the above, the extraction of tracers across capillary wall is described by the PS product. Only the effect of blood flow on PS was briefly discussed. There are many variables that could affect PS. To understand these effects, one needs to know the actual mechanism for tracer transport across the capillary wall. The transport mechanism could be quite different for different tracers. In general, there are two categories -- active transport and passive transport(57). Active transport requires energy(e.g., ATP), while passive transport does not. Active transport can transport a net flux of substance against a concentration gradient (i.e., from a lower concentration to a higher concentration). Examples of active transport are relatively few. The sodium potassium ion pump in neurons is a well known example(58). Other examples of active transport include the reabsorption of glucose and other nutrients by the proximal tubule in the kidney(59) and the absorption of nutrients by the intestinal epithelium cells(60).

Unlike active transport, the direction of net flux in passive transport is determined by the concentration gradient across the membrane. The transport characteristics are all bidirectional. In general, passive transport can be grouped into two categories-facilitated transport and passive diffusion. Passive diffusion is a basic physical property of molecules in liquids or gases. By random motions, molecules in the medium move about constantly. If there are different concentrations of a particular molecule in the medium, a net flux will diffuse from the high concentration region to the low concentration region. Allowing time, an equilibrium will be reached such that the concentration of the molecules throughout a confined region will be equal. The net flux of molecules from a high concentration region to a low concentration region is related only to the diffusion coefficient of the molecules in the medium and the concentration gradient(57). Many substances in the body (like water, oxygen, carbon dioxide, ammonia, ligands ets..., particularly compounds of small molecular sizes) depend on this diffusion mechanism for their transport between the vascular and tissue spaces. For this kind of transport mechanism, the diffusion coefficient divided by the separation distance between the two spaces is the permeability discussed earlier for extraction of tracers from the vascular space into the tissue(57).

Like passive diffusion, facilitated transport can only produce a net flux of transport from a high concentration to a low concentration region. However, in facilitated transport the movement of molecules across a membrane is assisted by enzymes in the membrane. Substances that rely on this kind of transport for extraction into the tissue include many important substrates, like glucose, free fatty acids, and amino acids. Although the exact mechanism of assistance in the transport depends on the substance and the membrane, the transport can usually be considered to consist of three steps, viz., the combination of the substrate molecule with some carrier molecule, the assisted movement of the substrate-carrier complex molecule, and the release of the substrate molecule on the other side of the membrane(57). The process is very similar to the enzyme catalyzed chemical reaction shown below

$$A + E \underset{k_2}{\overset{k_1}{\rightleftharpoons}} AE \xrightarrow{k_3} A + E$$

where A denotes the substrate and E the carrier molecule. The rate of transport of a facilitated transport is dependent on the characteristics of the substrate and the membrane carrier system, the number of membrane carrier molecules available for the transport of a particular substrate, and the membrane environment. Because the number of membrane carrier molecules is finite, a facilitated transport system is saturable (i.e., the flux of transport is dependent not only on the concentration difference between the two sides of the membrane but also on the absolute concentrations of the substrate on each side of the membrane) and displaceable (i.e., it can be affected by substances of similar molecular structures, as in competitive inhibition of enzyme catalyzed reactions). A facilitated transport system can usually be characterized by its maximal transport rate constant (V_m) and half saturation concentration (K_m), similar to the Michaelis-Menton constants for an enzyme catalyzed reaction. In other words, the uni-directional rate of a facilitated transport can be described by the following equation.

$$\text{(TRANSPORT FLUX)}=[A]\ V_m/([A]+K_m) \quad (4)$$

where [A] denotes the concentration of the transported substrate. This equation shows that as far as the substrate A is concerned the facilitated transport is not a linear process and can not be described by compartmental models. However, for the labelled tracer, which has a low concentration as compared to the natural substrate, the linearity still holds. This is similar to the case of modeling enzyme catalyzed reactions and will be discussed in more detail in the following subsection. The permeability-surface product of extraction for a facilitated transport is related to V_m, K_m and [A] as

$$PS=V_m/(K_m+[A]) \quad (5)$$

In addition to the active and passive transport mechanisms discussed above, substances can also cross the capillary wall in some tissues by bulk flow through the fenestrations(i.e., openings) in the capillary wall between the capillary endothelial cells(57). The extraction fraction due to this kind of transport is related to the amount of bulk flow across the capillary wall relative to the blood flow to the tissue. However, no bulk flow across cell membranes is known to exist. Also, the extraction of some substances could consists of a number of transport mechanisms. So, the permeability-surface product that is used to characterize the extraction of tracers into tissue could consist of a combination of the factors discussed above.

Competitive Enzyme Kinetics: Most chemical reactions in living tissues are enzyme catalyzed reactions. Generally, they can be represented as

$$A + E \underset{k_2}{\overset{k_1}{\rightleftharpoons}} AE \xrightarrow{k_3} P + E$$

where A denotes the substrate which is being converted to the product P through the catalytic action of the enzyme E. The k's are the rate constants for the reaction steps. The reaction could involve only a single substrate or multiple substrates. In the latter case, the concentrations of all other substrates not shown are assumed to be held constant. By assuming the enzyme concentration to be constant, the rate of reaction from A to P can be shown to be related to the concentration of A as

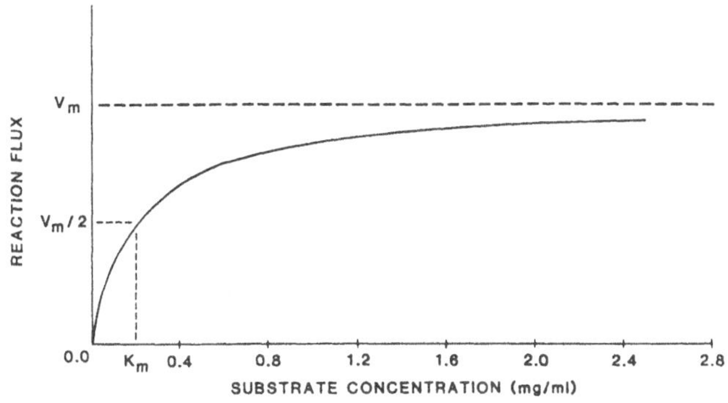

FIG. 8

Michaelis-Menton relationship between reaction flux and substrate concentration in an enzyme catalyzed reaction. The relationship is completely characterized by two parameters-K_m and V_m. V_m, the maximal reaction flux, which can only be approached at extremely high substrate concentrations, is dependent on the enzyme concentration. K_m is equal to the substrate concentration that has a flux of $V_m/2$ and is related to the association and dissociation rates between the enzyme and the substrate.

$$R = \frac{k_3\ C_0\ [A]}{(k_2+k_3)/k_1 + [A]} = \frac{V_m\ [A]}{K_m + [A]} \tag{6}$$

where C_0 is the total enzyme concentration. This equation is known as the Michaelis-Menton equation and the variables V_m and K_m that characterize the reaction rate are called the Michaelis-Menton constants(61). More specifically, V_m is called the maximal velocity for the reaction because it is the fastest rate possible (when [A] approaches infinity) for a given enzyme concentration. The value of K_m is equal to the concentration of A that would produce half the maximal rate and is called the half saturation concentration. Figure 8 shows the reaction rate as a function of concentration of A. The relationship is clearly not linear with respect to [A]. However, suppose a tracer A' is similar to A in its reaction with the enzyme E, i.e.,

$$A + E \rightleftharpoons AE \longrightarrow P + E$$

$$A' + E \rightleftharpoons A'E \longrightarrow P' + E$$

If the association and dissociation rates of the substrate-enzyme complex are much faster than the rate of variation in the concentration of A', the conversion fluxes from A and A' to P and P' can be shown to be

$$R = \frac{V_m[A]/K_m}{[A]/K_m + [A']/K_m' + 1}$$
$$R' = \frac{V_m' [A']/K_m'}{[A]/K_m + [A']/K_m' + 1} \qquad (7)$$

where V_m' and K_m' are the Michaelis-Menton constants of the enzymatic reaction for the tracer A'. If A' satisfies the tracer requirement that its concentration is much smaller than that of A (i.e., $[A'] \ll [A]$), then the above equations can be reduced to

$$R = \frac{V_m[A]}{[A] + K_m}$$
$$R' = \frac{V_m' K_m / K_m'}{[A] + K_m} [A'] \qquad (8)$$

The equation for the natural substrate, as expected, is the same as the one without the tracer added, because the tracer A' has a low concentration and is assumed to have a negligible effect on the steady state condition of the reaction. The equation for the tracer is similar to the one for the natural substrate , except that it is linear with respect to the concentration of the tracer. This is a critical relationship as far as tracer kinetic modeling is concerned. It is the fundamental basis for modeling enzyme catalyzed reactions with linear compartmental models.

From the above equations, the ratio of reaction fluxes between the tracer and the natural substrate is

$$R'/R = \frac{V_m' K_m}{V_m K_m'} \frac{[A']}{[A]} \qquad (9)$$

This equation shows that the ratio between the tracer and the natural substance in terms of reaction flux is only related to the basic characteristics of the enzyme and the concentration ratio of the tracer to the natural substrate. For example, for a labelled natural substrate, V_m' and K_m' are equal to V_m and K_m, and thus the reaction fluxes between the tracer and the natural substrate are only proportional to their chemical concentrations. In other words, the reaction rate constants for the tracer and the natural substrate are the same.

According to the above equation, the ratio of the reaction rate constants between an analog tracer and its corresponding natural substrate is only dependent on the relative activity of the enzyme for the tracer and the natural substrate which is usually expected to be constant and predictable. This relative activity is equivalent to a calibration constant for converting the reaction rate constants of the tracer, that are directly measurable, to the rate constants of the natural substrate. Thus, the reaction flux of the substrate can be obtained from that of the tracer. This property of the competitive enzyme kinetics is the basis that facilitates the use of analogs for measuring reaction rates of the natural substrates. For example, the FDG method for the measurement of glucose utilization rate requires the knowledge of the value of the lumped constant to convert the uptake flux of FDG to that of glucose. The relationship discussed above for competitive enzyme kinetics is one of the important theoretical bases that support the constancy and predictability of the lumped constant which are essential for the success of the method.

Chemical reactions in living tissues may be much more involved than the simple reaction model discussed above. However, if the reaction rate as a function of substrate concentration has the general relationship as shown in Figure 8, the reaction can be approximated as a simple reaction, as far as tracer kinetics is concerned. Even for reactions that do not have the exact relationship of Figure 8, the simple reaction can still be a good approximation, if the tracer is in low concentration relative to the natural substrate. That is, the reaction rate can still be characterized by a set of effective Michaelis-Menton constants V_m and K_m. However, for these reactions, the transport rate constants as a function of the concentration of the natural substrate will not follow the relationship of Equation 6.

Workable Models

As shown in Figure 5, a comprehensive model will consist of many separate compartments. Although compartmental models have good mathematical properties, the number of differential equations required goes up in parallel with the number of compartments, and the mathematical complexity could increase drastically. For example, analytical solutions for models of more than three compartments are possible only in rare cases. Also, the response function corresponding to the measured tracer kinetic data may consist of fewer exponential components than the number of compartments in the comprehensive model. In such cases, the set of model parameter values corresponding to the measured data is not unique and can not be determined with high certainty. Therefore, comprehensive models can only describe the tracer transport and reactions in qualitative terms and may only be sufficient for evaluating the effects on the tracer kinetics of certain transport and reaction steps. Furthermore, comprehensive models are usually too cumbersome to use for extracting physiological information from tracer kinetic data. Therefore, there is a need to reduce the comprehensive model to a simpler one having fewer compartments and parameters.

In the last section describing the building of comprehensive models, the physiological and biochemical information was only discussed for configuring the structure of a model. The a priori information about the size of the compartments or the magnitudes of the transport/reaction rates for a tracer at various steps has not been used. In general, there are two possible ways to incorporate this information. One approach is to reduce the number of compartments, by using the a priori information as a guide. The known physiological and biochemical information about the tracer and the process it traces can provide a general idea about the magnitude of the transport rate of each step in the model. From this information, the limiting steps (i.e., the slower steps in a chain of transport/reactions) can be identified. Separate compartments can then be combined to form a single compartment if the transport rates between them are not limiting (i.e., much faster than the other processes). This model reduction process can be most clearly understood by the use of an example.

The FDG model example shown in the last section has 4 compartments and 7 transport parameters. However, it is generally accepted that the transport of glucose as well as FDG across the cell membrane is very fast, especially as compared to the transport across the capillary wall and the phosphorylation reaction catalyzed by hexokinase(62). In other words, the concentration ratio between the interstitial space and the cellular space is nearly in equilibrium at all times. Therefore, the interstitial space and the cellular space can be approximated as a single compartment. The rate constants for the backdiffusion (tissue to plasma) and the phosphorylation reaction in the reduced model will have a slightly different meaning from the constants in the comprehensive model. In the reduced model, the rate constants refer to the fractions of the total tracer in the tissue space (including the interstitial and the cellular spaces) that are transported out from the space, while in the non-reduced model they are with respect to the individual spaces. Also, if the PS value is small compared to the blood flow, such that the plasma concentration of FDG along the capillary does not vary much due to the extraction of FDG into tissue or its backdiffusion, the transport of FDG into and out of tissue will be independent of the blood flow(19-21). In such a case, the blood flow can be eliminated completely, further simplifying the model. After these considerations, the FDG model is reduced basically to two compartments with four parameters, as shown in Figure 9. For such a model, not only is the mathematics much simpler, the estimated parameter values from the measured tracer kinetic data will also be more reliable and more easily obtained.

The second approach is to assign known values for the parameters in the model that do not have large variations or are predictable from other independent measurements. By doing so, the

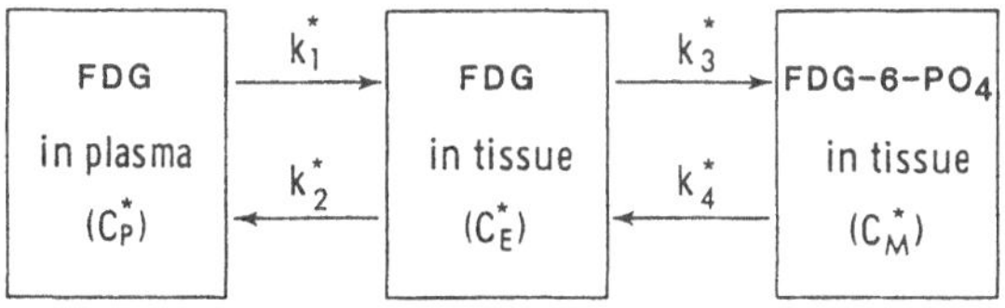

DIAGRAM OF THE THREE COMPARTMENTS IN FDG MODEL

FIG. 9

A workable model for FDG in cerebral and myocardial tissue. The model is reduced from the comprehensive model of Figure 5. The reduction is achieved by combining the interstitial and cellular spaces of free FDG into a single compartment and by neglecting the effect of blood flow on the extraction of FDG. This model has only four rate constants and the mathematics is easily manageable.

number of adjustable parameters in the model is reduced and the non-uniqueness problem is resolved by assigning a sufficient number of parameters to known/fixed values. The use of the equilibrium model and oxygen-15 water for the measurement of blood flow (63-66) is an example that has used such an approach.

The equillibrium technique relies on the balance between tracer delivery (by blood flow) and its clearance (by venous flow and by physical decay of ^{15}O). Based on Kety's single compartmental model(13), at equilibrium, the radioactivity(Q) in tissue is related to the blood flow (F) as

$$F = \lambda QV/(C_i V - Q), \qquad (10)$$

where V is the distribution volume of water in tissue, C_i is the arterial concentration of ^{15}O-water, and λ is the physical decay constant of ^{15}O. The values of Q and C_i can be measured and the value of λ is known. If the value of V is constant, then the blood flow can be calculated from the measurements Q and C_i. Normally, the distribution volume of water in tissue does not vary very much (i.e.,even gross edema will change the tissue water content by only about 5%). Thus, a constant value can be assigned to V and the accuracy of the result would still be within the tolerable limit(66). Because of the simplicity of the calculation, this equilibrium technique in combination with positron CT has been quite useful for providing local blood flows(65). The technique requires the short-lived tracer to be delivered to the subject at a constant concentration to maintain the equilibrium state during the measurement time. This could cause some practical problems if the isotope producing cyclotron is not very close to the study site.

Usually the problem of mathematical complexity in the solutions of these models is not alleviated by this second approach. Also, if the assigned values of the parameters differ from the true values of a particular study, the deviation could be reflected as errors in other parameters, resulting in potential errors in the parameters estimated from the tracer kinetic measurements. However, the two approaches for reducing the model structure have different characteristics. The approach of choice for a particular model depends on the individual situation. Also, the two approaches are not mutually exclusive. For some cases, the use of both approaches can provide the best workable model.

Validation of Models

In the development of a comprehensive model and in its reduction to a workable model, some assumptions and approximations have to be made. Whether these assumptions or approximations hold for a particular tracer is a major concern in tracer kinetic modeling. Therefore, after a workable model has been configured, it needs to be validated before it can actually be used. There are two major criteria for validating a tracer kinetic model. One is that the response from the model must be consistent with the kinetic measurements. This is usually referred to as the ability of the model to fit the measured data. To satisfy this criterion, the model should fit the data well and the model parameter values estimated from such a fit should be compatible with known physiological/biochemical knowledge. The method of curve fitting and parameter estimation in tracer kinetics will be discussed in the following subsection. The second validation criterion for tracer kinetic models is that the predictions from the model must match direct chemical measurements. This criterion is more stringent than the first one and is usually tested only after the fitting criterion is satisfied. This chemical validation criterion will be discussed after the discussion on the curve fitting methods.

Curve Fitting and Parameter Estimation: The first test of a tracer kinetic model is its ability to perform a good fit to experimental data. This section presents an overview of the procedures and assumptions associated with the regression, or fitting, of a set of experimental data to a model. A more complete and general discussion of regression topics can be found elsewhere (67,68). The primary goal of regression analysis is to produce estimates of each of the parameters of the model. An equally important aspect of regression is the calculation of a measure of how good each estimate is, i.e. the standard error of the estimate.

Assumptions of a regression analysis - A regression analysis assumes that each observation, can be directly predicted from the model. The difference between the observed and predicted values consists of a stochastic component, the random noise associated with the measurement process, and a deterministic part, the oversimplifications or missing components of the model. Standard regression assumes that the errors are zero mean, uncorrelated, normally distributed, their variance is known (and constant), and observation times and input functions are measured without error. A least squares regression analysis produces estimates of the model parameters by choosing those parameter values which minimize the sum of squared deviations between the observations and the model predictions.

Non-linear regression - If the model is linear in the parameters, best fit estimates can be computed in one step. However, tracer kinetic models generally have solutions which are non-linear in the parameters. In this case, finding the best-fit parameter estimates can be visualized as finding the point of lowest elevation of a multi-dimensional hilly terrain. Therefore an iterative procedure is required. A large set of techniques for estimating parameters in non-linear systems is available (See (69) and (70) for a review). The Gauss-Newton method, also called Ordinary Least Squares (OLS), and its common modifications comprise the most common set of algorithms. A starting value for the parameters must first be supplied, and each iteration step, equivalent to the one-step linear regression, proceeds as follows:

1. Determine the model's predicted values.
2. Calculate the sensitivity matrix of the model to the parameters.
3. Update the parameter estimates.

Iterations continue until the absolute change in each parameter over one iteration is smaller than some pre-determined criterion. The standard errors, a measure of the variation in the estimation from experiment to experiment, can then be calculated directly. Under the standard assumptions, the converged estimates will be unbiased, and will have minimum possible standard errors based on sample size. It is important to recognize that the computation of standard errors is based upon many approximations.

Implementation aspects of non-linear regression - To compute the predicted value from a tracer kinetic model, the differential equations must be solved, either analytically or by computer based numerical techniques (71). The second approach has the advantage of avoiding algebraic complexity but it requires substantially more computer time. To calculate sensitivity coefficients, there are three approaches: analytical specification of the derivatives (72), simultaneous numerical solutions for the derivatives of the function, or the simple secant approximation to derivatives. The modeler also has a choice whether to fit directly to the model's original, or micro-parameters, or the algebraically more convenient macro-parameters. There are also common extensions to the Gauss-Newton algorithm including step size modifications, such as step-halving and more elaborate schemes (73), and Marquardt-Levenberg algorithms(74,75) (for a review, see (69,70)).

Practical consideratons of non-linear regression: - All available information should be used to generate good initial values for the regression analysis, resulting in quicker convergence and avoiding unwanted solutions. In practice, it is often very difficult to supply good initial parameter estimates for a complicated model. One approach is to bootstrap parameter estimates from a simpler models. It is also useful to put a limit on the number of iterations permitted in the regression analysis, since a slowly converging regression may point to errors in the data or the specification of the model. Putting constraints on the parameters, e.g. bounding all rate constants to be non-negative, can also improve convergence.

In many applications, the error variance is not constant for all observations. Particularly, Poisson counting noise has a variance equal to its expectation. All information concerning the error variance can be used to improve the fitting via weighted least squares estimation (WLS). For region of interest values from positron CT images, the weights may depend primarily on the total coincidence events collected for the slice. Other sources of noise include patient movement during the scanning period, placement of the region of interest, calibration, etc. Unless these error sources are carefully analyzed, choosing the appropriate weights is not obvious. When the error variance is not constant, the use of OLS will produce unbiased parameter estimates, but they will not have the minimum possible variance.

Analysis of regression estimates and goodness of fit - Without critical examination of regression results, parameter estimates can easily be mis-interpreted. Analysis of Variance (76) provides a first test of the statistical significance of the fit, and can be extended to test for significant lack of fit when repeated observations at identical or nearly identical times are possible (68). Hypotheses concerning the parameters of a model and their differences between individuals and test conditions can be examined by using the standard errors with the T-test. The standard errors can also be used as weights for further statistical analyses of the parameter estimates. One of the best approaches for examination of the goodness of a fit is to examine the residuals. Any significant non-random nature to the residuals should be readily evident to the eye by plotting. (See (68), chapter 3, for a detailed discussion of residual analysis). Finally, it is important to compare a chosen model to simpler and more complex versions to test for a statistically significant change in the goodness of fit.

Direct Biochemical Validation: As mentioned earlier, the model corresponding to a tracer kinetic measurement is not unique. The use of curve fitting and parameter estimation techniques along with biochemical and physiologic information in the process of developing a model can exclude many unrealistic configurations. However, it still does not define a unique configuration. The ability of a model to fit the measured kinetic data is only a necessary condition and not a sufficient condition. In other words, a good fit alone does not prove that the model is valid. Direct chemical validation can check the validity of some of the assumptions and approximations made in the model. If the model predictions are found to be consistent with the direct chemical measurements, the model will be considered more valid and its predictions more reliable.

A direct chemical validation procedure in tracer kinetics involves performing a tracer kinetic study and a direct chemical assay experiment simultaneously. The independent results from the two experiments will be compared to assess the validity of the model. Although the tracer kinetic experiment is non-invasive, the direct chemical assay experiment involves traumatic interventions. The invasiveness of the procedure usually restricts the validation to a very limited number of studies. Also, when chemical assay of the tissue is required, the procedure can not be performed on man (except in cases where tissue samples are resected for clinical reasons), and animal experiments must be used. The choice of the animal model to use and the extrapolation of results from animal experiments to human subjects depend on many factors and need to be performed with extreme care. A full discussion of this is outside the scope of this chapter. Instead, an example of direct chemical validation of the model for FDG in myocardium is shown below to illustrate the procedures involved.

The workable model for FDG shown in Figure 9 has been found to fit the tracer kinetic data of myocardium quite well(77,45,46). In order to further test the validity of the model, chemical assay experiments have been performed in conjunction with the FDG tracer experiments. In these experiments, FDG was introduced as a step function to an isolately perfused rabbit heart septum. The ^{18}F radioactivity in the septum was monitored by a pair of coincidence detectors. At the end of the experiment which varied from 30, 60 and 90 min after the start of the FDG infusion, a tissue sample was taken from the septum. The tissue sample was homogenated and the chemical forms of the ^{18}F labelled compounds were determined by HPLC to be only FDG and FDG-6-PO_4 (46). This is consistent with the model. Also, the chemically determined fractions of FDG and FDG-6-PO_4 were compared with the predictions obtained from the tracer kinetic data (measured by the coincidence detectors) by the use of the model. The results from the kinetic data were found to match well with those by chemical assays, as shown in Table 1. Also, the utilization rate of glucose as predicted by the model and the tracer data was found to be equal to the value calculated from the arterial-venous difference by Fick's method. From these direct chemical validation results, the FDG model of Figure 9 is considered to be valid for the myocardium under the condition studied.

Extrapolation of the results from animal experiments needs to be examined carefully. Also, a tracer kinetic model is useful only if it is applicable to a wide range of physiological or pathological conditions. Therefore, a full validation of a model must be carried out for various conditions for which the model will be employed.

TABLE 1

PERCENT FDG-6-PO_4 IN MYOCARDIUM

	Time after infusion of FDG (min)		
	30	60	90
tissue assay	48.2$\pm$9.0	62.8$\pm$4.3	65.3$\pm$2.4
estimated by model	43.8$\pm$1.5	55.0$\pm$5.4	62.6$\pm$5.1

MODEL APPLICATIONS

After a model has been validated, it is ready to be used to extract physiological or biochemical information from the tracer kinetic data. The positron labelled tracer can be introduced to the subject and the radioactivity in tissue measured as a function of time by a positron CT scanner. The input function can be obtained from blood samples at various times after the tracer introduction as described above. By curve fitting these data with the model, estimates of the rate of the processes under study can be obtained. However, due to the limitation of positron CT scanners that only a few sections of an organ can be measured at a time, only a limited fraction of an organ can be studied at a time. Also, due to practical limitations, it may not be possible to carry out the study with the subject in the positron CT scanner continuously during the whole experimental period. Therefore, in practical application of the model, some adaptations are needed to make the procedure more convenient to apply and more comfortable for the subject. Especially if the procedure is going to be used clinically, not only does the convenience of the study need to be considered, but the data processing time for the parameter estimation should be minimized. Nonlinear regression with iterative methods is not the fastest in terms of computation. Efficient operational equations that are computationally fast and can provide good estimates of the physiological or biochemical information would be very desirable.

Even if the problems mentioned above are not critical for some situations, guidelines for selecting various variables (e.g., the length of the study) in the study procedure are needed to optimize the signal to noise ratio to give the most reliable results possible. In fact, all the problems mentioned above are interrelated and need to be considered at the same time. Because the overall problem involves selecting an optimal study procedure under some specific constraints, the problem is very much like experimental design in statistics. In order to solve this problem, one needs to understand first the characteristics of the model with respect to the various procedural variables. Sensitivity analysis is a general technique to provide this information. A full discussion of the technique can be found elsewhere(78,79,80). Basically, by examining the magnitude of the effect in the model response or in the operational equation that is due to a small change of a variable parameter, one can assess the significance or the expected accuracy of the parameter in the estimation process. Its use for guiding the study procedure to give an improved accuracy in the extracted information will be illustrated below with examples after a brief discussion of operational equations.

Operational Equations and Sensitivity Analysis

As mentioned earlier, iterative nonlinear regression for parameter estimation is not very fast. For positron CT, which involves a large volume of data for each single study, this could mean very long data processing (i.e., many hours or longer). Such long data processing times would hinder the use of a model in an environment that has daily positron CT studies. The development of equations that can calculate the estimates in a single step is essential for the application of the model. This can be illustrated by the operational equations for the calculation of blood flows using ^{15}O water.

Because of its inertness and its fast diffusion into tissue, ^{15}O water has been used for measurement of blood flows. There are a few different approaches, but all are based on the same single compartment model that Kety(13) had used many years ago. The approach that is used at UCLA is to collect the dynamics of the tracer delivery and clearance to determine the flow and the distribution volume of water simultaneously(81). Ordinarily, one would need to perform the CT image reconstruction for each temporal sampling point. The radioactivities at all temporal sampling points for each image pixel define the tracer dynamics for the corresponding tissue element. The model can then be used to fit these data to give estimates of flow and distribution volume. However, if the model equation is reformulated(81), the values of flow and distribution volume can be solved in terms of the time integrals of the decay corrected (with superscript *) and non-decay corrected activities(Q^* and Q), as

$$F = \frac{\lambda \int Q^* \, dt \int Q \, dt - Q^*(T) \int Q \, dt}{\int C_i \, dt \int Q^* \, dt - \int Q \, dt \int C_i^* \, dt}, \tag{11}$$

$$V = \frac{\lambda \int Q^* \, dt - Q^*(T)}{\lambda \int C_i^* \, dt - Q^*(T) \int C_i \, dt / \int Q \, dt}. \tag{12}$$

where C_i^* and C_i are decay corrected and non-decay corrected activities in the arterial blood. These operational equations not only eliminate the time consuming procedure of curve fitting but also reduce the number of CT image reconstructions required. The reason for the latter is that the time integrals of the activity can be obtained by CT reconstruction of the time integral of the projection measurements(81,82). Therefore, the data processing for the application of the model is incorporated directly into the image reconstruction of positron CT, thus greatly enhancing the usefulness of the model(81). Figure 10 shows an example of the reconstructed images of cerebral blood flow and mean transit time using these operational equations.

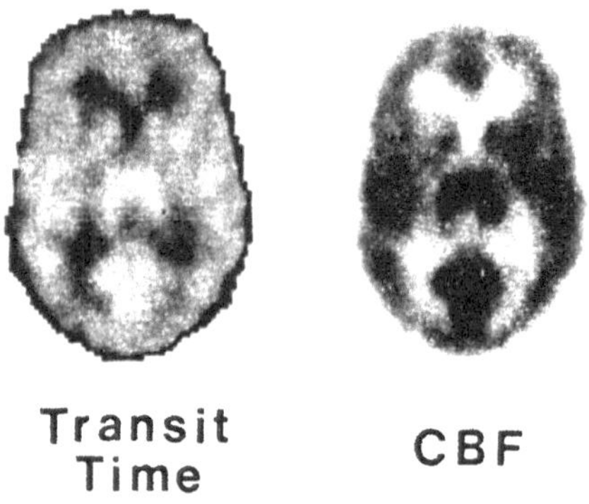

FIG. 10

Images of mean transit time and blood flow in a brain cross section(OM+4 cm) of normal subject. Intravenous bolus injection of ^{15}O-water was used and positron CT data were collected for 10 minutes after tracer administration. Operational equations 11 and 12 were used to generate images of flow and distribution volume(not shown) and image of transit time was obtained by the ratio of volume and flow images according to the central volume principle(Eq. 1).

The calculation of glucose utilization rate based on the FDG model is another example that demonstrates the usefulness of operational equations (19,20,21). Instead of using the full dynamics of FDG in tissue for estimating the glucose utilization rate, the operational equation formulates the calculation in terms of the FDG level in tissue at a single time. This approach is possible because the end product of the reaction sequence (FDG-6-PO_4) accumulates in the tissue with only a small dephosphorylation rate. In this case, not only is the data processing time much reduced, but the study procedure also becomes simpler and allows the whole organ to be studied with a single injection of FDG.

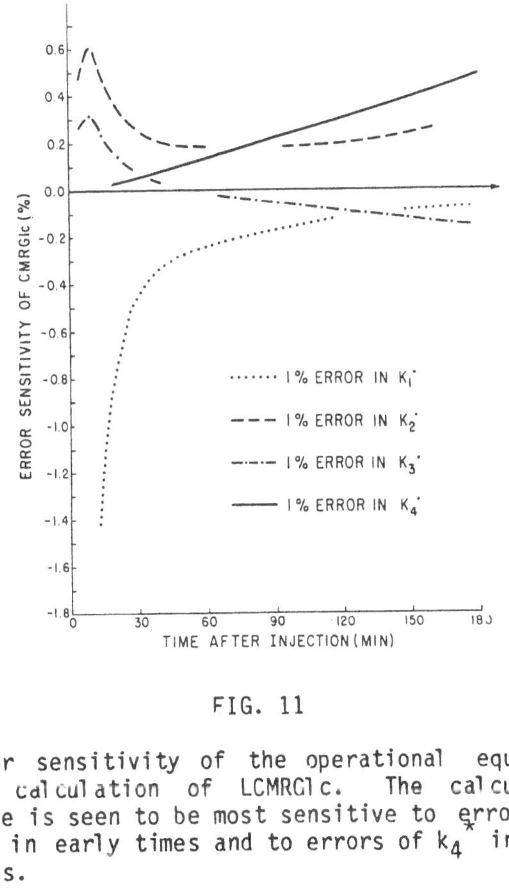

FIG. 11

Error sensitivity of the operational equation for calculation of LCMRGlc. The calculated value is seen to be most sensitive to errors of k_1^* in early times and to errors of k_4^* in late times.

In the above examples, the accuracy or reliability of the estimates obtained by the operational equations has not been discussed. An inaccurate estimate that can be calculated quickly will not be very useful. Fortunately, the accuracy or reliability can usually be improved by adjusting the time of measurement, the length of the study, or the shape of the input function which can be easily controlled. This is best illustrated by the analysis of the operational equation of the FDG method.

To avoid the use of the full dynamic measurements of radioactivity, the operational equation of the FDG method requires a "typical set" of values for the transport and reaction rate constants. For a particular study, the actual values are not likely to be equal to the values in the typical set. This discrepancy will introduce error in the calculations(20,83,84).

To understand this error, sensitivities of the operational equation with respect to each of the rate constants can be computed(20) and are shown in Figure 11. Also, if the range of variation of the rate constants are known, the expected overall error can be calculated(20,83) as shown in Figure 12. From this result, it is clear that if measurements with the positron CT scanner are taken at a time between 40 to 120 minutes after FDG injection, the expected error due to the use of the typical rate constants is the smallest (about 10 per cent). If the measurements are taken too early or too late, the potential error would be larger. Thus, through this analysis, the optimal time for the positron scans is determined and the expected accuracy of the calculated glucose utilization rate is known.

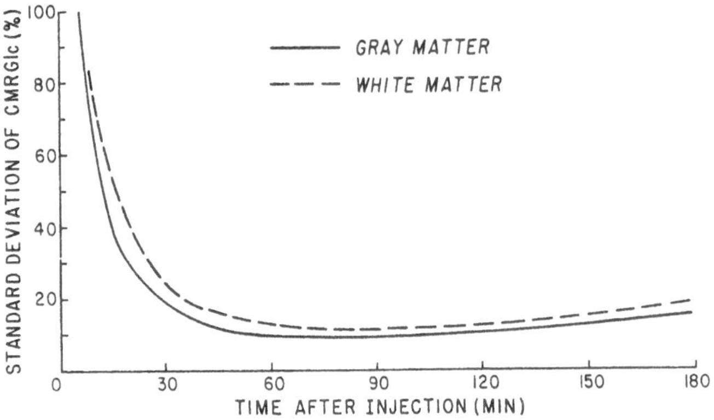

FIG. 12

Graph showing the expected error of the calculated LCMRGlc in gray and white matter of normal brain due to the use of a set of typical rate constants in the operational equation of the FDG method. The expected error is seen to be smallest when the tissue ^{18}F concentration is measured between 45 and 120 min.

If the sensitivity of an operational equation with respect to the measurements is calculated, the effect of the measurement error (i.e., statistical noise) can be evaluated. This effect usually is a function of other study parameters, and finding the minimum of this function with respect to these parameters can help in optimizing the signal to noise ratio of the operational equation. An example of such an analysis can be found in reference 64.

If the operational equation can not achieve the desired accuracy by adjusting the study variables, it will need to be reformulated. The results of the sensitivity analysis usually can provide some guides for the reformulation of a better operational equation. It is also likely that this formulation and evaluation process would go through a few iterations before a satisfactory operational equation can be obtained.

In the development of a practical study procedure, many other factors, like the radiation dose, the amount of computation and the convenience of the study procedure, all need to be considered. However, the accuracy of the operational equation will always be an important consideration. The sensitivity analysis can usually provide a basic framework for the design of a practical study procedure that can satisfy the overall objective.

AN INTERACTIVE MODELING ENVIRONMENT

Computer software is a necessity for the tracer kinetic modeler. A flexible, user-friendly system can provide substantial power in the design and verification of tracer kinetic models. The purpose of this section is to discuss the set of features necessary in computer software to produce a truly useful modeling tool. The subsequent section will describe BLD(85), a software system written by the authors, whose design is based upon these requirements.

Requirements of a Computer Modeling Tool

The specification of any computer software can be presented on two levels. The first level consists of a description of the available features - the modules or subroutines which perform the calculations and manipulations of interest. The second level is the packaging - the ease of its use, flexibility, transportability, etc. The requirements of a computer modeling software system will be discussed in this manner.

Essential Capabilities: The functional units required of modeling software are as follows:

Data entry, storage, and editing - A fundamental problem in the real world of data is the processing required to enter data into the computer, review the data for accuracy, and subsequently store it on magnetic media. In positron CT, some data, such as counts from a series of blood samples, may need to be entered manually, while other data may be extracted by image analysis programs directly onto disk. The modeling system should have very general facilities for data entry and storage. It should also give the user powerful features for data verification.

Capability for model definition - Most statistical packages require the definition of a model in terms of computer code, generally FORTRAN, to compute the terms of the differential equation or the analytical solution. A versatile modeling tool should provide this feature, but it should also have directly built-in a set of models which are in regular use. These should include an arbitrary sum of exponentials, arbitrary order polynomials, and multiple linear regression. A powerful feature is the capability to define a model system directly, without programming, using a model/function definition language. Such a language should resemble conventional mathematical notation as much as possible.

Model simulation - In order to study the behavior of a model under a variety of parameter values and input functions, the software should include the capability to perform numerical solutions to differential equations. The step size of the simulation should be variable, if necessary, and easily controllable. Initial conditions should also be easily modified. The model should be defineable in any of the forms mentioned above. Finally, there should be substantial power in the manipulation and display of the results.

Parameter estimation - The software requires the facility of linear and non-linear regression with the definition of the fitting function available in all of the above mentioned forms. There should be the capability to calculate sensitivity coefficients in a variety of ways, assign weights for weighted least squares(WLS), put constraints on the estimation, and limit the number of iterations. The routine should produce statistics including standard errors, F-test for significance of the fit, and R^2. Furthermore, the modeler should have flexibility in the examination of the residuals(the remaining deviations between data and the fitted curve).

Display and plotting capability - In order to examine data and analyze results, the software should provide means for both hard-copy and CRT production of plots. There should be sufficient flexibility to display entered data, simulated data, regression predictions, and residuals. For the hard copies, plots produce on a line printer are adequate, but the high resolution of electrostatic or pen plotters is far superior. Similarly for display, plots on a terminal screen are a poor substitute for a graphics display system.

User-friendly Features: The following features, when incorporated into a modeling system, turn a set of calculation facilities into a powerful tool for the modeler.

User orientation - The software should not require the user to have an extensive knowledge of the program. Brief, informative messages should be coordinated into a question and answer format. The system should be forgiving of the inevitable user errors and provide understandable error messages. Another useful feature is the capability to provide supplementary information to the user upon request, i.e. a help feature.

Power for the sophisticated user and ease of use for the novice - To be widely used, the software must be understandable to a novice computer user and modeler. Therefore reasonable defaults need to be applied, (e.g. the iteration limit for non-linear regression), and the number of questions should be kept to a minimum. However, the system must also provide the advanced modeler access to all the computation options mentioned previously, in a direct, interactive manner.

Flexibility - Many similar functions are required in different aspects of the modeling process, e.g. plotting is useful in data verification, simulation, and examination of regression residuals. The system should provide the user with flexible control of what functions can be carried out and in what order. This general-purpose feature will allow one modeling system to support the needs of many different projects.

Interactive and batch operation - An interactive environment is well suited to the process of physiological modeling. However, the system should have the capability to process a well defined sequence of operations with limited user interaction. For example, the modeler should not need to re-define a differential equation model from scratch at every terminal session. Ultimately, the modeling system could even be programmable.

Compatibility with mini-computer environment and portability - In the past few years, a large percentage of data handling has moved from the mainframe computer to the 16 bit mini. While a significant amount of statistical and modeling routines has been written, only some of these programs are available on smaller machines. Such a system needs to be modular in design to allow subroutine overlaying. Portability between systems is also a desirable trait in a software system. The program should be written in a readily available high level language, such as FORTRAN. ASCII format should be available for file input/ouput. All system dependent parameters and subroutines, particularly device dependent operations such as plotting, should be well isolated in the code.

BLD : A Software System for Data Handling and Model Analysis

A number of software packages have been written which handle some or all of the essential capabilities described above. These include commercially available statistical packages, such as BMD, SAS, and SPSS, software libraries such as IMSL, and more specialized modeling system, such as MLAB and NONLIN. Descriptions of additional software are available elsewhere (67,69). The BLD system, written by the authors, was designed and implemented to provide powerful modeling and statistical capabilities within a user-friendly environment.

BLD System Components: The BLD system is written entirely in FORTRAN and currently executes in our laboratory on a number of different DEC PDP 11 series computers. The name, BLD, originated from the use of the program to process time-activity curves of radioactive BLooD samples, and from the proclivity of computer operating systems to abbreviate. The system consists of two main divisions. First is an interpreter which acts on an internal workspace of variables constructed by the user. The second division, the bulk of the package, is the set of independent utilities which act on any subset of this data. Modules are available to handle all of the essential function capabilities of a modeling system, as described above.

The interpreter - This routine provides the user with a free-format language consisting of standard arithmetic operators, vector and matrix operations, and a set of built-in functions for logarithms, trigonometry, and random number generation. The interpreter can act as an online calculator as well as performing arbitrary mathematical transformations on inputted data, such as applying a scalar calibration to a curve, or performing decay correction. Model definition may be performed with the interpreter, either as an explicit function, or as a system of differential equations. The interpreter is loosely based on the APL programming language, but with only the essential operators, and without the need for a specialized keyboard. It uses a parallel mode of operation, i.e. a command need only be interpreted once to operate on an entire vector or matrix of data, thus the interpreter is quite efficient. Using the multi-tasking capability of the operating system, the interpreter can also pass data back and forth to user-written external programs. This provides a modeler with programming skill the ability to evaluate specialized functions (such as power series expansions) and decrease computation time by direct coding.

The utilities - A central module selector allows the BLD user to choose any utility in any order to operate on a current set of "selected" variables. Input/output modules allow data movement in ASCII or binary format to or from any device on the system. All terminal input is completely free-format, and these modules allow comment data to remain associated with the numeric data. A simple-minded pointwise data editor allows review and modification of data. Data entry and editing can also be performed with more power in the interpreter, but without the question and answer mode. Data may be plotted on a DEANZA image display system, or graphed on a GOULD electrostatic plotter. All display-related operations take place via a set of device-specific subroutines. The hard copy plotting module supplies the user with complete power in plot specification, but with default values suitable for standard X-Y plotting. Plotting is performed through a set of CALCOMP compatible subroutines running in background mode.

BLD performs numerical solutions of differential equations using a fourth order Runge-Kutta algorithm (71). The equations may be defined directly in the interpreter's language, or indirectly by an external program. The step size and initial conditions are easily controlled. Parameter estimation can be performed through linear, polynomial, and non-linear regresion modules. There are two built-in non-linear regression functions: a sum of exponentials, and the FDG compartment model (20,21). Fitting can also take place using a model defined through the interpreter. The non-linear regression algorithm of BLD is Gauss-Newton with step halving. The user can define a limit on the number of iterations and the extent of step halving, specify the technique by which the sensitivity coefficients are computed, and to define a vector of observation weights for weighted least squares. All regression routines produce a statistical summary and store the parameter estimates and their standard errors so as to be available through the interpreter. The user also has the ability to monitor visually the convergence of the regression, iteratively, on the graphics display system. Upon convergence, residuals are available for display and analysis. Other specialized calculation utilities available in BLD include

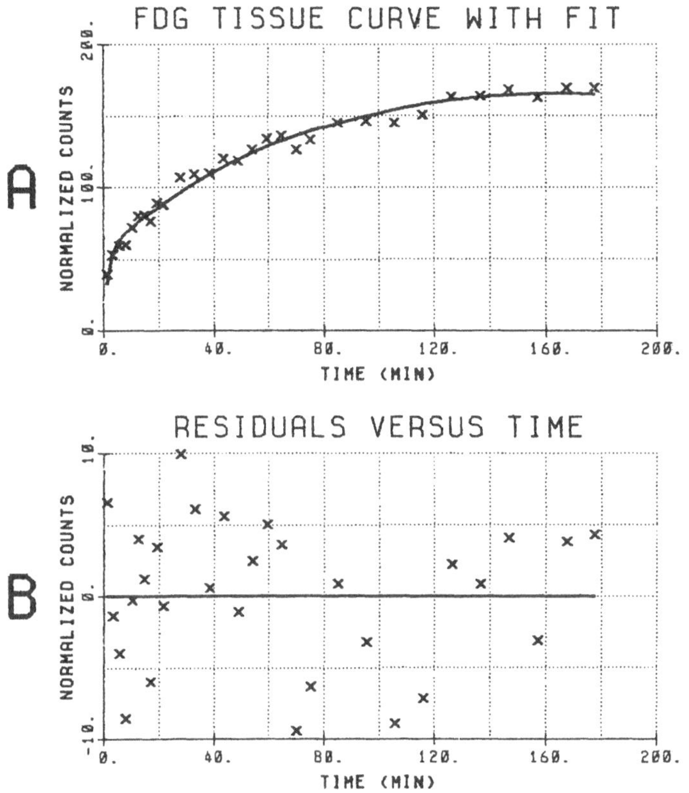

FIG. 13

Example of the parameter estimation procedure for FDG rate constants using the BLD program. A. Plot of FDG tissue activity (x) and fitted curve from the model (solid line). Sample points are measured from a region of interest in the left posterior temporal cortex (OM+5) from sequential FDG brain images collected by the NeuroECAT over 3 hours. The model calculation is based on the time-activity curve of FDG in plasma as measured by blood samples counted in a well counter. The parameter estimates (and standard errors) are k_1=.082 (.011), k_2=.194 (.050), k_3=.067 (.010), and k_4=.0055 (.0007). The standard error of the model's predicted value is 5.367 and R^2=.983. B. A residual plot depicting the difference between the measured data and the fitted values from A. The residuals appear to be randomly distributed about zero and to have constant variance over time. Note the change in plotting scale from A to B.

numerical integration of a sampled curve, cubic spline generation (86), and radioactive decay correction.

Miscellaneous features - BLD supports a generalized command file language, i.e. at any input request the user may specify the name of a file containing BLD responses. This file can request data from the user, perform conditional and un-conditional branching, and substitute values of internal variables into replies. In this manner, BLD "programs" can be written. This language is well suited to the complicated environment of a computer dedicated to physiological data handling and model analysis. Other useful features of BLD include the ability to save an entire workspace, i.e. all data and function definitions, to return to at a later time; substantial help information which is available at any terminal input request; and the capability to issue system commands, such as directory listings, while remaining in the BLD environment.

Experience and Performance: The BLD system has been in operation for three years, and is currently used regularly by modelers, programmers, physicists, chemists, engineers, physicians, and technicians. This system has integrated most of the data processing in the laboratory not directly related to image processing, and has dramatically reduced the need for new FORTRAN programming. BLD command files have been written for analysis of variance, stepwise linear regression, scanner calibration calculation, image histogram generation, detector resolution calculation, and cardiac scan segmental analysis, to name a few. Tracer kinetic models for measurement of local blood flow (using ^{15}O H_2O) glucose metabolism (^{18}F-FDG), oxygen metabolism (^{15}O-O_2), protein synthesis (^{11}C-leucine), fatty acid oxidation and esterification(^{11}C-palmitate), membrane permeability and receptor binding have all been formulated and studied using BLD. Figure 13 shows the typical results obtained in curve fitting a set of experimental kinetic data with the workable model of FDG (Figure 9). Both the fitting and the residuals are readily available for on-line inspection to assess the fitting between the model and the experimental data. The parameter values estimated from the curve fitting are always provided with the standard errors of the estimates, so the reliability of the estimated values can also be assessed. The BLD system has proven to be a powerful interactive facility for efficient data handling and model analysis. Its versatility has allowed it to go far beyond its original expectations.

SUMMARY

Modeling is a general technique of incorporating a priori knowledge to help extract useful and reliable information from observations. Using incorrect models is equivalent to giving wrong a priori information and leads to incorrect conclusions from acquired data. Also, cumbersome models can not be used conveniently. Therefore, modeling must be performed with care to be useful. In this chapter, the characteristics of modeling in tracer kinetics have been discussed, especially in the special environment of positron CT. The general procedures useful for the development and validation of models have been described and examples given to illustrate the basic procedural steps. Sensitivity analysis and the development of operational equations that are essential for the successful application of tracer kinetic models have also been discussed. The procedures involved in tracer kinetic modeling require a large effort of computer simulations, curve fittings, animal/chemical experiments, and mathematical analysis, in addition to the tracer kinetic experiments. Frequently, some of these procedures need to be repeated a number of times before a satisfactory result is obtained. Fortunately, many of these efforts can be accomplished with the use of a computer. An interactive computing environment that has been demonstrated to facilitate tracer kinetic modeling has also been described. This system is not simply an input/output processor. Rather it is an interactive tool which enhances the experimenter's ability to explore the mathematical descriptions of biological processes through the principles of tracer and competitive enzyme kinetics.

ACKNOWLEDGEMENTS

The authors appreciate the supports by DOE contract DE-AM03-76-SF-0012, NIH grant R01-GM-24839-01, USPH grant 515654-01, and donations form the Will's Foundation, Houston, Texas; Fritts Family Foundation, Bakersfield, California; the Hereditary Disease Foundation, Los Angeles, California; and Jennifer Jones/Simon Foundation, Los Angeles, California.

REFERENCES

1. Stewart GN, Researches on the circulation time and on influences which affect it, J. Physiology, 22:159-183, 1897

2. Hamilton WF, Moore JW, Kinsman JM, Spurling RG, Simultaneous determination of the pulmonary and systematic circulation times in man and of a figure related to the cardiac output, Am. J. Physiol. 84:338-344, 1928

3. Kety SS, Schmidt CF, The nitrous oxide method for the quantitative determination of cerebral blood flow in man: theory, procedure, and normal values, J. of Clin. Invest. 27:476-483, 1948

4. Von Hevesey G, Adventures in radioisotope research, In: The Collected Papers of G. Hevesey, Pergamon Press, London, 1962

5. Sheppard CW, Basic Principles of the Tracer Method, John Wiley, New York, 1962

6. Rescigno A, Segre G, Drug and Tracer Kinetics, Blaisdell, Waltham MA, 1966

7. Jacquez JA, Compartmental Analysis in Biology and Medicine, Amsterdam: Elsevier/North Holland, 1972

8. Shipley RA, Clark RE, Tracer Methods for In Vivo Kinetics, Academic Press, New York, 1972

9. Lassen NA, Pearl W, Tracer Kinetic Methods in Medical Physiology, Raven Press, New York, 1979

10. Phelps ME, Hoffman EJ, Mullani NA, Ter-Pogossian MM, Application of annihilation coincidence detection to transaxial reconstruction tomography. J. Nucl. Med. 16:210-224, 1975

11. Phelps ME, Positron computed tomography studies of cerebral glucose metabolism in man: theory and application in nuclear medicine, Semin. Nucl. Med. 11:32-49, 1981

12. Phelps ME, Mazziotta JC, Huang SC, Study of cerebral function with positron computed tomography, J. Cereb. Blood Flow Metabol. 2:113-162, 1982

13. Kety SS, The theory and applications of the exchange of inert gas at the lungs and tissues. Pharmacol. Rev. 3:1-41, 1951

14. Meier P, Zierler KL, On the theory of the indicator-ditution method for measurement of blood flow and volume, J. Appl. Physiol. 6:731-744, 1954

15. Stephenson JL, Theory of measurement of blood flow by dye dilution technique, IRE Trans. Medical Electronics, PGME-12:82-88, 1958

16. Zierler KL, Equations for measuring blood flow by external monitoring of radioisotopes, Circ. Res. 16:309-321, 1965

17. Bassingthwaighte JB, Ackerman FH, Mathematical linearity of circulatory transport, J. Appl. Physiol. 22:879-888, 1967

18. Carson ER, Jones EA, Use of kinetic analysis and mathematical modeling in the study of metabolic pathway in vivo, New Eng. J. of Med. 300:1016-1027, 1979

19. Sokoloff L, Reivich M, Kennedy C, Des Rosiers MH, Patlak CS, Pettigrew KD, Sakurada O, Shinohara M, The (^{14}C)-deoxyglucose method for the measurement of local cerebral glucose utilization: theory, procedure and normal values in the conscious and anesthetized albino rat. J. Neurochem. 28:897-916, 1977

20. Huang SC, Phelps ME, Hoffman EJ, Sideris K, Selin CJ, Kuhl DE, Non-invasive determination of local cerebral metabolic rate of glucose in man. Am. J. Physiol. 238:E69-E82, 1980

21. Phelps ME, Huang SC, Hoffman EJ, Selin C, Sokoloff L, Kuhl DE, Tomographic measurement of local cerebral glucose metabolic rate in humans with (F-18)2-fluoro-2-deoxy-D-glucose: validation of method. Ann. Neurol. 6:371-388, 1979

22. Phelps ME, Barrio JR, Huang SC, Keen R, MacDonald NS, Mazziotta JC, Smith C, Sokoloff L, The measurement of local cerebral protein synthesis in man with positron computed tomography and L-(1-^{11}C)Leucine, J. Nucl. Med. 23:p6, 1982

23. Barrio JR, Phelps ME, Huang SC, Keen RE, MacDonald NS, Smith C, Sokoloff L, Positron-emitting labeled L-amino acids for measurement of protein synthesis, Trans. Amer. Nucl. Soc. 41:17-18, 1982

24. Berman M, Schoenfeld R, Invariants in experimental data on linear kinetics and the formulation of models, J. Appl. Physiol. 27:1361-1370, 1956

25. Carson ER, Cobelli C, Finkelstein L, Modeling and identification of metabolic systems, Am. J. Physiol. 240:R120-R129, 1981

26. Welch TJC, Potchen EJ, Welch MJ, Fundamentals of the Tracer Method, Saunders, Philadelphia, 1972

27. Obrist WD, Thompson HK, Wang HS, Wilkinson WE, Regional cerebral blood flow estimated by ^{133}xenon inhalation, Stroke 6:245-256, 1975

28. Ter-Pogossian MM, Eichling J, Davis D, Welch M, Metzger J, Determination of regional cerebral blood flow by means of water labeled with radioactive oxygen-15, Radiology 93:31-40, 1969

29. Raichle ME, Larson KB, Phelps ME, Grubb RL Jr, Welch MJ, Ter-Pogossian MM, In vivo measurement of brain glucose transport and metabolism employing glucose-^{11}C. Am. J. Physiol. 228:1936-1948, 1975

30. Shepp LA, Logan BF, The Fourier reconstruction of a head section. IEEE Trans. Nucl. Sci. NS-21:21-43, 1974

31. Phelps ME, Emission computed tomography, Semin. Nucl. Med. 7:337-365, 1977

32. Hoffman EJ, Phelps ME, Huang SC, Kuhl DE, et al, A new tomograph for quantitative positron emission computed tomography of the brain. IEEE Trans Nucl. Sci. NS28:99-103, 1981

33. Bohm C, Eriksson L, Bergstrom M, Litton J, Sundman R, A computer assisted ring detector positron camera system for reconstruction tomography of the brain, IEEE Trans. Nucl. Sci. NS-25:624-637, 1978

34. Ter-Pogossian MM, Ficke DC, Hood JT, Yamamoto M, Mullani NA, PETT VI: a positron emission tomograph utilizing cesium fluoride scintillation detectors, J. Comput. Assist. Tomogr. 6:125-133, 1982

35. Derenzo SE, Budinger TF, Huesman RH, Cahoon JL, Vuletich T, Imaging properties of a positron tomograph with 280 BGO crystals, IEEE Trans. Nucl. Sci. NS-28:81-89, 1981

36. Brooks RA, Sank VM, DiChiro G, Friauf WS, Leighton SB, Design of a high resolution positron emission tomograph: the neuro-pet, J. Comput. Assist. Tomogr. 4:5-13, 1980

37. Phelps ME, Hoffman EJ, Huang SC, Kuhl DE, ECAT: A new computerized tomographic imaging system for positron-emitting radiopharmaceuticals. J. Nucl. Med. 19:625-647, 1978

38. Budinger TF, Derenzo SE, Gullberg GT, Greenberg WL, Huesman RG, Emission computer assisted tomography with single-photon and positron annihilation photon emitters. J. Comput. Assist. Tomogr. 1:131-145, 1977

39. Phelps ME, Huang SC, Hoffman EJ, Plummer D, Carson RE, An analysis of signal amplification using small detectors in positron emission tomography. J. Comput. Assist. Tomogr. 6:551-565, 1982

40. Webb JL, Enzyme and Metabolic Inhibitors, Vol. I, II, and III, Academic Press, New York, 1963

41. Barrio JR, Biochemical parameters in radiopharmaceutical design, In: Proceedings of the International symposium on Positron Emission Tomography of the Brain, Ed. WD Heiss, Springer-Verlag, New York, pp. 116-139, 1983

42. Reivich M, Kuhl D, Wolf A, Greenberg J, Phelps M, Ido T, Casella V, Hoffman E, Alavi A, Sokoloff, The F-18 fluorodeoxyglucose method for the measurement of local cerebral glucose utilization in man. Circ. Res. 44:127-137, 1979

43. Ido T, Wan CN, Casella V, Fowler JS, Wolf AP, Reivich M, Kuhl DE, Labeled 2-deoxy-D-glucose analogs: ^{18}F-labeled 2-deoxy-2-fluoro-D-glucose, 2-deoxy-2-fluoro-D-mannose, and ^{14}C-2-deoxy-2-fluoro-D-glucose, J. Label Compds. Radiopharm. 24:174-183, 1978

44. Gallagher BM, Fowler JS, Gutterson NI, MacGregor RR, Wan CN, Wolf AP, Metabolic trapping as a principle of radiopharmaceutical design: some factors responsible for the biodistribution of (F-18)-2-deoxy-2-fluoro-D-glucose. J. Nucl. Med. 19:1154-1161, 1978

45. Ratib O, Phelps ME, Huang SC, Henze E, Selin CE, Schelbert HR, Positron tomography with deoxyglucose for estimating local myocardial glucose metabolism. J. Nucl. Med. 23:577-586, 1982

46. Krivokapich J, Huang SC, Phelps ME, Barrio J, Watanbe C, Selin C, Shine K, Determination of myocardial metabolic rate for glucose from fluoro-18-deoxyglucose. Am. J. Physiol. 243:H884-H895, 1982

47. MacGregor RR, Fowler JS, Wolf AP, Shiue C-Y, Lade RE, Wan CN, A synthesis of ^{11}C-2-Deoxy-D-glucose for regional metabolic studies. J. Nucl. Med. 22:800-803, 1981

48. Oldendorf WH, Brain uptake of radiolabeled amino acids, amines, and hexoses after arterial injection. Am. J. Physiol. 221:1629-1639, 1971

49. McIlwain H, Bachelard HS, Biochemistry and the Central Nervous System, Willians and Wilkins, Baltimore, 1971

50. Schon HR, Schelbert HR, Robinson G, Najafi A, Huang SC, Hansen H, Barrio J, Kuhl DE, Phelps ME, C-11 labeled palmitic acid for the noninvasive evaluation of regional myocardial fatty acid metabolism with positron-computed tomography 1: kinetics of C-11 palmitic acid in normal myocardium. Am. Heart J. 103:532-547, 1982

51. Frost JJ, Pharmacokinetic aspects of the in vivo, noninvasive study of neuroreceptors in man, In:Receptor-Binding Radio Tracers, Vol II, Ed. WC Eckelman, CRC Press, Florida, 1982

52. Berman M, The formulation and testing of models. Ann. N. Y. Acad. Sci. 108:192-194, 1963

53. Renkin EM, Transport of potassium-42 from blood to tissue in isolated mammalian skeletal muscles. Am. J. Physiol. 197:1205-1210, 1959

54. Crone C, Permeability of capillaries in various organs as determined by use of the indicator diffusion method. Acta Physiol. Scan. 58:292-305, 1964

55. Phelps ME, Huang SC, Hoffman EJ, Selin C, Kuhl DE, Cerebral extraction of N-13 ammonia: its dependence on cerebral blood flow and capillary permeability-surface area product. Stroke 12:607-619, 1981

56. Yudilevich DL, Serial barrier to blood-tissue transport studied by the single injection indicator diffusion technique, In: Capillary Permeability, Ed. Crone C, Lassen NA, Academic Press, New York, pp.115-134, 1970

57. Brown AC, Passive and active transport, In: Physiology and Biophysics, Ed. Ruch TC and Patton HD, Saunders, Philadelphia, 1966

58. Woodbury JW, The cell membrane: ionic and potential gradients and active transport, In: Physiology and Biophysics, ed. Ruch TC and Patton HD, Saunders, Philadelphia, 1966

59. Koch A, The kidney, In: Physiology and Biophysics, ed. Ruch TC and Patton HD, Saunders, Philadelphia, 1966

60. Brown AC, Masoro EJ, Absorption from the gastrointestinal tract, In: Physiology and Biophysics, ed. Ruch TC and Patton HD, Saunders, Philadelphia, 1966

61. Mahler HR, Cordes EH, Biological Chemistry, Harper and Row, New York, 1966

62. Lund-Andersen H, Transport of glucose from blood to brain, Physiol. Rev. 59:305-352, 1979

63. Jones T, Chesler DA, Ter-Pogossian MM, The continuous inhalation of oxygen-15 for assessing regional oxygen extraction in the brain of man. Br. J. Radiol. 49:339-343, 1976

64. Huang SC, Phelps ME, Hoffman EJ, Kuhl DE, A theoretical study of quantitative flow measurements with constant infusion of short lived isotopes. Phys. Med. Biol. 24:1151-1161, 1979

65. Frackowiak RS, Lenzi GL, Jones T, Heather JD, Quantitative measurement of regional cerebral blood flow and oxygen metabolism in man using ^{15}O and positron emission tomography: theory, procedure and normal values. J. Comput. Assist. Tomogr. 4:727-736, 1980

66. Lammertsma AA, Jones T, Frackowiak FS, Lenzi GL, A theoretical study of the steady-state model for measuring regional cerebral blood flow and oxygen utilization using oxygen-15. J. Comput. Assist.Tomogr. 5:544-550, 1981

67. Beck, James V, Arnold, Kenneth, J, Parameter Estimation in Engineering and Science, John Wiley and Sons, New York, 1977.

68. Draper, NR, Smith, H, Applied Regression Analysis, John Wiley and Sons, Inc., New York, 1966.

69. Bard, Yonathan, Nonlinear Parameter Estimation, Academic Press, New York, 1974.

70. Jennrich, RJ, Ralston, ML, Fitting nonlinear models to data, Ann. Rev. Biophys. Bioeng., 8:195-238, 1979.

71. Gear, CW, Numerical Initial Value Problems in Ordinary Differential Equations, Prentice-Hall, Englewood Cliffs, NJ, 1971.

72. Jennrich, RI, Bright, PB, Fitting systems of linear differential equations using computer generated exact derivatives, Technometrics, 18:385-392, 1976.

73. Box, GEP, Kanemasu, H, Topics in model building, part II, On non-linear least squares, Tech. Rep. No. 321, University of Wisconsin, Dept. of Statistics, Madison, Wis., Nov., 1972.

74. Levenberg, Kenneth, A method for the solution of certain non-linear problems in least squares, Q. Appl. Math. 2:164-168, 1944.

75. Marquardt, Donald W, An algorithm for least squares estimation of nonlinear parameters, J. Soc. Indust. Appl. Math. 11:431-441, 1963.

76. Dixon, WJ, Massey, FJ, Introduction to Statistical Analysis, McGraw-Hill, New York, 1969.

77. Phelps ME, Hoffman EJ, Selin C, Huang SC, Kuhl DE, Investigation of (F-18)2-fluoro-2-deoxyglucose for the measurement of myocardial glucose metabolism. J. Nucl. Med. 19.1311-1319, 1978

78. Huang SC, Phelps ME, Hoffman EJ, Kuhl DE, Sensitivity analysis in physiological modeling, Proceedings of 2nd International conference in Mathematical Modeling, pp.883-892, 1980

79. Tomovic R, Vukobratovic M, General Sensitivity Theory, Elsevier, New York, 1972

80. Cruz JB(Ed), System Sensitivity Analysis, Dowden, Hutchinson and Ross, Stroudsburg, Pennsylvania, 1973

81. Huang SC, Carson RE, Phelps ME, Measurement of local cerebral blood flow and distribution volume with short-lived isotopes: a general input technique. J. Cereb. Blood Flow Metabol. 2:99-108, 1982

82. Tsui E, Budinger TF, Transverse section imaging of mean clearance time. Phys. Med. Biol. 23:644-653, 1978

83. Huang SC, Phelps ME, Hoffman EJ, Kuhl DE, Error sensitivity analysis of fluorodeoxyglucose method for measurement of cerebral metabolic rate of glucose. J. Cereb. Blood Flow Metabol. 1:391-401, 1981

84. Hawkins R, Phelps ME, Huang SC, Kuhl DE, Effect of ischemia on quantification of local cerebral glucose metabolic rate in man. J. Cereb. Blood Flow metabol. 1:37-52, 1981

85. Carson RE, Huang SC, Phelps ME, BLD: a software system for physiological data handling and model analysis. Proceedings of the Fifth Annual Symposium on Computer Applications in Medical Care. 562-565, 1981

86. Huang, SC, Phelps, ME, Hoffman, EJ, Kuhl, DE, Cubic splines for filter design in CT, IEEE Trans. Nucl. Sci. NS-27:1368-1374, 1980.

87. Klein MS, Goldstein RA, Welch MJ et al, External assessment of myocardial metabolism with [^{11}C] palmitate in rabbit hearts. Am. J. Physiol. 237:H51-H57, 1979

88. Reivich M, Alavi A, Wolf AP. Greenberg JH, Fowler JS, Christman DR, MacGregor R, Jones SC, London J, Shiue C-Y, Yonekura Y, The use of 2-Deoxy-D-[1-^{11}C]-Glucose for the determination of local cerebral glucose metabolism in humans: variation within and between subjects. J. Cereb. Blood Flow Metabol. 2:307-319, 1982

PHARMACOKINETIC MODELS AND POSITRON EMISSION TOMOGRAPHY: STUDIES OF PHYSIOLOGIC AND PATHOPHYSIOLOGIC CONDITIONS

Martin Reivich and Abass Alavi

University of Pennsylvania, Philadelphia, PA

INTRODUCTION

Because of the structurally and functionally heterogeneous nature of the brain, it is necessary to measure changes in physiologic and biochemical parameters in the human brain on a regional basis. Such information is important in furthering our understanding of the normal function of the brain and the derangements that occur in various pathologic conditions. The development of the Kety-Schmidt technique for the quantitative measurement of cerebral blood flow in man, made it possible to determine the average rates of glucose and oxygen utilization and blood flow in the brain as a whole (1). Using these same principles a method to measure hemispheric changes in these parameters has been developed (2). Regional methods for the determination of cerebral blood flow using diffusable tracers have also been developed (3-5). These methods, however, do not provide 3-dimensional resolution by which it is possible to determine the physiologic and metabolic parameters in specific structural and functional subunits of the brain. With the development of the ^{18}F-fluorodeoxyglucose technique it became possible to do this in terms of glucose metabolism in the human brain (6). The ability to detect alterations in local cerebral glucose metabolism in humans has become a valuable tool in advancing our understanding of brain function in various physiologic and pathologic states.

METHODOLOGY

Local Glucose Consumption

The ^{18}F-FDG technique is based on the (^{14}C)-2-deoxyglucose [(^{14}C)-DG] method for measuring LCMRgl autoradiographically in animals (7). In this method (^{14}C)-DG is used as a tracer for the exchange of glucose between plasma and brain and its phosphorylation by hexokinase in the tissues. This analogue of glucose is used because the labeled product, (^{14}C)-deoxyglucose-6-phosphate, is essentially trapped in the tissue over the time course of the measurement. Deoxyglucose has been shown to enter cells rapidly (8) to be phosphoralated by brain hexokinase (9) and not to be further metabolized (9-12). Deoxyglucose-6-phosphate is not a substrate for either phosphohexose isomerase or glucose-6-phosphate dehydrogenase (9). It is transported from the blood into the brain by the same saturable carrier that transports glucose (11-13). The activity of glucose-6-phosphatase, an enzyme that might be expected to hydrolyze deoxyglucose-6-phosphate, is reported to be very low in mammalian brain (14-16). Because of the low levels of phosphatase activity in the brain, its effect can be neglected for studies performed over a period of 50 minutes. The effect of phosphatase activity, however, can be taken into consideration if required in a particular instance (17).

A model was designed based on the assumptions of a steady state for glucose consumption, a first-order equilibration of the free (^{14}C)-DG pool in the tissue with the plasma level, and relative rates of phosphorylation of (^{14}C)-DG and glucose determined by their relative concentrations in the precursor pools and their respective kinetic constants for the hexokinase reaction (7).

In order to use this model to quantify the rate of local cerebral glucose utilization, the following assumptions in addition to those above are required: (1) the local region is homogeneous with respect to blood flow, rates of transport of glucose and (^{14}C)-DG between plasma and tissue, and rates of phosphorylation of glucose and (^{14}C)-DG; (2) these rates and the plasma glucose concentrations are constant during the period of measurement; (3) the (^{14}C)-DG and glucose are present in a single compartment in each homogeneous local region; (4) the (^{14}C)-DG and (^{14}C)-DG-6-P are present in trace amounts; and (5) the arterial plasma concentrations of glucose and (^{14}C)-DG are approximately equal to their capillary plasma concentrations. Since the cerebral extraction ratios of glucose and (^{14}C)-DG are normally about 10%, the mean capillary plasma concentrations are fairly well approximated by the arterial plasma concentrations. The operational equation for this model in terms of determinable variables (7) is:

$$R = \frac{C_T^*(T) - k_1^* e^{(k_2^*+k_1^*)T} \int_0^T C_p^* e^{(k_2^*+k_1^*)t}\, dt}{\left[\frac{\lambda \cdot V_{max}^* \cdot K_m}{\phi \cdot V_{max} \cdot K_m^*}\right] \left[\int_0^T (C_p^*/C_p)\, dt - e^{(k_2^*+k_1^*)T} \int_0^T (C_p^*/C_p) e^{(k_2^*+k_1^*)t}\, dt\right]} \quad (1)$$

where R = the calculated rate of glucose consumption per gram of tissue; C = the concentration of DG + DG-6-PO_4 in the tissue; C_p* and C_p = the arterial plasma concentrations of DG and glucose, respectively; k_1*, K_2*, k_3* are the rate constants for the transport from plasma to the tissue precursor pool, for the transport back from tissue to plasma and for the phosphorylation of DG in the tissue, respectively; λ = the ratio of the distribution volume of DG in the tissue to that of glucose; ϕ = the fraction of glucose that, once phosphorylated, continues down the glycolytic pathway; and K_m* and V_{max}* and K_m and V_{max} are the kinetic constants of hexokinase for DG and glucose, respectively. The latter six constants can be combined into one constant, which has been designated the lumped constant ($\lambda \cdot V_{max}^* \cdot K_m/\phi \cdot V_{max} \cdot K_m^*$). The lumped constant is essentially an isotope correction factor arising because of the use of an analogue of glucose instead of labeled glucose itself.

The extension of this method to man (6) requires the use of a tracer that satisfies the following criteria: (a) The tracer must be taken up by the brain at a rate proportional to that of glucose and its metabolic products must remain within the tissue in a known form, as is the case with DG. (b) The tracer must be labeled with a γ- emitting radionuclide which is chemically stable in vivo and which can be detected through the skull using emission tomography. (c) The radiation exposure resulting from the use of this tracer must be safe.

(^{18}F)-FDG is a labeled analogue to DG which satisfies these requirements. FDG, like DG, is a good substrate for yeast hexokinase (18). This was confirmed by in vitro incubation studies of (^{14}C)-fluorodeoxyglucose (6). The substitution of a fluorine atom for a hydrogen atom on the second carbon of the deoxyglucose molecule does not alter its metabolic fate significantly. (^{18}F)-FDG in a manner similar to (^{14}C)-DG is phosphorylated by hexokinase to 2-deoxy-2-fluoro-D-glucose-6-phosphate which is a relatively poor substrate for either glucose 6-phosphate-dehydrognease or phosphohexose isomerase (19-20). Although there is some evidence suggesting that fluorodeoxyglucose is a non-reversible inhibitor of glucose phosphorylation (21), this is not likely to cause a significant effect on glucose metabolism in the present method in which fluorodeoxyglucose is used in tracer amounts. Fluorine-18 decays by positron emission, upon annihilation produces two 511-keV photons and has a short half-life (110 minutes), thereby meeting the requirements for external detection and acceptable radiation dosimetry (6).

(^{18}F)-FDG was produced by the direct fluorination of 3,4,6-tri-*O*-acetyl-D-glucal with high specific activity (^{18}F)-fluorine to give (^{18}F)-3,4,6-tri-*O*-acetyl-2-deoxy-2-fluoro-D-glucopyranosyl fluoride, which was hydrolyzed to (^{18}F)-FDG (22). With the utilization of this agent for the first time it became possible to determine the regional metabolic rate for glucose in humans non-invasively (6).

In order to determine the regional metabolic rate for glucose, one must measure, as indicated in Eq. 1, the distribution of the ^{18}F-activity in the brain, the time course of arterial plasma ^{18}F-FDG and glucose concentrations and know the values of the rate constants and lumped constant for FDG in humans.

The 3-dimensional distribution of ^{18}F-activity in the brain is determined with a positron emission tomographic scanner. Such an instrument consists of an array of scintillation detectors positioned around the subject's head. The detectors are mounted on a gantry capable of rectilinear and/or rotatory motion. Collimation is achieved by measuring only positron annihilation radiation, by having each detector in coincidence with the detectors on the opposite side of the array. With translation and/or rotation of the gantry, the radioactivity in the brain tissue is measured from a number of angles. From the measured data, transverse sections through the brain are calculated using a filtered, back-projection reconstruction technique (23).

In addition to the determination of the distribution of brain ^{18}F-activity, knowledge of both the arterial blood plasma glucose and ^{18}F-FDG concentrations as a function of time following the intravenous administration of ^{18}F-FDG is required. In order to minimize the amount of free ^{18}F-FDG in the precursor pool, the ^{18}F-FDG is administered as a bolus and then 30 minutes are allowed to elapse before the brain distribution of ^{18}F-activity is determined. Thus, most of the ^{18}F-activity in the section scan is in the form of ^{18}F-FDG-6-P. Correction is made for the small amount of free ^{18}F-FDG present from knowledge of the arterial plasma ^{18}F-FDG time course and the turnover rate of the precursor pool.

It can be demonstrated (7) that the rate constants are mathematically related to the time course of the total concentrations of ^{18}F-activity in a region in the brain and the time course of the arterial plasma ^{18}F-FDG concentration by the following equation:

$$C_1^*(\tau) = k_1^* e^{-(k_2^*+k_3^*)\tau} \int_0^\tau C_p^* e^{(k_2^*+k_3^*)dt} + k_1^* k_3^* \int_0^\tau [e^{-(k_2^o+k_3^o)\tau} \int_0^t C_p^* e^{(k_2^*+k_3^*)dt}]dt \qquad (2)$$

where $C_1^*(\tau)$ equals the brain ^{18}F-activity at time τ . The other terms are as defined above.

Thus, by determining the brain and arterial plasma concentrations of ^{18}F as a function of time following the intravenous administration of a bolus of ^{18}F-FDG, it is possible to determine the values of k_1^*, k_2^*, k_3^* using an iterative least-squares fitting technique. The arterial plasma ^{18}F concentration is measured in blood samples obtained from the radial artery while the brain ^{18}F concentration time course is obtained by making repeated section scans at various times after ^{18}F-FDG administration. From these scans, the time course of ^{18}F activity in gray matter and white matter structures is determined. Using Eq. 2 and these arterial and brain tissue time course data, a best-fit of values for k_1^*, k_2^*, k_3^* for various gray and white matter structures are determined. This is done as follows: the plasma data are first fitted to an empirical exponential expression relating C_p to time. The paramters of this expression are calculated using a function minimization procedure (24). This explicit expression is then used to represent C_p^* in Eq. 2. The integration method of Gear (25) can be used to solve this differential equation, with the Fletcher-Powell (24) minimization procedure selecting the best-fit rate constant values. Table 1 contains the rate constants for various glucose analogues which have been determined by use of Eq. 2.

Table 1. Glucose analogue rate constants

Constant (min^{-1})	Deoxyglucose: Rat, Sokoloff et al (7), Gray Matter	Rat, Sokoloff et al (7), White Matter	Monkey, Kennedy et al (26), Gray Matter	Monkey, Kennedy et al (26), White Matter	Human, Reivich et al (27), Gray Matter	Human, Reivich et al (27), White Matter	Fluorodeoxyglucose: Human, Phelps et al (17), Gray Matter	Human, Phelps et al (17), White Matter
k_1^*	0.189 ±0.012	0.079 ±0.008	-	-	0.090 ±0.006	0.057 ±0.004	0.102 ±0.029	0.054 ±0.015
k_2^*	0.245 ±0.040	0.133 ±0.046	-	-	0.221 ±0.018	0.109 ±0.015	0.130 ±0.066	0.109 ±0.044
k_3^*	0.052 ±0.010	0.020 ±0.020	-	-	0.105 ±0.009	0.078 ±0.021	0.062 ±0.019	0.045 ±0.006
Half life of * precursor pool	2.38 ±0.40	4.51 ±0.90	2.00	4.81	2.37 ±0.20	3.29 ±0.40	4.25 ±1.78	5.30 ±2.49
Distribution Volume +	0.647 ±0.073	0.516 ±0.171	-	-	0.238 ±0.029	0.234 ±0.033	0.593 ±0.230	0.383 ±0.137

Values are means ± SE.
* $\ln 2/(k_2^* + k_3^*)$ (min)
\+ $k_1^*/(k_2^* + k_3^*)$ (ml/g)

It can be shown that following a step change in arterial plasma ^{18}F-FDG concentration the lumped constant is equal to the asymptotic value of the ratio of the extraction fractions of ^{18}F-FDG and glucose, multiplied by the ratio of the arterial blood to plasma-specific activities (7). The value of the lumped constant for ^{18}F-FDG in man has been obtained in a series of normal subjects in which a programmed infusion was used to produce a step change in arterial plasma ^{18}F-FDG concentration over a period of 50-60 minutes during which time arterial and cerebral venous blood samples were obtained and analysed for their ^{18}F-FDG and glucose concentrations. From these data the ratio of the cerebral extraction of ^{18}F-FDG and glucose can be calculated. The lumped constant has been determined in a series of normal subjects (28).

With this information it is possible to calculate the metabolic rate for glucose in any region of the brain with a resolution of 8 to 12 mm depending upon the resolution of PET scanner used. The above values for the rate constants and lumped constant have been determined for normal physiologic states. There is evidence in the literature that these parameters may be altered under some conditions (29,30,31). Therefore, caution must be exercised in applying these values in pathological states. The model is relatively insensitive to changes in the rate constants (32) but this is not true for the lumped constant.

More recently we have used ^{11}C-deoxyglucose as the tracer for the measurement of local cerebral glucose consumption (27). This tracer has the advantage that a repeat measurement can be made within a period of two hours due to the 20 minute half-life of the carbon-11. This allows a subject to serve as his own control and by reducing inter-subject variability allows smaller changes in regional glucose metabolism to be detected with confidence.

The coefficient of variation of LCMRgl for different gray matter structures varies from 20 to 26% (33). By performing two measurements in the same subject 2 hrs. apart the coefficient of variation of repeated measurements for these structures ranges from 5 to 9% (27). Thus, the reliability of the measurement can be increased by making a control and experimental measurement in the same subject over a brief time interval.

Local Blood Flow and Oxygen Consumption

A method has been developed for the quantitative measurement of regional cerebral blood flow and oxygen metabolism using ^{15}O and positron emission tomography (34-36). The continuous inhalation of ^{15}O in the form of $C^{15}O_2$ results in an equilibrium being attained when the continuous arrival of ^{15}O to the brain is balanced by its rate of washout and rate of radioactive decay. The ^{15}O in the brain is in the form of $H_2{}^{15}O$ which is produced in the lung when the ^{15}O is transferred from carbon dioxide to water. This reaction is catalized by carbonic-anhydrase (37). The following equation describes this equilibrium:

$$C_t = \frac{C_a \cdot F}{(F/pV) + \lambda} \qquad (3)$$

where C_t is the regional brain tissue $H_2{}^{15}O$ concentration and C_a is the arterial concentration of $H_2{}^{15}O$ when breathing $C^{15}O_2$, F is the blood flow through a region of volume V, p is the partition coefficient of water between brain and blood and λ is the radioactive decay constant for ^{15}O. C_a is determined by measuring the ^{15}O activity in arterial blood samples while C_t is obtained from the PET image. Rearranging Eq. 3 above and solving for cerebral blood flow yields the following equation:

$$CBF = {}^{F}/_{V} = \frac{\lambda}{C_a/C_t - 1/p} \qquad (4)$$

During the continuous inhalation of oxygen 15 labeled molecular oxygen the total activity in the brain at equilibrium is the sum of 3 components: a) oxygen-15 labeled water of metabolism produced in the tissues from molecular oxygen-15 extracted from the arterial blood, b) recirculating oxygen-15 labeled water of metabolism and c) oxygen-15 labeled molecular oxygen attached to hemoglobin in the vascular compartment. The volume of the vascular compartment can be considered negligible in relation to the total brain tissue volume and can, therefore, be neglected. During $^{15}O_2$ inhalation the total arterial oxygen concentration at equilibrium, C_a, is equal to the sum of the ^{15}O concentration in the form of water, C_{aw}, and the ^{15}O concentration in the form of hemoglobin-bound molecular oxygen, C_{ao}'. The brain ^{15}O activity at equilibrium C_t' is described by the following equation:

$$C_t' = \frac{F(C_{ao}' \; OER + C_{aw}')}{(F/pV) + \lambda} \qquad (5)$$

Dividing the cerebral activity obtained during $^{15}O_2$ inhalation, by that obtained during $C^{15}O_2$ inhalation and assuming that the ratio of water in the arterial whole blood to that in the plasma is the same during $^{15}O_2$ and $C^{15}O_2$ inhalation, we obtain an expression for oxygen extraction (OER).

$$OER = \frac{C_t'/C_t \cdot C_a/C_p' - C_a/C_p}{C_a'/C_p' - C_a/C_p} \qquad (6)$$

where subscription p' refer to arterial plasma.

Finally, the cerebral metabolic rate for oxygen ($CMRO_2$) can be calculated from the following equation: $CMRO_2$ = CBF x OER x arterial blood oxygen content.

Thus, CBF, OER and $CMRO_2$ can be calculated by measuring ^{15}O concentrations in brain slices during $C^{15}O_2$ and $^{15}O_2$ inhalation by positron emission tomography, by measuring arterial whole blood and plasma ^{15}O concentrations, and arterial oxygen content.

Normal values for CBF, $CMRO_2$ and OER in gray (temporal) and white (central) matter in a series of 14 normal subjects (3 female and 11 male) of average age 48 years (range 26-74) is shown in Table 2.

TABLE 2

	rCBF (ml/100ml/min)	$rCMRO_2$ (mlO_2/100ml/min)	rOER
Gray	65.3 ± 7.2	5.9 ± 0.59	0.49 ± 0.02
White	21.4 ± 1.9	1.8 ± 0.22	0.48 ± 0.04

(Values are mean ± S.D., from Frackowick, et al (34)).

Repeat measurements at intervals on the order of 30 minutes demonstrated a variation of less than 5% in all cases. Long term variability in these parameters was studied over a period of 4 to 6 months in 4 subjects. The mean changes for rCBF, $rCMRO_2$ and rOER in gray matter were +15.0(range -0.2 to +39.0 ml/100ml/min), 0.0(range -0.6 to +0.8 mlO_2/100ml/min), and -0.10(range -0.20 to +0.02) respectively.

Several difficulties with this method for measuring rCBF have been pointed out. The sensitivity of this blood flow technique to changes in flow at high flow rates, (i.e. greater than 80ml/100ml/min) is reduced (36,38-40). In addition, the model assumes 100% extraction of water which is assumed to be freely diffusible. At high flow rates studies have shown that the extraction is less than 100% (41-42). Another potential source of error is variation in the partition coefficient of water in various disease states.

A statistical study of the propagation of errors in the ^{15}O equilibrium method for measuring rCBF and $rCMRO_2$ has been performed using phantoms (43). The coefficient of variation (COV) in rCBF increases linearly being about 5.5% for a rCBF of 17ml/100ml/min and 16.5% for a rCBF of 114ml/100ml/min. The COV in rOER is 3 to 7% in the range of rOER's between 0.3 and 0.7. In a group of 17 normal subjects, mean COV's in rCBF and $rCMRO_2$ were 10 and 15%, respectively, in gray matter and 7 and 12% in white matter. These values compare very well with theorectical predictions (38-39).

PHYSIOLOGIC STUDIES

Visual Stimulation

The effect of visual hemifield stimulation on LCMRgl has been investigated in 10 normal male volunteers (44). Either the left (N = 4) or right (N = 6) visual hemifield was stimulated. The subject was instructed to fixate on a small light which was dimmed at random located at the center of a 46 cm diameter hemisphere positioned 70 cm from him. The luminance of the fixation stimulus was adjusted so as to be detectable only by foveal vision. Thus, the subject's hemifields could be defined relative to the hemisphere and stimulation could be limited to the desired hemifield. Subjects reported greater than 95% of the dimming events, indicating good visual fixation. One half of the hemisphere was painted black and the space around the painted side was darkened with black cloth to eliminate all visual input from that hemifield. The stimulus consisted of a well-illuminated, slowly moving, high-contrast black-and-white pattern of small lines at various orientations as well as abstract color images presented to one visual hemifield. The subjects wore earplugs.

This visual stimulus caused the visual cortex contralateral to the stimulated hemifield to become 8 $\pm$ 3.0% (mean $\pm$ standard deviation) more active than the ipsilateral visual cortex. This asymmetry was significant in comparison with the controls ($t(14) = 4.06$, $P < .01$), who showed a left-right asymmetry of only 0.5 $\pm$ 3.0%.

These data conform well to what is known about the visual system from human clinical, anatomical and electrophysiological data (45-50). It is known that each visual hemifield projects to the opposite calcarine cortex. The effect was clearly demonstrated in each subject.

In another study the effect of stimulation as well as deprivation on the visual system was examined (51). The visual stimulation was carried out at several levels of intensity. The first consisted of a bright, white light. The next was a two cycle per second alternating black and white checkerboard pattern. The third and most complex visual stimulation was produced by allowing the subjects to view an outdoor scene.

Stimulation with white light resulted in an increase in LCMRgl in the primary visual cortex (PVC) of the order of 12% and in the associative visual cortex (AVC) of 6%. The use of the alternating black and white checkerboard pattern resulted in a larger increase in metabolic activity in both the PVC and the AVC, 29 and 27%, respectively. When one eye checkerboard stimulation was compared to two eye stimulation, the one eye stimulation response was 37% less in the PVC and 18% less in the AVC. It is not clear why the decrease is substantially less than the expected 50% decline. The left to right ratios in LCMRgl for homologous regions of the visual cortex appear to be symmetric in unstimulated subjects as well as in one eye and two eye stimulation studies. These data confirm that half of the input to each human visual cortex comes from each eye.

When the subjects were stimulated by the outdoor scene the largest increase in metabolic rate was seen compared to eyes closed controls (average rise of 45% in PVC and 59% in AVC).

These investigators also studied patients with homonymous hemianopsia. In these subjects the visual cortex appeared to be anatomically normal on CT scans. Two clinically blind subjects were included in this series. Additionally, a man with visual auras and partial complex seizures was studied both intra- and interictally.

All patients with hemianopsia showed reduced LCMRgl in the visual cortex contralateral to the visual field defects. The average decline of LCMRgl with respect to the contralateral side was $32 \pm 7\%$ (in the PVC) and $44 \pm 6\%$ (in the AVC). In subjects who were visually stimulated the metabolic rates in the affected visual cortex showed no increase.

In one of the blind subjects, during stimulation with the alternating checkerboard pattern, the LCMRgl in the visual cortex was the same as in normal subjects with eyes closed. In the other blind subject, the checkerboard stimulation resulted in an increase of 13% in LCMRgl in the anterior portion of the PVC. This was attributed to retained scattered peripheral vision in one eye.

In the patient with visual aura the interictal study showed decreases in LCMRgl of 55% in the AVC and 47% in the PVC on the side of the EEG abnormality compared to the contralateral side. The LCMRgl in the AVC and PVC were significantly lower in this subject compared to the eyes closed controls. Also these values were lower than in the hemianoptic patients which may reflect functional damage of the visual cortex from the repeated seizure activity. Ictal study showed increased LCMRgl of 167 and 247% for the PVC and AVC respectively when compared to the contralateral side. The active area appeared to extend beyond the AVC to include the posterior temporal region. This metabolic activation site corresponded to the focal EEG abnormalities.

We have examined local cerebral glucose metabolism during visual stimulation in seven patients with various visual field defects due to vascular disease (52). The metabolic data were compared with Goldman perimetry and CT scans. These patients were stimulated with a full-field reversing pattern checkerboard presented on a hemisphere by rear projection with 3° check size at a 2 per second reversal rate. They all had had a sudden onset of their visual symptoms. In five patients with stable visual field defects perimetry demonstrated the following visual field abnormalities, all of which were congruous: (1) a right inferior quadrantanopsia without macular sparing; (2) a left superior quadrantanopsia without macular sparing; (3) a left inferior quadrantanopsia with macular sparing; (4) a right homonymous hemianopsia with macular sparing; and (5) a left homonymous hemianopsia with macular sparing. The lesion was complete in all patients except patient number 3. The CT scan revealed an appropriate lesion in only three of the five patients whereas the metabolic PET scan revealed marked asymmetry in the metabolic rate for glucose in the visual cortex in four of the five patients. These were the four patients with complete lesions. In the patient with the incomplete lesion the PET scan did not show such asymmetry.

These data demonstrate the ability of metabolic mapping to subdivide the occipital cortex into distinct regions. Within striate cortex, eight subdivisions were demarcated. These units comprise right or left hemisphere, superior or inferior calcarine bank and posterior (macular) and anterior (peripheral) visual cortex. Diminished metabolic activity in the thalamus, not suspected from clinical or CT data, was noted on two occasions. These metabolic changes in the thalamus may be related to the fact that the pulvinar is heavily interconnected with striate and extrastriate visual cortical areas (53-55). The large size of the macular representation, as evaluated in patients with macular sparing, is quiet striking on the metabolic scan.

Success of this pilot study in mapping stable lesions of the visual cortex led us to extend the investigation to an additional two patients with changing visual deficits. One patient was scanned close to the time of occipital infarction. The CT scan showed no lesion acutely. Metabolic scan at 96 h following onset disclosed grossly diminished glucose metabolism in the inferior calcarine bank, appropriate to the superior quadrant field defect. A second patient had regained perception of movement in an inferior quadrant field defect a month following onset. No defect appeared on the metabolic scan. These findings support the observation that metabolic scanning can reveal alterations of cortical function not detectable by CT scan and suggest that metabolic measurements may anticipate the course of visual recovery.

Auditory Stimulation

The auditory system has been studied by means of metabolic mapping by a number of investigators. In one study (44) the subjects listened to a tape recorded facutal story presented through earphones to only one ear. To reduce ambient noise both ears of the subject were covered by earphones housed in auditory enclosures which produced a 32-35 dB attenuation. Attentiveness to the story was assessed by testing the subject's recall at the end of the study. In addition, they were told that they would be paid in proportion to how much detail they could remember. These subjects were also blindfolded to reduce visual input during the study. The monaural auditory stimulation elevated the metabolic rate in the temporal cortex contralateral to the stimulated ear in each subject. This region had a metabolic rate 7 $\pm$ 2.5% higher than in the ipsilateral temporal cortex. This asymmetry was significant in comparison with control subjects ($p < .001$) who showed a left-right asymmetry of only 1 $\pm$ 2%. These data are consistent with studies in the literature suggesting the predominance of the crossed pathways in the human auditory system (56). These data are also in agreement with neurophysiologic studies in animals (57).

In another study (58) the cerebral metabolic response to a verbal auditory stimulus consisting of a factual story was studied in 4 subjects, 2 with left ear and 2 with right ear stimulation. Significant activation was seen in the left frontal cortex

(6+8%) and bilaterally in the posterior (left=11+7%, right=5.9+ 10.1%) and transverse (left=25+7%, right=17+19%) temporal cortices. A small but significant (6+ 14%) activation also occurred in the left thanamus. It was found that the cortical response to verbal stimulation was predominately left sided regardless of the ear stimulated. The tonal memory test and timbre test were also administered to a series of subjects (59). In the tonal memory test significant increases above hemispheric mean were found in right posterior superior (16+11.8%) and middle (27.3+5.8%) temporal cortices. Those subjects employing a nonanalytic strategy for remembering the sequence of tones had higher metabolic rates in the right frontal and parieto-temporal regions. In those subjects using an analytic approach, higher metabolic rates occurred in the left posterior superior temporal cortex. The metabolic changes observed were a function of the strategy employed rather than the side of stimulation. In the timbre test right greater than left asymmetries occurred in the frontal regions as well as diffusely in the posterior temporal and temporo-occipital junction. These changes were of the order of 5 to 13%. These results suggest that the metabolic responses to auditory stimuli are determined by the content of the stimulus and analysis strategy of the subject. Asymmetries were generally left greater than right for verbal, and right greater than left for non-verbal auditory stimuli. The stimuli used were complex and involved mulitple cognitive functions, making interpertation of specific cognitive processes difficult.

Tactile Stimulation

An investigation of the somatosensory system has been performed (44). The tactile stimulus consisted of rapid but light stroking (2 to 3Hz) of the volar and dorsal surface of the fingers and hand of one arm (left, N=2; right, N=3) with a hand-held brush, which was just stiff enough to cause an apprecialbe stimulus without causing any discomfort. Subjects were blindfolded to eliminate visual input and wore earplugs to minimize auditory input.

This somatosensory input caused the postcentral gyrus contralateral to the stimulus to become metabolically more active (9 $\pm$ 10.2%) than the homologous area in ipsilateral cortex. This was not significantly different from the controls (1+6.8%, t(9)=1.5, P>.1) due to the large variance in the control subjects at the level of the postcentral gyrus.

Little information is available concerning the function and anatomical organization of the somatic sensory cerebral cortices of humans (60-63). Localization of asymmetrical LCMRgl at 8 and 9 cm above the OM plane (OM+8 and OM+9), after vigorous unilateral brush stroking of the hand and fingers, is in agreement with topographical maps of the postcentral gyrus (60-63) as well as with other functional studies (64-65). Although more extensive areas than the postcentral gyrus were activated in these studies, more ventral portions of the postcentral gyrus (presumptive face and lip area) were not asymmetrically labeled.

Pilot studies in which light unilateral brush stroking of the face and lip was performed showed asymmetrical labeling in the parietal cortex at levels OM + 6 and OM + 7, with the contralateral cortex exhibiting higher glucose metabolism than the ipsilateral cortex.

Cognitive Activity

We have examined the effects of performance of cognitive tasks, verbal-analytic and spatial on LCMRgl in eight right-handed male subjects. Each task produced a specific pattern of lateralized metabolic activity. The subjects were randomly assigned to one of two stimulation conditions, with 4 subjects in each condition. Stimuli were either verbal analogies taken from the Miller Analogies Test (66) or spatial stimuli adapted from Benton's Line-Orientation Test (67), with lines made shorter and hence more difficult to solve.

Regions of interest (ROI) were defined on the PET images and rates of glucose metabolism were calculated in two primary target regions, the superior temporal (ST) and inferior parietal (IP) cortices, and in three adjacent control regions, the inferior temporal (IT), auditory (AUD) and visual association (VA) cortices. ST and IP were selected on the basis of clinical evidence implicating these regions in higher verbal-analytic functions in the left hemisphere (Wernicke's area) and spatial orientation functions in the right hemispheric homologues (68-70). In addition, metabolic rates were calculated for the frontal eye fields (FEF) and two adjacent control regions, the frontal pole (FP) and inferior frontal (IF) cortices. FEF was chosen due to evidence from conjugate lateral eye movement studies suggesting increased leftward orientation during cognition involving spatial tasks and increased rightward orientation for verbal tasks (71-74).

These data were examined by means of an analysis of variance. The two groups (verbal vs. spatial task) did not differ in overall metabolic rates ($F(1,6) = 1.17$, n.s.). However, there was significantly ($F(1,6) = 23.25$, $p < .01$) higher right-hemispheric metabolism across groups. The findings of increased overall right hemispheric metabolism during the performance of cognitive tasks is consistent with earlier findings in right-handed males (75). It may be due to right-hemispheric predominant involvement in attentional processes (76,77). There was also a significantly ($F(1,6) = 24.75$, $p = .0025$) different effect of the two tasks on hemispheric metabolism. The regions also differed significantly ($F(7,42) = 12.97$, $p < .001$) and a hemisphere - region interaction ($F(7,42) = 3.84$, $p < .005$) indicated variability in laterality of metabolic activity as a function of brain region.

To examine the task effects on laterality of metabolic rates in each region, laterality scores were calculated as $(R-L/R+L) \times 100$ where R and L are the metabolic rates in the region on the right and left respectively.

The two groups differed in laterality of metabolism in the two primary target regions ST ($p < .05$, 1-tailed) and IP($p < .001$ 1-tailed), with laterality scores being higher (greater right hemispheric metabolism) for the spatial compared to verbal task conditions. The two groups of subjects also differed in laterality scores for FEF ($p < .025$, 1-tailed) and the effect was in the same direction. The differences between the groups were not significant in any of the control regions.

The three regions in which the verbal and spatial tasks produced opposite lateralized effects on local metabolism were ST, IP and FEF. These regions had higher metabolism in the left for subjects performing the verbal task and higher metabolism in the right for subjects performing the spatial task. The effects in areas ST and IP are consistent with clinical evidence concerning the role of these regions in verbal-analytic and spatial cognitive processing. These results provide an experimental confirmation of a hypothesis generated by clinical observation.

Regarding the frontal eye fields, a hypothesis was suggested by Trevarthen (78) that in a functionally asymmetric brain "cognitive" or other internally generated activation will mimic the effects of lateralized sensory stimulation and produce a contralateral orienting response. This hypothesis has thus far been tested indirectly by correlating direction of lateral head and eye movements with type of cognitive stimulation (e.g. verbal and spatial) and the evidence in favor of the hypothesis (71-74) has been contested (79; but c.f. (80)). Our results for the FEF provide the first experimental demonstration that lateralized metabolic activity, produced by different types of cognitive tasks (verbal and spatial), also produces similarly lateralized metabolic activity in a motor region.

Vigilance

Basic hemispheric asymmetries have been revealed in vigilance capacity (81-85). These studies suggest a greater right hemispheric involvement in the capacity to maintain attentiveness to stimuli in a vigilance situation.

The unique role of the inferior parietal lobe in regulating sensory integration and attention in primates has been suggested by ablation studies (86,87) axonal tracing investigations (88,89) and single cell recordings (90,91). These studies indicate that the inferior parietal lobe mediates the integration of multimodal sensory information with internal drive states and has extensive connections with regions controlling motor orientation (88-91). Clinical data suggest that lesions in the right inferior parietal lobe are more likely to be associated with unilateral attentional neglect (88,89,92-95) and that the right hemisphere predominates in vigilance performance (96-97).

To test the hypothesis that this region would be preferentially activated during an attentional task we examined the data from 24 young (age 18-24) right-handed male volunteers. They were studied under one of two conditions. 1) Stimulated: visual (N=8) or auditory (N = 7) attentional tasks. 2) Unstimulated: no visual or auditory input (N = 9).

Subjects in the unstimulated conditions were fitted with blindfolds and ear plugs throughout the experimental procedure.

In the visual stimulation condition, a light emitting diode was placed in central fixation and the subject's task was to indicate changes in its intensity. Light dimming occurred at random with a mean interval of 30 sec. In the auditory stimulation condition a verbal discourse was presented in a language unfamiliar to the subjects (Hungarian), whose task was to indicate the occurrence of a prespecified word (vonat) embedded in the text. The word appeared randomly with a mean interval of 2 minutes. The subjects in both conditions responded by pressing a lever with both hands. Attentional performance was monitarily rewarded following the study.

Three regions of interest (ROI) were selected for quantification of local cerebral glucose metabolism. The inferior parietal lobe (IP) was the target ROI. The superior parietal lobe (SP) was selected as a control region because it contains adjacent sensory cortex (somatosensory assoication) that has not been implicated in lateralized attentional processing. The cerebellum (CR) served as a second control region because it is involved in sensory and motor aspects of the tasks but not in attentional functions (98-99).

Metabolic rates in each region were the dependent measures in a 2 (stimulated, unstimulated) x 2 (left, right) analysis of variance, with the first factor (Condition) testing between-group effects and second factor (Hemispheres) yielding within group comparisons. Stimulated subjects were included as one group since neither side nor modality of stimulation had significant effects on laterality of metabolism (both Fs $(1,13) < 1$). For IP, the significant effect was a Condition X Hemisphere interaction, $F (1,22) = 9.89$, $p < .005$. Metabolic rates in stimulated subjects were higher in the right IP ($p < .005$) whereas nonstimulated subjects did not show significant metabolic asymmetry in this region For SP, no effects reached statistical significance. For CR, there was a marginally significant main effect for Condition, $F (1,22) = 4.27$, $p = .051$, with stimulated subjects manifesting higher cerebellar metabolism.

The only region in which laterality of metabolism differed significantly between stimulated and unstimulated subjects was IP, ($t (22) = 3.85$, $p < .001$), reflecting relatively greater right metabolism in stimulated subjects.

Our findings indicate asymmetrically increased neuronal activity in the right IP of humans directing attention to external sensory stimulation. This asymmetry was independent of modality and side of stimulation. Since a major component of the difference between the stimulated subjects and controls was the requirement to attend to external stimulation, the results experimentally support the clinical evidence suggesting right parietal predominance in directed attention.

There is considerable evidence for right hemispheric predominance in spatial perceptual synthesis(100-104).The IP possesses a uniquely elaborate representation of the external sensory environment due, presumably, to the extensively processed sensory information it receives from multimodal sensory cortices (88-89). This raises the possibility that the very presence of sensory stimulation may contribute to the observed parietal asymmetry. Further research is necessary to determine the separate contributions of the attentional and perceptual components.

Anxiety

Observation of subjects undergoing positron emission scanning for measurement of local cerebral glucose metabolism suggested that many of these subjects are under considerable anxiety evidently produced by the arterial and venous catheterization, the injection of the isotope and the scanning itself.

In order to evaluate the effect of this inadvertently produced anxiety on LCMRgl we have administered Spielberger's State-Trait Anxiety Inventory (STAI) to a group of 18 right-handed males with no left-handed first degree relatives. The STAI was administered immediately following catheterization and again after the LCMRgl measurement was completed.

Data from brain stimulation, psychosurgery and measurement of electrocortical activity suggest a major involvement of the fronto-cortical regions in the regulation of anxiety and negative affect. These data are consistent with anatomical findings suggesting that the limbic system has major projections to the posterior fronto-orbital and to the middle frontal regions (105).

Metabolic rates were calculated for homotopic regions in the two cerebral hemispheres that contain the primary cortical projections of the limbic system i.e. the posterior fronto-orbital and the middle frontal regions. When these rates were evaluated as a function of trait-anxiety and state-anxiety, the scatter plot suggested a curvilinear relationship between anxiety and fronto-cortical metabolic rates. Indeed, a quadratic function fit the data for state-anxiety significantly better than a linear function ($F\ (15,16) = 11.05\ p < .001$). A cubic function did not significantly improve this fit in comparison to the quadratic function. Thus, it appears that metabolic rates in these regions increase as a function of anxiety up to a point, after which greater anxiety is associated with decreased metabolic activity. This pattern was not observed in control regions not hypothesized to include significant limbic projections.

In order to evaluate the data as they bear on a hypothesized right-hemispheric involvement in negative affect, the subjects were divided by the median anxiety score into High-Anxious and Low-Anxious groups and an analysis of variance was performed. The two groups did not differ in overall metabolic rates ($F\ (1, 16)<1$) but the interaction between anxiety and metabolic rates in the two hemispheres was significant ($F\ (1,16) = 6.64$, $p = 0.21$). This interaction indicates that the high-anxiety group had higher metabolic rates in the right relative to the left hemisphere to a significantly greater extent than the low-anxiety group.

These findings underscore the role of the frontal projections of the limbic system in mediating anxiety and support the hypothesis of greater right hemispheric involvement in high anxiety states.

PATHOPHYSIOLOGIC STUDIES

Stroke

Metabolic and blood flow studies in patients with cerebrovascular disease have been performed using positron emission tomography. In one report ten patients with clinical evidence of completed stroke were studied (106). A majority of these patients had evidence of thrombotic or embolic infarctions in the distribution of the middle cerebral artery. In each patient paired $^{13}NH_3$ and (^{18}F)-FDG scans were performed.

In acute infarcts $^{13}NH_3$ uptake was very low during the first two days. Only during the first two weeks was the uptake of this radiopharmaceutical increased in the infarct margins. This is probably due to local reactive hyperaemia. In three patients who demonstrated an hyperaemic pattern with $^{13}NH_3$, pertechnetate flow studies confirmed this finding. $^{13}NH_3$ uptake was significantly decreased in chronic infarcts that measured larger than 2 cm on the CT scan.

There was uncoupling of glucose and $^{13}NH_3$ uptake within the infarct in the first two weeks after stroke. The gluocse utilization was less impaired than the perfusion in this early period, possibly due to transient enhancement of anaerobic glycolysis (107, 108, 109). It has been shown in animals that cerebral glucose utilization is increased immediately after the onset of hypoxia but little is known concerning LCMRgl within the infarct in the first few days after stroke in human beings (110-111). In animal experiments marked uptake of (^{14}C)-DG has been shown in discrete areas immediately after an ischaemic insult. Ginsberg et al. (107) found enhanced glucose consumption 90 minutes after focal ischaemia in cats in a rim surrounding an area of markedly decreased glucose utilization. In another investigation significantly increased glucose metabolism was seen in subcortical white matter 10 minutes following a diffuse ischaemic insult to the rat brain (108).

In chronic stable infarcts in man metabolism and perfusion were coupled (106). The areas seen as permanent infarcts on the CT scan had local cerebral metabolic rates 62% below normal.

Both the (^{18}F)-FDG and $^{13}NH_3$ scans consistently demonstrated hypofunctional zones in remote cerebral cortex, striatum and thalamus that appeared structurally normal on the CT scans. $^{13}NH_3$ appeared to be a less sensitive indicator of this decreased function than (^{18}F)-FDG. This may be due to a non-linear response of $^{13}NH_3$ trapping in response to changes in LCBF.

These studies indicate that PET may be quiet useful in defining the location and extent of disordered function following stroke. The findings on the scan may also aid in early identification of tissue with potential for recovery and in the estimation of surviving tissue in the chronic state.

Changes in rCBF and $rCMRO_2$ in patients with strokes have also been studied using positron emission tomography (112). In the region of the infarct $rCMRO_2$ was found to be reduced. In the first two weeks after the infarct, patients with a good final clinical outcome had a $rCMRO_2$ in the infarcted region that never fell below 40% of the contralateral value. The maxium depression in $CMRO_2$ occurred between 5 and 7 days following the stroke. The pattern of rCBF changes was found to be less predictable due to the development of luxury perfusion. This phenomenon was observed mainly between the 6 and 21 day after infarction. In the first two weeks after stroke an absolute decrease of rCBF below 20ml/100ml/min seemed to correlate with a poor clinical outcome. In the first two weeks, rOER is decreased indicating an uncoupling between flow and metabolism. Thereafter, rOER tended to return toward normal but remained in general lower in patients with a poor clinical outcome and a larger area of infarction. In the tissue bordering the infarct the depression of oxygen consumption and rCBF was not as marked as in the lesion itself.

A decrease in oxygen metabolism and flow was detected in the homologous contralateral cerebral region. This was present in the first 2 weeks in about 1/3 of the cases. Oxygen consumption and flow were 70% or less than the values in the adjacent regions.

Cerebral hemisphere infarcts produced a parallel decrease in $rCMRO_2$ and rCBF in the contralateral cerebellar hemisphere of 16% and 19% respectively in the early phase of the infarction. This increased in the stablized phase of the stroke to 25% for $rCMRO_2$ and 27% for rCBF. There was no correlation between the degree of crossed cerebellar diaschisis and the general clinical outcome of the patients. When the infarct predominately involved the parietal lobe the crossed cerebellar diaschisis was 50% greater than in cases where the lesion effected anterior regions only.

Crossed cerebellar diaschisis was first noted with PET studies of LCBF and $LCMRO_2$ by Barron et al (113). They found the phenomenon to be significantly correlated with the presence of hemiparesis. It was not observed later than 2 months after the ischemic insult.

We have noted abnormal glucose metabolism in the cerebellum in studies of unilateral supratentorial lesions using positron emission tomography (114). Nine patients with acute ischemia of the anterior circulation, 2 with initially presenting astrocytoma, and 8 normal controls were studied. Local metabolic rates for glucose were calculated in the cerebellum, and these data were used to express a left-to-right metabolic ratio for the cerebellar hemispheres (0.99 ± 0.05 in controls). Within the lesion group this ratio showed a significant asymmetry (10% or greater difference) in 5 cases (3 strokes, 2 tumors); in each case, the lower metabolic rate lay in the cerebellar hemisphere contralateral to the cerebral lesion ($p < 0.05$ by sign test). Although this ratio was not significantly asymmetrical in the other 6 patients with lesions, the lesser metabolism also lay contralateral to the cerebral lesion. When compared to control values, the lesion ratios showed significantly greater asymmetry ($p < 0.02$ by Mann-Whitney U test). A cerebellar abnormality tended to occur when the PET images showed widespread depression of cerebral metabolism. The presence of a cerebellar abnormality on PET did not appear to be influenced by either the degree of motor weakness or the presence of a cerebellar syndrome.

These data indicate that a mechanism exists whereby unilateral cerebral dysfunction may influence contralateral cerebellar metabolism, possibly by disruption of descending tracts that are destined to modulate activity in the cerebellum.

In a preliminary report of measurements of rCBF, $rCMRO_2$ and rCMRgl in two stroke patients the data suggested the presence of enhanced anaerobic glycolysis (115).

The combined utilization of the PET techniques for measuring LCBF, $LCMRO_2$ and LCMRgl should improve our understanding of the sequence of events following a stroke and its response to therapeutic intervention.

Seizures Disorders

It is well established that seizures (generalized and focal) are associated with increases in CBF and metabolism and both are decreased immediately after the ictus (116-119). Other investigators using the ^{14}C-DG autoradiographic technique have been able to demonstrate changes in glucose metabolism associated with penicillin-induced seizures in the rat and monkey (120-121). In man regional increases in CBF have been demonstrated by the ^{133}Xe CBF technique during the ictal state (117, 122-125). Kuhl et al studied 17 patients with partial epilepsy using ^{18}F-FDG and $^{13}NH_3$ with positron emission tomograph (126).

All patients underwent scalp EEG recording at the time of imaging. Recordings from sphenoidal and intracerebral depth electrodes were also made in some patients.

One very important factor should be taken into consideration in the interpretation of results obtained with the ^{18}F-FDG technique, which is applicable more to seizure disorders than to other less transient dysfunctions of the brian. If events are to be detected and quantified, they must occur simultaneously with tracer fixation. The majority of the ^{18}F-FDG is trapped in the tissue during the first 10 to 15 minutes after injection. Consequently, the method underestimates transient increases in metabolic rate that may be associated with neuronal activities of shorter duration.

Interictal Findings: ^{18}F-FDG scans obtained interictally were able to detect dysfunctional brain zones considered more likely to be responsible for seizures in patients with partial epilepsy. These areas usually appeared normal on the CT scan. In 12 of 15 patients who had focal or unilateral EEG abnormalities, broad regions of cortical hypometabolism and hypoperfusion were demonstrated on the PET scans. These areas corresponded well to the EEG lateralization and localizations. In five of six patients who underwent temporal lobectomy, the ^{18}F-FDG scan correctly detected the pathologically confirmed lesion as a hypometabolic region, and the surgical removal of the lesion resulted in marked clinical improvement.

Considering the nonlinear relationship between $^{13}NH_3$ trapping and flow (127), the data demonstrated coupling of LCMRgl and LCBF within the zone of dysfunction. There are reports both in favor of and against these findings. Some investigators have shown decreased LCBF in the interictal state by the ^{133}Xe techniques (117, 123) and others have found increases in regional perfusion (122,125). No patient was noted to have increased local perfusion in the interictal state by means of the PET measurements. In four patients who underwent repeated interictal studies no change in distribution and magnitude of relative perfusion and metabolism was found. This was interpreted to indicate permanent brain damage undetectable by CT rather than transient supressed function alone. This is supported by the loss of neurons, impairment in local circulation and glial cell proliferation found in experimental epileptic foci (128). In addition, biochemical studies in the regions of an epileptic focus have shown impaired energy metabolism (129). It is not certain yet whether the local hypofunction in these cases represents structural damage alone or a combined effect including neuronal inhibition during the interictal period (130).

In this study only five of 17 epileptic patients had abnormalities seen on the CT scans. All were atrophic abnormalities. In only three patients did the atrophic lesions seen on the CT scan coincide with both EEG and PET localization. In the other two patients, while the abnormalities on the EEG and PET were shown in the temporal lobe, the CT atrophy was seen in the frontal region. In both patients the presence of a lesion in the anterior temporal lobe was confirmed after temporal lobectomy.

Ictal Findings: When studied during an active seizure, the metabolism and perfusion in the cortical epileptic focus were found to increase to about twice normal. These same areas were hypometabolic and hypoperfused in the interictal state. It has been shown that in humans during seizure activity, increased neuronal metabolism is accompanied by a rise in regional CBF (130-133). Increases in CBF of 2 to 10 times normal in the epileptic focus during spontaneous seizures in humans have been recorded (117,122,123). Also, a corresponding rise in the metabolic rates using the Kety-Schmidt technique has been shown in the whole brain (131,133). The PET techniques indicate that both metabolism and perfusion are coupled during partial seizures. In one patient decreases in both metabolism and perfusion in the area surrounding the seizure focus were noted. These depressed values were attributed to "surround inhibition", which has been defined electrophysiologically for the penicillin-induced focus (130).

In approximately 20% of patients with partial epilepsy who are uncontrolled by medication, additional information is usually required (other than clinical evaluation, surface EEG recording, and CT scan) if surgery is being contemplated (134-137). Depth electrodes, although valuable in these patients, may not be successful in localizing the primary epileptogenic focus in every patient (134,135,137). The PET can be used in the assessment of local cerebral function complementary to EEG findings and with better spatial resolution. The data from the PET scan are especially useful when EEG abnormalities are bilateral or confusing. For example, the scan may help distinguish a frontal site of origin from a temporal site in those instances when it is difficult to differentiate on EEG a primary temporal lobe onset from a secondary onset propagated at a site distant from the recording electrode (138-139). With the scan a more exact localization of the site of seizure can also be accomplished. It is conceivable that with a combination of a surface EEG and an interictal ^{18}F-FDG scan, the need for depth electrode studies will be obviated in patients for whom surgery is planned.

Aging and Dementia

Studies of the effect of aging on cerebral circulation and metabolism started very soon after the introduction of the nitrous oxide technique by Kety and Schmidt (1). It was shown that patients with senile dementia had markedly reduced CBF and $CMRO_2$ compared with young men (140). Later it was found that all types of dementia led to reductions in CBF and $CMRO_2$ (141,142). In one study the effects of normal aging on CBF, $CMRO_2$ and cerebral glucose utilization were determined (143). No significant difference in CBF and $CMRO_2$ was found between the young controls and normal old subjects. However, a significant difference was found between these two groups and patients with Alzheimer's disease. On the other hand, cerebral glucose consumption was significantly lower in normal old subjects than normal young controls, and lower in demented patients than in the elderly normal subjects. In other words, there occurs a dissociation between $CMRO_2$ and glucose utilization with aging. This dissociation is even more pronounced in patients with dementia. It may be partly related to the use of substrates other than glucose (e.g. ketone bodies) in the aging brain (144).

Following the introduction of the intracarotid ^{85}Kr and ^{133}Xe techniques to measure CBF, it became possible to measure local cerebral function although with poor resolution in man (3,4). Obrist et al (145) found an overall reduction in CBF in senile dementia with greater decline in prefrontal and anterior temporal regions. Similar work by Ingvar and Gustafson (146) and Simard et al (147) extended this work and confirmed these findings. The latter investigators found a good correlation between the rCBF pattern and clinical symptomatology, as well as with the autopsy findings. These studies showed a decrease in mean hemispheric blood flow grossly proportional to the intellectual decline (148). They also noted a relationship between the memory disturbance and the reduction of flow in the temporal region (149). Agnosia and confusion correlated with a drop in flow to temporo-occipito-parietal regions (146, 148). Patients with expressive aphasias showed low flows in regions related to Wernicke's and Broca's areas (150).

The use of noninvasive rCBF techniques (5, 151), either by inhalation or intravenous administration of ^{133}Xe, has permitted the measurement of regional flow on a routine basis. With this technique, Obrist et al (5) and Wang and Busse (152) have shown a significant difference between the normal elderly group and young controls. They also demonstrated significant flow reductions in demented patients compared with a normal age-matched group. Using Obrist's technique, Baer et al (153) and Levy et al (154) have shown a decline in CBF with aging and a further reduction with both presenile and senile dementias. These investigators speculated that similar underlying morphological changes may be responsible for the decrease in CBF in both groups with more dramatic alteration in patients with dementia.

We have recently determined the effects of aging and dementia on cerebral glucose metabolism using the ^{18}F-FDG technique(155-156). In this study we examined nine young normal male volunteers (mean age, 22; range 19 to 26) and 12 elderly subjects. The normal young controls were free of mental and physical disorders. The elderly subjects were evaluated by a battery of psychometric tests (Guild Memory Scale and WAIS vocabulary subtest) and were categorized as being either elderly normal or having senile dementia. Based on the psychological testing, each subject was assigned a Global Deterioration Scale (GDS) rating of 1 to 7 as follows: 1 = normal, 2 = very mild, 3 = mild, 4 = moderate, 5 = moderately severe, 6 = severe, 7 = very severe. There were four elderly normal subjects (mean age, 72; range 60 to 86) and eight patients with dementia (mean age 72; range 64 to 78) in this group.

The mean rates of glucose consumption for various areas of the brain were determined in all three groups. In the young subjects the metabolic rates ranged from 4.1mg/100g/min (frontal cortex) to 14.2mg/100g/min (visual cortex). The metabolic rates ranged from 3.1mg/100g/min (frontal cortex) to 6.9mg/100g/min (visual cortex) in elderly controls and from 2.1mg/100g/min (frontal cortex) to 6.3mg/100g/min (visual cortex) in patients with senile dementia. The mean cortical value (average metabolic rates for frontal, auditory and visual cortices) was 6.5 ± 2.9mg/100g/min for the young controls, 4.8 ± 1.0mg/100g/min in the elderly control, and 3.7 ± 0.9mg/100g/min in the demented patients. There was a significant difference between the mean cortical values obtained in young controls and patients with dementia ($p < 0.05$). However, no significant difference in metabolic rates was found between this group and old controls or between old controls and patients with dementia. In general the metabolic activity appeared symmetric in all three groups. No significant correlation was noted between the mean cortical metabolic rates and the Global Deterioration Scale rating as determined by psychometric studies in either elderly controls or patients with dementia. No attempt was made to correlate the regional metabolic rates with a specific psychometric measurement.

Recently Kuhl et al studied the effects of aging on LCMRgl in 40 normal subjects aged 18-78 years (157). On the average, at age 78, mean LCMRgl was 26% less than at age 18. This is of the same order as the variance among subjects at any age. Their data indicated that the gradual decline of mean LCMRgl with aging occurred at a faster rate than was reported for cerebral oxygen utilization. This was attributed to increasingly altered pathways for glucose utilization, or to increasing utilization of ketone bodies or alternate substrates. Glucose utilization in the hemispheres was symmetrical in every age group. However, the ratio of metabolic rates of the superior frontal cortex to superior parietal cortex declined with age, possibly due to selective degeneration of the superior frontal cortex or differences in response to sensory and cognitive input between the young and the aged.

Frackowiak et al have studied aging (34) and dementia (158-159)using the ^{15}O equilibrium technique. These authors report a progressive fall with age of both CBF and $CMRO_2$.

A much greater decline of $CMRO_2$ and CBF was demonstrated in the demented patients over a period of 6 months. The declines were approximately 30% for both variables. The couple between flow and metabolism remained intact. There was a progressive coupled fall in blood flow and oxygen consumption with increase in severity of dementia. Both the vascular (multi-infarct) and degenerative (Alzheimer) dementia groups showed this coupled depression of flow and oxygen consumption of approximately equal severity. There was no significant elevation of OER in either group thus providing no evidence for ongoing ischemia in the vascular patients.

The parietal $CMRO_2$ was most markedly depressed in early dementia of both the degenerative and vascular types and in severe vascular dementia. The severe degenerative group showed a marked depression of frontal $CMRO_2$, this agrees with the known pattern of pathological damage in Alzheimer's disease. These focal abnormalities occur in the context of a general reduction in $CMRO_2$ in all areas in both vascular and degenerative dementia.

Recently, another group has attempted to measure the parameters governing brain protein synthesis in normal aging and in patients with senile dementia (160). These investigators used ^{11}C L-methionine as an indicator of protein synthesis. This amino acid shares with many other neutral amino acids the same facilitated transfer system through the blood-brain barrier. Most of this tracer is rapidly incorporated into proteins after its penetration into the brain and only a negligible amount of this substance follows the transmethylation pathway. A three-compartment linear model (cerebral blood pool, brain free methionine, and protein incorporated methionine) was used for curve fitting and calculation of the following parameters: methionine input and output, brain free methionine half-life, protein incorporation, brain free methionine concentration, methionine volume of distribution, single pass extraction and equilibrium extraction. Brain activity curves were corrected for blood and skull radioactivity. This approach was used in four aged normal subjects and nine patients with differing stages of senile dementia. In dementia the methionine brain input and the protein incorporation were decreased as compared with normals of the same age group. An increase in the biologic half-life of brain free methionine was also observed in these patients. On the basis of these preliminary data the investigators propose the use of this technique in the diagnosis and understanding of the pathophysiology of dementia and other disorders that may include impaired amino acid metabolism.

Schizophrenia

Farkas et al (161) studied a patient with a diagnosis of schizophrenia according to Research Diagnosis criteria who had never been treated with psychoactive medication. A PET scan using ^{18}F-FDG revealed a 39% depression in LCMRgl in the frontal lobe. When the subject was on perphenazine medication, LCMRgl rose to 76% of normal, whereas after withdrawal of this medication, LCMRgl returned to the depressed level observed prior to drug therapy. In 13 patients with schizophrenia studied by this group a uniform depression of frontal lobe metabolic activity has been noted (Farkas, unpublished data).

Similarly, Buchsbaum et al (162, 163) have noted that patients with schizophrenia have lower metabolic activity (using ^{18}F-FDG) in the frontal cortex compared to age matched controls. In the normal subjects the LCMRgl in the frontal cortex was 12.5% higher than the average for the whole slice, whereas, in the patients with schizophrenia it was only 6.4% higher. This difference between the two groups was significant ($t = 2.40$, $p < .05$). In the schizophrenic patients LCMRgl in the left central gray matter area (mainly caudate) was 6% lower than the average for the whole slice while in the control subjects it was 3% higher. The relatively reduced metabolic activity in the frontal regions in these patients may be related to the reduced motor output and lack of goal-directed behavior that are characteristic of schizophrenia (164).

The reduced metabolism in the left central gray matter may be related to evidence implicating the basal ganglia in the generation of both perceptual-cognitive and motor-behavioral symptoms in schizophrenia (165, 166). The low central gray matter metabolism is also of interest in view of the reports of increased dopamine receptors in the caudate nucleus in schizophrenia (167-169).

Brain Tumor

DiChiro et al (170, 171) have reported the use of ^{18}F-FDG imaging in the evaluation of cerebral gliomas. These authors have shown a positive correlation between the ^{18}F-FDG activity as measured by PET and the histologic grade of the gliomas. The metabolic activities for high-grade tumors generally were significantly higher than for low-grade tumors. Since the value for the lumped constant in these tumors is not known, absolute quantification of LCMRgl was not possible. Therefore, they have used the terms "hot" and "cold" to indicate the relative metabolic activity of these lesions. High-grade gliomas appear to be "hot" and low-grade tumors appear to be "cold" on these images. These authors have studied glucose utilization in cultured human glioma cells and found values similar to measured metabolic rates in tumors in vivo by the ^{18}F-FDG technique. They indicate that the ^{18}F-FDG technique may be of help in the early detection and recognition of recurrence and changes in the growth rate of brain tumors.

Recently Patronas et al (172) reported their data using ^{18}F-FDG and PET in five patients who had undergone radiation therapy for cerebral tumors. All five cases had similar clinical and CT findings. In contrast the ^{18}F-FDG scan was able to distinguish radiation necrosis in two patients from recurrent tumor in the remaining three cases. The metabolic rates in the brain were elevated in patients with recurrent tumor and markedly reduced in those with radiation necrosis. The accuracy of the diagnoses was confirmed by either biopsy or autopsy.

Lammertsma et al (173) made measurements of $LCMRO_2$ and LCBF in a series of eight patients with brain tumors. A decrease in LCBF in gray matter was found in both the affected and contralateral hemispheres. LCBF in the solid part of the tumors was comparable to white matter values. A relative uncoupling between LCBF and $LCMRO_2$ was observed in all tumors as indicated by a decreased rOER. The reduced OER suggests that the solid tumor tissue has a sufficient blood flow to match a low oxygen demand or that the tumor cells have significant anaerobic glycolysis to match a limited blood supply. Since tumors are thought to contain significant numbers of hypoxic cells (174) the latter may be the more correct interpretation.

Huntington's Disease

Kuhl et al (175, 176) have studied 13 patients with Huntington's Disease ranging in age from 28 to 71 with a duration of their disease of 1 to 15 years. The ^{18}F-FDG studies were correlated with the findings on the CT scans and clinical presentations. Although the severity of choreoathetosis and dementia correlated well with the duration of the illness, no correlation was noted between these manifestations and global or regional glucose utilization. The most severely demented patients had marked cortical and central atrophy, but some patients with the worst atrophy had the least dementia. Not all patients had caudate atrophy; when present, striatal atrophy was greater in those with longer duration of the disorder.

A decrease in glucose utilization in the caudate and putamen was observed which appeared early and preceeded bulk tissue loss. In this study a caudate metabolic index was used as it was difficult to measure LCMRgl in the hypometabolic caudate nuclei of Huntington's patients. This index will be elevated from normal by caudate hypometabolism but also by any abnormal increase in inter-caudate distance caused by caudate atrophy or by ventricular dilatation. Glucose utilization was normal throughout the rest of the brain regardless of the severity of symptoms and in spite of apparent shrinkage of brain tissue. In contrast to the ventricular CT index, mean LCMRgl did not correlate with the severity of symptoms. In asymptomatic patients at risk for Huntington's Disease the data suggests the possibility that the caudate may be hypometabolic in some of these patients.

The finding of a nearly normal cortical metabolic rate in demented Huntington's patients is in agreement with both clinical and biochemical data suggesting that the primary dementing process in this disease may be subcortical (177). In Huntington's Disease there is a normal cortical level of choline acetyltransferase, the marker enzyme for cholinergic neurons (178), whereas this enzyme is decreased in Alzheimer's Disease (179).

REFERENCES

1. Kety, SS, Schmidt, CF: The nitrous oxide method for the quantitative determination of cerebral blood flow in man: Theory, procedure and normal values. J Clin Invest 27:476-483, 1948.

2. Meyer, JS, Shinohara, Y: A method for measuring cerebral hemispehric blood flow and metabolism. Stroke 1:419-431, 1970.

3. Lassen NA, Ingvar DH: Regional cerebral blood flow measurement in man. Arch Neurol 9:615-622, 1963.

4. Lassen NA, Ingvar DH: The blood flow in the cerebral cortex determined by radioactive krypton-85. Experientia 17:42, 1961.

5. Obrist WD, Thompson HK, Wang HS, Wilkinson WE: Regional cerebral blood flow estimated by ^{133}Xe inhalation. Stroke 6: 245-256, 1975.

6. Reivich M, Kuhl D, Wolf A, Greenberg G, Phelps M, Ido T, Casella, V, Fowler, J, Hoffman, E, Alavi, A, Som, P and Sokoloff, L: The (^{18}F) Fluorodeoxyglucose method for the measurement of local cerebral glucose utilization in man. Circ Res 44:127-137, 1979.

7. Sokoloff L, Reivich M, Kennedy C, DesRosiers MH, Patlak CS, Pettigrew, KD, Kakurada, D, Shinohara, M: The (^{14}C) Deoxyglucose method for the measurement of local cerebral glucose utilization: Theory, procedure and normal values in the conscious and anesthetized albino rat. J Neurochem 28:897-916, 1977.

8. Wick AN, Drury DR, Morita TN: 2-Deoxyglucose-A metabolic block for glucose. Proc Soc Exp Biol Med 89:579-582, 1955

9. Sols A, Crane RK: Substrate specificity of brain hexokinase. J Biol Chem 210:581-595, 1954.

10. Tower DB: The effects of 2-deoxy-D-glucose on metabolism of slices of cerebral cortex incubated in vitro. J Neurochem 3: 185-205, 1958.

11. Bachelard HS: Specificity and kinetic properties of monosaccharide uptake into guinea pig cerebral cortex in vitro. J Neurochem 18:213-222, 1971.

12. Horton RW, Meldrun BS, Bachelard HS: Enzymic and cerebral metabolic effects of 2-deoxy-D-glucose. J Neurochem 21:507-520, 1973.

13. Bidder TG: Hexose translocation across the blood brain interface: Configurational aspects. J Neurochem 15:867-874, 1968.

14. Hers HG, DeDuve C: Le systéme hexose phosphatasique: Repartition de l'activité glucose-6-phosphatasique dans les tissus. Bull Soc Chim Biol 32:20-29, 1950.

15. Raggi F, Kronfeld DS, Kleiber M: Glucose-6-phosphatase activity in various sheep tissues. Proc Soc Exp Biol Med 105:485-486, 1960.

16. Prasannan KG, Subrahmanyan D: Effect of insulin on the synthesis of glycogen in cerebral cortical slices of alloxan diabetic rats. Endocrinology 82:1-6, 1968.

17. Phelps ME, Huang SC, Hoffman EJ, Selin C, Sokoloff, L, Kuhl DE: Tomographic measurement of local cerebral glucose metabolic rate in humans with (F18)2-fluoro-2-deoxy-D-glucose: Validation of method. Ann Neurol 6:371-388, 1979.

18. Bessell EM, Foster AB, Westwood JH: The use of deoxyfluoro-D-glucopyranoses and related compounds in a study of yeast hexokinase specificity. Biochem J 128:199-204, 1972.

19. Bessel EM, Courtenay VD, Foster AB, Jones M, Westwood JH: Some in vivo and in vitro antitumor effects of deoxygluoro-D-glucopyranoses. Eur J Cancer 9:463-470, 1973.

20. Gallagher BM, Fowler JS, Gutterson NJ, MacGregor RR, Wan CN and Wolf AP: Metabolic trapping as a principle of radiopharmaceutical design: some factors responsible for the biodistribution of (^{18}F)2-deoxy-2-fluoro-D-glucose. J Nucl Med 19: 1154-1161, 1978.

21. Coe EL: Inhibition of glycolysis in ascites tumor cells preincubated with 2-deoxy-2-fluoro-D-glucose. Biochem Biophys Acta 264:319-327, 1972.

22. Ido T, Wan CN, Casella V, Fowler JS, Wolf AP, Reivich M and Kuhl D: Labeled 2-deoxy-D-glucose analogs. ^{18}F-labeled 2-deoxy-2-fluoro-D-glucose, 2-deoxy-2-fluoro-D-mannose and ^{14}C-2-deoxy-2-fluoro-D-glucose. J Labeled Comp Radiopharmaceut 14:175-183, 1978.

23. Herman GT: Image Reconstruction from Projections: The Fundamentals of Computerized Tomography. New York, Academic Press. 1980.

24. Fletcher R, Powell MJD: A rapid descent method for minimization. Comp J 6:163-168, 1963

25. Gear CW: The automatic integration of ordinary differential equations. Comm Assoc Comput Mach 14:176-179, 1971.

26. Kennedy C, Sakurada O, Shinohara M, Jehle J, Sokoloff L: Local cerebral glucose utilization in the normal conscious macaque monkey. Ann Neurol 4:293-301, 1978.

27. Reivich M, Alavi A, Wolf A, Greenberg JH, Fowler J, Christman D, MacGregor R, Jones SC, London J, Shiue C and Yonekura Y: Use of 2-deoxy-D-(1-^{11}C) Glucose for the determination of local cerebral glucose metabolism in humans: variation within and between subjects. J CBF & Metab 2:307-319, 1982.

28. Greenberg J, Reivich M, Alavi A, Goldberg H: Evaluation of the lumped constant and the kinetic constants for fluorodeoxyglucose in man. Stroke 10:485, 1979.

29. Sunda S, Shinohara M, Miyaoka M, Kennedy C and Sokoloff L: Local cerebral glucose utilization in hypoglycemia. J Cereb Blood Flow Metab 1:Suppl. 1:S62, 1981.

30. Schuier F, Orzi F, Suda S, Kennedy C and Sokoloff L: The lumped constant for the (^{14}C) deoxyglucose method in hyperglycemic rats. J Cereb Blood Flow Metab 1:Suppl 1:S63, 1981.

31. Ginsberg MS and Reivich M: Use of the 2-deoxyglucose method of local cerebral glucose utilization with abnormal brain. Evaluation of the lumped constant during ischemia. Stroke 10:4-83, 1981.

32. Sokoloff L: Localization of Functional Activity in the Central Nervous System by Measurement of Glucose Utilization with Radioactive Deoxyglucose J of CBF and Metab 1:7-36, 1982.

33. Reivich M, Alavi A and Greenberg J: Unpublished observations.

34. Frackowiak RSJ, Lenzi GL, Jones T and Heather JD: Quantitative Measurement of Regional Cerebral Blood Flow and Oxygen Metabolism in Man Using ^{15}O and Positron Emission Tomography: Theory, Procedure and Normal Values. J of Computer Asst Tomograph 4:727, 1980.

35. Jones T, Chesler DA, Ter-Pogossian MM: The continuous inhalation of oxygen-15 for assessing regional oxygen extraction in the brain of man. Br J Radiol 49:339-343, 1976.

36. Subramanyan R, Alpert NM, Hoop B Jr, Brownell GL, Taveras JM: A model for regional cerebral oxygen distribution during continuous inhalation of $^{15}O_2$, $C^{15}O$ and $C^{15}O_2$. J Nucl Med 19:48-53, 1978.

37. West JB, Dollery CT: Uptake of oxygen-15 labeled CO_2 compared with carbon-11-labeled CO_2 in the lung. J Appl Physiol 17:9-13, 1962.

38. Jones SC, Reivich M, Greenberg JH: Error propagation in the determination of cerebral blood flow and oxygen metabolism with the inhalation of $C^{15}O_2$ and $^{15}O_2$. Acta Physiol Scand 60:Suppl 72:228-229, 1979.

39. Jones SC, Greenberg JH and Reivich M: Error Analysis for the Determination of Cerebral Blood Flow with the Continuous Inhalation of ^{15}O-Labeled Carbon Dioxide and Positron Emission Tomography. J of Computer Asst Tomography 6:116-124, 1982.

40. Huang SC, Phelps ME, Hoffman EJ, Kuhl DE: A theoretical study of quantitative flow measurements with constant infusion of short lived isotopes. Phys Med Biol 24:1151-1161, 1979.

41. Eichling JO, Raichle ME, Grubb RL Jr, Ter-Pogossian MM: Evidence of the limitations of water as a freely diffusible tracer in brain of the rhesus monkey. Circ Res 35:358-364, 1974

42. Raichle ME, Eichling JO, Straatmann MG, Welch MJ, Larson KB Ter-Pogossian MM: Blood-brain barrier permeability of ^{11}C-labeled water. Am J Phsyiol 230:543-552, 1976.

43. Lammertsma AA, Heather JD, Jones T, Frackowiak RSJ, Lenzi GL: A Statistical Study of the Steady State Technique for Measuring Regional Cerebral Blood Flow and Oxygen Utilization Using ^{15}O. J Comput Assist Tomogr 6:566-573, 1982.

44. Greenberg J, Reivich M, Alavi A, Hand P, Rosenquist A, Rintelmann W, Stein A, Tusa R, Dann R, Christman D, Fowler J, MacGregor B and Wolf A: Metabolic mapping of functional activity in human subjects with the (^{18}F)-fluorodeoxyglucose technique. Science 212:678-680, 1981.

45. Holmes G: Disturbances of vision by cerebral lesions. Br, J Ophthal 2:353-384, 1918.

46. Spaldins JMK: Wounds of the visual pathway. J Neurol Neurosurg Psychiat 15:99-109, 169-183, 1952.

47. Teuber NG, Battersby WS and Bender MD: Visual field defects after penetrating missile wounds of the brain, pp 89-98. Harvard University Press, Cambridge MA, 1975.

48. Polyak S: The vertebrate visual system. Univeristy of Chicago Press. 1957.

49. Brindley GS and Lewis WS: The sensations produced by electrical stimulation of the visual cortex. J Physiol Lond. 196: 479-493, 1968.

50. Dobelle WH, Mladejavk MF and Girvin JP: Artificial vision for the blind. Electrical stimulation offers hope for functional prosthesis. Science 183:440-444, 1974.

51. Phelps ME, Mazziotta JC, Kuhl DE, Nuwer M, Packusood J, Metter J and Engel J: Tomographic mapping of human cerebral metabolism: Visual stimulation and deprivation. Neurology: 31:517-529, 1981.

52. Reivich M, Cobbs W, Rosenquist A, Stein A, Schatz N, Savino P, Alavi A and Greenberg J: Abnormalities in local cerebral glucose metabolism in patients with visual field defects. J Cereb Blood Flow Metab 1:Suppl 1:S471-472, 1981.

53. Benevento LA and Rezak M: The cortical projection of the inferior pulvinar and adjacent lateral pulvinar in the rhesus monkey. An autoradiographic study. Brain Res 108:1-24, 1976.

54. Clark WE and LeGross M: The structure and connections of the thalamus. Brain 55:406-70, 1932.

55. Trojanowski J and Jacobson S: Areal and laminar distribution of some pulvinar cortical efferents in the rhesus monkey. J Comp Neurol 169:371-392, 1976.

56. Cullen, JD, Berlin CI, Hughes LF et al: Proceedings of a Symoposium on Central Auditory Processing Disordres: University of Nabraska Medical Center, Omaha, 1975, 108-127.

57. Aetken LM and Webster WR: Medial geniculate body of the cat: organization and responses to tonal stimuli of neurons in ventral division. J Neurophysiol 35:365-380, 1972.

58. Mazziotta JC, Phelps ME, Carson RE and Kuhl DE: Tomographic mapping of human cerebral metabolism. Auditory Stimulation. Neurol 32:921-937, 1982.

59. Seashore CE, Lewis D and Sactveit JG: Seashore measures of musical talents. Psychological Corp New York, series B, 1960.

60. Penfield WF and Rasmussen AT: The cerebral cortex of man: a clinical study of localization of function. Macmillan, NY. 1950.

61. Mountcastle VB: Modality and topographic properties of single neurons of cats' somatic sensory cortex. J Neurophysiol 20: 408-435, 1957.

62. Powell TPS and Mountcastle VB: Some aspects of the functional organization of the cortex of the postcentral gyrus of the monkey: a correlation of findings obtained in a single unit analysis with cytoarchitecture. Bull Johns Hopkins Hosp 105: 133-162, 1959.

63. Whitsel BD, Dreyer DE and Roppolo JR: Determinants of body reprsentataion in postcentral gyrus of macaques. J Neurophysiol 34:1018-1034, 1971.

64. Penfield WG and Boldray E: Somatic motor and sensory representation in the cerebral cortex of man as studied by electrical stimulation. Brain 60:389-443, 1937.

65. Woolsey CN, Erickson TC, Gilson WG: Localization in somatic sensory and motor areas of human cerebral cortex as determined by direct recording of evoked potentials and electrical stimulation. J Neurosurg 51:476-506, 1979.

66. Turner DR: Miller Analogies Test. Arco, New York. 1973.

67. Benton Al, Varney WR and Hamsher K: Judgement of line orientation, Form V University of Iowa Press, 1975, Iowa City.

68. Levy-Agresti J, Sperry RW: Differential Perceptual Capacities in major and minor hemispheres. Proc Natl Acad: Science 61:1151, 1968.

69. Benton AL: "The Minor Hemisphere". Journal Hist Med All Sci 27:5-14, 1972.

70. Hecaen H and Albert ML: Human Neuropsychology. Wiley, New York 1978.

71. Kinabourne M: Eye and Head Turning Indicates Cerebral Lateralization. Science 176:539-541, 1972.

72. Bakan P, Srorad D: Resting EEG Alpha & Asymmetry of Reflecting lateral eye movements. Nature 223:975-976, 1969.

73. Gur RE, Gur RC and Harris LJ: Cerebral Activation as measured by subjects' lateral eye movements, is influenced by Experimenter location. Neuropsychol 13:35-44, 1975.

74. Gur RC and Reivich M: Cognitive task effects on hemispheric blood flow in humans: evidence for individual differences in hemispheric activation. Brain Lang 9:78-93, 1980.

75. Gur RC, Gur RE, Obrist WD, Hungerbuhler JP, Younkin D, Rosen AD, Skolnick BE and Reivich M: Sex and Handedness Differences in Cerebral Blood Flow During Rest and Cognitive Activity. Science 217:659-661, 1982.

76. Heilman KM and Van Dea A: Right hemispheric dominance for mediating cerebral activation. Neuropsychol 17:315-321, 1979.

77. Mesulam MM: A cortical network for directed attention and unilateral neglect. Ann Neurol 10:309-325, 1981.

78. Trevarthen C: In: Cerebral Interhemispheric Relations (eds.) Cernacvek J and Podivinsky F. Publishing House Solvak Academy Sciences, 1972.

79. Ehrlichman H and Weinberger A: Psych Bull 85:1080-1101, 1978.

80. Gur RE and Gur RC: Letter to the Editor: Reply-regarding Cerebral Activation, as measured by subjects' lateral eye movements, is influenced by experimenter location. Arch Gen Psych 36:493-494, 1973.

81. DeRenzi E and Faglioni P: The comparative efficiency of intelligence and vigilance tests detecting hemispheric damage. Cortex 1:410-433, 1965.

82. Diamond S: Depletion of attentional capacity after total commissurotomy in man. Brain 99:347-356, 1976.

83. Diamond S: Performance by split-brain humans on lateralized vigilance tasks. Cortex 15:43-50, 1979.

84. Murphy EH and Venables PH: Ear asymmetry in the threshold of fusion of two clicks: A signal detection analysis. Q J of Experimental Psychology 22:288-300, 1970.

85. Heilman KM, Schwartz HD and Watson RT: Hypoarousal in patients with the neglect syndrome and emotional indifference. Neurology 28:229-232, 1978.

86. Denny-Brown D and Chambers RA: The parietal lobe and behavior. In: The Brain and Human Behavior. Research Publications of the Association for Research of Nervous and Mental Diseases 36:35-117. Baltimore: Williams & Wilkins, 1958.

87. Heilman KM, Pandya DN and Geshwind N: Trimodal Inattention following Parietal Lobe Ablations. Trans Am Neurol Assoc 95:259, 1970.

88. Mesulam MM, Van Hoesen GW, Pandya DN, Geschwind N: Limbic and sensory connections of the inferior parietal lobule (area PG) in the rhesus monkey: A study with a new method for horseradish peroxidase histochemistry. Brain Res 136: 393-414, 1977.

89. Mesulam MM: A cortical network for directed attention and unilateral neglect. Annals of Neurology 10:309-325, 1981.

90. Mountcastle VB, Lynch JC, Georgopoulos A, Kakata H, Acuna C: Posterior Parietal Association Cortex of the Monkey: Command Functions for Operations Within Extrapersonal Space. J Neurophys 38:871-908, 1975.

91. Mountcastle VB: Brain mechanisms for directed attention. J R Soc Med 71:14-28, 1978.

92. Brain WR: Visual disorientation with special reference to lesion of the Right Cerebral Hemisphere. Brain 64:244, 1941.

93. Hecaen H, Penfield W, Bertrand C and Malmo R: The syndrome of apractognosia due to lesions of the minor cerebral hemisphere. AMA Archives of Neurology and Psychiatry 75:400-434, 1956.

94. DeRenzi E, Faglioni P and Scotti G: Hemispheric contribution to exploration of space through the visual and tactil modality. Cortex 6:191-203, 1970.

95. Gainotti G, Messerli P, Tissot R: Qualitative analysis of unilateral spatial neglect in relation to laterality of cerebral lesions. J Neurol Neurosurg Psychiat 35:545-550, 1972.

96. Diamond S: Depletion of attentional capacity after local commissurotomy in man. Brain 99:347-356, 1976.

97. Diamond S: Performance by split brain humans on lateralized vigilance tasks. Cortex 15:43-50, 1979.

98. Brodal A: Neurological Anatomy in Relation to Clinical Medicine Oxford University Press, New York, 1981.

99. Williams PL and Warwick R: Functional Neuroanatomy of Man. WB Saunders, Philadelphia, 1975.

100. Hecaen H and Albert ML: Human Neuropyschology, John Wiley & Sons, New York, Chichester Brisbone, Toronto, 1978.

101. Levy-Agresti J and Sperry RW: Differential Perceptual Capacities in Major & Minor hemispheres. Proc Natl Acad Sci 61: 1151, 1968.

102. Levy J, Trevarthen CB and Sperry RW: Perception of Bilateral Chemeric figures following hemispheric deconnexion. Brian 95:61-78, 1972.

103. Bogen JE: The other side of the brain IV; The AIP ratio. Bull Los-Angeles Neurol Soc 34:135, 1969.

104. Benton AL: The "minor" hemisphere. J Hist Med Allied Sci 27: 5, 1972.

105. Nauta WJH: Connections of the frontal lobe with the limbic system In: Surgical Approaches in Psychiatry. (Eds) LV Laitenen and KE Livingston. Baltimore, MD, University Park Press, 1972.

106. Kuhl DE, Phelps ME, Kowell AP, Metter EJ, Selin C and Winter J: Effects of stroke on local cerebral metabolism and perfusion: mapping by emission computed tomography of ^{18}FDG and $^{13}NH_3$. Ann Neurol 8:47-60, 1980.

107. Ginsberg MS, Reivich M, Giandomenico A and Greenberg JH: Local glucose utilization in acute focal cerebral ischemia; local dysmetabolism and diaschisis. Neurology 27:104-148, 1977.

108. Pulsinelli WA and Duffy TE: Local cerebral glucose metabolism during controlled hypoxemia in rats. Science 204:626-629, 1979.

109. Spatz M, Mrsulja BB, Micic D, Mrsulja BJ and Klatzo J: Ischemic and postischemic effects on 2-deoxy-D-(H) glucose uptake in cerebral capillaries. Brain Res 120:141-145, 1977.

110. Cohen PJ, Alexander SC and Smith TC: Effects of hypoxia and normocarbia on cerebral blood flow and metabolism in conscious man. J Appl Physiol 23:183-189, 1967.

111. Norberg K and Siesjo BK: Cerebral metabolism in hypoxic hypoxia. I. Pattern of activation of glycolysis: a re-evaluation. Brain Res 8:31-44, 1975.

112. Lenzi GL, Frackowiak RSJ and Jones T: Cerebral Oxygen Metabolism and Blood Flow in Human Cerebral Ischemic Infarction Cerebral Ischemic Infarction. Journal of CBF and Metab 2: 321-335, 1982.

113. Baron JC, Bousser MG, Comar D, Castaigne P: "Crossed Cerebellar Diaschisis" in Human Supratentorial Brian Infarction. Trans Neurol Assoc 105:459-461, 1980.

114. Kushner M, Reivich M, Alavi A, Dann R, Hurtig H and Greenberg J: Contralateral Cerebellar Hypometabolism following Cerebral Hemispheric Insult: A Positron Emission Tomographic Study. Ann Neurol 12:88, 1982.

115. Baron JC, Lebrun-Grandie Ph, Collard Ph, Crouzel C, Mestelan G and Bousser MG: Noninvasive Measurement of Blood Flow, Oxygen Consumption and Glucose Utilization in the Same Brain Regions in Man by Positron Emission Tomography: Concise Communication. J Nucl Med 23:391-399, 1982.

116. Howse DC, Caronna JJ, Duffy TE, Plum F: Cerebral energy metabolism, pH and blood flow during seizures in the cat. Am J Physiol 227:1444-1451, 1974.

117. Ingvar DH: Regional cerebral blood flow in focal cortical epilepsy. Stroke 4:359-360, 1973.

118. Plum F, Posner JB, Troy B: Cerebral metabolic and circulation responses to induce convulsions in animals. Arch Neurol 18: 1-13, 1968.

119. Plum F, Howse DC, Duffy TE: Metabolic effects of seizures. In Plum F (Ed.) Brain Dysfunction in Metabolic Disorders. New York, Raven, 1974, 53:141-157.

120. Collins RC, Kennedy C, Sokoloff L, Plum F: Metabolic anatomy of focal motor seizure. Arch Neurol 33:536-542, 1976.

121. Kennedy C, DesRosiers MH, Jehle J, Reivich M, Sharp F and Sokoloff L: Mapping of functional neural pathways by autoradiographic survey of local metabolic rate with (14C) deoxyglucose. Science 187:850-853, 1975.

122. Hougaard K, Oikawa T, Sveinsdottir E, Skinhøj E, Ingvar DH, Lassen NA: Regional cerebral blood flow in focal cortical epilespy. Arch Neurol 33:527-535, 1976.

123. Ingvar DH: rCBF in focal cortical epilepsy. In Langfitt TW, McHenry LC, Jr, Reivich M, Wollman H (Eds.) Cerebral Circulation and Metabolism. New York, Springer-Verlag, 1975, 361-363.

124. Lavy S, Melamed E, Portnoy Z, Carmon A: Interictal regional cerebral blood flow in patients with partial seizure. Neurology 26:418-422, 1976.

125. Sakai F, Meyer JS, Naritomi H, Hsu MG: Regional cerebral blood flow and EEG in patients with epilepsy. Arch Neurol 35:648-657, 1978.

126. Kuhl DE, Engel J, Phelps ME, Selin C: Epileptic patterns of local metabolism and perfusion in humans determined by emission computed tomography of ^{18}FDG and $^{13}NH_3$. Ann of Neurol 8:348-360, 1980.

127. Phelps ME, Hoffman EJ, Raybaud C: Factors which affect cerebral uptake and retention of $^{13}NH_3$. Stroke 8:694-702, 1977.

128. Pope A: Perspectives in neuropathology. In Jasper AS, Ward HH, Pope A (Eds.) Basic Mechanisms of the Epilepsies. Boston, Little Brown, 1969, 773-781.

129. Woodbury DM, Kemp JW: Initiation, propagation and arrest of seizure. In Mrsulja BB, Rakic ZM, Klatzo I (Eds.) Pathophysiology of cerebral energy metabolism. Plenum, NY, 1967, 313-351.

130. Prince DA, Wilder BJ: Control mechanisms in cortical epileptogenic foci. Arch Neurol 16:194-202, 1967.

131. Meyers JS, Gotoh F, Favale E: Cerebral metabolism during epileptic seizures in man. Electroencephalogr Clin Neurophysiol 21:10-22, 1966.

132. Penfield W, Von Santha K, Cirriani A: Cerebral blood flow during induced epileptiform seizures in animals and man. J Neurophysiol 2:257-267, 1939.

133. Posner JB, Plum F, Van Posnak A: Cerebral metabolism during electrically induced seizures in man. Arch Neurol 20:388-395, 1969.

134. Engel J, Rausch R, Leib J, Kuhl DE, Crandall PE: Re-evaluation of criteria for localizing the epileptic focus in patients considered for surgical therpay of epilepsy. Epilepsia 21:184-185, 1980.

135. Crandall PH: Developments in direct recordings from epileptogenic regions in the surgical treatment of partial epilepsies. In Brazier MAB (Ed.) Epilepsy, Its Phenomena in Man. New York, Academic Press, 1973, 287-310.

136. Falconer MA, Davidson S: The rationale of surgical treatment of temporal lobe epilepsy with particular reference to childhood and adolescence. In Harris P, Mawdsley C (Eds.) Epilepsy, Proceedings of the Hans Berger Centenary Symposium. Edinburgh, London, New York/Livingstone, 1974.

137. Walter RD: Tactical considerations leading to surgical treatment of limbic epilepsy. In Brazier MAB (Ed.) Epilepsy, Its Phenomena in Man. New York, Academic Press, 1973, 99-119.

138. Falconer MA, Driver MV and Serafetinides EA: Temporal lobe epilepsy due to distant lesions; two cases revealed by operation. Brain 85:521-534, 1982.

139. Ludwig GI, Ajmone-Marsan C: Clinical ictal patterns in epileptic patients with occipital electroencephalographic foci. Neurology 25:463-471, 1975.

140. Freyhan FA, Woodford RB, Kety SS: Cerebral blood flow and metabolism in psychosis of senility. J Nerv Ment Dis 113: 449-456, 1951.

141. Lassen NA, Munck O, Tottery ER: Mental function and cerebral oxygen consumption in organic dementia. Arch Neurol Pyschiat 77:126-133, 1957.

142. Lassen NA, Feinberg I, Lane MH: Bilateral studies of cerebral oxygen uptake in young and aged normal subjects and in patients with organic dementia. J Clin Invest 39:491-500, 1960.

143. Sokoloff L: Cerebral circulartory and metabolic changes associated with aging. Res Publ Assoc Ment Dis 41:237-254, 1966.

144. Gottstein U, Held K, Muller W, Berghoff W: Utilization of ketone bodies by the human brain. In Meyer JS, Reivich M, Lechner H (Eds.) Research on the Cerebral Circulation, 5th International Salzburg Conference. Springerfield, IL, 1970, 137-145.

145. Obrist WD, Chivian E, Cronquvist S, Ingvar DH: Regional cerebral blood flow in senile and presenile dementia. Neurology 20:315-322, 1970.

146. Ingvar DH, Gustafson L: Regional cerebral blood flow in organic dementia with early onset. Acta Neurol Scand 43:42-73, 1970.

147. Simard D, Olesen J, Paulson OB, Lassen NA, Skinhøj E: Regional cerebral blood flow and its regulation in dementia. Brain 94:273-288, 1971.

148. Hagberg B, Ingvar DH: Cognitive reduction in presenile dementia related to regional abnormalities of the cerebral blood flow. Br J Psychiat 128:209-222, 1976.

149. Hagberg B: Defects of immediate memory related to the cerebral blood flow distribution. Brain Lang 5:366-377, 1978.

150. Gustafson L, Hagberg B, Ingvar DH: Speech disturbances in presenile dementia related to local cerebral blood flow abnormalities in the dormant hemisphere. Brain Lang 5:102-118, 1978.

151. Obrist WD, Thompson HK, King CH, Wang HS: Determination of regional cerebral blood flow by inhalation of ^{133}Xe. Circ Res 20:124-135, 1967.

152. Wang HS, Busse BW: Correlates of regional cerebral blood flow in elderly community residents. In Harper AM, Jennett WB, Miller JD, Rowan JO (Eds.) Blood Flow and Metabolism in the Brain. London: Chruchill/Livingstone, 1975, 817-818.

153. Baer PE, Faibish GM, Meyer JS, Mathew NT and Rivera VM: Neuropsychological correlates of hemispheric and regional cerebral blood flow in dementia. In Meyer JS, Lechner H and Reivich M (Eds.) Cerebral Vascular Disease. 7th Int. Conf. Salzburg. Theieme, Stuttgart, 1976, 100-106.

154. Lavy S, Melamed E, Benton S, Cooper G, Rinot Y: Bihemispheric decreases of regional blood flow in dementia: correlates with age-matched normal controls. Ann Neurol 4:445-450, 1978.

155. Alavi A, Ferris S, Wolf A, Reivich M, Farkas T, Dann R, Christman D, Fowler J: Determination of cerebral metabolism in senile dementia using F-18-deoxyglucose and positron emission tomography. J Nucl Med 21:21, 1980.

156. Alavi A, Ferris S, Wolf A, Christman D, Fowler J, MacGregor R, Farkas T, Greenberg J, Dann R, Reivich M: Determination of cerebral metabolism in dementia using F-18 deoxyglucose and positron emission tomography. Satellite-symposium on physiological and pathophysiological aspects of the aging brain. Experimental Brain Research, Springer-Verlag, Heidelberg, 1982.

157. Kuhl DE, Metter EJ, Riege WH and Phelps ME: Effects of human aging on patterns of local cerebral glucose utilization determined by the (^{18}F) fluorodeoxyglucose method. J CBF and Metab 2:163-171, 1982.

158. Frackowiak RSJ, Pozzilli C, Legg NJ, DuBoulay GH, Marshall J, Lenzi GL, Jones T: A prospective study of regional cerebral blood flow and oxygen utilization in dementia using positron emission tomography and oxygen-15. J CBF and Metab 1:(Suppl 1):S453, 1981.

159. Frackowiak RSJ, Pozzilli C, Legg NJ, DuBoulay GH, Marshall J, Lenzi GL and Jones T: Regional Cerebral Oxygen Supply And Utilization In Dementia. Brain 104:753-778, 1981.

160. Bustany P, Sargent T, Suadubray JM, Henry JF, Cumar D: Regional human brain uptake and protein incorporation of ^{11}C-L-Methionine studied in vivo with PET. J CBF and Metab 1:(Suppl 1):S17, 1981.

161. Farkas T, Reivich M, Alavi A, Greenberg J, Fowler J, MacGregor R, Christman D, Wolf A: The application of ^{18}F-2-deoxy-2-D-glucose and positron emission tomography in the study of psychiatric conditions. In Passoneau JV, Hawkins RA, Lust WD, Welsh FA (Eds.) Cerebral Metabolism and Neurological Function. Williams and Wilkins, Balitmore, 1980, 403-408.

162. Buchsbaum MS, Kessler R, Bunney WE, Cappelletti J, Coppolo R, Van Kammen DP, Rigal F, Waters R, Sokoloff L, Ingvar D: Simultaneous electroencephalography and cerebral glucography with positron emission tomography (PET) in normals and patients with schizophrenia. J CBF and Metab 1:(Suppl 1):S457, 1981.

163. Buchsbaum MS, Ingvar DH, Kessler R, Waters RN, Cappelletti J, Van Kammen DP, King CA, Johnson JL, Manning RG, Flynn RW, Mann LS, Bunney WE, Jr, Sokoloff L: Cerebral Glycography With Positron Tomography Use in Normal Subjects and in Patients With Schizophrenia. Arch Gen Psychiatry 39: 251-259, 1982.

164. Ingvar D: Abnormal distribution of cerebral activity in chronic schizophrenia: A neurophysiological interpretation. In Baxter CF and Melnechuck T (Eds.) Perspectives in Schizophrenia Research. New York, Raven Press, 1980, 107-125.

165. Lidsky T, Weinhold P, Levine F: Implications of basal ganglionic dysfunction for schizophrenia. Biol Psychiatry 14: 3-12, 1979.

166. Bowman M, Lewis MS: Sites of subcortical damage in disease which resembles schizophrenia, Neuropsychologia 18:597-601, 1980.

167. Lee T, Seeman P: Elevation of brain neuroleptic/dopamine receptors in schizophrenia. Am J Psychiatry 137:191-197, 1980.

168. Lee T, Seeman P, Farley IJ, Hornydeiwicz O: Binding of ^{3}H-apomorphine in schizophrenic brains. Nature 274:897-900, 1978.

169. Owen F, Crow TJ, Poulter M, Cross AJ, Longden A, Riley GJ: Increased dopamine-receptor sensitivity in schizophrenia. Lancet 1:223-226, 1978.

170. DiChiro G, DeLapaz R, Smith B, Kornblith P, Sokoloff L, Brooks R, Blasberg R, Cummins C, Kessler R, Wolf AP, Fowler J, London W, Sever J: ^{18}F-2-fluoro-2-deoxyglucose positron emission tomography of human cerebral gliomas. J CBF and Metab 1:(Suppl 1):S11, 1981.

171. DiChiro G, DeLaPaz RL, Brooks RA, Sokoloff L, Kornblith PL, Smith BH, Patronas NJ, Kufta CV, Kessler RM, Johnston GS, Manning RG, Wolf AP: Glucose Utilization of Cerebral Gliomas Measured by (^{18}F) Fluorodeoxyglucose and Positron Emission Tomography. Neurology 32:1323-1329, 1982.

172. Patronas NJ, DiChiro G, Brooks RA, DeLaPaz RL, Kornblith PL, Smith BH, Rizzoli HV, Kessler RM, Manning RG, Channing M, Wolf AP, O'Connor CM: Work in Progress: (^{18}F)fluorodeoxyglucose and positron emission tomography in the evaluation of radiation necrosis of the brain. Radiology 144:885-889, 1982.

173. Lammertsma AA, Ito M, Wise RSJ, Bernardi S, Frackowiak RSJ, Heather JD, McKenzie CG, Thomas DGT and Jones T: Measurement of Regional Cerebral Blood Flow and Oxygen Utilization in Patients with Cerebral Tumours Using ^{15}O and Positron Emission Tomography: Analytical Techniques and Preliminary Results. Neuroradiology 23:63-74, 1982.

174. Withers HR, Peter LJ: Biological aspects of radiation therapy. In Fletcher GH (Ed.) Textbook of radiotherapy, 3rd ed. Lea & Febiger, Philadelphia, 1980, 103-179.

175. Kuhl DE, Markham Ch, Phelps ME, Winter J, Metter J: Local cerebral glucose metabolism in Huntington's disease determined by emission computed tomography of ^{18}F-fluoro-deoxyglucose. J Nucl Med 22:15, 1981.

176. Kuhl DE, Phelps ME, Markham CH, Metter EJ, Riege, WH, Winter J: Cerebral Metabolism and Atrophy in Huntington's Disease Determined by ^{18}FDG and Computed Tomographic Scan. Ann Neurol 12:425-434, 1982.

177. Albert ML: Subcortical dementia. In Katzman R, Terry RD, Bick KL (Eds.) Alzheimer's Disease: Senile Dementia and Related Disorders (Aging Vol 7). New York, Raven, 1978, 173-180.

178. Spokes EGS: Neurochemical alterations in Huntington's chorea. A study of post-mortem brain tissue. Brain 103:179-210, 1980.

179. Bowen DM, Smith CB, White P, Davison AN: Neurotransmitter related enzymes and indices of hypoxia in senile dementia and other abiotrophies. Brain 99:459-496, 1976.

KINETIC ANALYSIS OF THE UPTAKE OF GLUCOSE AND SOME OF ITS ANALOGS IN THE BRAIN USING THE SINGLE CAPILLARY MODEL: COMMENTS ON SOME POINTS OF CONTROVERSY

Niels A. Lassen and Albert Gjedde

Bispebjerg Hospital and Copenhagen University,
Copenhagen, Denmark

INTRODUCTION

In 1961 Crone (1) demonstrated that the glucose transport across the blood-brain barrier occurs by facilitated diffusion. Since then, many studies with a variety of techniques have confirmed this observation and extended our knowledge of the process in details (2, 3, 4, 5, 6, 7, 8). In particular, the finding that glucose analogs share the facilitated transport mechanism has proven fertile. It forms the basis for Sokoloff's ingenious autoradiographic method of determining the local rate of glucose metabolism (lCGU) in animals by measuring the rate of phosphorylation of the analog 2-deoxyglucose (2DG) which is trapped in brain (9). Using positron-emitting derivatives, this method has even been applied to man, yielding spectacular maps of the local rates of metabolism, the intensity of which change during changes of brain activity of motor, sensory, or mental type (10). It is perhaps worth noting, however, that the facilitated diffusion of glucose, one of the major prerequisites of the model on which the method is based, never has been documented in man. The use of positron emission technology would be one approach to the solution of this problem.

Clinical studies with the 2DG-method appear at a rapid rate. This paper reviews the kinetics of the uptake and phosphorylation processes, confining the treatment to the single capillary model: Each brain area studied is considered homogenous with respect to capillary uptake and tissue concentration of glucose (for a discussion of the effect of heterogeneity, see the paper by Bass in this volume). A tracer of glucose is supplied to the capillary at time zero. The tracer represents a second species of glucose besides native glucose itself, but the actual concentration of the tracer is so low that its mass can be ignored, and also so low that its concentration is insignificant when compared to native glucose.

THE EXTRACTION FRACTION

Tracer and Native Glucose Concentration Profiles in the Capillary

The brain is modelled as a capillary with its surrounding brain tissue mantle. With the transit time denoted by τ, consider a small volume of source fluid (plasma water in lower mammals, whole-blood water in humans), dV, crossing a cross-section during a differential element of time $d\tau$. During $d\tau$, the distance travelled by the volume element is dL cm. Since the volume element travels the total capillary length L in τ seconds,

$$\frac{dV}{V} = \frac{d\tau}{\tau} = \frac{dL}{L} = dx \qquad (1)$$

where x is the fractional length dV has travelled in t seconds.

Now consider the process as dV travels down the capillary in a sequence of discrete jumps of fractional length dx. At the fractional distance x from the arterial inlet, the capillary blood has the glucose concentration C(x) mmol/l, and at the fractional distance x+dx the concentration C(x+dx) mmol/l. The difference between the two is due to the transcapillary transport of glucose in and out of the capillary section of length dx.

Assuming saturation kinetics of the Michaelis-Menten-kind, the fluxes through the capillary wall in both directions are,

$$dJ_1(x) = \frac{T_{max}\, C_1(x)}{K_t + C_1(x)}\, dx \quad \text{(influx to brain)} \qquad (2)$$

and

$$dJ_2(x) = \frac{T_{max}\, C_2}{K_t + C_2}\, dx \quad \text{(efflux from brain)} \qquad (3)$$

where T_{max} and K_t are the Michaelis-Menten constants, the maximal transport capacity and the concentration at a flux half the maximal flux. The term $C_1(x)$ represents the concentration at the fractional length x, C_2 the interstitial concentration assumed to be constant.

For the tracer glucose, the fluxes are calculated by multiplying with the specific activity on the right hand side, i.e. by multiplying with C_1^*/C_1 or C_2^*/C_2, respectively, the asterisk denoting the tracer.

In order to obtain a practical solution to the differential equation based on the fluxes (eqs. 2 and 3), the influx equation is simplified by substituting $C_1(x)$ in the denominator by $C_1(0) = C_a$, the arterial source fluid concentration. The error incurred by this step was discussed by Gjedde(11) who derived an exact solution for the unidirectional flux case, i.e. for $C_2 = 0$, without this simplification. He found that the fractional error involved was less than 1/1000 for realistic values of the variables involved.

With the simplification mentioned, the terms $T_{max}/(K_t+C_a)$ and $T_{max}/(K_t+C_2)$ may be considered apparent permeability-surface-area products, P_1A (for influx, i.e. flux in the direction from compartment "1"). and P_2A (for efflux, i.e. flux in the direction from comparrment "2"). The mass balance for dV yields the differential equation to be solved to find the longitudinal gradient in the capillary:

$$F\, C_1(x) + P_2A\, C_2\, dx = F\, C_1(x + dx) + P_1A\, C_1(x)\, dx \qquad (4)$$

The solution of equation (4) is,

$$C_1(x\ ) = C_a\, e^{-(P_1A/F)x} + C_2 \frac{P_2A/F}{P_1A/F}\left(1 - e^{-(P_1A/F)x}\right) \qquad (5)$$

where F is the flow of source fluid from which the glucose is extracted (see discussion below).

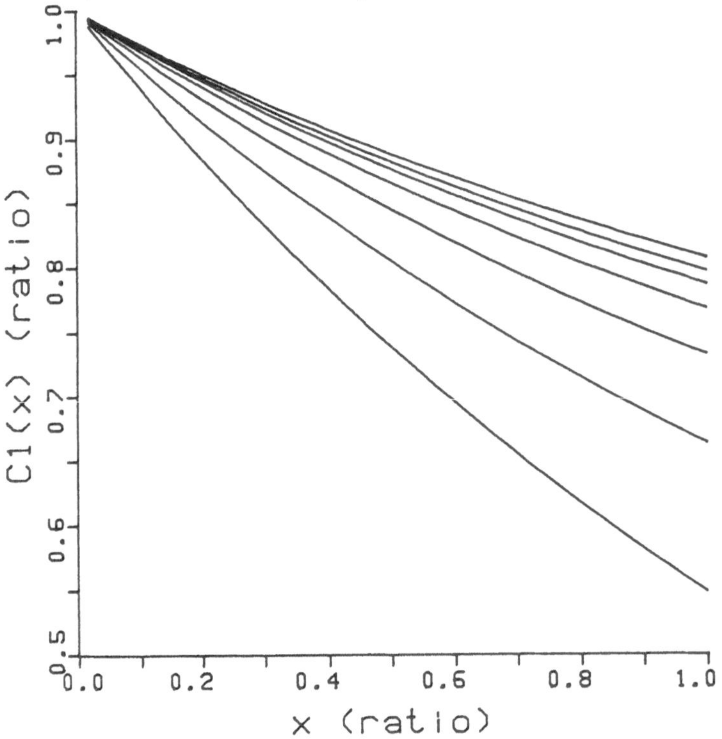

Figure 1: Concentration profile in capillary of tracer glucose for T_{max} = 400 and CMR = 70 µmol/hg/min, C_a = 9 mM, K_t = 7 mM, and F = 40 ml/hg/min (7,8). The lines (from the bottom) represents the times '0', 1, 2, 3, 4, 5, and 45 min.

From equation 5, the end capillary concentration C_v is obtained by setting the fractional length x equal to 1. The average capillary concentration $\bar{C}_1 = \int_0^1 C_1(x)dx$ is obtained by appropriate integration,

$$\bar{C}_1 = C_a\,(1 - e^{-P_1A/F})\,\frac{1}{P_1A/F} + C_2\,\frac{P_2A/F}{P_1A/F}\,\left(1 - \frac{1}{P_1A/F}\,(1 - e^{-P_1A/F})\right) \qquad (6)$$

This can be used to calculate the total in- and efflux and net influx $J_1 - J_2$:

$$J_1 = P_1A\,\bar{C}_1 = C_a\,(1 - e^{-P_1A/F})\,F + C_2\,P_2A\,\left(1 - \frac{1 - e^{-P_1A/F}}{P_1A/F}\right) \qquad (7)$$

$$J_2 = P_2A\,C_2 \qquad (8)$$

or

$$J_1 - J_2 = K_1\,C_a - k_2\,M_2 \qquad (9)$$

where $K_1 = F\,(1 - \exp(-P_1/F))$ and $M_2 = C_2V_d$, V_d being the volume of distribution in the brain. Costumarily F, the source fluid flow rate, is expressed in milliliters per 100 g per minute. In that case, V_d is the volume of distribution in ml per 100 g of brain tissue. We will, however, for practical reasons, both use 100 grams (also written "hectogram" = hg) and 1 gram as the unit of brain weight in the following text. K_1 has the dimension of a clearance (ml per 100 g brain per minute), whereas k_2 has the dimension of a fractional clearance (fraction per minute).

The extraction fraction E, defined as $(C_a - C_v)C_a$, is obtained by appropriate use of equation 5:

$$E = (1 - e^{-P_1A/F}) - \frac{C_2}{C_a}\,\frac{P_2A/F}{P_1A/F}\,(1 - e^{-P_1A/F}) \qquad (10)$$

The Tracer Extraction Fraction at Very Short Times, E*(0)

When the tracer is injected and first arrives in the capillary, C_2^* is zero. Assuming adequate mixing in V_d, the amount leaving the capillary during a short time is too small to augment C_2^* significantly. Hence, the tracer goes through the capillary wall only by unidirectional transport. This crucial point will be analyzed in the discussion on the basis of some experimental results. Assuming it to be fulfilled that $C_2^* \sim 0$ for the first seconds (20 seconds in the experiments to be discussed), equation 10 yields:

$$E^*(0) = 1 - e^{-P_1A/F} \qquad (11)$$

The variable $E^*(0)$ is subject to experimental determination. It contains the variable P_1A, defined by $T_{max}/(K_t + C_a)$ and the term F, representing the flow rate of "source fluid".

Glucose is not extracted from the erythrocytes during a single capillary transit in lower mammals while it is so extracted in man. Thus, in rats, F is the flow of plasma water, in man the blood water flow. To illustrate the relevance of this point, it may be mentioned that the rate of source fluid flow is about the same in the two species (50 ml plasma water in rats, and 50 ml blood water in man per 100 g and per minute). The net removal of glucose is almost twice as high in rat as in man due to the higher metabolic rate of the brain; and the rats' apparent permeability-surface area product P_1A is also about twice as high as that in man (20 ml/100g/min in rats, Gjedde 1983 (8)) vs. 10 ml/100g/min in man (10). Thus, the concentration profile falls more steeply along the capillary in the plasma of rats compared to whole blood (and plasma) in man. Had F erroneously been equated with the blood water flow in the rat, the concentration drop would be underestimated.

The Steady-State of Tracer Glucose

The steady-state of tracer glucose is defined as a state of equal specific activity at all sites. In this state, equation 5 describes the concentration profile of native and tracer glucose. The ratio C_2/C_a (and hence the ratio C_2^*/C_a^*) assumes the value determined by the variables discussed above and by the rate of metabolism $J_1 - J_2$ (see below).

Under most circumstances, i.e. with normal, elevated or slightly subnormal F (see Fig. 1), the steady-state equation for $C_1(x)$ can be simplified to a linear function,

$$C_1(x) = C_a - ax \qquad (12)$$

where a equals $(J_1-J_2)/F$, the metabolic net uptake per ml of source fluid. It implies that the steady-state $\bar{C}_1$ is the arithmetic mean of inlet and outlet concentrations,

$$\bar{C}_{1\,steady\text{-}state} = \frac{C_a + C_v}{2} \qquad (13)$$

In this case, the unidirectional influx of native glucose (and tracer glucose in the steady-state) becomes simply:

$$J_1 = P_1A \; \frac{C_a + C_v}{2} \qquad (14)$$

The simplification of equation 13 over equation 6 introduces an overestimation of $\bar{C}_1$ of approximately 2/1000 for realistic values of the variables.

With K_t = 7 mM, Ca = 8 mM, C_2 = 2 mM; $P_2/P_1 \sim 2$. Hence with the extraction fraction of steady-state of equation 10 set at .10, and with $1 - \exp(-P_1A/F) = E^*(0)$, equation 10 yields, $.10 = E^*(0) - .50\,E^*(0)$ or $E^*(0) = .20$ and, by equation 11,

$P_1A/F = .223$

Thus, equation 6 yields,

$$\frac{\bar{C}_1}{C_a} = .20\,\frac{1}{.223} + .25 \times 2\left(1 - \frac{.20}{.223}\right) = .50 + .10/.223 = .948$$

while equation 13 yields $\bar{C}_1/C_a = .950$.

Experimental Determination of the Tracer Extraction Fraction

The tracer extraction fraction is the ratio between the mass of the tracer transported into the tissue and the mass of the tracer supplied by the arterial circulation,

$$E^*(0) = \frac{M^*('0') - V\,\bar{C}_1^*('0')}{F\int_0^{'0'} C_a^*(t)\,dt} \tag{15}$$

where V is the source fluid volume in the brain, and $\bar{C}_1^*('0')$ the tracer concentration in the source fluid at the end of the experiment. $M^*('0')$ is the total radioactivity of the tissue, including the activity in the blood vessels. The concentration $\bar{C}_1^*('0')$ can be considered to be close to the concentration $C_a^*('0')$, if the concentration curve in the arterial circulation has reached the point where it falls only moderately with time. After an intravenous bolus injection into a rat, this point is reached at about 15 seconds, from which moment and onwards the approximation can be considered to be valid.

The extraction fraction can be determined directly if the flow of the source fluid is known, and if the input integral and the transported mass can be measured simultaneously before there is significant loss of tracer by back-diffusion to the circulation (integral method of Gjedde (12) and Ohno et al. (13)). According to equation 15, $E^*(0)$ can be measured by a single determination of $M^*('0')$ when V and F are known. If V and F are both unknown, equation 15 can be given a linear form,

$$\frac{M^*('0')}{C_a^*('0')} = E^*(0)\,\frac{F\int_0^{'0'} C_a^*(t)\,dt}{C_a^*('0')} + V \tag{16}$$

where $E^*(0)$ F is the slope and V the ordinate intercept of a series of measurements performed at different times '0'. This is the form first suggested by Blasberg et al. (14). It readily yields the vascular (i.e. "initial") volume of distribution of the tracer by retropolation. In a sample of brain cortex stripped of large vessels and the pial membrane, the thus determined blood volume is close to 1 ml per 100 g of tissue, and the plasma volume appr. .7 ml/hg (15). In the light of these findings, recent reports of a blood volume of close to 7% in the cortical brain tissue of the rat (16) must be viewed with considerable doubt.

The "integral method" has received considerable attention lately because of its simplicity and accuracy. It can be applied successfully to substances of low, intermediate, or high permeability. In the case of substances of very high permeability, the method yields blood flow (17,18,19). The method has also been applied to the study of glucose transport through the blood-brain barrier (11). However, in the case of the facilitated transport of substances that compete for transport with other substances in plasma (e.g. amino acids), the method is of limited value (20) because it is difficult to separate the influences of many competitors for the same transport mechanism.

In these cases, the Brain Uptake Index method of Oldendorf(21) is helpful. In this method, the tracer extraction fraction is evaluated by comparison to a substance of known extraction fraction. Thus, using equation 15 and neglecting the term for the amount of tracer inside the vascular bed at time '0',

$$BUI = \frac{\dfrac{M^*('0')}{M_{ref}('0')}}{\dfrac{C^*}{C_{ref}}} \sim \frac{\dfrac{M_2^*('0')}{M_{2\,ref}('0')}}{\int_0^{'0'} C_a^*(t)dt \Big/ \int_0^{'0'} C_{a\,ref}(t)dt} = \frac{E^*('0')}{E_{ref}('0')} \tag{17}$$

where the subscript "ref" refers to a reference substance. The ratio between the injected concentrations, C^*/C_{ref}, is assumed to equal the ratio of the amounts reaching the brain, cf. the denominator in equation 15. Hence, if the numerator is corrected for the amounts remaining in the vascular bed at the end of the experiment, the BUI of Oldendorf equals the ratio of the extraction fractions. The intracarotid injection permits a brief but complete replacement of the blood in the brain vasculature by the injectate, thus clearing the transport sites of competing substances that are not present in the injectate. The reference is usually water or a completely flow-limited compound, for which the initial extraction fraction is close to unity. However, in cases of high perfusion rates, the wash-out of the reference in combination with possibly incomplete initial extraction as in the case of tritiated water may give values of BUI that are much lower than that of $E^*(0)$. An additional disadvantage is the absence of simultaneous blood flow measurement, particularly since the rate of perfusion during the intracarotid injection may differ from the normal rate of source fluid flow.

If the reference substance is impermeable and the amount of test substance extracted is calculated from measurements of effluent venous concentrations, the method is known as the "indicator diffusion" method of Crone (22) (see also 5).

TABLE 1

Methods of Measuring Initial Extraction Fractions, Their Advantages and Disadvantages

Method	Disadvantages	Application
Integral	Invalidated by competiting substances in plasma	Measurements of low permeability, facilitated diffusion, blood flow measurements, possible application in man (see below)
BUI	Perfusion rate not known	Amino acids, rapid screening
Indicator diffusion	Insensitive to high and low permeabilities, no regional application	Human studies (limited application), repetitive measurements in animals

The integral method can be applied to human studies by means of detection of single or double photon emission from suitable labeled tracers. The accumulation of the tracer would be recorded continuously by one or more detectors and the ratio between the accumulated amounts and the value of the input integral calculated for as many points as desired. The value of the input integral could be determined either by continuous withdrawal of arterial blood at a known rate.

THE TRANSFER CONSTANTS

The clearance of native glucose in the steady-state is the difference between the fluxes in the directions blood-to-brain and brain-to-blood, i.e., where K is the net clearance, defined by $E(\infty)\ F = ((C_a - C_v)/C_a\ F$. Thus, the object of the 2DG-method can be briefly stated to be the measurement of K locally. By multiplication with C_a, the steady-state glucose concentration in arterial plasma, we obtain $J_1 - J_2$, the net glucose transfer or local metabolic rate (ICGU or CMR),

$$J_1 - J_2 = K\ C_a \tag{18}$$

TABLE 2

Comparison of the transfer constants for glucose, 2DG, and 3-O-methylglucose (3OMG). The values are based on the model discussed by Gjedde (7), using values for CMR, C_a, T_{max}, and F of 70 µmol/hg/min, 9 mM, 400 µmol/hg/min, and 40 ml/hg/min. The hexose volume of distribution in brain was assumed to be 0.77 ml/g.

Analog	Michaelis' Affinity Constant	Transfer Constants		
	K_t (mM)	K_1 (ml/g/min)	k_2 (min^{-1})	k_3 (min^{-1})
glucose	6.8	0.19	0.37	0.26
2DG	2.2	0.34	0.69	0.08
3OMG	9.6	0.15	0.29	0

The Basic Equations Expressed for 2DG (denoted by ")

As shown by Gjedde (7), equation 9 describes the net flux of tracer, analog, or native glucose across the endothelium at all times. For 2DG we have

$$J_1''(t) - J_2''(t) = K_1'' C_a''(t) - k_2'' M_2''(t) \tag{19}$$

where

$$k_2'' = \frac{P_2 A'' K_1''}{P_1 A'' V_d} \tag{20}$$

The term V_d represents the volume of distribution of the compound in brain common to all glucose analogs. The product k_2'' $M_2''(t)$ does not equal the efflux. In fact, since the difference always equals the net transport, the product k_2'' $M_2''(t)$ is as much lower than the rate of efflux as the product K_1'' $C_a''(t)$ is less than the rate of influx (see the term containing C_2 in equation 7).

The fractional rate of metabolism of the tracer is a function of the hexokinase reaction for which the rate constant, in the irreversible case, assumes a form dependent on competition kinetics, as known from enzymology (23),

$$k_3'' = \frac{K_m \, V''_{max}}{K''_m \, (K_m + C_2) \, V_d} \tag{21}$$

where K_m is the affinity of native glucose for hexokinase, and K_m'' the affinity of the tracer 2DG with which native glucose competes. V''_{max} is the maximal hexokinase reaction rate for 2DG, probably equal to V_{max}, the maximal reaction rate for glucose. Thus defined, the rate of metabolism of the tracer is,

$$J_3''(t) = k_3'' \, M_2''(t) \tag{22}$$

where $M_2''(t)$ is the brain tissue's content of un-metabolized tracer.

We are now in a position to estimate the accumulation of tracer in the brain. Using equation 19 and subtracting the metabolized amount represented by $J_3''(t)$ in equation 22, the accumulation rate of un-metabolized tracer $dM_2''(t)/dt$ is given by $J_1''(t) - J_2''(t) - J_3''(t)$, i.e.

$$\frac{dM_2''(t)}{dt} = K_1'' \, C_a''(t) - (k_2'' + k_3'') \, M_2''(t) \tag{23}$$

or

$$\frac{M_2''(T)}{K_1''} = \int_0^T C_a''(t)dt - \frac{k_2'' + k_3''}{K_1} \int_0^T M_2''(t) \, dt \tag{24}$$

while the accumulation of metabolized tracer is given by,

$$\frac{dM_3''(t)}{dt} = k_3'' \, M_2''(t) \tag{25}$$

or

$$M_3''(T) = k_3'' \int_0^T M_2''(t)dt \tag{26}$$

where $M_3''(t)$ represents the accumulated metabolic product.

The Operational Equations of the 2DG Method

In the steady-state, 2DG obeys equations 9 and 18. Hence,

$$J_1''(\infty) - J_2''(\infty) = K'' C_a''(\infty) = K_1'' C_a''(\infty) - k_2'' M_2''(\infty) \quad (27)$$

As $J_3''(\infty) = J_1''(\infty) - J_2''(\infty)$, equation 22 yields,

$$J_1''(\infty) - J_2''(\infty) = k_3'' M_2''(\infty) \quad (28)$$

From these two equations it follows that

$$K'' = K_1'' \frac{k_3''}{k_2'' + k_3''} \quad (29)$$

Inserting equation 26 into equation 24, and using equation 29, as well as the substitution that $M''(T) = M_2''(T) + M_3''(T)$, we obtain the fundamental equation of Sokoloff et al. (9),

$$K'' = \frac{M_3''(T)}{\int_0^T C_a''(t)dt - \frac{M_2''(T)}{K_1''}} \quad (30)$$

or

$$K'' = \frac{M''(T) - \frac{k_2''}{k_2'' + k_3''} M_2''(T)}{\int_0^T C_a''(t)\, dt} \quad (31)$$

Equations 30 and 31 are the operational equations of the 2DG-method. In equation 30, originally developed by Sokoloff (9), $M_3''(T)$ is calculated as the difference between $M''(T)$ and $M_2''(T)$. $M_2''(T)$ is the solution of equation 23 with the transfer constants being assumed to be known, viz.

$$M_2''(T) = K_1'' e^{-(k_2''+k_3'')T} \int_0^T C_a''(t)\, e^{(k_2''+k_3'')t}\, dt \quad (32)$$

Equation 31, first developed by Gjedde (7), is simpler to use because $M_2''(T)$ in the steady-state is given by a rearrangement of equation 27, after inserting the expression for K" from equation 29, viz.

$$M_2''(\infty) = \frac{K_1''}{k_2'' + k_3''} C_a''(\infty) \qquad (33)$$

in which case, if sufficiently long time has passed ($T \rightarrow \infty$), the integral of the arterial plasma concentration in equation 31 may be determined directly and the amount to be subtracted from M"(T) calculated as,

$$\frac{K_1'' \, k_2''}{(k_2'' + k_3'')^2} C_a''(\infty) \qquad (34)$$

which only requires measurement of the final plasma concentration of the tracer when the constants are known, just as they must be for using the Sokoloff equation 30.

The Variability of the Transfer Constants

The transfer constants are functions of variables that change with changes of the condition of the experimental subject. The transfer constants determine the amount to be subtracted from the total radioactivity of the brain at the end of the experiment. This amount is quite small (approximately 10% of the numerator) when the experiment is carried out to 30 or 45 minutes as is typically done. Accurate correction for this amount demands, however, in principle the measurement of the transfer constants in a given situation. In discussing this point, it is necessary to distinguish between regions in the brain under physiological conditions and pathological states.

In physiologic conditions, there is evidence to support the notion that K_1'', k_2'', and k_3'' tend to change in parallel due to proportional changes of A (the surface area of the endothelium) or P_1'', and of F and V_{max} (15, 24). This is in agreement with the recent finding of capillary recruitment in the brain (25). Then, since the value of $C_a''(T \rightarrow \infty)$ is common to all regions in the brain, the amount to be subtracted from $M''(\infty)$ cannot vary much regionally.

In severe hypoglycemia, k_3'' does not vary in parallel with K_1'' and k_2'' since the blood flow may go up but the metabolic rate go down, and the correction is therefore uncertain (26). But in this state, as in ischemia, the brain glucose concentration is probably very low and hence the omission of a correction for M_2'' probably results in no grave error. In other pathological conditions, such as halothane anesthesia, and hypo- or hypercapnia, blood flow and metabolic rate do not vary in parallel so that K_1'', k_2'', and k_3'' cannot be expected to be proportional to their values determined under physiologic conditions.

The Apparent Volumes of Distribution

The ratio K_1/k_2 is common to all glucose analogs, including the native glucose itself, because it equals V_d, the physical (actual) volume of distribution of hexoses in brain, multiplied by the ratio P_1/P_2 (see equation 20). The latter ratio equals $(K_t + C_2)/(K_t + C_a)$ (see equations 2 and 3). Thus, denoting K_1/k_2 by V_e,

$$V_e = \frac{K_1}{k_2} = \frac{P_1}{P_2} V_d = \frac{K_t + C_2}{K_t + C_a} V_d \qquad (35)$$

As seen from equation 9, in the case of an analog with no metabolic breakdown (i.e. with $J_1 - J_2 = 0$ in the steady-state), V_e represents an apparent volume of distribution since $V_e = K_1/k_2 = M_2(\infty)/C_a(\infty)$. This suggests that the steady-state ratio between the amount of 3-O-methylglucose in the brain and reference fluid can be employed to calculate the amount to be subtracted from M"(T).

The volume V_e changes when the ratio between C_2 and C_a changes. Because of the terms K_t, V_e is in a sense a "damped" index of the ratio C_2/C_a. Therefore, when C_2/C_a changes, V_e changes but to a lesser degree. Knowing K_t, V_e allows the calculation of the steady-state C_2/C_a ratio.

The virtual volume of distribution of a metabolizable analog, V_f, is lower than V_e (because of the addition of k_3 to k_2), and equations 31 and 34 show that the apparent volume of the precursor "pool", V_g, is even lower. These volumes and their calculation are shown in Table 3.

TABLE 3

Apparent Volumes of Distribution Calculated from Table 2

Term	Unit	Formula	GLC	2DG	3OMG
V_d	ml/g	(water volume)	0.77	0.77	0.77
V_e	-"-	K_1/k_2	0.50	0.50	0.50
V_f	-"-	$K_1/(k_2+k_3)$	0.30	0.45	0.50
V_g	-"-	$K_1k_2/(k_2+k_3)^2$	0.18	0.40	0.50

THE "LUMPED CONSTANT"

The Meaning of the "Lumped Constant"

If the tracer 2DG had the same constants as glucose, K" would equal K, and K could then be determined directly from equations 30 or 31. As it is, the net clearance of 2-deoxyglucose is less than that of glucose. For this reason, the ratio between the K" of the tracer and the K of native glucose must be known. This ratio is the "lumped constant" (LC). According to equation 29, LC equals

$$LC = \frac{K''}{K} = \frac{E''(\infty)}{E(\infty)} = \frac{K_1'' \, k_3'' \, (k_2 + k_3)}{K_1 \, k_3 \, (k_2'' + k_3'')} \qquad (36)$$

In the past, LC was determined from the ratio of the net clearances which also equals the ratio between the extraction fraction in the steady-state.

The Variability of the "Lumped Constant"

While the LC was determined for whole-brain only in several species, including man, in the normal state and in certain experimental states, its regional variability must be assessed from a combination of equations 33 and 36,

$$LC = \frac{k_3''}{k_3} \; \frac{\dfrac{M_2''(\infty)}{C_a''(\infty)}}{\dfrac{M_e}{C_a}} = \frac{k_3''}{k_3} \; \frac{V_f''}{V_f} \qquad (37)$$

where $M2''(\infty)/C_a''(\infty)$ and M_2/C_a are the apparent (rather than actual) volumes of distribution of 2-deoxyglucose and glucose. Sokoloff et al. (9) symbolized the ratio V_f''/V_f by the term λ. If the k_3''/k_3 is considered constant, equation 37 expresses the proportionality of LC to the ratio between the apparent volumes of distribution of 2DG and native glucose.

The analog and the native glucose compete for the transport mechanism in the endothelium as well as for the hexokinase reaction. If the ratio between brain and plasma glucose changes, the apparent volume of the tracer will change in the opposite direction due to the competition which will inhibit transport of tracer in the direction in which the transport of native glucose is favored. Hence, if the brain glucose concentration falls (e.g. because of increased brain glucose consumption or because of hypoglycemia) the LC will increase (27, 28). On the other hand, if brain glucose increases because of decreased brain glucose consumption or hyperglycemia, the LC will fall and approach the ratio k_3''/k_3 which has been found to lie somewhere between .3 and .4 (28, 24).

The first question we ask is, whether the LC will vary regionally if regional rates of glucose consumption vary? The answer depends on the regional variation of the relationship between tissue and plasma glucose. Usually, the regional rates of glucose consumption, blood flow, and glucose transport are so well adjusted, as mentioned previously, that regional tissue glucose levels are expected not to vary much (24). Calculation of the regional variation of the value of the LC, based on measurements of the regional distribution of labeled 3-O-methylglucose (see below) gave no evidence of significant regional variation within grey matter in normal rats (29).

The second question regards the influence of regional increases of the glucose consumption rate, in seizures for instance. Figure 2 shows the estimated change of the LC in a theoretical case of a change of glucose consumption from 10 to 175 µmol/100g/min with no change of the variables T_{max}, K_t, F, and C_a. Figure 2 confirms that mismatches between the demand and supply of glucose that cause the brain glucose content to fall will cause the LC to rise. Again, the important variable is the relationship between the brain and plasma glucose levels.

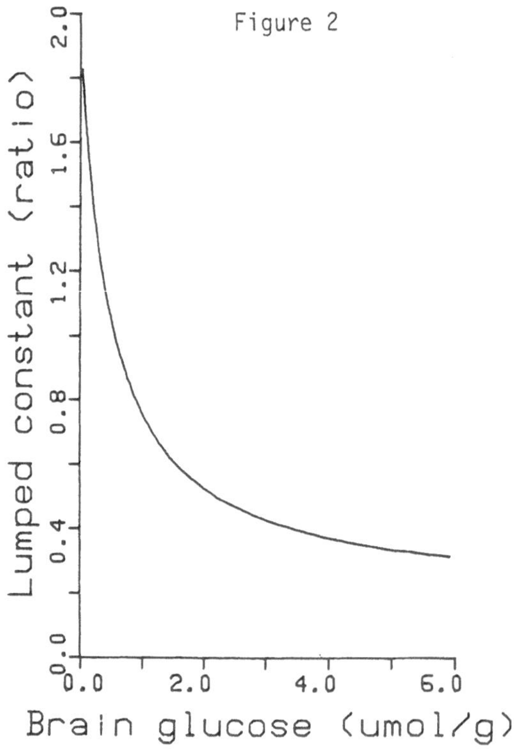

If we were in a position to know the apparent regional volumes of distribution of tracer 2DG (which is chiefly a function of the brain glucose concentration), as well as the tissue and plasma glucose concentrations, we would be able to calculate the LC (assuming the ratio k3"/k3 to be known) of the same regions.

Equation 35 shows that measurement of the tissue glucose represents an approach to the problem of the apparent volume of distribution of the tracer in experimental animals, since the values of V_d and K_t can be assumed to be known and constant. However, the tissue glucose level of the human brain is unknown and this poses a problem for the human studies with 2DG. All human studies have used the same LC for the entire brain, based on measurements of the whole-brain LC.

The Radiographic Determination of Regional Brain Glucose by 3-O-Methylglucose

As discussed above, the problem of the LC can be reduced to the problem of knowing the brain glucose concentration (more correctly the content) when the plasma glucose concentration is known. The regional brain glucose concentration can be measured in experimental animals, and nomograms have been constructed showing the relation between the "lumped constant" and the brain and plasma glucose concentrations (30) (see also figure 2).

Figure 3

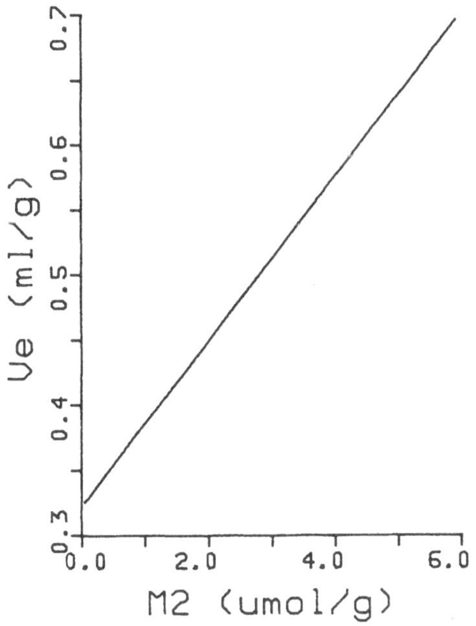

The relationship between the brain glucose content and the apparent distribution volume V_e that equals the steady-state distribution volume of 3-O-methylglucose, calculated during a change of the glucose consumption rate from 10 to 175 µmol/100g/min. The other variables (kept constant in this example) included C_a = 9 mM, F = 40 ml/100g/min, and T_{max}= 400 µmol/100g/min.

Another approach is to proceed from equation 37. This equation expresses that the LC is proportional to the ratio between the apparent volumes of distribution of tracer 2DG and native glucose. The apparent volume of distribution of native glucose is the ratio between brain and plasma glucose, and the apparent volume of distribution of tracer 2-deoxyglucose is likewise the ratio between the brain and plasma contents of the unmetabolized tracer in the steady-state. The latter volume can be measured only following separation of phosphorylated and non-phosphorylated tracer in brain (which is impossible in humans, of course). However, above we recognized that this volume is not very different from the apparent volume of distribution of an inert (non-metabolizable) hoxose like 3-O-methylglucose (Table 2). The hexokinase reaction constant k_3'' is zero for such a substance. Thus, since we noted above that the k_3'' of 2-deoxyglucose is small compared to k_2'', the value of V_f'' will be close to the ratio K_1''/k_2'' which, as also noted above, is identical for all hexoses competing with native glucose for transport. As a consequence, equation 35 expresses the apparent volume of distribution of 3-O-methylglucose and may be used for two purposes, first to calculate brain glucose according to the equation,

$$C_2 = \frac{V_e}{V_d}(K_t + C_a) - K_t \qquad (38)$$

and then to calculate the LC according to the equation

$$LC = \frac{k_3''}{k_3} \cdot \frac{V_f''}{V_f} \sim \frac{k_3''}{k_3} \cdot \frac{V_e''}{V_f} = \frac{k_3''}{k_3} \cdot \frac{\dfrac{K_t + C_2}{K_t + C_a} V_d}{\dfrac{C_2}{C_a} V_d} \qquad (39)$$

Measurements with 3-O-methylglucose have been made in rats but not yet in humans. In rat, a pathological distribution of regional brain glucose is shown in figure 4, along with the calculation of the distribution of the LC (31). Figure 4 shows the distribution of the LC in kainic acid induced seizures in which the glucose content of the hippocampal region falls. Calculation of the LC based on autoradiographic measurements of brain glucose confirmed that the LC of the hippocampal area exceeded in whole-brain average by 50%.

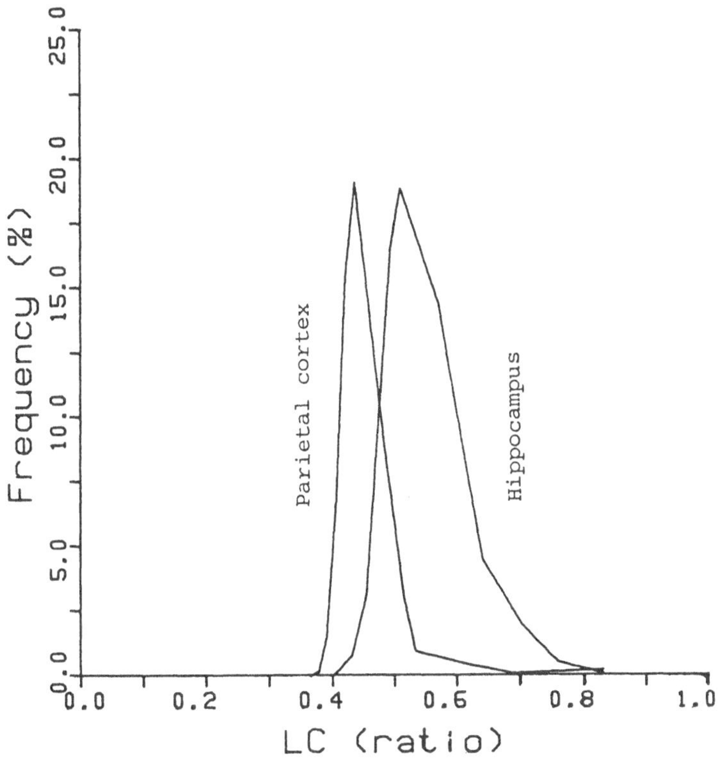

FIG. 4

Calculation of the "lumped constant" in two regions of the brain during kainic acid-induced saizures. The graph to the left shows the distribution of LC-values in the parietal cortex, the average value being close to .4, corresponding to a glucose content of 6.3 μmol/g. The graph to the right shows the distribution of LC-values in the hippocampus, the average value being close to .6, corresponding to a glucose content of 3.6 μmol/g. The plasma glucose level was elevated in this animal (31).

Several pieces of fundamental evidence are still missing for human studies of cerebral glucose metabolic rate to rest on as sound a foundation as the comparable studies in rats. As alluded to previously, the facilitated diffusion of hexoses has not yet been documented in humans. Second, the human brain glucose concentration is unknown, and the relationship between influx and efflux of glucose cannot therefore be determined with certainty. In fact, available evidence (5, 6) suggests that the brain glucose concentration in humans could be relatively much lower than that in rats, because the extraction fraction of net transport is only slightly lower than the extraction fraction for unidirectional transport. Third, the regional variability of the "lumped constant" is unknown, although the whole-brain value of the "lumped constant" is not different from that of the rat (10).

Under normal circumstances, including activation studies, these problems probably play a minor role when judged from the comparable situations in the rat, where tissue glucose concentrations are remarkably constant.

In pathological states, however, we know nothing of the tissue glucose concentration in man. In fact, in situations in which the glucose approaches zero, the "lumped constant" may rise so much that despite a fall of glucose consumption, the tissue 2DG accumulation increases. In these situations, the regional "lumped constant" must be measured. Note also that in such states the glucose uptake (K) is no longer necessarily proportional to the energy metabolism.

We suggest the following studies: First, it is necessary to measure the T_{max} and K_t of blood-brain glucose transport in humans. The most practical method for this purpose is the integral method, adapted for use with detection of single or double photon emission. The uptake of labeled glucose or glucose analogs is followed over some time, and the values of K_1 computed from the initial influx rates at different plasma glucose concentrations. For 2-deoxyglucose and 3-O-methylglucose, the uptake curves also yield k_2 and k_3. For glucose, the determination of k_2 and k_3 is difficult, but not quite necessary, because the ratio k_3''/k_3 can be assumed to be constant regionally.

When the T_{max} and K_t are known, the steady-state distribution of 3-O-methylglucose can be determined, also by single or double photon emission detection, and most practically as the termination of an uptake experiment. From the steady-state distribution, the human brain glucose concentration can be calculated as described above.

Finally, from the distribution of the brain glucose concentration the variability of the "lumped constant" can be calculated regionally, and in various experimental situations, always assuming the ratio k_3''/k_3 to be constant.

A Comment on the Significance of k_4''

The hexokinase reaction was originally thought to be irreversible for 2DG although allowance was made for some phosphatase activity for glucose-6-phosphate (9). In the original formalism, the phosphatase activity was represented by the greek letter Φ This ambiguity has caused problems for the proper interpretation of 2DG-6-phosphate accumulation: Is or isn't some phosphatase activity permissible, and is it fully accounted for?

The phosphatase activity has been represented by the rate constant k_4'' which was shown to be substantial in humans (10). The problem is in some ways similar to the problem of unidirectionality of blood-brain transport. In case of significant phosphatase activity, the steady-state accumulation of the non-metabolizable product 2DG-6-phosphate will represent the apparent volume of distribution rather than the phosphorylation rate, just as the steady-state accumulation of 3/MG in brain represents its apparent volume of distribution rather than blood-brain transport. If there is <u>any</u> phosphatase activity, the steady-state extraction fraction for 2DG and the steady-state "lumped constant" must be zero.

In the practical application of the 2DG method the importance of the problem depends on a consideration of the time-course of equilibration and the importance of the metabolic "back-flux" at the particular experimental times chosen, just as one needs to consider the problem of blood-brain-barrier back-flux in relation to the chosen period of experimentation.

After administration of 2DG, the combined apparent volume of distribution of 2DG, M_2'', and 2DG-6-P, M_3'', in brain $(M_2'' + M_3'')/C_a''$ will rise and then slowly approach the steady-state apparent volume of distribution given by $J_1'' + J_2'' = K_1'' C_a'' - k_2'' M_2'' = 0$ and $dM_3''/dt = k_3'' M_2'' - k_4'' M_3'' = 0$, yielding $(M_2'' + M_3'')/C_a'' =$

$$\frac{K_1'' (k_3'' + k_4'')}{k_2'' k_4''} \tag{40}$$

It follows from the above considerations, that the value of the "steady-state" clearance K" depends on the time chosen for termination of the experiment, if there is a significant phosphatase activity.

To some extent the "lumped constant" determined experimentally for the whole brain, as the ratio between the quasi steady-state extraction fractions determined at 45 minutes reflects the loss of label from the 2DG-6-P pool, if there is some phosphatase activity. Thus, this experimentally determined "lumped constant" tends to minimize the error incurred by metabolic "back-flux". This is not true of the "lumped constant" calculated from the constants K_1'', k_2'', and k_3'', nor of the "lumped constant" estimated from the steady-state distribution of 3OMG.

The presence of significant phosphatase activity can be determined by long time measurements of 2DG distribution in brain, and from the long-time "steady-state" extraction fractions, e.g. as measured beyond the customary 45 minutes. If the latter does not reach zero within a reasonable period of time, then there is no significant phosphatase activity. It may be concluded that the absence of significant phosphatase activity is an important assumption for the 2DG method. No method has been devised to correct for its presence in regional studies in animals. Fitting procedure has been used to obtain approximate values of k_4'' based on a series of positron tomograms using F-18-2DG (10). Similar studies have not been reported in rats, but preliminary estimates of the 24 hour distribution volume of 2DG-label in brain suggest that k_4'' is close to 0.0042 min^{-1} and that the hexokinase reaction rate may be underestimated by 10% at 45 minutes. This is illustrated in fig. 5 based on the values of K_1'', k_2'', and k_3'' from Table 2, and the k_4'' mentioned just above.

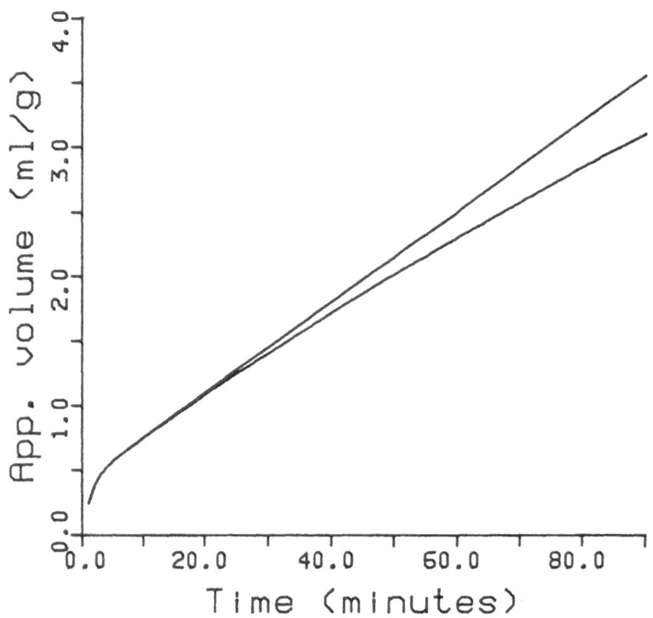

FIG. 5

Estimates of the brain uptake the sum of 2DG and 2DG-6-phosphate in rat using the values of K_1, k_2'', k_3'', and k_4'' given in the text. Abscissa: time (min). Ordinate: Total amount of label in brain, normalized against final arterial tracer concentration (ml/g). The upper curve represents zero phosphatase activity, the lower curve a k_4'' of 0.0042 min^{-1}.

The uptake curves in fig. 5 were constructed from a constant arterial concentration of tracer, unlike an intra-venous bolus experiment in which the tracer concentration falls. Hence a real study performed at 45 minutes should be compared to the 90 minute point on fig. 5, i.e. it shows a 10% effect of k_4''.

REFERENCES

1. Crone C: Om diffusionen af nogle organiske non-elektrolyter fra blod til hjernevæv. Thesis, University of Copenhagen 1961. Munksgaard Publ., Copenhagen.

2. Oldendorf WH: Brain uptake of radiolabeled amino acids, amines, and hexoses. Am J Physiol 221:1629-1639, 1971

3. Pardridge WM & Oldendorf WH: Kinetics of blood-brain barrier transport of hexoses. Biochim Biophys Acta 382:377-392, 1975

4. Lund-Andersen H: Transport of glucose from blood to brain. Physiol Rev 59:305-352, 1979

5. Hertz MM, Paulson OB, Barry DI et al.: Insulin increases glucose transfer across the blood-brain barrier in man. J Clin Invest 67:597-604, 1981

6. Hertz MM & Paulson OB: Transfer across the human blood-brain barrier: Evidence for capillary recruitment and for a paradox glucose permeability increase in hypocapnia. Microvasc Res 24:364-376, 1982

7. Gjedde A: Calculation of cerebral glucose phosphorylation from brain uptake of glucose analogs in vivo: A re-examination. Brain Res 4:237-274, 1982

8. Gjedde A: Modulation of substrate transport to the brain. Acta Neurol Scand 67:3-25, 1983

9. Sokoloff L, Reivich M, Kennedy C et al.: The (^{14}C)deoxy-glucose method for the measurement of local cerebral glucose utilization: Theory, procedure, and normal values in the conscious and anaesthetized albino rat. J Neurochem 28:897-916, 1977

10. Phelps ME, Huang SC, Hoffman EJ et al.: Tomographic measurement of local cerebral glucose metabolic rate in humans with (F-18)2-fluoro-2-deoxy-D-glucose: Validation of method. Ann Neurol 6:371-388, 1979

11. Gjedde A: Rapid steady-state analysis of blood-brain glucose transfer in rat. Acta Physiol Scand 108:331-339, 1980

12. Gjedde A: High and low affinity transport of D-glucose from blood to brain. J Neurochem 36:1463-1471, 1981.

13. Ohno K, Pettigrew KD, Rapoport SI: Lower limits of cerebrovascular permeability to non-electrolytes in the conscious rat. Am J Physiol 235:H299-H307, 1978

14. Blasberg RG, Patlak CS, Jehle JW & Fenstermacher JD: An autoradiographic technique to measure the permeability of normal and abnormal brain capillaries. Neurology 28:363, 1978

15. Gjedde A & Rasmussen M: Pentobarbital anesthesia reduces blood-brain glucose transfer in the rat. J Neurochem 35:1382-1387, 1980

16. Hossmann K-A: Treatment of experimental cerebral ischemia. J Cerebr Blood Flow Metab 2:275-298, 1982

17. Schaefer JA, Gjedde A, Plum F: Regional cerebral blood flow using n-(^{14}C)-butanol. Neurology 26:392, 1976

18. Van Uitert RL & Levy DE: Regional brain blood flow in the conscious gerbil. Stroke 9:67-72, 1978

19. Gjedde A, Hansen AJ, Siemkowicz E: Rapid simultaneous determination of regional blood flow and blood-brain glucose transfer in brain of rat. Acta Physiol Scand 108:321-330, 1980

20. Sage JI, Van Uitert RL, Duffy TE: Simultaneous measurement of cerebral blood flow and unitirectional movement of substances across the blood-brain barrier: Theory, method and application to leucine. J Neurochem 36:1731-1738, 1981

21. Oldendorf WH: Measurement of brain uptake or radiolabeled substances using a tritiated water internal standard. Brain Res 24:372-376, 1970

22. Crone C: The permeability of capillaries in various organs as determined by use of the "indicator diffusion" method. Acta Physiol Scand 58:292-305, 1963

23. Dixon M & Webb EC: Enzymes. 2nd Ed, London, Longmans Green, 1964, p. 84

24. Cremer JE, Ray DE, Sarna GS & Cunningham VJ: A study of the kinetic behavious of glucose based on simultaneous estimates of influx and phosphorylation in brain regions of rats in different physiological states. Brain Res 221:331-342, 1981

25. Weiss HR, Buchweitz E, Murtha TJ & Auletta M: Quantitative regional determination of morphometric indices of the total and perfused capillary network in the rat brain. Circ Res 51:494-503, 1982

26. Ingvar M, Nevander G, Gjedde A & Siesjö BK: Unidirectional glucose transport into the brain during bicuculline induced status epilepticus. Correlation with local cerebral blood flow and glucose utilization. J. Cerebr Blood Flow Metab 3: suppl. 3, 1983 (in press)

27. Suda S, Shinohara M, Miyoka M et al.: Local cerebral glucose utilization in hypoglycemia. J Cerebr Blood Flow Metab 1, suppl. 1:S62, 1981

28. Crane P, Pardridge WM, Braun L et al.: The interaction of transport and metabolism on brain glucose utilization: Re-evaluation of the lumped constant. J Neurochem 36:1601-1604, 1981

29. Gjedde A & Diemer NH: Autoradiographic determination of regional brain glucose content. J Cerebr Blood Flow Metab, 1983 (in press)

30. Pardridge WM, Crane PD, Mietus LJ & Oldendorf WH: Kinetics of regional blood-brain barrier transport and brain phosphorylation of glucose and 2-deoxyglucose in the barbiturate-anesthetized rat. J Neurochem 38:560-568, 1982

31. Diemer NH & Gjedde A: Autoradiographic determination of brain glucose content and visualization of the regional lumped constant. J Cerebr Blood Flow Metab 3, suppl. 3, 1983 (in press)

THE USE OF ^{11}C-METHYL-D-GLUCOSE FOR ASSESSMENT OF GLUCOSE TRANSPORT IN THE HUMAN BRAIN; THEORY AND APPLICATION

Karel Vyska, Miroslav Profant, Franz Schuier, C. Freundlieb, Anton Höck, Hans-U. Thal, Veit Becker, Ludwig E. Feinendegen

Nuclear Research Center Jülich, University of Dusseldorf and University of Duisburg, F.R.Germany

INTRODUCTION

Imbalance between perfusion, transport and metabolism may determine the ultimate damage in ischemic brain disease (1,2). Therefore, for the quantitative assessment of ischemic brain disorders the knowledge of at least two parameters is necessary. One is local perfusion. The second parameter should relate to tissue metabolism, for example, to the glucose utilisation rate (3,4,5) or to the local unidirectional glucose transport rate (6,7,8,9).

In the present study, for the determination of the unidirectional glucose transport rate, ^{11}C- methyl-D-glucose (CMG) was used.

CMG is an analogue of glucose, which is transported across the blood brain barrier (BBB) by the same carrier as glucose (10,11, 12,13,14,15,16,17,18), yet it does not enter cellular metabolism (12,17). It returns to the circulating blood. The CMG technique, used in this study, is based on the concomitant evaluation of time dependent changes of CMG blood and CMG tissue concentrations.

The present paper demonstrates that by means of the CMG technique the rate constants for glucose influx (κ_1) and glucose efflux (k_2) may be determined in any selected brain area. It will be shown that these parameters permit the determination of the local unidirectional glucose transport rate (LUGTR); moreover, it is proposed to extend the method to measure simultaneously the local perfusion rate (LPR).

In the first part of the contribution, the theoretical aspects of the CMG technique are discussed. In the second part, the examples of the application of this theory in clinical practice are presented.

MATERIAL AND METHODS

In the present studies, 2-5 mCi of CMG were injected into an antecubital vein of the patient, and the transaxial activity distribution in one selected slice of brain was registered with the ECAT II scanner at 2-minute intervals for 40 minutes. Medium re-resolution shadow shields and high resolution data collection were used. The measured attenuation correction was applied for image reconstruction.

At different regions of brain scans ROIs were selected and the activity curves created. Since the blood volume in brain is very small (cortex ∿4%, white matter ∿2%) the time activity curves registered over brain were considered as a measure for the brain CMG concentration, c_2^* .

As estimate for the capillary blood CMG concentration, c_B^*, either the arterial or venous CMG concentrations can be used. According to Sokoloff et al. (3), the cerebral extraction ratio of the labeled glucose is very low (approximately 5 %). This means that the mean capillary plasma concentration cannot differ from the arterial or venous plasma level by more than 5 %. Therefore, it can be assumed that the arterial as well as venous blood concentrations are approximately equal to, or bear a constant relationship to, the capillary blood concentration (3).

In the present study the activity registered over the superior longitudinal sinus (SLS) was taken as an estimate for the CMG venous concentration. This approach seems acceptable since by the use of the CMG technique the following conditions are fulfilled:

1.) The non-metabolizable CMG is slowly eliminated from the blood pool, so that its concentration in blood remains relatively high during the whole measurement period; it is of the same magnitude as that in brain cortex,

2.) according to our model, not the absolute CMG concentrations in blood and in tissue but their ratios are needed, and

3.) from the spatial point of view the SLS can be considered as being integrated in the body of the brain cortex.

Under these conditions and ROIs SLS and brain cortex being of comparable size, the partial volume as well as crossover effects are nearly the same and they would practically cancel out in the ratio of the ROI tissue and ROI SLS activities. Consequently the accuracy of the determination of the ratio tissue over blood CMG concentration would be higher than the accuracy of the determination of the absolute concentrations in the corresponding areas.

For the analysis of regional distribution of CMG in brain tissue the sum of the first 6 images registered in the dynamic study was used. For the analysis of time activity curves usually 6 ROIs were selected in cortex and 2 in white matter.

Thus far, four healthy volunteers and 50 patients suffering from ischemic stroke (two of them before and after an extra-intracranial bypass operation) have been examined. In all cases a CT investigation was performed before the CMG study. In this paper several of these cases were selected in order to demonstrate the applications of the CMG-technique.

MODEL

In the present study for the determination of the unidirectional glucose transport rate the ^{11}C-methyl-D-glucose (CMG) synthesized by Kloster et al.(7) was used. The CMG is a glucose analogue in which the hydrogen atom of the hydroxyl group at carbon-3 is replaced by ^{11}C-methyl group .

CMG is transported across the blood brain barrier by the same carrier as glucose, but it is not phosphorylated or further metabolized (10,18). In the model presented in Fig. 1 c_B^* is the concentration of CMG in blood; c_2^* is the CMG concentration in brain tissue; κ_1^* is the observed rate constant for CMG influx and k_2^* is the rate constant for CMG efflux.

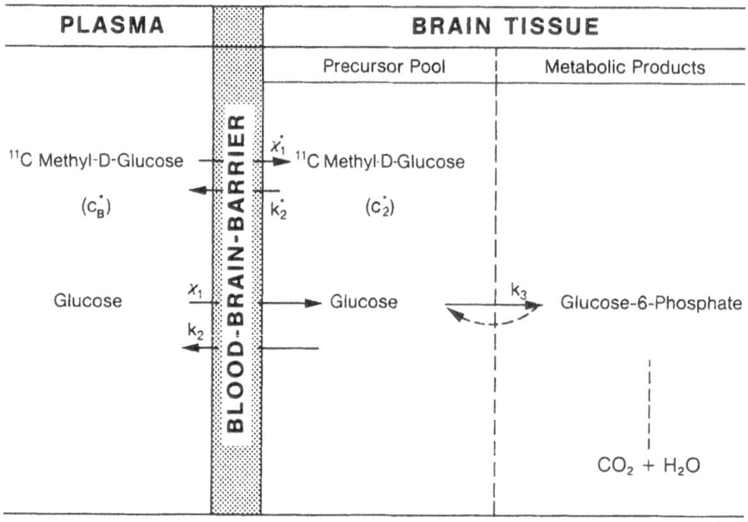

FIG. 1

The model used for interpretation of CMG measurements (modified according to Sokoloff et al.(3))

In plasma, CMG competes with glucose for a common carrier for transport into a primary precursor pool in brain tissue. The rate of CMG accumulation in brain tissue is equal to the difference between the rate of CMG influx ($\kappa_1^* . c_B^*$) and CMG efflux ($k_2^* . c_2^*$) :

$$dc_2^*/dt = \kappa_1^* \cdot c_B^* - k_2^* \cdot c_2^* . \qquad (1)$$

As demonstrated by Sokoloff et al (3), under the conditions of:

1.) steady state of cerebral glucse utilization during the period of measurement,
2.) a constant plasma glucose concentration,
3.) symmetry of glucose transport across BBB and
4.) application of CMG in tracer amounts,

the rate constants for CMG influx and efflux may be considered as true first order constants, which are independent of the plasma CMG concentration.

The formal solution of eq. (1) is

$$c_2^*(t) = \kappa_1^* \cdot \int_0^t c_B^*(\tau) \cdot e^{-k_2^*(t-\tau)} . d\tau + c_2^*(0) \cdot e^{-k_2^* t} . (2)$$

where $c_2^*(0)$ is the tissue CMG concentration at time t=0.

If $c_2^*(t)$ and $c_B^*(t)$ are known, κ_1^* and k_2^* can be calculated from eq. (1) or eq. (2) by various numerical methods (for example the least square method).

In the case that the elimination of the non-metabolizable CMG from the blood pool is so slow that it can be neglected and the mixing of the indicator in the blood is practically instantaneous so that the CMG blood concentration $c_B^*(t)$ can be considered to be constant, the rate constants κ_1^* and k_2^* can be determined from steady state concentrations of CMG in blood and tissue and from the slope of the approach of CMG tissue concentration to the steady state (see Fig.2).

In this case, in steady state ($dc_2^*/dt = 0$) the influx is equal to efflux i.e.:

$$\kappa_1^* \cdot c_{Bss}^* = k_2^* \cdot c_{2ss}^* \quad \text{and} \quad \kappa_1^*/k_2^* = c_{2ss}^*/c_{Bss}^* \qquad (3)$$

where c_{2ss}^* and c_{Bss}^* are the CMG concentrations in brain tissue and blood at steady state respectively.

This means that in steady state the ratio κ_1^*/k_2^* is equal to the ratio of tissue and blood CMG concentrations.

Because the CMG influx is directly proportional to the blood CMG concentration, the CMG influx is constant, when blood CMG concentration is constant. In this case the equation (1) can be written as follows:

$$\frac{dc_2^*}{dt} = \kappa_1^* \cdot c_B^* - k_2^* \cdot c_2^* = \text{const} - k_2^* \cdot c_2^* = k_2^* . (\text{const}/k_2^* - c_2^*) \; . \qquad (4)$$

If in eq. (4) the term const/k_2^* is designated as const_1 this equation can be rearranged as follows:

$$\frac{1}{\text{const}_1 - c_2^*} \cdot \frac{d(\text{const}_1 - c_2^*)}{dt} = -k_2^* \; . \qquad (5)$$

This means that in the case of $c_B^*(t)$ being constant the slope of approach of CMG tissue concentration to the steady state is equal to k_2^*.

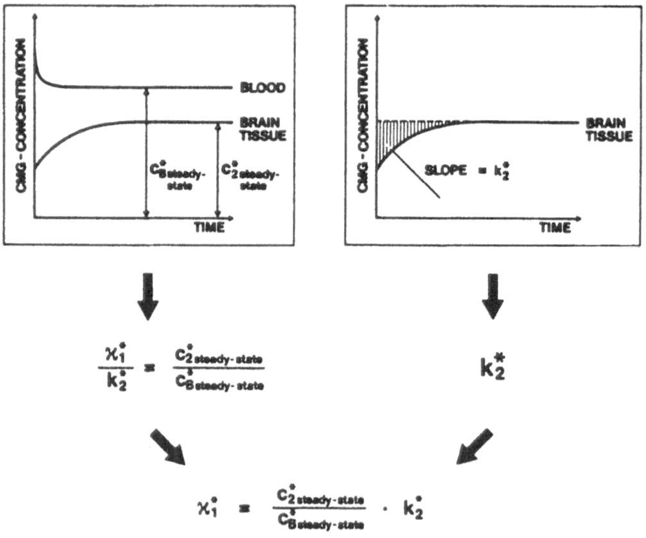

FIG. 2
Schematic representation of the evaluation of CMG data in the theoretical case that the blood CMG concentration is constant i.e. $c_B^* = \text{const.}$

Usually, however, the c_B^* is not constant. In most cases the CMG elimination from the blood could be approximated either by one or by two exponential functions (see Fig. 3):

$$c_B^*(t) \;=\; a_1^* \cdot e^{-\lambda_1^* t} + a_2^* \cdot e^{-\lambda_2^* t} \qquad (6)$$

Under these conditions, on the basis of eq. (2) the tissue concentration c_2^* must be expected to be described by the sum of three exponential functions

$$c_2^*(t) \;=\; b_1^* \cdot e^{-\lambda_1^* t} + b_2^* \cdot e^{-\lambda_2^* t} + b_3^* \cdot e^{-k_2^* t} \qquad (7)$$

In this case the rate constants κ_1^* and k_2^* can be obtained from experimental data as described in Appendix I.

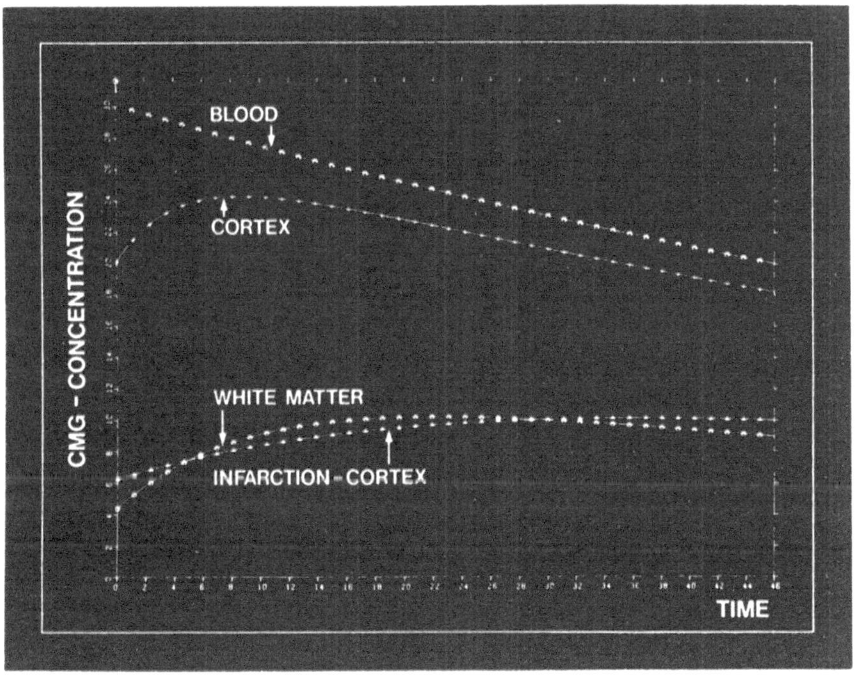

FIG. 3

Normalized, smoothed, and interpolated time activity curves registered over different brain regions after CMG injection (CMG concentration [cpm/pixel], time [min]).

Determination of local unidirectional glucose transport rate Φ_i (LUGTR). The glucose influx rate Φ_i is given by

$$\Phi_i = \kappa_1 \cdot c_B, \qquad (8)$$

where κ_1 is the rate constant for the glucose influx and c_B is the blood concentration of the glucose which is available for transport.

Using argumentation similar to that of Sokoloff et al.(3) it can be demonstrated that the rate constant for the glucose influx κ_1 relates to the rate constant for the CMG influx κ_1^*, as follows:

$$\frac{\kappa_1}{\kappa_1^*} = \frac{V_M}{V_M^*} \cdot \frac{K_M^*}{K_M}, \qquad (9)$$

where V_M, V_M^* and K_M, K_M^* are the maximal velocities and Michaelis-Menten constants for glucose and CMG influx respectively.

Therefore,

$$\Phi_i = \frac{V_M}{V_M^*} \cdot \frac{K_M^*}{K_M} \cdot \kappa_1^* \cdot c_B . \qquad (10)$$

Since, practically, only the glucose in the plasma and not that in the erythrocytes is available for transport across the BBB[+], the available blood- (c_B) and plasma- (c_p) glucose concentrations are related to each other by

$$c_B = (1-H_t) \cdot c_p, \qquad (11)$$

with H_t being the hematocrit[++].

Thus,

$$\Phi_i = \frac{V_M}{V_M^*} \cdot \frac{K_M^*}{K_M} \cdot \kappa_1^* \cdot (1-H_t) \cdot c_p. \qquad (12)$$

This is the algorithm used for the determination of LUGTR in the present study.[+++]

Proposal for the determination of the local perfusion rate LPR. Available data (20,21) suggest that the rate constant for the glucose influx, observed under in vivo conditions, κ_1 is not only proportional to the rate constant characterizing the catalytic activity of the carrier system for glucose influx (k_1) but also to the flow (f), i.e. that

$$\kappa_1 = m.f.k_1,$$

where m is the proportionality constant having the dimension min^*. In analogy to this we assumed that also the rate constant for the

CMG influx observed under in vivo conditions κ_1^* is given by

$$\kappa_1^* = m \cdot f \cdot k_1^*,$$

where k_1^* is the rate constant characterizing the catalytic activity of the carrier system for the CMG influx.

Since in brain tissue the transport of glucose due to the movement of the extravascular fluid is negligible, the rate constant characterizing the CMG efflux from the brain tissue, k_2^*, is determined only by the catalytic activity of the carrier system. Therefore, the ratio κ_1^*/k_2^* can be expressed as follows:

$$\frac{\kappa_1^*}{k_2^*} = m \cdot f \cdot \frac{k_1^*}{k_2^*} . \qquad (13)$$

This equation indicates that the ratio κ_1^*/k_2^* can be expected to be directly proportional to the local perfusion rate and to the ratio of the rate constants characterizing the catalytic activity of the carrier system for CMG influx and efflux (k_1^*/k_2^*).

After rearranging of eq. (13) one obtains:

$$f = \frac{1}{m} \cdot \frac{k_2^*}{k_1^*} \cdot \frac{\kappa_1^*}{k_2^*} . \qquad (14)$$

In this relationship the value of κ_1^*/k_2^* can be obtained from CMG-dPET data. The ratio k_1^*/k_2^* is not known. However, as discussed in Appendix II there are theoretical reasons which suggest that $k_1^* = k_2^*$. Therefore, we assumed that the ratio $k_1^*/k_2^* = 1$. (The validity of this assumption has yet to be proven by independent measurements of local flow).

Under these conditions,

$$f = \frac{1}{m} \cdot \frac{\kappa_1^*}{k_2^*} . \qquad (15)$$

This is the algorithm used in this study for the determination of the local perfusion rate.

In order to determine the value of the constant m, we substituted in eq. (15) for the ratio κ_1^*/k_2^* the average value of κ_1^*/k_2^* determined in this study by the CMG technique in gray matter (κ_1^*/k_2^* = 0.88). As an estimate for the local perfusion rate, f, the average value for the perfusion in gray matter, that was observed by Obrist et al. (23) in normal humans by the use of Xe-133 inhalation and blood sampling technique, was used (f = 0.88 ml/min g).

Under these conditions, the value of m appears to be 1 min. This value was used for all perfusion determinations in the present study.

RESULTS AND DISCUSSION

Using the approach described above the values of κ_1^*/k_2^* in normal cortex were determined to be 0.80 - 0.98. In normal white matter values of 0.3 - 0.4 were observed. These values agree favourably with the data reported in the literature for the measurements in vivo (3,4,24).

The average value of k_2^* was determined to be 0.235 min^{-1} in normal cortex and 0.121 min^{-1} in normal white matter. These values are in good agreement with the data reported by Sokoloff et al. (3) with ^{14}C-deoxyglucose and by Pardridge et al. (17) with ^{14}C-methylglucose for rat brains and by Reivich et al. (24) with ^{11}C-deoxyglucose for human brain. They are, however, higher than the values reported for humans by Phelps et al. (4) with ^{18}F-deoxyglucose.

The value of k_2^* in cortex is approximately twice the value in white matter. This may be expected since the measured k_2^* is not only determined by the catalytic activity of the carrier system but also influenced by the total area of exchange surface, and it is known that the total capillary surface in the cortex is approximately twice as high as in white matter.

The local unidirectional glucose transport rate (LUGTR) was calculated to be 0.43 - 0.6 μmol/min g in normal cortex and 0.09 - - 0.12 μmol/min g in white matter. These values are higher than the values reported with ^{18}F-deoxyglucose (FDG) (4,25,26). This is expected, because CMG measures the glucose influx and not the net glucose transport rate, as does FDG.

The ratio of the glucose influx rate in cortex to that in white matter was approximately 4 . This value is in good agreement with data reported by Kennedy et al. (27), who used FDG in monkeys. It is, however, higher than the ratio measured with FDG in humans by Phelps et al. (4).

The local perfusion rate calculated according to equation (15) was 0.8 - 0.98 ml/min g in normal cortex and 0.3 - 0.4 ml/min g in white matter. These data are slightly higher than the values reported by Ingwar et al. (28), who used ^{133}Xe injected into the internal carotid artery. The values for the white matter are higher than those determined by ^{133}Xe (23). This is probably due to the inclusion of larger vessels in the ROIs white matter in the present study.

The CMG was found to be effectively accumulated in normal brain cortex; significantly lower accumulation was observed in normal white matter (see Fig. 4).

The data obtained in stroke patients demonstrate that the accumulation defects in CMG scintigrams are frequently larger than the hypodense zones in CT. This finding is in close agreement with observations made by others (5,29) using the FDG technique.

In the areas of accumulation defects, which were observed in morphologically intact cortex (cortex areas interpreted as "normal" on CT scan), the changes of LPR were either parallel to or significantly different from the relative changes of LUGTR.

Parallel changes of LPR and LUGTR could be observed, for example in a patient with left homonymous hemianopia caused by infarction in the distribution area of the right middle cerebral artery, but with intact posterior cerebral artery. The CMG image, which was taken 5 - 6 cm above the orbitomeatal line clearly showed two accumulation defects. One of them, a large frontotemporal area extending from the surface into the depth of the brain,

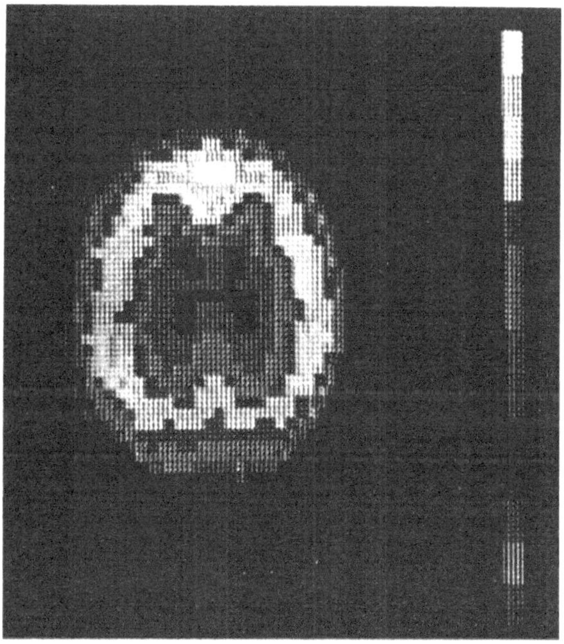

FIG. 4

CMG distribution pattern in normal brain.

closely correlated with CT findings (30). The second was in the occipital lobe, where CT did not show any abnormality. In this area both the LPR (0.68 ml/min g) and LUGTR (0.38 μmol/min g) were 22 % lower than the corresponding values in the opposite hemisphere. The rate constant characterizing the glucose carrier system (k_2^*) in this area was, however, the same as that in the opposite hemisphere. This suggests that the reduction of LUGTR in morphologically intact visual cortex was solely due to the reduction of the LPR. Reivich et al. (31), Phelps et al. (32) and Kuhl et al. (5), observed in normals a similar degree of decrease in glucose net flux into the visual cortex when visual stimulation was shut off. The similarity of data suggests that the accumulation defect observed in the visual cortex results from transport and perfusion response of the morphologically intact cortex to the destruction of visual pathways.

In another patient (a 43 years old male with symptoms of prolonged reversible ischemic neurological deficit) the neurological symptoms (sensory loss) suggested an alteration of corresponding brain tissue, but there were no CT findings. In CMG scans a clear accumulation defect in the temporoparietal cortex was recognized. In this area, the LPR (0.93 ml/min g) was normal. The LUGTR was, however, 40 % lower when compared with the opposite hemisphere. This reduction was solely due to 40 % reduction of the rate constant for the glucose carrier system. Also this observation is in a close agreement with observations of Kuhl et al. (5) and indicates that residual impairment of the glucose transport systems may follow transient ischemia and should be discussed as one of the reasons for deactivation of a morphologically intact cortex.

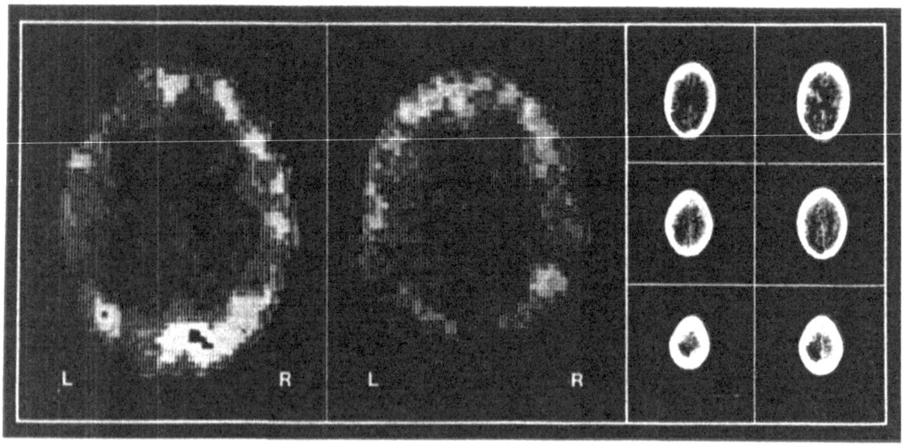

FIG. 5

CMG distribution and CT findings from a patient with moya-moya disease.

The results obtained in a patient with moya-moya disease (a 22 year old female) are demonstrated in Fig. 5. The only neurological finding in this case was homonymous hemianopia. The CT showed a hypodense area in the left occipital lobe indicating an old cerebral ischemic damage. Angiographically, a stenosis of the left internal carotid artery and of the left middle cerebral artery, associated with formation of a fine network of abnormal collateral vessels as well as a mild stenosis of the right middle cerebral artery, were demonstrated. In CMG scans the activity accumulation defects could be recognized in both the left and the right hemisphere at different levels. These defects were significantly larger than the hypodense areas in CT. In the residual non-infarcted left cortex that corresponded to the distribution of the left middle cerebral artery, the LPR (0.7 ml/min g) was reduced to 79 % when compared with the opposite non-affected hemisphere (0.88 ml/min g). The LUGTR, however, was practically the same as that in the opposite hemisphere. This was due to the significant increase of the rate constant for the glucose carrier system (140 % when compared with the opposite hemisphere). This probably reflects a mechanism compensating for a slowly developing perfusion deficit.

The results of a study done before and after extra-intracranial bypass surgery are demonstrated in Fig. 6. This study was carried out on a 72 year old female patient. In this case the initial

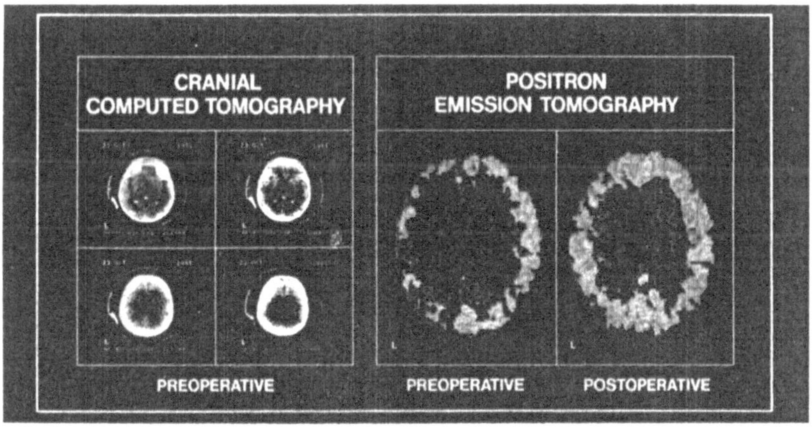

FIG. 6
CMG distribution images from a patient with occlusion of the left middle cerebral artery before and after extra-intracranial bypass operation.

symptom was a sudden onset of aphasia which, at first, lasted some minutes. In the following 4 months, 7 attacks were registerec In the later attacks the aphasia lasted up to one hour. Angiographically, a "kinking" of the left internal carotid artery without hemodynamic significance in the Dopplersonogram and a severe stenosis of the left middle cerebral artery were demonstrated. The CT-scan was normal. In a preoparative CMG scintigram large accumulation defects in the left cortex were evident. In this area, the local perfusion rate (0.79 ml/min g) was 10 % lower when compared with the contralateral hemisphere (0.88 ml/min g). The LUGTR in this area was 44 % lower than that in the opposite hemisphere. This disproportionally lower LUGTR was due to a lower value of the rate constant for the glucose carrier system. Subsequent to the CMG scintigraphy, an extra-intracranial bypass was performed. Postoperatively, a minor aphasic episode appeared for two days and diminished. A Dopplersonogram and an-angiography indicated that anastomosis was patent. The LPR in the treated hemisphere became normal (0.93 ml/min g) and was practically the same as LPR in the opposite hemisphere (0.96 ml/min g). Also the LUGTR increased. It did not, however, achieve the values observed in the opposite hemisphere. The persistently lower value of LUGTR (18 % reduction when compared to the opposite hemisphere) was due to a persistently lower value of the rate constant for the glucose carrier system.

APPENDIX I

For the quantitative evaluation of the data, all time activity curves were first normalized by dividing them by the number of pixels in ROI. The normalized time activity curves ($y(t)$) are directly proportional to the tissue or blood CMG concentration ($c(t)$), i.e.

$$c(t) = \beta \cdot y(t), \qquad (16)$$

where β is the proportionality factor relating CPM per pixel to concentration.

The normalized time activity curve from ROI sup. long. sinus ($y_B(t)$) was fitted with two exponential functions:

$$y_B(t) = A_1^* \cdot e^{-\lambda_1^* t} + A_2^* \cdot e^{-\lambda_2^* t} \qquad (17)$$

The intercepts A_1^* and A_2^* and slopes λ_1^* and λ_2^* were determined by the least square method.

The normalized time activity curve from blood was used as input function to express the time course of CMG concentration in brain tissue $c_2^*(t)$. After substituting eq. (17) in eqs. (16) and (2) the following expression is obtained:

$$c_2^*(t) = \beta \cdot \frac{\kappa_1^* \cdot A_1^*}{k_2^* - \lambda_1^*} \cdot e^{-\lambda_1^* t} + \beta \cdot \frac{\kappa_1^* \cdot A_2^*}{k_2^* - \lambda_2^*} \cdot e^{-\lambda_2^* t} + \quad (18)$$
$$+ \beta \cdot (y_2^*(0) - \frac{\kappa_1^* \cdot A_1^*}{k_2^* - \lambda_1^*} - \frac{\kappa_1^* \cdot A_2^*}{k_2^* - \lambda_2^*}) \cdot e^{-k_2^* t}$$

This equation demonstrates that the concentration of CMG in the brain tissue ($c_2^*(t)$) is described by the sum of three exponential functions.

Consequently, the time activity curve over the ROI brain ($y_2^*(t) = c_2^*(t)/\beta$) must also be expected to be described by the sum of three exponential functions.

$$y_2^*(t) = \frac{c_2^*(t)}{\beta} = B_1^* \cdot e^{-\lambda_1^* t} + B_2^* \cdot e^{-\lambda_2^* t} + B_3^* \cdot e^{-k_2^* t} \quad (19)$$

where

$$B_1^* = \frac{\kappa_1^* \cdot A_1^*}{k_2^* - \lambda_1^*} , \quad (20)$$

$$B_2^* = \frac{\kappa_1^* \cdot A_2^*}{k_2^* - \lambda_2^*} \quad \text{and} \quad (21)$$

$$B_3^* = (y_2^*(0) - B_1^* - B_2^*) \quad (22)$$

The time activity curves from different brain regions were fitted with three exponential functions by the least square method. (By this approximation, the slopes λ_1^* and λ_2^*, determined from the blood curve, were taken as fixed values.) This fitting provides the intercepts B_1^*, B_2^*, B_3^* and slope k_2^*.

Determination of κ_1^*. The value of κ_1^* can be determined from eq. (21):

$$\kappa_1^* = \frac{B_2^*}{A_2^*} \cdot (k_2^* - \lambda_2^*). \quad (23)$$

APPENDIX II

The carrier-mediated transport of glucose across the BBB has been demonstrated by several investigators. As summarized by Pardridge and Oldendorf (17), the blood-brain barrier hexose carrier exhibits properties compatible with those of mobile carrier including saturable uptake, stereospecificity, competitive inhibition with other hexoses and transport counterflow. Therefore, the glucose transport across the BBB is generally assumed to be comparible with a reversible unimolecular enzyme catalyzed reaction (33,34) i.e.

$$S_1 + C_1 \rightleftarrows (SC)_1 \rightleftarrows (SC)_2 \rightleftarrows C_2 + S_2 , \qquad (24)$$

where S_1 is the sugar in blood, S_2 is the sugar in tissue, C_1 is the carrier when it is on blood side, C_2 is the carrier on the tissue side, $(SC)_1$ is the complex of sugar and carrier on the blood side, and $(SC)_2$ is the complex of sugar and carrier on the tissue side (33). The rate of such a reaction is described by the general form of the rate equation and not by simple Michaelis-Menten equation (35,36). In the general form of the rate equation, the rate constant which characterize the catalytic activity of the carrier system for glucose influx, k_1, is described by the following expression (33):

$$k_1 = \frac{V_{M_1}}{K_{M_1} \cdot (1 + S_1/K_{M_1} + S_2/K_{M_2})} \qquad (25)$$

The rate constant which characterizes the catalytic activity of carrier system for glucose efflux, k_2 is given by:

$$k_2 = \frac{V_{M_2}}{K_{M_2} \cdot (1 + S_1/K_{M_1} + S_2/K_{M_2})} \qquad (26)$$

In these equations K_{M_1}, V_{M_1}, K_{M_2} and V_{M_2} are kinetic constants for glucose influx and efflux respectively.

According to experiments of Pardridge and Oldendorf (17), which were carried out on rat brains, the kinetic constants (K_{M_1}, V_{M_1} and K_{M_2}, V_{M_2}) for glucose influx and efflux are the same i.e.

$$K_{M_1} = K_{M_2} = K_M \text{ and } V_{M_1} = V_{M_2} = V_M .$$

Consequently the equations (25) and (26) can be written as follows:

$$k_1 = k_2 = \frac{V_M}{K_M(1 + S_1/K_M + S_2/K_M)} \qquad (27)$$

This means that the rate constant characterizing the catalytic activity of the carrier system for glucose influx can be expected to be the same as that for glucose efflux.

This conclusion is in close agreement with the experimental data of Lund-Andersen et al. (22), who found that the ^{14}C labelled 3-O-methyl glucose equilibrates in thick rat brain cortex slices at a concentration which relates to concentration of methyl glucose in the incubation medium in a ratio of 0.95 to 1.

FOOTNOTES

+ The experiments of Whitfield et al. (19) demonstrated that the half time for glucose influx in erythrocytes is more than 40 minutes. This observation indicates that in capillaries the exchange of glucose between blood plasma and erythrocytes cannot significantly influence the rapid exchange of glucose between blood plasma and brain tissue.

++ In our calculations we used the large vessel hematocrit as an estimate for the capillary hematocrit. This was based on the observation of Larsen and Lassen (37) who found that the average cerebral hematocrit is 92.2 % of the large vessel hematocrit. Against this assumption it might be argued that according to Eke (38), the optical hematocrit in superficial cortex capillaries is only 50 % of the large vessel hematocrit. However, according to Klitzman and Duling (39) (who observed the similary low values of microvascular hematocrit in striated muscle) by the evaluation of optical hematocrit it must be considered that

a.) the hematocrit in small arteries (100 - 200 μ) and in small veins (measured by the withdrawing and centrifuging of a blood sample) is 94 % of the hematocrit in the large vessels,

b.) the arteriovenous shunting of blood around the capillary bed is less than 2.5 % of the total blood flow to the examined capillary bed and

c.) the dilution of capillary blood by the fluid absorbed from the environment is less than 1 % of the measured flow.

Based on these data, the authors have concluded that the low values of the optical hematocrit in a capillary bed are due to the presence of a very slow moving plasma boundary layer in the capillaries. This means that the plasma in capillaries must be considered as consisting of at least two compartments: a "stationary" and a "dynamic" one. According to Klitzman and Duling (39), the values of the capillary hematocrit, when related to the dynamic component of plasma, are very similar to that of large vessels. Since the utilisation of glucose in the stationary component of the plasma is, if at all, very low, it becomes evident that, for the determination of the available glucose in the capillary network, not the stationary but the dynamic plasma component is relevant. Consequently, for the calculation of the glucose influx rate, the effective hematocrit (hematocrit related to the dynamic component of plasma in capillaries) and not the optical hematocrit, should be considered, Therefore, the use of the large vessel hematocrit in our calculations is throughout justifiable.

+++ If the values K_M^*, V_M^*, K_M and V_M determined by Pardridge et al. (17) in rat brains are considered, the value of $(V_M/V_M^*).(K_M^*/K_M)$ is 1.11.

* With respect to the meaning of m, the eqs. (3) and (13) were considered. According to these

$$\frac{k_1^*}{k_2^*} = \frac{m.f.k_1^*}{k_2^*} = \frac{c_{2ss}^*}{c_{Bss}^*} . \qquad (28)$$

In this relationship f is equal to F_i/W_i, where F_i is the flow perfusing W_i cm^3 of tissue; thus, eq. (28) can be rearranged as follows:

$$\frac{m.F_i}{W_i} . \frac{k_1^*}{k_2^*} = \frac{c_{2ss}^*}{c_{Bss}^*} . \qquad (29)$$

If, as discussed above k_1^*/k_2^* in normal cortex is assumed to be 1, one obtains:

$$\frac{m.F_i}{W_i} = \frac{c_{2ss}^*}{c_{Bss}^*} . \qquad (30)$$

In this relationship, the ratio $m.F_i/W_i$ represents the ratio ratio of two volumes. The term $m.F_i$ [cm^3] expresses the volume of blood passing W_i cm^3 of tissue in m minutes and W_i represents the tissue volume being perfused by this blood volume. The term c_{2ss}^*/c_{Bss}^* represents the partition coefficient of CMG. The eq. (30) thus indicates that the partition coefficient of CMG in vivo is proportional to flow with m being the proportionality constant and that the term $m.F_i$ [cm^3] probably represents the blood volume which actually serves as the relative intravascular distribution space for CMG.

ACKNOWLEDGEMENTS

The authors appreciate the discussions with Prof. L. Sokoloff, NIH, Bethesda, MD, Prof. M.E. Phelps and Dr. S.C. Huang, University of California, Los Angeles, CA, Prof. W. Shreeve, State University of New York, Stony Brook, NY, and Dr. L. Commerford, presently

Institute of Medicine, Nuclear Research Center Jülich, F.R.Germany.

REFERENCES

1. Mies G, Hossman KA: Double tracer autoradiographic investigation of regional blood flow and glucose metabolism during spreading depression. J Cereb Blood Flow Metabol 1, Suppl 1: 94-95, 1981

2. Pulsinelli W, Brierley J, Duffy T, Levy D, Plum F: Ischemic neuronal damage, postischemic regional blood flow and glucose metabolism in rat brain. J Cereb Blood Flow Metabol 1, Suppl 1: 166-167, 1981

3. Sokoloff L, Reivich M, Kennedy C, Des Rosiers MH, Patlak CS, Pettigrew KD, Sakurada O, Shinohara M: The ^{14}C deoxyglucose method for the measurement, of local cerebral glucose utilisation: Theory, procedure, and normal values in the conscious and anesthetized albino rat. J Neurochem 28: 897-916, 1977

4. Phelps ME, Huang SC, Hoffman EJ, Selin C, Sokoloff L, Kuhl DE: Tomographic measurement of local cerebral glucose metabolic rate in humans with ^{18}F-Fluoro-2-deoxy-D-glucose: Valididation of method. Ann of Neurol 6: 371-388, 1979

5. Kuhl DE, Phelps ME, Kowell AP, Metter EJ, Selin C, Winter J: Effects of stroke on local cerebral metabolism and perfusion: Mapping by emission computed tomography of ^{18}F-FDG and ^{13}N-NH_3. Annals of Neurol 8: 47-60, 1980

6. Vyska K, Freundlieb C, Höck A, Becker V, Feinendegen LE, Kloster G, Stöcklin G, Traupe H, Heiss WD: The assessment of glucose transport across the blood brain barrier in man by use of 3-^{11}C-methyl-D-glucose. J Cereb Blood Flow Metabol 1, Suppl 1: 42-43, 1981

7. Kloster G, Müller-Platz C, Laufer P: 3-^{11}C-methyl-D-glucose a potential agent for regional cerebral glucose utilisation. Synthesis, chromatography, and tissue distribution in mice. J Lab Comp Radiopharm 18: 855-863, 1981

8. Vyska K, Höck A, Freundlieb C, Feinendegen LE, Kloster G, Stöcklin G: 3-(C-11)-methyl glucose a promising agent for in vivo assessment of function of myocardial cell membrane. J Nucl Med 21: P56-P57, 1980 (Abstr.)

9. Heiss WD, Kloster G, Vyska K, Traupe C, Freundlieb C, Becker V, Feinendegen LE, Stöcklin G: Regional cerebral distribution of ^{11}C-methyl-D-glucose compared with CT perfusion patterns in stroke. J Cereb Blood Flow Metabol 1: Suppl 1: 506-507, 1981

10. Betz AL, Gilboe DD, Drewes LB: Effects of anoxia on net uptake and unidirectional transport of glucose into the isolat-

ed dog brain. Brain Research 67: 307-316, 1974

11. Bidder TG: Hexose translation across the blood-brain interface: configurational aspects. J Neurochem 15: 867-874, 1968

12. Cutler RWP, Sipe JC: Mediated transport of glucose between blood and brain in the cat. Am J Physiol 120: 1182-1186, 1971

13. Oldendorf WH: Brain uptake of radiolabeled amino acids, amines and hexoses after arterial injection. Am J Physiol 221: 1629-1639, 1971

14. Agnew WF, Crone C: Permeability of brain capillaries to hexoses and pentoses in the rabbit. Acta Physiol Scand 70: 168-175, 1967

15. Betz LA, Gilboe DD: Kinetics of cerebral glucose transport in vivo. Inhibition by 3-O-methyl-glucose. Brain Res 65: 368-372, 1974

16. Buschiazzo PM, Terrell EB, Regen DM: Sugar transport across the blood brain barrier. Am J Physiol 219: 1505-1513, 1970

17. Pardridge WM, Oldendorf WH: Kinetics of blood brain barrier transport of hexoses. Biochim Biophys Acta 22: 185-186, 1956

18. Czaky TZ, Wilson JE: The fate of 3-O-$^{14}CH_3$-glucose in the rat. Biochim Biophys Acta 382: 377-382, 1975

19. Whitfield CF, Rames RS, Morgan HE: Acceleration of sugar transport in avian erythrocytes by catecholamines. J Biol Chem 249: 4181-4188, 1974

20. Betz LA, Gilboe DD, Yudilevich DL, Drewes L: Kinetics of unidirectional glucose transport into the isolated dog brain. Am J Physiol 225: 586-592, 1973

21. Vyska K, Kloster G, Feinendegen LE, Heiss WD, Stöcklin G, Höck A, Freundlieb C, Aulich A, Schuier F, Thal HU, Becker V, Schmid A: Regional perfusion and glucose uptake determination with ^{11}C-methyl-glucose and dynamic positron emission tomography. In Heiss WD, Phelps ME, Eds. Positron emission tomography of the brain. Springer-Verlag Heidelberg (In press)

22. Lund-Andersen H, Kjeldsen CS: Kinetical analysis of the uptake of glucose analogs by rat brain cortex slices from nornormal and ischemic brain. In Levi G, Battistin L and Lajtha A, Eds. Transport phenomena in the nervous system: Physiological and pathological aspects. New York, London, Plenum Press, 1976, pp 265-272

23. Obrist WD, Thompson HK, King CH, Wang HS: Determination of

regional cerebral blood flow by inhalation of ^{133}Xe. Circ Res 20: 124-135, 1967

24. Reivich M, Alavi A, Wolf A, Greenberg JH, Fowler J, Christman D, MacGregor R, Jones SC, London J, Schiue C, Yonekura Y: Use of 2-deoxy-D(1-^{11}C)-glucose for the determination of local cerebral glucose metabolism in humans: Variation within and between subjects. J Cereb Blood Flow Metabol 2: 307-319, 1982

25. Phelps ME, Mazziotta JC, Huang SC: Study of cerebral function. J Cereb Blood Flow Metabol 2: 113-162, 1982

26. Huang SC, Phelps ME, Hoffman EJ, Sideris K, Selin CJ, Kuhl DE: Noninvasive determination of local cerebral metabolic rate of glucose in man. Am J Physiol 238: E69-E82, 1980

27. Kennedy C, Sakurada O, Shinohara M, Jehle J, Sokoloff L: Local cerebral glucose utilisation in the normal conscious macaque monkey. Ann Neurol 4: 293-301, 1979

28. Ingwar DA, Cronquist S, Ekberg R, Risberg J, Hoedt-Rasmussen K: Normal values of regional cerebral blood flow in man including flow and weight estimates of gray and white matter. Acta Neur Scand 41, Suppl 14: 72-84, 1965

29. Ackerman RH, Correia JA, Alpert NM, Baron JD, Gouliamos A, Grotta JC, Brownell GL, Taveras JM: Positron imaging in ischemic stroke disease using compounds labeled with ^{15}O. Arch Neurol 38: 537-543, 1981

30. Heiss WD, Vyska K, Kloster G, Traupe H, Freundlieb C, Höck A, Feinendegen LE, Stöcklin G: Demonstration of decreased functional activity of visual cortex by ^{11}C-methylglucose and positron emission tomography. Neuroradiol 23: 45-47, 1982

31. Reivich M, Greenberg J, Alavi A: The use of fluorodeoxy-glucose technique for mapping of functional neural pathways in man. Acta Neurol Scand 60, Suppl 72: 198-199, 1979

32. Phelps ME, Mazziotta JC, Kuhl DE, Nuwer M, Packwood J, Metter J, Engel J Jr: Tomographic mapping of human cerebral metabolism, visual stimulation and deprivation. Neurology 31: 517-529, 1981

33. Narahara HT, Özand P, Cori CF: Studies of tissue permeability VII. The effect of insulin on glucose generation and phosphorylation in frog muscle. J Biochem 235: 3370-3378, 1960

34. Macey RI: Mathematical models of membrane transport processes. In Andreoli TE, Hoffman JF and Fanestil DD, Eds. Physiology of membrane disorders. New York, London, Plenum Medical Book Company, 1979, pp 125-146

35. Mahler HR, Cordes EH: Biological Chemistry 2nd Edition, New York, Evanston, San Francisco, London, Harper and Row Publishers, 1971, pp 267-325

36. Segel IH: Enzyme kinetics. New York, London, Sydney, Toronto, Wiley - Interscience Publication, John Wiley, 1975, pp 34-39

37. Larsen OA, Lassen NA: Cerebral hematocrit in normal man. J Appl Physiol 19: 571-574, 1964

38. Eke A: Reflectometric mapping of microregional blood flow and blood volume in the brain cortex. J Cereb Blood Flow Metabol 2: 41-53, 1982

39. Klitzman B, Duling BR: Microvascular hematocrit and red cell flow in resting and contracting striated muscle. Am J Physiol 237: H481-H490, 1979

THE INDICATOR DILUTION METHOD: ASSUMPTIONS AND APPLICATIONS TO BRAIN UPTAKE

Olaf B. Paulson and Marianne M. Hertz

State University Hospital, Copenhagen, Denmark

INTRODUCTION

Evaluation of vascular permeability can be made using intra-arterial injection of two tracers, i.e. a test and an impermeable reference substance, and measurements of their concentrations in the venous outflow following a single passage through the organ, as first introduced by Chinard and co-workers (1,2). In his careful evaluation of this method, Crone made quantitative measurement possible and applied this to studies of blood-brain barrier glucose permeability (3,4).

The method has since been used in a number of clinical studies. The lack of extracerebral contamination and the larger circulation time in man compared to experimental animals made it possible to further evaluate and develop the indicator dilution method. Thus Lassen and co-workers and Bolwig and co-workers drew attention to pitfalls which might result from different intravascular behaviour of the reference and test substance (5,6). The method assumes homogeneity of the microcirculation, as it is based on a single capillary model. This assumption cannot quite be met in the brain: Hertz and Paulson showed that the shape of the venous outflow curves gave strong evidence for heterogeneity of the cerebral microcirculation (7). But, with appropriate precautions, the method can still be used for quantitative measurement of blood-brain permeability as discussed and illustrated in this chapter.

A problem which has not quite been solved as yet, is that of back-diffusion of tracer from brain to the blood during a single passage through the organ. Martín and Yudilevich have made corrections for it based on analysis of the shape of the outflow curves (7). However, especially in man, heterogeneity makes calculation of back-diffusion rather difficult. Furthermore, back-diffusion may be different for different substances, even if they have the same extraction.(8).

The present paper deals with the above mentioned methodological aspects of the tracer dilution method for evaluation of blood-brain barrier permeability. In addition a model for cerebral upta-

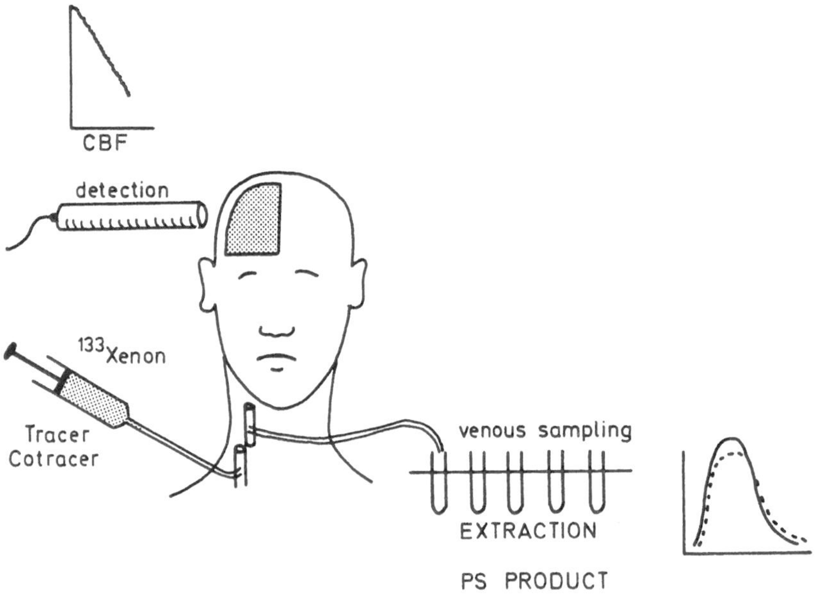

FIG. 1

Schematic illustration of the indicator dilution method in man, combined with measurement of cerebral blood flow.

ke rate of drugs is described.

THE INDICATOR DILUTION METHOD

The indicator dilution method consists of an intraarterial bolus injection (injection time c. 1 sec) of a test and an impermeable reference substance, immediately followed by serial venous outflow sampling (Fig. 1). The method measures unidirectional transcapillary loss during a single vascular transit in a non-steady state: it is assumed that the extracapillary test substance concentration is minimal, i.e. that no back-diffusion takes place until after the period of measurements.

In human studies, undertaken in connection with cerebral angiography, small catheters are placed in the internal carotid artery, supplying only the brain, and in the internal jugular vein, draining cerebral tissue.

Extracerebral contamination

In animal studies conditions are less advantageous than in man, because the vascular supply and drainage is less selective. Precautions must therefore be taken to ensure that only brain tissue is studied and that no extracerebral contamination occurs from facial muscles etc. An internal indicator for the degree of contamination can be used, as the cerebral extraction (fractional transcapillary loss) of small ions is extremely low (1%) compared to that in muscle tissue (50%); Thus the extraction of $^{24}Na^{+}$ will be a sensitive indicator of extracerebral contamination (9).

Calculation of extraction

The concentrations of test and reference substance in the venous samples divided by their concentrations in the injectate ($C_{ref}(t)$ and $C_{test}(t)$) give the outflow curve (Fig. 2) and allow calculation of the fractional transcapillary loss of test molecules (E) at any time (t):

$$E(t) = \frac{C_{ref}(t) - C_{test}(t)}{C_{ref}(t)} \qquad (1)$$

Intravascular separation of test and reference substance

The impermeable reference substance (e.g. albumin or labelled red cells) which stays in the vascular bed throughout the vascular transit allows calculation of the dilution of injectate until sampling. This, however, assumes identical intravascular behaviour of test and reference substance and such ideal conditions seldom exist. Two important phenomena, interlaminar diffusion and red cell carriage result in intravascular separation of test and reference substance, influencing considerably both the shape of the E(t) curve (Eq. 1) and the calculation of average E.

Interlaminar diffusion (also called Taylor's phenomenon) is the result of differences in the diffusibility of the test and reference substance, yielding a U-shaped E(t) curve and, when E is low, two cross-over points between the outflow curves (Fig. 3) (5,10). Labelled Na^{+} diffuses more rapidly than albumin away from the fast-moving axial core of the blood stream into the slowly moving peripheral parts. Thus immediately after the bolus injection, the Na^{+} curve lies below that of albumin and E(t) for Na^{+} is positive. On the first part of the downslope the Na^{+} curve lies above that of albumin as diffusion of labelled Na^{+} is now reversed: Na^{+} comes from the peripheral stream back into the axial stream and E(t) is now negative. Later, when the slow peripheral parts of the blood stream reach the venous outflow, Na^{+} has been washed out and its curve again lies below that of albumin.

Red cell carriage (precession) also influences the shape of the E(t) curve. A tracer which penetrates into the red cells has a shorter transit time than a pure plasma tracer because the ery-

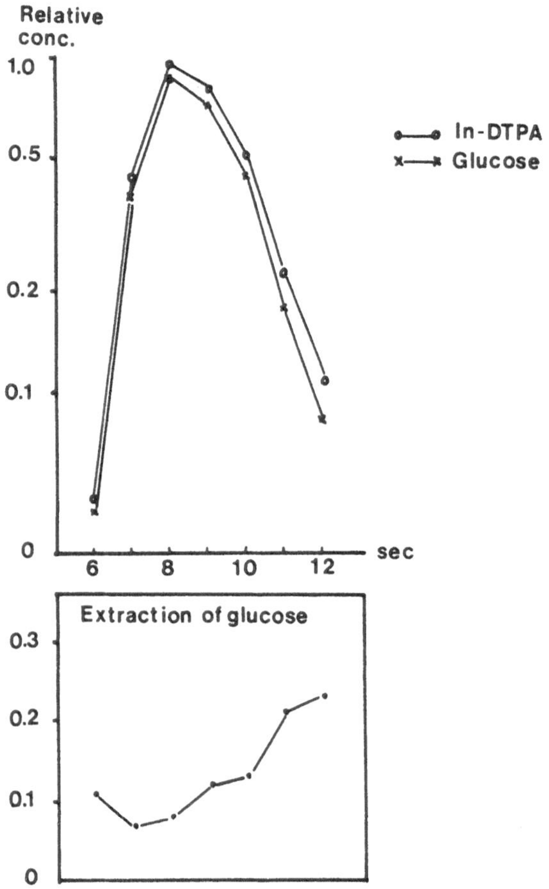

FIG. 2

Venous outflow curves in man for ^{14}C-D-glucose and reference substance, ^{113m}In-DTPA. Note E(t) increases with time as sign of heterogeneity (correction for intravascular separation does not change this shape).

throcyte transit time through the cerebral vascular bed is shorter than that of plasma (11). Fig. 4 illustrates how the outflow curve of Cl^-, which penetrates red cells, is displaced to the left of, but parallel to, the curve of Na^+ which remains in plasma.

To obtain a true E value, attention must be paid to these intravascular phenomena by matching test and reference closely or by the use of multiple references and by integrating appropriate parts of the venous outflow curves. Thus if interlaminar diffusion is present, E, when low, is best calculated by integrating Eq. 1

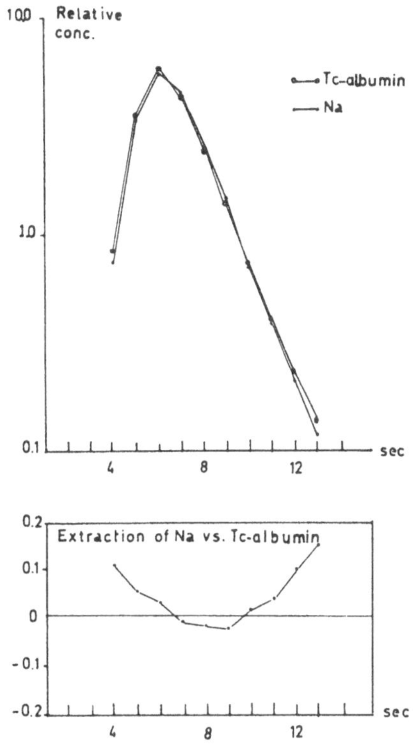

FIG. 3

Venous outflow curves in man for $^{24}Na^{+}$ and ^{99m}Tc-albumin. Note the two cross-over points and the U-shaped E(t) curve as evidence of interlaminar diffusion.

from time zero to a time on the downslope between the two cross-over points of the tracer dilution curves where the reference curve has reached 40% of its peak value. At this point the false negative and false positive E(t) values balance each other out (5). If red cell carriage is present and E very low, then it is best calculated by integrating Eq. 1 from zero to infinity after extrapolation (6). When E is larger, the tail part of the venous outflow curve of test substance will be influenced by back-diffusion from the brain to the tissue; then the mentioned integrations of Eq. 1 for the calculation of E, and especially the last mentioned with extrapolation to infinity, will no longer be meaningful. In such instances the E value is best calculated by integrating Eq. 1 over a short interval (a few sec in man) around the top of the venous outflow curve of the reference substance (7). The latter mode of calculating E will be commented upon in the following paragraph.

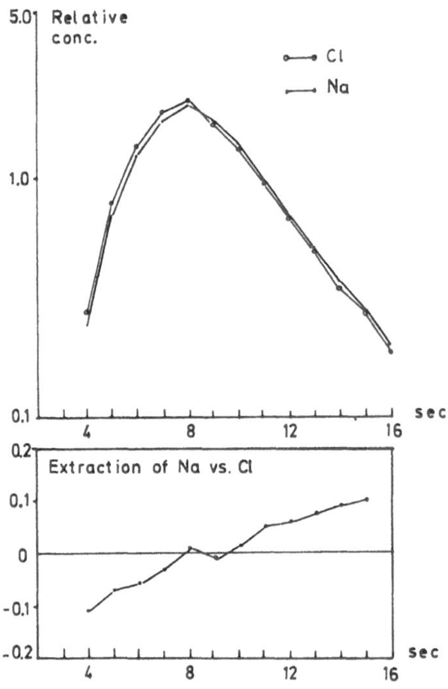

FIG. 4

Venous outflow curves in man for $^{36}Cl^-$ and $^{24}Na^+$. Note the shorter transit time of $^{36}Cl^-$ and increase of E(t) as evidence of $^{36}Cl^-$ penetration into the red cells.

Heterogeneity of capillary flow

The final assumption of the method in its classical form is that the vascular bed is homogeneous, i.e. as it is derived from a single capillary model it applies strictly to a capillary bed of equal lengths, flows and permeabilities.

The assumption is not valid for the brain in general. Thus, a human study has shown the presence of microvascular heterogeneity, i.e. capillaries with short transit times have lower extractions than capillaries with longer transit times (7). In this case the true extraction increases with time as does the apparent extraction until back-diffusion sets in (Fig. 2). This can also be shown by theoretical modelling (12). When a large part of the curve is integrated (see above) the calculated average E will be a good estimate of the true value. However, for substances with high E and high back-diffusion the tail of the curve can be heavily influenced by the back-diffusion and cannot be used for the calculations. To avoid underestimation of E due to heterogeneity, it is better to calculate average E from a short part of the curves around the peak - and not from the whole upslope. The influence of intravascular separation phenomena is also less pronounced around the peak. Thus, the above mentioned problems can be minimized and a good estimation of true average E obtained (see Hertz and Paulson (7) for details).

PERMEABILITY SURFACE AREA PRODUCT (PS)

Above we have discussed the determination of the extraction (E) using the indicator dilution method with a single injection of test and reference substance into the arterial inlet. We will now consider the calculation of the permeability-surface area product (PS), firstly under conditions of microvascular homogeneity, i.e. for an organ built up as a classical single capillary model where all capillaries have the same P, S and E values. Thereafter, conditions of microcirculatory heterogeneity will be dealt with. We will not consider P and S separately, but only mention that S, the capillary surface area in the human brain based on Cobb's observations is about 190 cm^2/g in grey matter and about 57 cm^2/g in white matter (13). In the following, E, unless otherwise stated, is considered to be the true unidirectional fractional extraction of the substance during its passage through the organ.

PS under conditions of microvascular homogeneity

Under these conditions, as shown by Crone (3) the PS product is determined by the equation

$$PS = - F' \ln(1-E) \quad \text{or} \quad E = 1 - e^{PS/F'} \qquad (2)$$

where F' is the solvent flow through the organ, i.e. the fraction of the blood flow in which the test substance equilibrates often the plasma flow. E is the unidirectional extraction of the test substance as discussed earlier. This equation and its derivation is analogous to the one derived for lung diffusion by Bohr (14), for inert gasses by Kety (15), and for indicator diffusion with steady arterial infusion by Renkin (16). The equation can be made more general so as to apply also to substances such as drugs which are protein bound and carbon dioxide which, in the blood, is in essentially instantaneous equilibrium with a much larger bicarbonate pool (17,18). The equation then becomes:

$$PS = - \phi F \ln(1-E) \quad \text{or} \quad E = 1 - e^{-PS/\phi F} \qquad (3)$$

where ϕ is the apparent volume of distribution of the substance in whole blood, given below by Eq. 8. F is the total blood flow through the organ. In the present model with zero brain concentration the derivation of Eq. 3 is as follows:

The unidirectional flux (J) across the blood-brain barrier can be expressed as

$$J = PS\ \bar{C}_{cp,free} \qquad (4)$$

when $\bar{C}_{cp,free}$ is the average capillary free plasma concentration of the substance. J can also be expressed as:

$$J = F\ E\ C_{ab,total} \qquad (5)$$

where $C_{ab,total}$ is the arterial total blood concentration of the substance.

In order to compare these two equations we want to use the mean capillary total blood concentration, $\bar{C}_{cb,total}$ in Eq. 5 instead of the value for arterial blood. This can be calculated from the arterial and venous concentrations as the fractional extraction in the single capillary model is the same in all segments of the capillary, i.e. $dC_{cb,total}(x)/dx = \text{constant} \cdot C_{cb,total}(x)$, where $C_{cb,total}(0)$ = the arterial concentration $C_{ab,total}$ and $C_{cb,total}(1)$ = the venous concentration $C_{vb,total}$. Integration gives

$$\bar{C}_{cb,total} = (C_{vb,total} - C_{ab,total})/\ln(1-E) \qquad (6)$$

where E is the extraction corresponding to the whole blood concentrations, $E = (C_{ab,total} - C_{vb,total})/C_{ab,total})$.

Inserting Eq. 6 and the expression for E into Eq. 5 one obtains:

$$J = F\ \bar{C}_{cb,total}\ \ln(1-E) \qquad (7)$$

and from Eq. 4 and 7:

$$PS = -\frac{\bar{C}_{cb,total}}{\bar{C}_{cp,free}}\ F\ \ln(1-E)$$

which is Eq. 3 with:

$$\phi = \frac{\bar{C}_{cb,total}}{\bar{C}_{cp,free}} = K\ \left(\frac{\bar{C}_{cp,free}}{\bar{C}_{cp,total}}\right)^{-1} \qquad (8)$$

In the case that conversion between the free plasma fraction and the non-free whole blood fractions is rapid compared to the transit through the cerebrovascular bed, then the ratio in Eq. 8 for capillary concentrations will be equal to the corresponding ratio for arterial blood (It is here assumed that the extraction in the capillaries have not changed the equilibrium ratio). Under such conditions it is evident that the middle part of Eq. 8 directly express the apparent volume of distribution of the substance in whole blood, e.g. for carbon dioxide the whole blood concentration of bicarbonate + carbon dioxide divided by the carbon dioxide concentration in plasma. The right side of Eq. 8 expresses that ϕ is a constant divided by the free fraction of the plasma concentration, e.g. a constant divided by the non protein bound fraction of the plasma concentration of a drug. The constant is one with which the total plasma concentration has to be multiplied in order to get the total blood concentration. But, ϕ may in any instance be estimated from known steady state values in blood. The crucial point is then whether the thus determined ϕ will be representative for average capillary blood, i.e. whether the conversion from the non-free to the free fraction is rapid enough. Experimental results have shown that this is the case both for carbon dioxide and for several drugs (17,18).

The indicator dilution method has been modified using a hyperosmolar bolus to measure not only diffusion (P_d) across the blood-brain barrier, but also water filtration (P_f) across it (9).

PS under conditions of microvascular heterogeneity

The single capillary model seems not to be valid for the brain as a whole organ, but this problem can be circumvented by calculation of average E with integration of parts of the outflow curves as discussed previously in this chapter.

Another, and mathematically more correct, calculation of E under these circumstances has recently been proposed by Bass and Robinson (20) who in principle weighted the extraction of each part of the outflow curves by the frequency function of the transit times of the intravascular reference substance ($h(t) = C_{ref}(t)/\int_0^\infty C_{ref}(t)dt$) and obtained:

$$PS = - \phi F \int_0^\infty h(t) \ln(1-E(t))dt \qquad (9)$$

ϕ has been added to the equation to make it comparable to our Eq.3. It appears that if E(t) is constant, the equation is simply reduced to Eq. 3 as $\int_0^\infty h(t)dt = 1$.

Bass and Robinson also considered another type of heterogeneity where the capillaries delivering tracer in each time interval are heterogeneous, i.e. have not extracted equally (20). Here there need not be a time dependence of E(t), since this heterogeneity may affect all consecutive samples equally. If this type of heterogeneity is present in addition to the above mentioned heterogeneity the equation for PS becomes:

$$PS = - \phi F \int_0^\infty h(t) [\ln(1- E(t)) + \tfrac{1}{2} \varepsilon^2[\ln(1-E(t))]^2]dt \qquad (10)$$

ε is here the coefficient of variation of the distribution of PS/F over the capillaries in the tracer delivering suborgan, i.e. a term which increases with increasing heterogeneity. It appears that the introduction of the term ε increases the PS value, and that disregarding this type of heterogeneity would result in an underestimation of PS. The correction introduced by the ε term is, however, small (20). It also appears that the ε correction becomes relatively less important at small E values and thus very small $[\ln(1-E(t))]^2$ values. If only the last mentioned type of heterogeneity is present, and E(t) is constant, Eq. 10 is reduced and the integral sign and h(t) function disappear as for Eq. 9.

Although matematically more correct, limitations in the use of Eq. 9 and 10 are also present as the whole venous outflow curves have to be used, including the tail part which is influenced by back-diffusion of test substance from the brain to the blood. Thus, using these equations one obtains PS values which may underestimate the true PS values, especially when the extraction is high. At present we still prefer to calculate the PS values using the more simple estimation described above, of the average E value because all PS calculations have limitations and deviation from the true PS values is in any case rather small.

Physiological modulation of PS

Much attention has been focused on measurement of exact transfer parameters which in turn allow calculations of kinetic values for transport across the blood-brain barrier. However, it is worth noting that transfer is not a fixed entity but subject to a variety of modulations by different physiological conditions, e. g. hormonal and by pH (21,22). First and foremost, blood flow changes have been shown to influence the size of the PS product (22,23). Non-uniform circulation, probably in the form of capillary intermittency where more vascular channels open up at high flows, can explain the PS increase with flow. A larger surface is then available for diffusional exchange.

BACK-DIFFUSION

During transit through the cerebrovascular bed the test substance diffuses from the blood to the cerebral tissue. But, once it has crossed the blood-brain barrier it may not only remain in the cerebral tissue but may also diffuse back to the blood. This back-diffusion becomes relatively more marked at the tail part of the tracer dilution curves when more substance has crossed from the blood to the cerebral tissue and when the capillary concentration of test substance is rapidly falling. Back-diffusion is different for different substances, e.g. much more marked for amino acids than for glucose (7), probably depending on diffusion constants and volumes of distribution in different compartments of the tissue (Paulson, Patlak and Hertz, under preparation).

For substances with low or medium extractions the influence of back-diffusion can be minimized, although not eliminated, by integrating appropriate parts of the venous outflow curves (7). For substances with very high extraction, such as water, we have previously used a correction where the tail part of the curve representing pure back-diffusion was extrapolated back to the top of the curve and subtracted from it (19). This might be an overcorrection as not all tracer particles have been available for diffusion across the blood-brain barrier at the peak of the tracer dilution curve and as the peak of "vascular concentration of extracted substance" will first be reached later on (24). On the other hand it might also be an undercorrection as the venous outflow curve initially is higher than expected due to shunting by diffusion, i.e. test molecules leaving the vascular volume near the arteriolar end diffuse through the tissue to the nearest venule more rapidly than intravascular reference molecules which are carried by the capillary blood flow. However, shunting by diffusion mainly influences the very first part of the venous outflow curve (24,25). Thus, this simple correction still seems suitable albeit a little rough.

In their description of the method, Martîn and Yudilevich used a derivation which allowed correction for back-diffusion based on the actually measured venous outflow curves of test and reference substance (8). The analysis, however, was based on the assumption of homogeneity with a constant true E value and therefore strongly weighted the E value corresponding to the initial part of the venous outflow curves. The analysis will therefore underestimate the average E if heterogeneity is present with an increasing E(t).

CEREBRAL UPTAKE RATE OF DRUGS

The cerebral uptake rate or the cerebral concentration of a drug as a function of time can be calculated if the arterial concentration profile is known, if the distribution ratio between blood and tissue at equilibrium is known, and if its extraction across the blood-brain barrier and the cerebral blood flow are known (17,26). For the derivations given below it is furthermore assumed that the drug reaches and leaves the cerebral tissue by diffusion across the blood-brain barrier, i.e. either the drug is not metabolised in the brain or the rate of metabolism is negligible compared to the transfer rate across the blood-brain barrier, and the exchange between brain tissue and cerebrospinal fluid is negligible compared to the transfer across the blood-brain barrier. Finally, it is assumed that the permeability of the drug is the same in both directions across the blood-brain barrier.

In the following, C_a, C_c, $\bar{C}_c$, C_v, and C_{br} designate the drug concentrations in total arterial, total capillary, mean total capillary and total venous blood and in the brain tissue respectively. ϕ designates the apparent volume of distribution of the drug in total blood as given by Eq. 8. λ designates the brain-to-blood concentration ratio at equilibrium, i.e. $\lambda\phi$ is the apparent volume of distribution of the drug in the cerebral tissue. $\bar{C}_c(t)/\phi$ and $C_{br}(t)/\lambda\phi$ are then the free concentration fractions available for diffusion.

The change in drug concentration in the brain will be determined by

$$dC_{br}(t) = \left(\frac{\bar{C}_c(t)}{\phi} - \frac{C_{br}(t)}{\lambda\phi}\right)PS\ dt \qquad (11)$$

In order to express the mean capillary drug concentration by the arterial one, we consider a segment dx of a capillary with the length l. In any segment of the capillary the diffusion across the blood-brain barrier will be determined by:

$$F\ dC_c(t,x) = -\ PS\ \left(\frac{C_c(t,x)}{\phi} - \frac{C_{br}(t)}{\phi\lambda}\right)dx$$

Integration with regards to x yields:

$$C_c(t,x) - \frac{C_{br}(t)}{\lambda} = \left(C_c(t,0) - \frac{C_{br}(t)}{\lambda}\right)\ e^{-(PS/\phi F)x} \qquad (12)$$

Inserting $C_c(t,0) = C_a(t)$, integrating this equation from $x = 0$ to $x = 1$, and dividing by the integral $\int_o^l dx = l$ gives the mean capillary concentration:

$$\bar{C}_c(t) = \frac{\phi F}{PS}\left(C_a(t) - \frac{C_{br}(t)}{\lambda}\right)\left(e^{-PS/\phi F} - 1\right) + \frac{C_{br}(t)}{\lambda} \qquad (13)$$

Inserting Eq. 13 into 11, and Eq. 3 into this new equation one obtains:

$$dC_{br}(t) = FE\ \left(C_a(t) - \frac{C_{br}(t)}{\lambda}\right)dt$$

or integrating

$$C_{br}(t) = e^{-FEt/\lambda}\ [C_{br}(0) + FE \int_o^t e^{FE\tau/\lambda}\ C_a(\tau)d\tau] \qquad (14)$$

which has to be solved for any particular $C_a(t)$ function.

Most often $C_a(t)$ can be described as a constant and a sum of exponential functions (each of which may be zero):

$$C_a(t) = b + \sum_{i=1}^{n} a_i\ e^{-\alpha_i t} \qquad (15)$$

where b, a_i and α_i are constants.

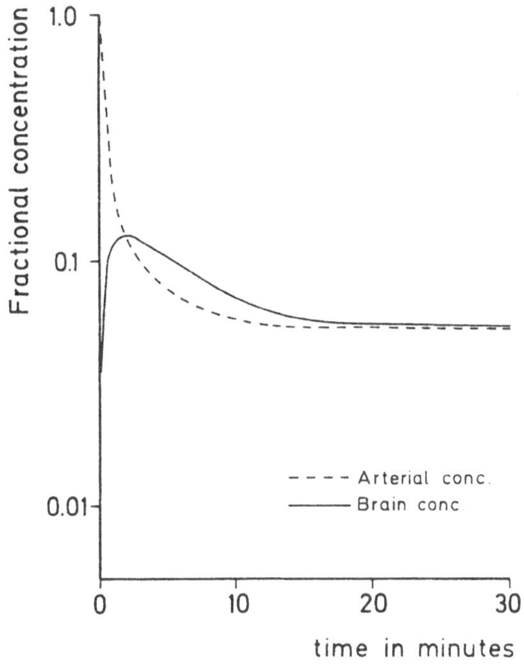

FIG. 5

Arterial and cerebral grey matter concentrations of clonazepam following a rapid intravenous injection.

Inserting 15 into 14 and assuming $C_{br}(o)$ = yields

$$C_{br}(t) =$$

$$\lambda b - \lambda b e^{-FEt/\lambda} + \sum_{i=1}^{n} \frac{FE\lambda a_i}{FE - \lambda\alpha_i} (e^{-\alpha_i t} - e^{-FEt/\lambda}) \quad (16)$$

This equation, 16, has been used to evaluate the cerebral uptake rate of antiepileptic drugs (17). For clonazepam, the arterial concentration profile following an intravenous injection of drug was determined experimentally and found to be a sum of three exponential functions: $Ca(t) = a_1 e^{-\alpha_1 t} + a_2 e^{-\alpha_2 t} + a_3 e^{-\alpha_3 t}$ where $a_1 = 0.85$, $a_2 = 0.12$, $a_3 = 0.33$, $\alpha_1 = 3.0$, $\alpha_2 = 0.14$ and $\alpha_3 = 1.1 \times 10^{-3}$. The unbound plasma fraction, according to the literature, is 0.53 and ϕ was set to 1/0.53. For cerebral cortical tissue (grey matter) λ was set to 1. E and F, determined experimentally, were 0.42 and 0.52 ml g^{-1} min^{-1} respectively. The resulting cerebral concentration curve calculated by Eq. 16 reached equilibrium with the arterial concentration already 2 min after maximal arterial concentration as illustrated in Fig. 5.

SUMMARY

The indicator dilution method is described. A bolus containing a test substance and an impermeable reference substance which remains in the vascular bed is injected into the arterial inlet to the organ and blood samples are simultaneously collected from the venous outflow. Intravascular phenomena (interlaminar diffusion and red cell carriage) have to be taken into account when evaluating the venous outflow curves. Analysis of the shape of the cerebral venous outflow curves reveals that microvascular heterogeneity is present. The permeability surface area product (PS) is calculated as $-\phi F \ln(1-E)$ where ϕ is the volume of distribution of the test substance in blood, F the blood flow and E the fractional extraction of the test substance during the single passage through the organ as calculated from the venous outflow curves. PS is influenced by several physiological factors, and among these especially by the blood flow level. Influence on the calculated extractions of back-diffusion of test substance from the tissue can be minimized by evaluating appropriate parts of the venous outflow curve, but back-diffusion deserves further evaluation. Knowledge of the extraction of a substance, of the cerebral blood flow, and of some other physiological variables allows to calculate the cerebral uptake rate or cerebral concentration as function of time when the arterial concentration profile is known.

REFERENCES

1. Chinard FP, Flexner LB: Capillary permeability. Bull Johns Hopkins 88:489-492,1951

2. Chinard FP, Vosburgh GJ, Enns T: Transcapillary exchange of water and of other substances in certain organs of the dog. Amer J Physiol 183:221-234,1955

3. Crone C: The permeability of capillaries in various organs determined by use of the indicator diffusion' method. Acta Physiol Scand 58:292-305,1963

4. Crone C: Facilitated transfer of glucose from blood into brain tissue. J Physiol 181:103-113,1965

5. Lassen NA, Trap-Jensen J, Alexander SC, Olesen J, Paulson OB: Blood-brain barrier studies in man using the double-indicator method. Amer J Physiol 200:1627-1633,1971

6. Bolwig TG, Hertz MM, Paulson OB, Spotoft H, Rafaelsen OJ: The permeability of the blood-brain barrier during electrically induced seizures in man. Europ J Clin Invest 7:87-93, 1977

7. Martín P, Yudilevich D: A theory for the quantification of transcapillary exchange by tracer-dilution curves. Am J Physiol 207:162-168,1964

8. Hertz MM, Paulson OB: Heterogeneity of cerebral capillary flow in man and its consequences for estimation of blood-brain barrier permeability. J Clin Invest 65:1145-1151,1980

9. Hertz MM, Bolwig TG: Blood-brain barrier studies in the rat: an indicator dilution technique with tracer sodium as an internal standard for estimation of extracerebral contamination. Brain Research 107:333-343,1976

10. Crone C, Lassen NA: The extraction fraction of a capillary bed to hydrophilic molecules. In Crone C and Lassen NA, Eds. Capillary Permeability. New York, Academic Press, 1970, pp 48-59

11. Larsen OA, Lassen NA: Cerebral hematocrit in normal man. J Appl Physiol 19:571-574,1964

12. Levitt DG: Quantification of error of the E_0 method of measurement of capillary permeability for certain capillary and organ models. In Crone and Lassen NA, Eds. Capillary Permeability. New York, Academic Press, 1970, pp 81-103

13. Cobb S: The cerebrospinal blood vessels. In Penfield E, Ed. Cytology and Cellular Pathology of the Nervous System. New York, Hoeber, 1932, pp 575-610

14. Bohr C: Über die spezifische Tätigkeit der Lungen bei der respiratorischen Gasaufnahme und ihr Verhalten zu der durch die Alveolarwand stattfindenden Gasdiffusion. Scand Arch Physiol 22:221-280,1909

15. Kety SS: The theory and application of the exchange of inert gas at lung and tissues.Pharmaco Rev 3:1-41,1951

16. Renkin EM: Transport of potassium-42 from blood to tissue in isolated mammalian skeletal muscles. Amer J Physiol 197:1205-1210,1959

17. Paulson OB, Györy A, Hertz MM: Blood-brain barrier transfer and cerebral uptake of antiepileptic drugs. Clin Pharmacol Ther 32:466-477,1982

18. Friis ML, Paulson OB, Hertz MM. Carbon dioxide permeability of the blood-brain barrier in man. Microvasc Res 20:71-80, 1980

19. Paulson OB, Hertz MM, Bolwig TG, Lassen NA: Filtration and diffusion of water across the blood-brain barrier in man. Microvasc Res 13:113-124,1977

20. Bass L, Robinson PJ: Capillary permeability of heterogeneous organs: A parsimonious interpretation of indicator diffusion data. Clin Exp Pharmacol Physiol 9:363-388,1982

21. Hertz MM, Paulson OB, Barry DI, Christensen JS, Svendsen PA. Insulin increases glucose transfer across the blood-brain barrier in man. J Clin Invest 67:597-604,1981

22. Hertz MM, Paulson OB. Transfer across the human blood-brain barrier: Evidence for capillary recruitment and for a paradox glucose permeability increase in hypocapnia. Microvasc Res 24:364-376,1982

23. Phelps ME, Sung-Cheng Huang, Hoffman EJ, Selin C, Kuhl DE: Cerebral extraction of N-13 ammonia: its dependence on cerebral blood flow and capillary permeability - surface area product. Stroke 12:607-619,1981

24. Perl W. An interpolation model for evaluating permeability from indicator dilution curves. In Crone C and Lassen NA, Eds. Capillary Permeability. New York, Academic Press, 1970, pp 185-201

25. Brodersen P, Sejrsen P, Lassen NA. Diffusion bypass of Xenon in brain circulation. Circ Res 32:363-369,1973.

26. Rapoport SU, Ohno K, Pettigrew K: Drug entry into the brain. Brain Res 172:354-359,1979

MEASUREMENT OF RECEPTOR-LIGAND BINDING: THEORY AND PRACTICE

David E. Schafer

Veterans Administration Medical Center, West Haven, CT

1. INTRODUCTION

1.1. Scope of the Subject

1.1.1. What Is a Receptor? The word "receptor" may seem at times to mean something different to almost everyone; this is not particularly surprising, since investigators in a wide variety of separate fields routinely employ the term to refer to something they work with. They may use it to refer to cellular components that specifically bind neurotransmitters; classical hormones; other hormone-like agents, such as paracrines, growth factors, and interferons; plant and bacterial toxins; lectins; antigens; antibodies; transported molecules and ions; second messengers; and ultimately the entire spectrum of drugs and poisons. In short, the concept of a "receptor" is truly protean (some might prefer to call it lipoprotean).

The elementary theoretical description outlined in this chapter can be applied with minimal changes to all, or almost all, these systems. Therefore, although in any given field the precise definition of the object of study is usually critical, for our present purpose a "receptor" may be virtually anything anybody calls a receptor. Let us say that a receptor is any biomolecule whose (a) specific (b) binding of (c) a chemical agent ("ligand") from either inside or outside the cell (d) initiates, or prevents the initiation of, (e) a biological response. Some of the possibilities are suggested in Fig. 1.

This working definition is deliberately vague. The ligand may be almost any kind of substance, physiological, pathological, or synthetic, from almost any source. The specificity of binding may be high, but is rarely absolute. With a bit of caution, most of the material in this chapter can apply equally to receptors in the extracellular compartments, plasma membrane, or cytosol. The "response" may be, and usually is, a complex chain of events in the cell; the chain, which may be branched, usually culminates in one or more classical "responses"--events, such as secretion or contraction, that can be observed from outside the cell.

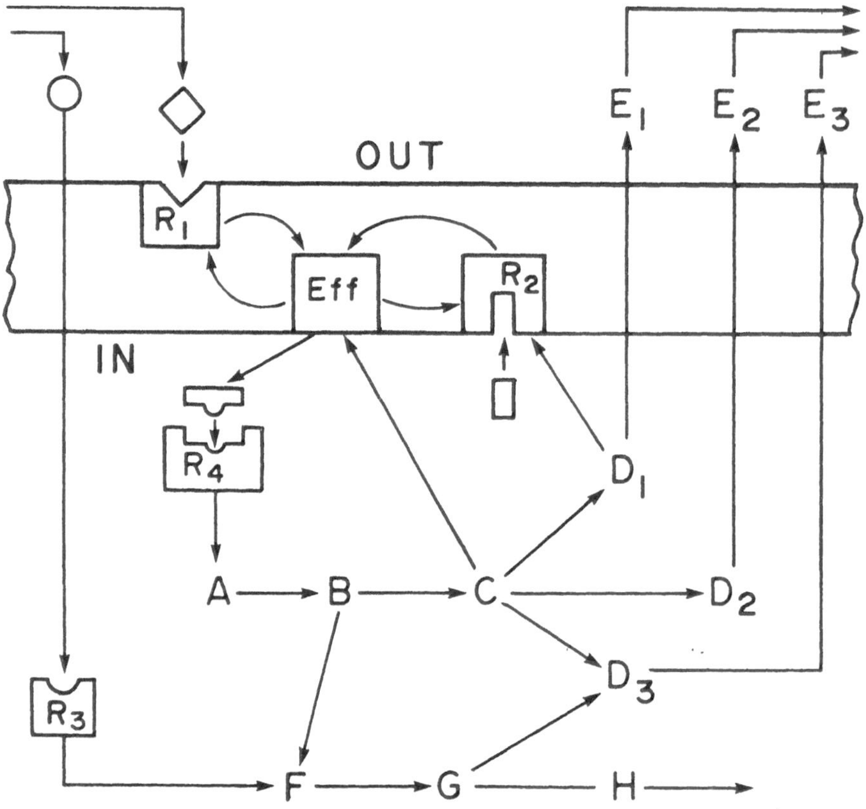

FIG. 1

Generalized concept of a "receptor" as any cell molecule (R_1, R_2, R_3, R_4) whose specific binding to an ion or another molecule ("ligand") leads to one or more "responses" (A, B, etc.). R_1 and R_2 are "coupled" to an effector in the membrane. One or more "classical responses" (E_1-E_3) are observable outside the cell. One must not read too much into this figure; it is intended only to suggest the possibility of multiple series and parallel effects, feedback loops, and intracellular interactions between systems. The arrows represent either stimulatory or inhibitory actions. The result can be both a mathematician's paradise and an experimenter's nightmare. The ultimate fates of the ligands and receptors are not even hinted at here.

1.1.2. The Nature and Uses of Receptor Binding Studies: The methodology of experiments on the binding of radioactive ligands to receptors naturally depends on the questions to be answered. According to this criterion, receptor studies fall broadly into two main classes: (a) those intended to characterize the receptor or ligand and the relation of ligand binding to other events, including the "biological response," and (b) those intended to exploit binding as a specific marker of cell types, and as a measure of changes in different functional states and in disease.

In the first type of study, for example, there is often particular emphasis on the effects of various conditions upon the relation of binding at equilibrium to ligand concentration, for different ligands and for different combinations of ligands, and on the speed of association and dissociation of the ligand-receptor complex (see Sections 2 and 3). It is of great interest to observe and understand any changes taking place in these characteristics when the tissue is altered enzymatically, or the cell is disrupted, or the receptor is purified. The time course of binding, and the effect of ligand concentration on binding, are closely correlated with specific responses in an effort to establish quantitative causal relationships.

In the second type of study, major emphasis is usually placed on ensuring that the ligand selected as a marker is highly selective for the cell and receptor to be labeled and has maximal affinity for the receptor. Often, especially in human investigations, minimum intensity and duration of functional effects may be an important consideration. In both types of receptor research, determination of the number of binding sites is a conspicuous goal. The present chapter, therefore, is intended especially as an introduction to current practices in assessing the numbers of receptor sites and the manner in which their association with particular ligands varies with time and ligand concentration.

1.1.3. Scope of This Chapter: It will be clear from later paragraphs that there is no dearth of excellent introductions to the methodology of ligand-receptor binding. I have tried to avoid unnecessary duplication. Instead, it is my intention to bridge what I see as a small but significant gap between the less quantitative and more quantitative treatments in the literature, supplementing the former and providing an introduction to the latter, particularly for readers who may lack either the time or the inclination to explore between the lines in the available presentations. I hope thereby to impart a degree of insight into the bases for several generalizations commonly encountered, and a corresponding level of self-sufficiency for those intending to delve further into the subject.

My approach will be to start from the fundamental equation of bimolecular reactions and develop the elementary theory of bimolecular equilibrium in a somewhat leisurely and detailed fashion, first for one ligand and then for two. I shall then consider some situations where the system is not at equilibrium. Finally, I shall conclude where many authors begin, with an outline of the practical application of the theory.

1.2. Origins of Ligand-Receptor Binding Kinetics

1.2.1. Introduction: The analysis of interactions between receptors and their ligands has its principal roots in studies of four rather distinct topics: (a) specific biological responses to chemical agents; (b) the binding of ligands to proteins in solution; (c) the kinetics of enzyme reactions; and (d) the use of isotopes as tracers. While ultimately all these disciplines originated in the late nineteenth and early twentieth centuries, it is only within roughly the past decade that technical advances in many supporting fields have brought them together in the separate and rapidly growing quantitative science of receptors.

1.2.2. The Development of Receptor Theory: The notion of a receptor began to take shape toward the end of the nineteenth century. In 1878, in the maiden volume of the Journal of Physiology (London), J.N. Langley introduced the concept that atropine and pilocarpine form "compounds" with "some substance or substances" in the cells, in order to explain the antagonistic effects of these agents on salivary secretion (1). He applied this concept of a "receptive substance" over some thirty years, e.g., in his studies of the effect of curare on the stimulation of skeletal muscle by nicotine (2,3). In 1906, H.H. Dale invoked a similar interpretation to explain his observations on the ergot alkaloids (4).

During much the same period, in Germany, Paul Ehrlich was developing a virtually identical idea, namely, that chemical agents exert their effects on living cells only after binding to specific cell "side-chains" (5). Ehrlich is said to have been the first to use the term "receptor." He summarized his views in the dictum, corpora non agunt nisi fixata ("particles must be attached to something to have an effect"), a generalization which he applied to many different systems, particularly in two fields closely associated with his name, immunology (for which he shared the Nobel prize in 1908) and chemotherapeutics.

The first important attempt to apply quantitative concepts of molecular binding to a receptor came many years later, when A.J. Clark, studying the effects of acetylcholine on muscle cells, offered a theoretical explanation of his dose-response curves in terms of a bimolecular binding reaction between the drug and the binding site (6,7). Not long afterward, Gaddum expanded Clark's quantitative treatment to include the possibility that some inhibitors act by successfully competing with the agonist for binding to the site (8), and he and his associates applied this analysis, for example, to the actions of serotonin (9). To a large degree, the equations and concepts used by Clark, Gaddum, and their successors form the basis for those in this chapter.

Until the late 1960's, in the absence of direct methods for measuring binding of hormones and transmitters to receptors, quantitative development of the receptor concept, at least as applied to such substances and their inhibitors, continued to rest mainly on the analysis of curves describing the relationship of biological responses to the concentration of agents, and comparison of such curves between structural analogs in the same and different biological systems. During this period, Clark's theory was remarkably successful in explaining a great variety of observations, but of course it was impossible to correlate biological responses with specific binding of ligands, or even to confirm that such binding actually occurred.

A major problem for receptor research, recognized almost from the beginning, was the fact that receptors must be present in extremely small numbers within the cell. The comparative novelty of such small numbers just a few years ago is illustrated by the fact that the reference just cited (9), published in 1955, contains a footnote explaining what a "nanogram" is*. We now know that receptor populations per cell are typically of the order of hundreds or thousands, though in a few cases they run as high as a million or so (10). To study such small quantities of any structure of molecular dimensions required the development of new techniques, especially in the use of radioisotopes.

1.2.3. Ligand Binding to Proteins in Solution: The fact that many proteins are capable of binding small molecules in specific fashion engaged the attention of biochemists from the earliest days of biochemistry. In particular, the specific binding of oxygen to hemoglobin and myoglobin was extensively investigated, and the cooperative nature of this process was analyzed prior to 1925 by a number of outstanding workers, notably A.V. Hill (11,12) and G.S. Adair (13). Since 1925, the theory of ligand binding to proteins has undergone extensive development, particularly in connection with such problems as multivalency and positive and negative cooperativity, in the hands of Klotz (14,15), Scatchard (16,17), and many others. Often the results can be applied directly to receptors.

From the standpoint of cell function, several specialized subtopics, such as the binding of antigens to antibodies; sugars, amino acids, and other metabolic substrates and regulators to enzymes; and ions, sugars, amino acids and other substances to transport proteins have been of supreme interest, not just to protein chemists but to investigators in many areas of physiology as well. An extensive literature has sprung up in each of these fields, much of which clearly reveals their common theoretical basis despite their special, even unique methodological features.

In particular, the development of the radioimmunoassay by Yalow and Berson (18) and their successors in the 1960's led to the application of earlier protein-ligand binding theories to this new field, and its further growth into a sophisticated quantitative discipline, notably in the hands of Rodbard et al; for representative references see (19). In turn, Rodbard applied the results of these analyses to ligand-receptor binding with only minor changes (19), and he and his colleagues contributed a number of significant refinements over the next decade (20,21).

The subject of enzyme kinetics, another highly developed offshoot of the theory of binding to proteins, is important enough in the present context to merit a separate paragraph.

1.2.4. Enzyme Kinetics: The growth of enzyme kinetics began around the turn of the century and proceeded rapidly. A.J. Brown

(1892) and Victor Henri (1901-3) first proposed that the rate-determining step in the action of certain enzymes is an initial bimolecular binding reaction between the enzyme and its substrate (22,23). In 1913, L. Michaelis and M.L. Menten published their widely influential theory (24) applying essentially the same hypothesis, in the form of a quantitative relation, since universally known as the "Michaelis-Menten equation," between substrate concentration x and reaction velocity v, formally identical to the equation of ideal receptor binding:

$$v = Vx/(K + x). \qquad (1)$$

Three years afterward, I. Langmuir described the adsorption of molecules to surfaces in terms of a similar equation (25).

The reaction velocities for some enzymes did not obey the Michaelis-Menten equation, but could still be explained by relatively straightforward extensions of the theory (26). The actions of competitive and other inhibitors could also be explained in terms of similar reaction schemes (27). Within a few years it became possible to study a host of enzyme systems using highly purified enzymes, substrates, and reaction products and intermediates. The systems investigated displayed a great variety of reaction patterns, and correspondingly varied kinetics.

Around all these enzyme investigations there has grown up a very sizable body of theoretical literature, well summarized in several outstanding texts and references (e.g., 27,28,29). Some of this theory has formed the basis for the elementary theory of receptor-ligand interactions and is particularly relevant to this chapter. On the other hand, much of the detailed theory of individual enzyme reactions in solution is not yet applicable to receptors, perhaps in part because of experimental complexities, and it is too soon to estimate its future relevance to this field.

1.2.5. Tracers: The introduction of isotopic tracers into biomedical research is closely associated with the names of G. Hevesy and E. Segre. Starting in the early 1930's, they and their colleagues prepared radioactive phosphorus and used it and various "labeled" substances to follow physiological changes in living organisms (30,31). Tracer techniques were developed with great rapidity (32). The spectacular success of the method in elucidating transport and metabolic processes is well known.

The application of tracer methods to receptor studies had to await not only the synthesis of suitably labeled compounds of high specific activity, but also, in many cases, the development of methods for such syntheses. It was not until almost 1970, for example, that the availability of ^{3}H-ouabain made possible the the first direct observation of ouabain binding to Na^+,K^+-ATPase in mammalian cell membranes (33), and the availability of ^{125}I-ACTH and ^{125}I-angiotensin made possible the first direct study of hormone binding to specific membrane sites (34,35).

1.2.6. Radioactivity and concentration: Despite inevitable delays, it was clear from the outset that tracer methods must eventually play a major role in receptor research. One of the main reasons for the importance of radioactive tracer methods in general is their sensitivity, which makes it possible under suitable conditions to detect and accurately measure, locate, and identify extremely small amounts of material.

To appreciate the small quantities of radionuclides needed for tracer studies, consider the relationship between the half life of a radioactive substance and the quantity of the substance needed to obtain a certain number of disintegrations per minute. This relationship is particularly simple when the half life is expressed in _minutes_ and the amount of the substance as the number of radioactive _atoms_ present.

The number of disintegrations per minute, D (i.e., the number of atoms destroyed or decaying per minute), is a fixed fraction, k, of the total number, A, of atoms present,

$$D = -dA/dt = kA \qquad (2)$$

k being the _fractional turnover number_ or _rate constant_ for the process. It follows that

$$A = A_0e^{-kt} \qquad (3)$$

and

$$D = kA_0e^{-kt} \qquad (4)$$

where A_0 is the value of A at any time arbitrarily designated as t = 0. When t = (ln 2)/k,

$$A = A_0e^{-\ln 2} \qquad (5)$$

$$= (1/2)A_0$$

thus the half life of the decay process is just the time interval

$$t_{1/2} = (\ln 2)/k = (0.693...)/k \qquad (6)$$

If we now substitute k from Eq. 6 into Eq. 2, in the form A = D/k, we get the simple relationship

$$A = (t_{1/2}/\ln 2)D \qquad (7)$$

$$= (1.44...)t_{1/2}D$$

Equation 7 says that the number of _atoms_ required to obtain a given number of disintegrations per _minute_ is roughly 44% greater than the product of the given number of disintegrations _per minute_ times the radioactive half life _in minutes_.

In the case of ^{11}C, which has a half life of 20.3 min, 1 dpm would correspond to only about 1 atom per min x 20.3 min x 1.44 = _29.3 atoms_, or 48.6 x 10^{-24} mol; for ^{32}P, with a half life of 20,600 min, the values are approximately 1000 times as large. To look at the matter another way, the equation says that if any radioactive sample were to continue to decay at a constant rate equal to the initial rate (which is physically impossible, of course) it would all be used up in 1.44 x the half life (Fig. 2).

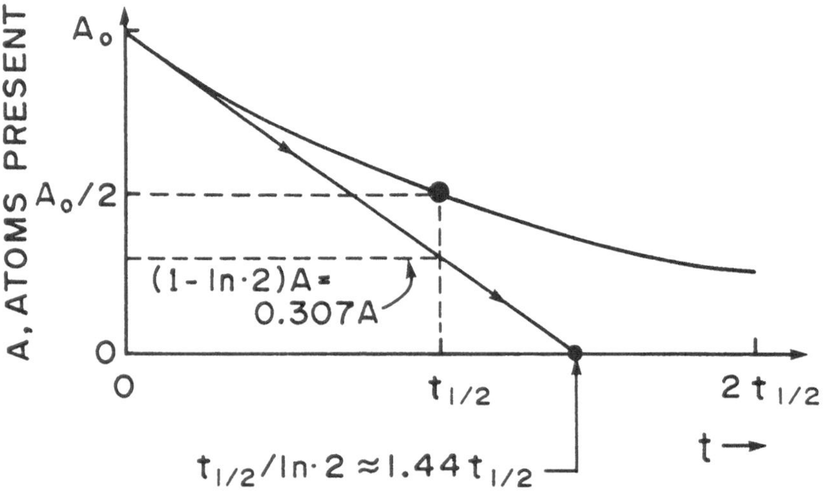

FIG. 2

Decay of a population of radioactive atoms. If we project the initial decay rate (dpm) forward it is evident that if decay could proceed at a constant rate from t = 0, all the atoms would disappear at about 1.44 times the half life (Eq. 7). This fiction enables us to calculate the atoms/dpm ratio easily from the half life.

1.2.7. Application--some useful nuclides: The quantitative relationship between half life, radioactivity, and total amount of a radionuclide is further illustrated in Table 1, which lists the half life of several nuclides important in receptor and pharmacokinetic studies, along with the amount of each nuclide needed to produce 1000 disintegrations per minute, quite enough for accurate counting in a conventional tracer experiment.

Three points are borne out by the information in Table 1. First, as Eq. 7 predicts, the number of moles of radionuclide required to give any specified number of disintegrations per minute is exactly proportional to the half life of the nuclide. Second, the range of values for the nuclides shown in the table is truly enormous; the half life of ^{14}C is about 140,000,000 times that of ^{11}C. Third, as was illustrated above for the case of ^{11}C, the absolute amount of material required for binding experiments is extremely small, particularly for a nuclide with a very short half life.

1.3. A Short Guide to the Literature

1.3.1. Introductions to Binding Methodology: For readers who want to learn more about the quantitative methodology of

TABLE 1

Readily Detectable Amounts of Some Radionuclides Used in Pharmacokinetic and Receptor Studies

Radio-nuclide	Half life (minutes)	Amount/1000 dpm (atoms)	Amount/1000 dpm (moles)
^{14}C	3.01×10^{9}	4.35×10^{12}	7.22×10^{-12}
^{3}H	6.46×10^{6}	9.31×10^{9}	15.5×10^{-15}
^{22}Na	1.37×10^{6}	1.97×10^{9}	3.28×10^{-15}
^{57}Co	$389. \times 10^{3}$	$561. \times 10^{6}$	$931. \times 10^{-18}$
^{45}Ca	$235. \times 10^{3}$	$339. \times 10^{6}$	$562. \times 10^{-18}$
^{35}S	125.8×10^{3}	$182. \times 10^{6}$	$302. \times 10^{-18}$
^{125}I	86.7×10^{3}	$125. \times 10^{6}$	$208. \times 10^{-18}$
^{51}Cr	39.9×10^{3}	57.5×10^{6}	95.5×10^{-18}
^{32}P	20.6×10^{3}	29.7×10^{6}	49.3×10^{-18}
^{131}I	11.58×10^{3}	16.7×10^{6}	27.7×10^{-18}
^{111}In	4.05×10^{3}	5.84×10^{6}	9.69×10^{-18}
^{77}Br	3.43×10^{3}	4.94×10^{6}	8.21×10^{-18}
^{99m}Tc	361.2	$519. \times 10^{3}$	$862. \times 10^{-21}$
^{18}F	109.7	$158. \times 10^{3}$	$263. \times 10^{-21}$
^{75}Br	102.0	$147. \times 10^{3}$	$244. \times 10^{-21}$
^{11}C	20.3	29.3×10^{3}	48.6×10^{-21}

receptor-ligand binding, I list here some materials which, in my judgment, may be particularly helpful at the outset. It might be useful to start with Waud's 1968 review (36) of pharmacological receptors, based on analyses of dose-response relationships. This is an excellent summary of the field immediately before the advent of hormone binding studies, and includes many references to earlier reviews. It is valuable not only for the perspective it indirectly provides on the revolution in receptor research brought about by binding measurements, but also for its rational treatment of receptor concepts that are no less relevant today.

In the 15 years since Waud's review, general introductions to the quantitative study of receptors have appeared at intervals; they reflect changing emphases to an extent, while at the same time they reaffirm some constant themes. One of the first of these, and in my judgment still one of the best, is the 1973 chapter by Rodbard mentioned above (19). A paper by Rodbard and Weiss on the theory of immunoradiometric assays, published the same year, is also fundamental (37). An early methodological chapter still frequently cited, and not overly theoretical, is that of Kahn (38).

Among later general presentations of the subject, I have found the following to be helpful at one time or another: a chapter on principles of steroid hormone receptors by Clark and Peck (39); relevant portions of reviews on adrenergic receptors by Maguire et al (40) and by Williams and Lefkowitz (41); and an article on gastrointestinal hormone receptors by Gardner (42).

The most recent additions in this category include an admirably concise summary of quantitative aspects of ligand binding by Levitzki (43). There are also two excellent general introductions to receptors, with few equations and numerous illustrations, by Jones (44) and by Blecher and Bar (45).

1.3.2. Other Basic Source Materials; It is hardly necessary to point out that in the past 15 years, scientific publications concerned with receptor-ligand interactions have appeared at a steadily increasing rate. Among these are several monographs, series, and symposia that are convenient sources of information about actual binding studies. Several of the chapters cited above (19,20,39-41,43-45) are contained in larger works, and these references may be consulted for such information. Among them, the volume edited by O'Brien (20) contains several first-rate articles pertinent to quantitative methodology.

In addition to those works already mentioned, several others, some of which will be cited later in specific contexts, should be noted here. The series Receptors and Recognition, edited by Cuatrecasas and Greaves (46), comprises two continuing subseries: Series A contains review articles of general interest, and Series B consists of monographs on specific topics. Other useful books published between 1978 and 1982 include those edited by Bolis and Straub (47), Smythies and Bradley (48), Leavitt and Clark (49), Jacob (50), Middlebrook and Kohn (51), and Kohn (52). Numerous symposia have appeared in journals; among those in recent years of most general interest have been three published in Federation Proceedings (53,54) and the American Journal of Physiology (55).

Finally, to be sure, there are individual journal articles. As of December, 1982, listings of receptor-related titles in Current Contents Life Sciences were averaging in the neighborhood of 50 per week, and a substantial proportion of these had to do with direct measurement of ligand binding. A significant fraction of articles in this area appear in such heavily read periodicals as the Proceedings of the National Academy of Sciences, USA and the Journal of Biological Chemistry, but they are found all over. Journals devoted exclusively to receptors may confidently be expected to proliferate; the first volume of the Journal of Receptor Research, published by Marcel Dekker, appeared in 1981.

2. THE "IDEAL" RECEPTOR

2.1. Introduction

2.1.1. Definition of "Ideal" Receptor: By far the largest part of receptor literature up to the present time has been based on a very simple model of the interaction between ligand and receptor. This model assumes that there is a single species of receptor site, and a single form of ligand-receptor interaction, and that the receptor molecules do not interact with each other. The properties of such systems have been extensively investigated in the literature mentioned in the preceding section, and they are reasonably well understood, if not always fully utilized.

Even where more complex models have been developed, the simple model is usually fundamental to understanding them, and in fact, the complex models can almost always be thought of as perturbations or combinations of the simple model. Therefore, the present chapter will be concerned in the main with some of the characteristics of this "ideal" receptor.

2.1.2. About Notation: The reader will quickly become aware that there is no completely uniform notation in the receptor field. Often the notation used is completely appropriate for the author's immediate purpose but less so for others. In deciding upon a notation for this chapter, I have been influenced by pedagogical considerations, especially the need for clarity, by the capabilities of the available word processor, and by a personal preference for mathematical "elegance," i.e., formal simplicity. The present system borrows features from those of Haldane and Stern (26), Dixon and Webb (27), and Rodbard (19).

In an effort to keep things as simple as possible, both for the typist and for the reader, I have generally avoided brackets and double symbols (such as LR and K_d), though subscripts are used sparingly. Potentially ambiguous symbols, such as I, l, and o, are excluded. Throughout the chapter, in keeping with familiar conventions, lower-case letters from a to n and capital letters in general refer to constants, and lower-case letters from p to z for variables. Dimensionless quantities are represented by a few of the more common Greek letters. I believe that the resulting simplicity of notation will repay any extra moments a reader may spend fixing each definition clearly in mind before proceeding.

Since the success of my notational system depends in part on instant recognition, I shall resort to a Shameless Device. To represent the unoccupied receptor site, I shall use the symbol Y--what symbol is more appropriate? Y has everything required: a notch at the top for the ligand to fit into, and a tail to couple it to a response. So, Y it shall be (Fig. 3). Then, to represent the free ligand, I have chosen X, partly because X represents the "unknown" (which it frequently is), and partly in deference to a tradition going back at least to Haldane and Stern (26). (If it seems that V might fit better into the notch of the Y, consider the following quantitative argument: As the inventor of Roman numerals realized, a V ("5") is half an X ("10"); it clearly follows that X is twice as suitable as V for our present purpose.) With X as the free ligand and Y as the unoccupied receptor, the choice of symbol for the ligand-receptor complex was, I am afraid, inevitable. Notice that both ligand and receptor undergo a rather large conformational change on binding.

2.1.3. The Association-Dissociation Reaction: In general, the binding of a ligand X to its receptor Y can be treated as a two-way ("reversible") exchange of ligand between the free state and the ligand-receptor complex Z ("bound ligand" or "bound receptor"). If the receptor itself is bound in a membrane, the ligand is exchanged between the medium and membrane phases. The exchange can be analyzed in terms of two fundamental molecular

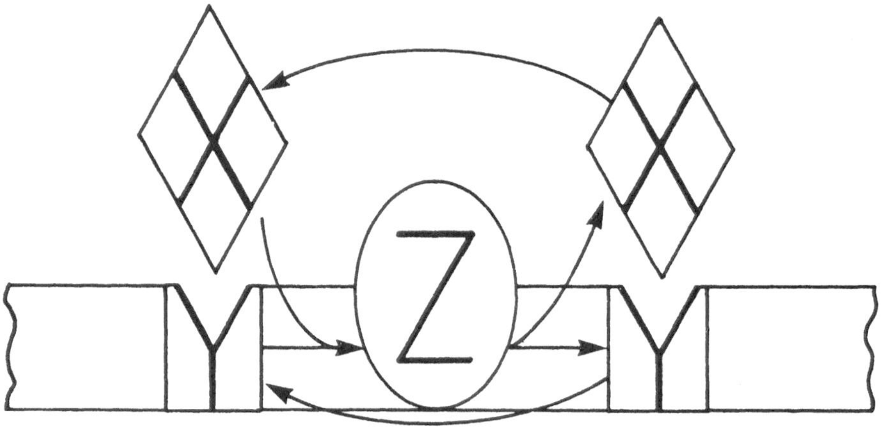

FIG. 3

Reversible association of ligand and receptor

processes, the association of X and Y and the dissociation of Z.

I shall represent the concentrations of X, Y, and Z, respectively, by the lower-case letters x, y, and z:

$$X + Y \underset{k_d}{\overset{k_a}{\rightleftharpoons}} Z$$

$$x \quad y \qquad z$$

2.1.4. Practical Variables: Often it is more convenient to describe the system in terms of the total concentrations (free plus bound) of receptor and ligand. Both receptor and ligand are conserved in the exchange process; that is, their total amounts are constant with time (though they may vary between experiments, and may be changed during a single experiment). Thus, if L and R, respectively, represent total concentrations of ligand and receptor and all concentrations are referred to the same volume,

$$L = x + z \tag{8}$$

and

$$R = y + z \tag{9}$$

and L and R are usually constants within a given experiment.

The concentrations employed here and below are concentrations per unit volume of reaction medium--extracellular fluid if the binding study is done with intact cells, and total volume if with isolated membranes. Since one is ordinarily more interested in the amount of receptor per cell or per unit of cell membrane than in some arbitrarily chosen fluid volume in which the binding experiment is performed, it has become customary in the receptor literature to express total receptor concentrations, R, and concentrations of bound ligand, z, in terms of number of sites or dpm per mg of cells, cell protein, or membrane protein. It is usually possible to calculate one concentration from another by multiplying by an appropriate conversion factor, e.g., mg of protein per ml of volume. If one wishes to make maximum use of those relationships described below which depend on Eqs. 8 and 9, it is important to make this conversion. Unfortunately, authors do not always report this factor for their experiments.

2.2. The differential equation of exchange

2.2.1. Dissociation: I shall work backward, and begin with dissociation of the complex, a bit simpler than association of two molecules. Dissociation of the complex Z can be described by the equation, exactly analogous to Eq. 2 for radioactive decay,

$$(dz/dt)_{dissoc} = - k_d z \qquad (10)$$

where k_d is considered to be a constant in the ideal case. If this were the only process taking place, it would therefore be described by an "exponential-decay" curve (see Section 7).

As for radioactivity, the constant k_d represents simply the fraction of molecules of Z dissociating (or "decaying") per unit time (the "fractional turnover"), and it has the dimensions of $(time)^{-1}$. Thus, the value of k_d is independent of the units of concentration in the system, and the way concentrations are defined. Because the rate of dissociation is proportional to one concentration, z, the reaction is said to be "first-order."

2.2.2. Association: The formation of Z by association of X and Y clearly depends on both x and y; it is, in fact, described by the equation

$$(dz/dt)_{assoc} = k_a xy \qquad (11)$$

where k_a is again considered a constant in the ideal case. In contrast to k_d, the numerical value of k_a does depend on the units and definition of concentration in the system, since k_a has the dimensions of $(concentration \times time)^{-1}$. Because the rate of association is proportional to the product of two concentrations, the reaction is said to be "second-order."

2.2.3. Two-Way Exchange: The complete process of exchange is the sum of the processes of association and dissociation, and may therefore be described by the differential equation

$$dz/dt = k_a xy - k_d z \qquad (12)$$

As it stands, Eq. 12 is useless, but it can be solved under a variety of conditions where suitable relationships can be found among the four variables x, y, z, and t. In the next six sections I shall introduce some of the applications of Eq. 12 most commonly encountered in discussions of ideal binding.

3. BINDING EQUILIBRIUM (I): THE BINDING ISOTHERM

3.1. Significance of Equilibrium

3.1.1. Existence of Equilibrium Solutions: It may seem "intuitively" obvious that, left to itself, an ideal ligand-receptor system will eventually approach a state of equilibrium, in which the velocities of association and dissociation will become equal, and no further change will occur with time. The time-dependent solution in Section 7 will show how this comes about. At equilibrium, $dz/dt = 0$, and the relationships between the other variables will not include the time explicitly.

3.1.2. Practical Importance: It quite often happens, especially in preliminary studies, that the investigator is content to determine only certain properties of the system that are accessible under equilibrium conditions. Being independent of time, equilibrium measurements are comparatively easy to make and interpret--often deceptively so. To date, the great majority of studies on ligand-receptor interactions have been conducted under conditions where the system had reached, or was assumed to have reached, such an equilibrium.

3.2. Mathematical Representation of Equilibrium

3.2.1. The Equilibrium Equation: At equilibrium, $dz/dt = 0$, and Eq. 12 reduces to

$$k_a xy = k_d z \tag{13}$$

It is clear that at equilibrium we no longer need two constants to describe the system. Introducing the definition

$$K = k_d/k_a \tag{14}$$

we may write the equilibrium equation in the form

$$xy = Kz \tag{15}$$

3.2.2. The Dissociation Constant: The constant K defined in the preceding paragraph is an "equilibrium constant." Moreover, it is a dissociation constant. This fact is easy to remember, since K is proportional to the dissociation rate constant k_d in Eq. 14 and to the dissociation product xy in Eq. 15. It will turn out that K is exactly analogous to the "Michaelis constant" K in Eq. 1.

K must always be carefully distinguished from its reciprocal, the association or affinity constant, used by Rodbard (19) and various other authors:

$$K_{assoc} = 1/K \tag{16}$$

The choice of K vs. K_{assoc} depends solely on the purposes and preference of the chooser. In this discussion I shall employ the dissociation constant exclusively, mainly because, as will be clear from Eq. 15, it has the dimensions of concentration and may, in fact, be thought of as a concentration (below). It also gives a simpler form of some of the equations I want to use.

3.2.3. Interpretation of K: One of the commonest ways of looking at K becomes apparent if we write Eq. 15 in the form

$$z = (x/K)y \tag{17}$$

The dimensionless ratio x/K in this equation can be thought of as "x, expressed in terms of K."

The value of x can vary from zero to infinity. In particular, if x = K, then z = y = R/2. In other words, K is just the free ligand concentration at which the concentrations of free and bound receptor will be equal to each other and to half the total receptor concentration. Thus we may say that "K represents the concentration of free ligand at half-saturation." Remember that we are discussing the ideal receptor with a single ligand; for other situations the interpretation is likely to be incorrect.

Of course, we could equally well have written

$$z = (y/K)x \tag{18}$$

and could then have concluded that K represents the concentration of free receptor at which the concentrations of free and bound ligand are equal to each other; but since it has been more common for the receptor concentration to be held constant in experiments while the ligand concentration is varied, this interpretation of K has received comparatively little emphasis.

3.2.4. Dimensionless Concentration of Free Ligand: It will be convenient to introduce the symbol

$$\alpha = x/K \tag{19}$$

for the dimensionless ratio in Eq. 17, and write the equilibrium equation in the form

$$z = \alpha y \tag{20}$$

3.3. The "binding isotherm"

3.3.1. Dimensionless Concentration of Bound Ligand: From Eq. 9, which describes the conservation of receptor, it is clear that, qualitatively, the concentration of bound ligand, z, has to lie somewhere between zero and R, the total concentration of receptor. The value of z approaches R when x (and therefore α) becomes very large. This fact suggests that it might be useful at times to express z as a fraction of R.

In partial analogy with Eq. 19, then, we can express the

concentration of bound ligand, z, as a fraction of R (not K!),

$$\phi = z/R \tag{21}$$

where the dimensionless quantity ϕ varies between 0 and 1 as z varies between 0 and R.

3.3.2. Derivation of the Binding Isotherm: By means of Eq. 9 (conservation of receptor) and Eq. 20 (equilibrium), we can now obtain a quantitative relationship between the concentrations of free and bound ligand, x and z, in a simple and mathematically "elegant" form, in terms of the dimensionless variables α and ϕ. This relationship, known as the binding isotherm, is one of a class of isotherms, so called because they refer to measurements generally made at constant temperature.

Using Eq. 20, then, we first write Eq. 9 as

$$R = y + \alpha y \tag{22}$$

Dividing Eq. 20 by Eq. 22 to eliminate y, we directly obtain a dimensionless (or "normalized" or "reduced") version of the binding isotherm,

$$\phi = \alpha/(1 + \alpha) \tag{23}$$

or its inverse,

$$\alpha = \phi/(1 - \phi) \tag{24}$$

Comparison of Eqs. 23 and 24 suggests still another equivalent and sometimes useful form,

$$(1 + \alpha)(1 - \phi) = 1 \tag{25}$$

Equations 23-25 are fundamental throughout receptor theory. They express a very simple but extremely powerful relationship between the equilibrium concentration of bound ligand, z (as a fraction of R, its maximum value) and that of free ligand, x (in terms of K, the dissociation constant).

3.3.3. Graphic Representation of the Isotherm. The relationship represented in Eqs. 23-25 is said to be hyperbolic, because the graph of the function, shown in Fig. 4, is that of the rectangular hyperbola

$$(\alpha)(-\phi) = 1 \tag{26}$$

in which both axes have been shifted by one unit. Only the first quadrant, in which both variables are positive, has any physical meaning, however. Some representative values of the function are given in Table 2.

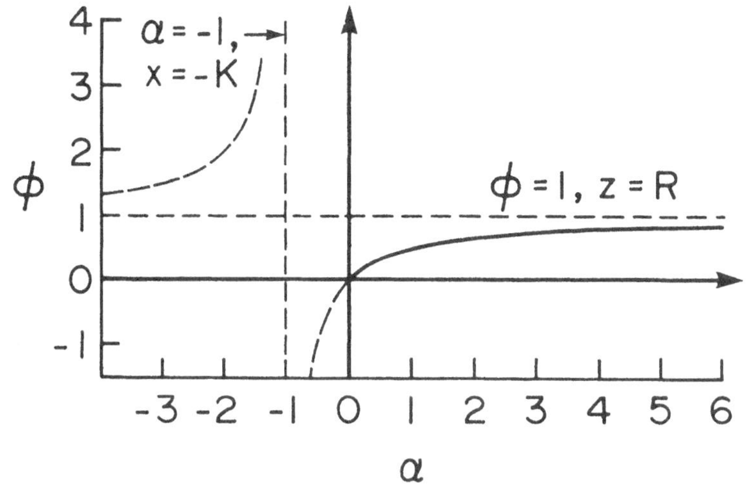

FIG. 4

Hyperbolic form of the binding isotherm (Eqs. 23-25). The broken and solid curves make up a rectangular hyperbola (Eq. 26 in the coordinate system represented by the broken axes). Only the solid curve has physical significance.

3.3.4. Characteristics of the Isotherm: Five properties of the binding isotherm are of practical importance:

1. When $\alpha = 0$, $\phi = 0$. As long as there is any free ligand present at equilibrium, there is some bound ligand present--and, perhaps more important, whenever bound ligand is present at equilibrium, there must also be free ligand.

2. When α becomes very large, ϕ approaches 1. The concentration of bound ligand, z, approaches a maximum value equal to the total concentration of receptor, R. Thus the isotherm shows "saturation."

3. When $\alpha = 1$, $\phi = 0.5$ ("half-saturation").

4. The initial slope of the curve is 1. When α is much less than 1, ϕ is approximately equal to α.

5. One of the most useful properties of the binding isotherm is that reciprocal values of α yield values of ϕ that add up to 1, expressed symbolically by the relationship

$$\phi(1/\alpha) + \phi(\alpha) = 1 \qquad (27)$$

or

$$\phi(1/\alpha) = 1 - \phi(\alpha) \qquad (28)$$

The reader can easily verify this algebraically. This property, illustrated by several values in Table 2, causes the isotherm to be antisymmetric in a semi-logarithmic plot (see section 3.3.6).

TABLE 2

Quantitative Comparison
of Binding Isotherm and Exponential Rise Functions

α or τ	$\phi = \alpha/(1+\alpha)$	$\psi = 1 - 2^{-\tau}$
0.000	0.000	0.000
0.1	0.0909...	0.067
0.2	0.166...	0.129
0.333...	0.25	0.206
0.4	0.28571...	0.242
0.5	0.333...	0.293
0.6	0.375	0.340
0.8	0.444...	0.426
1.000	0.500	0.500
1.25	0.555...	0.580
1.666...	0.625	0.685
2.0	0.666...	0.750
2.5	0.71428...	0.823
3.0	0.75	0.875
5.0	0.833...	0.969
10.0	0.90909...	0.999

3.3.5. Comparison with Exponential Decay: To fix the properties of the binding isotherm more firmly in one's mind, it may also be instructive to compare it with another dimensionless function often encountered in receptor theory,

$$\psi = 1 - 2^{-\tau} \tag{29}$$

This comparison is displayed numerically in Table 2, and also graphically in Fig. 5.

If Eq. 29 is not immediately familiar, it is probably because we more commonly see it in the form

$$\psi = 1 - e^{-kt} \tag{30}$$

where the rate constant k has the same significance as in Eq. 2. But if we define the dimensionless ratio

$$\tau = t/(t_{1/2}) \tag{31}$$

since

$$2^{-\tau} = e^{-(\ln 2)\tau} \tag{32}$$

and, from Eq. 6,

$$k = (\ln 2)/(t_{1/2}) \tag{33}$$

we then can see that the dimensionless form, Eq. 29, not only is equivalent to the more common form with e (Eq. 30), but in fact

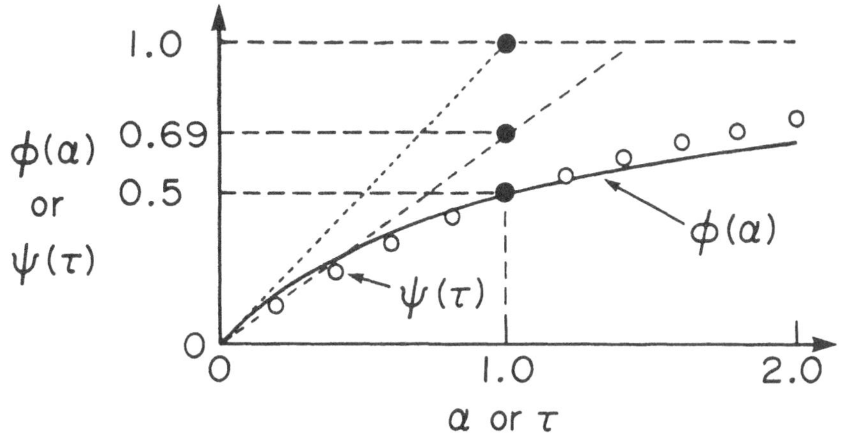

FIG. 5

Dimensionless form of the binding isotherm (solid curve) compared with the dimensionless function $\psi = 1 - 2^{-\tau}$ (open circles). The initial slopes are 1.0 and ln 2 = 0.693..., respectively. The two curves intersect at the origin and again at (1.0, 0.5); both approach 1.0 as the independent variable becomes large.

is the form most of us more or less unconsciously substitute when we describe exponential processes in terms of multiples of the half life, i.e., in terms of the dimensionless variable τ.

The two functions compared in Table 2 and Fig. 5 are exactly equal when the value of the independent variable is 0 and again when it is 1. They also approach the same limiting value, 1.0, when the independent variable becomes very large, but also have similar values (within 20% of each other) over the entire range of the independent variable. Their initial slopes are different, however; the initial slope of ψ is not 1, but ln 2 = 0.693...

3.3.6. Logarithmic Coordinates: Binding data are often plotted in logarithmic or semi-logarithmic form. It will be clear from the preceding discussion that the isotherm rises relatively rapidly near the origin, but plateaus above $\alpha = 1$ and rises more and more slowly thereafter. Consequently, the amount of useful information that is obtained about ϕ per unit of α is much greater at low than at high concentrations.

In an actual experiment, therefore, the concentration of free ligand may vary over several orders of magnitude, making it difficult to represent on a conventional graph but easy on a semi-logarithmic one. In addition, valuable information may sometimes be obtained more directly from semi-logarithmic or logarithmic plots than by other means. The reasons for this are suggested by Fig. 6, where the isotherm is plotted in conventional coordinates (a) and in five other coordinate systems (b-f).

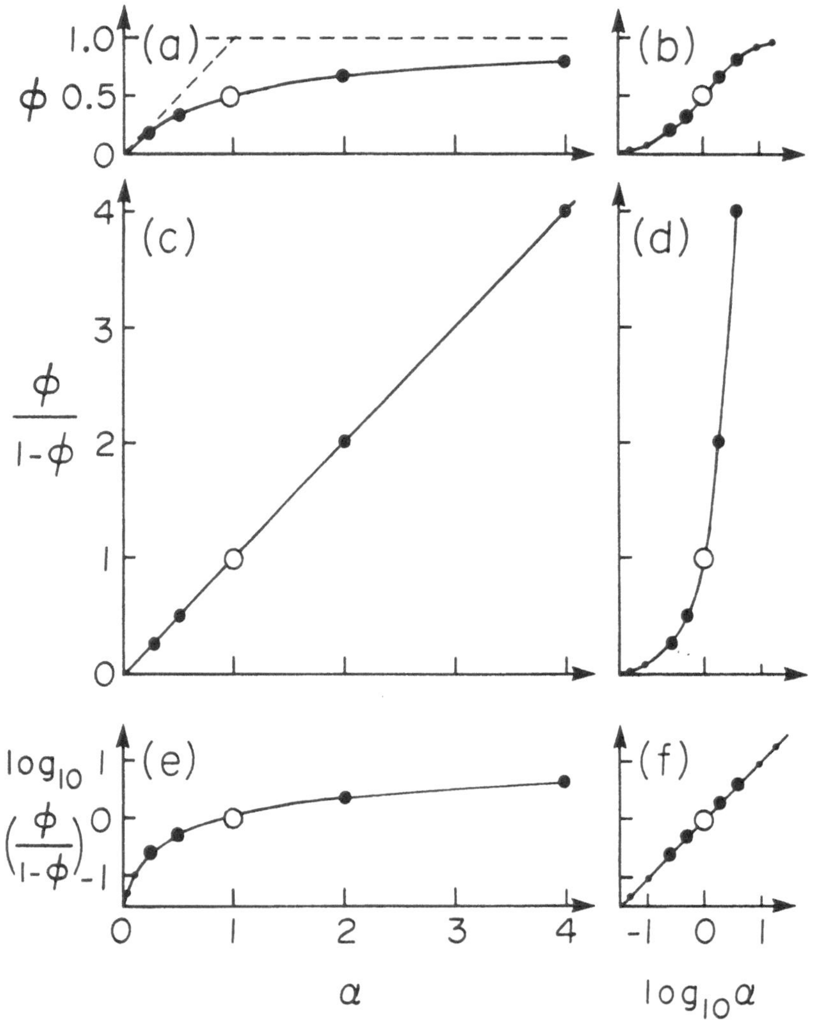

FIG. 6

The binding isotherm in various coordinate systems. In each graph half-saturation is represented by the open circle; the points corresponding to α = 1/4, 1/2, 2, and 4 are closed circles. Axis labels, and points on curves, correspond vertically and horizontally to those in adjacent graphs. (a) hyperbolic; (b) sigmoid (semi-logarithmic); (c) and (f) are identities for an ideal receptor; (f) is a form of "logit-log" or "Hill" plot; in (d) and (e), rarely used, the axes are interchanged.

3.3.7. The Sigmoid Curve: As I mentioned above (section 3.3.4), the binding isotherm is antisymmetric about the midpoint in a semi-logarithmic plot (Fig. 6,b). That is, the curve is not changed by rotating it 180° around the midpoint. The logarithm can be taken to any base, of course; in Fig. 6 the base is 10. In these coordinates the isotherm is S-shaped, or sigmoid.

The reason for this is not hard to see. In the coordinate system of Fig. 6,b, the half-saturation point is at (0,0.5). Any two reciprocal values of the independent variable, a and 1/a, will lie at equal distances on either side of this point, at $\pm$ log a. Because of Eq. 27, the points at a and 1/a are also equidistant vertically from the midpoint at (0,0.5).

3.3.8. The "Logit" Function: From Eq. 24 we know that the relationship shown in Fig. 6,c is an identity, a straight line at a 45° angle. When actual data are plotted in this way, we should expect a straight line if the receptor is "ideal." From a statistical standpoint, however, this is often undesirable, because such a plot gives greater weight to large errors at the upper end of both scales.

For this reason, it may be advantageous to plot the logarithms of both variables in Fig. 6,c (log-log plot), rather than the variables themselves. Fig. 6,f shows such a plot. Because such graphs are often used, the "logit" function has been introduced:

$$\text{logit } n = \ln \frac{n}{1 - n} = 2.3 \log_{10} \frac{n}{1 - n} \qquad (34)$$

In this terminology, Fig. 6,f is a plot of (logit ϕ)/2.3 vs. $\log_{10} \alpha$. It illustrates that such a plot is not only linear, with a slope of 45°, but also weighted so that equal relative errors at the high and low ends of the scale weigh equally.

The type of graph shown in 6,f, essentially a "logit-log" plot, is often used to linearize binding curves, and is quite popular for radioimmunoassay. It can also be thought of as the "Hill plot" (Section 8) for the case of the ideal receptor.

4. BINDING EQUILIBRIUM (II): DETERMINATION OF K AND R

4.1. Transition to Physical Variables

4.1.1. Role of Dimensionless Equations: Dimensionless relationships like Eqs. 23 and 29 are enormously helpful in dealing with all sorts of processes, including binding processes, because they are relatively simple, and therefore relatively easy to manipulate, visualize, and remember. They are also universal; their validity does not depend on any particular physical magnitudes. The physical quantities they represent may be very large or very small; for example, in the present instance, it is completely immaterial whether K and R are in, say, the picomolar or the millimolar range, or in the same or different ranges.

On the other hand, for practical applications it is usually necessary to restore the original variables, partly because

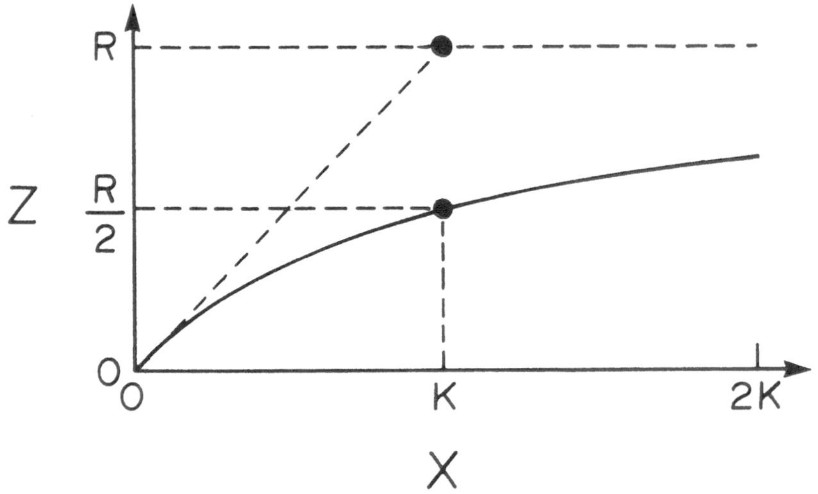

FIG. 7

How K and R are derived from the binding isotherm. The maximum value of z is R. When z = R/2, x = K. The initial slope is R/K.

actual physical variables have dimensions, and partly because we often do not know the values of the reference constants, in this case K and R--and, in fact, may be carrying out the experiments and the analysis in order to determine them.

4.1.2. Practical Form of the Binding Isotherm: Substituting Eqs. 19 and 21 into Eqs. 23 and 24, we obtain the much-desired "Michaelis-Menten" form (24), analogous to Eq. 1,

$$z = Rx/(K + x) \tag{35}$$

and its inverse

$$x = Kz/(R - z) \tag{36}$$

The relationship in this form is depicted graphically in Fig. 7, which also illustrates how it is possible to estimate K and R from the shape of the binding isotherm. The height of the curve gives R; the concentration at half-saturation gives K; and the initial slope of the curve gives R/K.

4.2. Linearized Binding Isotherms

4.2.1. Rationale: Because the isotherm is curved, it may not be a simple matter to evaluate the initial slope or the midpoint. The curve rises excruciatingly slowly at higher concentrations. In many cases--when the ligand is expensive, for example--it may not be possible to work at the comparatively high concentrations, 10-100 times K, required to "reach" z = R.

For such reasons it is often desirable to transform the data into the form of a simple straight line, when we wish to find K, R, or both directly from the graph. Equations 23-25 are not in linear form, but the binding isotherm can readily be changed into many different linear forms. We have already seen that in Fig. 6, both (c) and (f) are linear versions of the isotherm, involving logarithmic transformations of the data.

4.2.2. Non-Logarithmic Linear Forms: The isotherm can also be written in various simple equivalent linear forms that do not require the use of logarithmic coordinates:

$$1/\phi = 1 + 1/\alpha \tag{37}$$

$$\alpha/\phi = 1 + \alpha \tag{38}$$

and

$$\phi/\alpha = 1 - \phi \tag{39}$$

Graphs of Eqs. 37-39 are shown on the left in Fig. 8 (a,c,e). All these lines intercept the vertical axis at 1, and all have slopes of ± 1.

In each of these three graphs, the five data points shown correspond to the same data points used in Fig. 6. The direction of increasing concentrations is different in the three plots; it is indicated by the arrow at the half-saturation point. Notice that (a) and (c) are identical in form, but the points in one are reciprocals of those in the other, and the arrow is reversed. Graph (e) has two characteristics which set it apart from the other two: first, it is bounded by the horizontal and vertical axes, and second, points corresponding to reciprocal x values (a, 1/a) are symmetrically distributed about the midpoint.

4.2.3. Terminology: According to Haldane (56), all three linear transformations described above were first suggested by Barnett Woolf. Thus they might all be correctly termed "Woolf plots," were it not that distinctive names have been needed in order to tell them apart. Since each type of graph has been used in different contexts over the years, they are known by many names, chiefly in honor of persons who promoted their use.

The plot shown in (a) and (b) is generally referred to as a double reciprocal or Lineweaver-Burk (57) plot. That shown in (c) and (d), the one least commonly encountered, is called a Hanes (58) or Wilkinson (59) plot. The most popular type of plot for receptor studies has been the third type, shown in (e) and (f), which is usually known as the Scatchard (16) plot, less commonly as the Hofstee (60) or Eadie (61) plot. For mnemonic purposes, and to save paper, the three types of graphs may be designated as LIB, HOW, and SHE, respectively. Quite often the horizontal and vertical axes are interchanged in relation to those shown here, but interchanging the axes obviously has no effect whatever, except on the appearance of the graph.

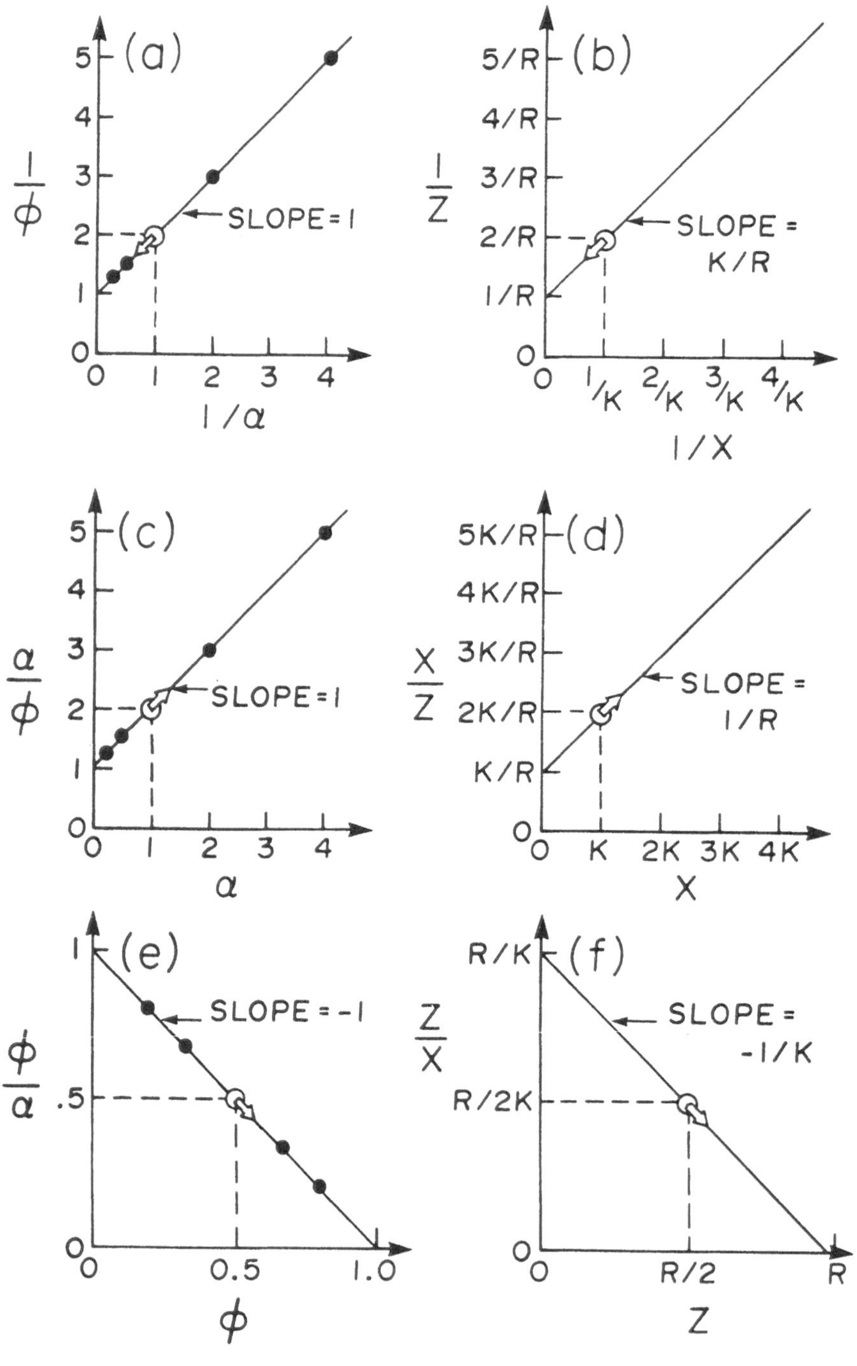

FIG. 8

Linearized forms of the binding isotherm (for explanation see text).

4.2.3. Linear plots in z and x: For practical use, e.g., when data are to be plotted linearly in order to estimate K and R, the equations must contain x, z, K, and R explicitly. In Fig. 8, immediately to the right of each dimensionless graph (a,c,e) is the corresponding graph (b,d,f) derived directly from values of z, x, z/x, and x/z, in coordinates explicitly based on K and R. The forms of Eqs. 37-39 that correspond to these graphs are:

Fig. 8,b $1/z = 1/R + (K/R)(1/x)$ (LIB) (37a)

Fig. 8,d $x/z = K/R + (1/R)x$ (HOW) (38a)

Fig. 8,f $z/x = R/K - (1/K)z$ (SHE) (39a)

In each case, we can estimate K and R, as shown, from the slope of the straight line and the point where the straight line intercepts one or both of the axes ("slope-intercept method"). In actual practice, of course, axes are laid out, not in terms of K and R, but in whatever concentration units are appropriate to the experiment, since K and R are usually not known in advance.

Which type of plot is chosen for the analysis is immaterial. All these equivalent linear forms may legitimately be used as the basis for practical methods of data analysis (below), so long as the statistical analysis is adequate (19) and Eqs. 23-25 describe the data accurately, i.e., the receptor is in fact ideal.

5. BINDING EQUILIBRIUM (III): PRACTICAL VARIABLES

5.1. Transition to "Practical" Variables--L vs. x

5.1.1. Rationale: The description of equilibrium in Sections 4 and 5 is always valid for the ideal receptor, but is frequently inadequate for actual experiments. In a typical equilibrium experiment, the investigator adds a known amount of radioligand (L) to a suspension containing a known amount of receptor (R), waits an infinite time (i.e., a decent interval), separates the bound ligand (z) from the medium, and measures z.

TABLE 3

Dependence of Bound Ligand Concentration (z) on Concentrations of Free Ligand (x) and Total Ligand (L)

x (free)	z (bound)	L (total)
K/3	R/4	K/3 + R/4
K/2	R/3	K/2 + R/3
K	R/2	K + R/2
2K	2R/3	2K + 2R/3
3K	3R/4	3K + 3R/4

Thus the concentration of free ligand, x, the variable we have used in the preceding sections, is usually not measured directly, though heaven knows it should be easy enough to calculate it from the relationship x = L - z, if L and z are known.

The problem is that when x is not measured, but inferred as L - z, the mathematical form of the isotherm becomes completely different (below). This difference affects the variability of the data, because errors in z occur two or three times in the equation. Worse yet, if L is erroneously taken as equivalent to x, serious errors may result under conditions which can readily be specified. Since the use of straight-line graphic methods to estimate constant parameters is endemic in the receptor field, the nature of this problem must be clearly recognized.

An additional reason for introducing the "practical" variable L at this stage is that the mathematics is fundamental to the following sections of this chapter, including those having to

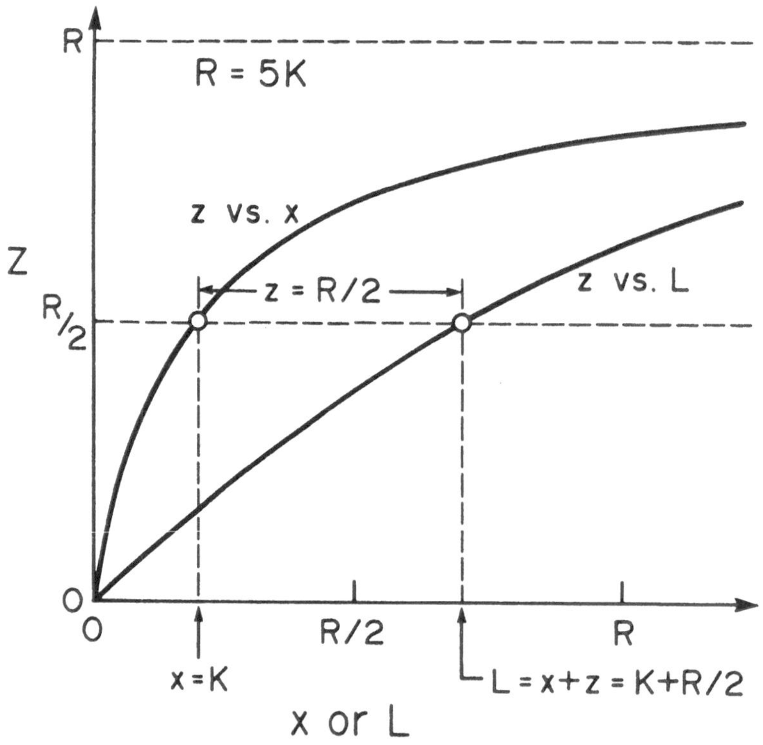

FIG. 9

Dependence of bound ligand concentration (z) on concentrations of free ligand (x) and total ligand (L). Since L is the sum of x and z, the curve of z vs. L is shifted to the right by the amount z. At the half-saturation point x = K, z = R/2, and L = K + R/2.

do with competing ligands and the approach to equilibrium.

5.1.2. The Isotherm in Terms of z and L: The contrasting dependence of bound ligand (z) on concentrations of free and total ligand (x and L) around the half-saturation point is shown in Table 3. The effect on the shape of the isotherm of plotting z against L rather than x is illustrated in Fig. 9, where the displacement of the half-saturation point to the right has been emphasized. Of course, when the curve is plotted in absolute concentration units, rather than in terms of K and R, the shape of the curve will depend completely on the values of K and R.

5.2. Calculating Bound Ligand (z) in Terms of Total Ligand (L)

5.2.1. The Equilibrium Equation in Practical Variables: We can readily obtain explicit equilibrium expressions for z (and by extension x and y), in terms of the constant concentrations L and R and the dissociation constant K. From these we can calculate equilibrium values of x, y, and z for any values of L, R, and K.

With the help of Eqs. 8 and 9, the equilibrium equation, Eq. 15, can be written as

$$(L - z)(R - z) = Kz \qquad (40)$$

which expands to the general expression

$$z^2 - (L + R + K)z + LR = 0 \qquad (41)$$

Equation 41 is the practical form of the equilibrium equation, on which much of the rest of this chapter will be based. Note that, in contrast to the hyperbolic binding isotherms discussed up to now, Eq. 41 is quadratic in form.

5.2.2. Solution of the Equilibrium Equation. Equation 41 can be written in the (simplified) "standard" quadratic form

$$z^2 - bz + c = 0 \qquad (42)$$

where $b = L + R + K$

and $c = LR$

This "standard" quadratic equation has the familiar solution

$$2z = b \pm (b^2 - 4c)^{1/2} \qquad (43)$$

If we substitute our values of b and c into Eq. 43 and expand, it will turn out that the solution can be written in a particularly compact form if we define the quantities

$$D = L - R \text{ ("Difference")} \qquad (44)$$

and

$$S = L + R \text{ ("Sum")} \qquad (45)$$

The equilibrium solution of Eq. 41 then becomes:

$$z = (S + K \pm F)/2 \qquad (46)$$

where $$F = (D^2 + 2SK + K^2)^{1/2}$$

(Notice that the parenthesis in F is similar in form to the square of S + K, except that S^2 is replaced by D^2.)

With Eq. 46 we can now calculate the equilibrium value of z for any desired values of L, R, and K. From the equilibrium value of z we can also calculate the equilibrium values of x and y, using Eqs. 8 and 9. Thus, for practical work, where x, the concentration of free ligand is unknown, Eq. 46 replaces the hyperbolic form of the isotherm (Eqs. 23 and 35).

5.2.3. Interpretation of the Equilibrium Solution: Some interesting features of Eq. 46 may be of practical importance:

(1) The equilibrium values of z (and therefore the values of x and y calculated from Eq. 46) do not depend on the initial concentrations of free and bound ligand and receptor, x, y, and z, so long as the total amounts of ligand and receptor present, L and R, are specified.

(2) At equilibrium, z depends only on the sum and difference of L and R. It is unnecessary to specify L and R separately.

(3) The solution depends on D^2 rather than D. It is therefore the same when D is negative as when it is positive--i.e., whether ligand or receptor is in excess.

(4) Both values of z are always real, since D^2, SK, and K^2 are all positive. As will become clearer in section 7, below, in connection with transient solutions, only the root containing - F yields a physically meaningful value, namely, the value of z at infinite time. As it happens, the root with + F represents the value of z at infinite negative time--a concept which is probably more stimulating to the imagination than to the progress of receptor research. Moreover, while both roots yield positive values of z, the root with + F yields negative values of x and y, an event to which we may assign a vanishingly small probability.

Since both roots turn out to be important for the transient solution, however, I shall designate the two roots of z as

$$P = (S + K - F)/2 \qquad (47)$$

and

$$Q = (S + K + F)/2 \qquad (48)$$

(where P and Q can be remembered, perhaps, as the Physical and Queer roots of Eq. 41, respectively). P is always less than Q.

5.2.4. Graphs of Bound vs. Total Ligand (z vs. L): With Eq. 46 one can readily plot graphs of z (or z/R) vs. L (or L/K, or L/R, as convenient). A graph of z vs. L, like a graph of z vs. x, depends on R and K. From Eq. 46 one can show that such a graph will have the characteristics of the function illustrated in Table 3 and Fig. 9. In addition, from Eq. 46 it is not hard to show that a graph of z/R vs. L/K will depend only on the ratio

R/K. (This can also be seen from the values in Table 3.)

It is probably obvious that if R is very small in relation to K, the concentration of bound ligand will generally be small in relation to the concentration of free ligand, and therefore the difference between x and L is less important, and may be quite negligible. On the other hand, if R is large in relation to K the concentration of bound ligand may greatly exceed that of free ligand, and the effect may be large. The importance of R/K is illustrated in Fig. 10, showing plots of z/R vs. x/K, calculated from Eq. 46 for three different values of R/K (0.1, 1, and 10). The curve for R/K = 0 (no effect) is not shown, because it is too close to the curve for R/K = 0.1 to be clearly drawn.

5.2.5. A Hypothetical Experiment. Let us suppose an investigator, unhappily (or is it happily?) ignorant of the

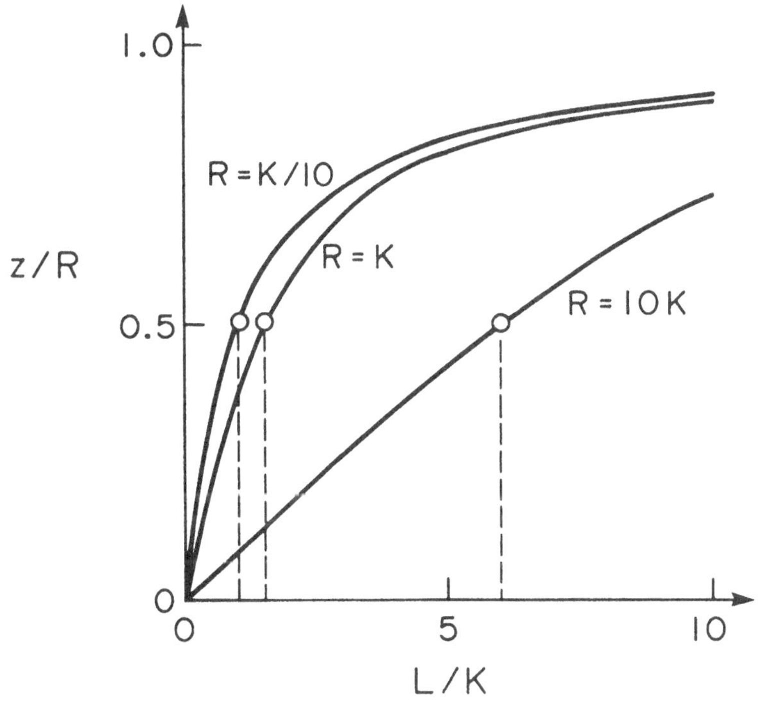

FIG. 10

Effect of the relative magnitudes of R and K on the curve of bound ligand z (expressed as z/R) vs. total ligand L (expressed as L/K). Curves for three values of the ratio R/K are shown: 0.1 (upper left), 1 (middle), and 10 (lower right). The curve for P/K = 0.1 is very close to the limiting curve for R/K = 0 (not shown).

effects just described, performs an experiment in which R/K is too large to be neglected. Let us suppose this person, assuming that L is equivalent to x, attempts to analyze the data by drawing a "linear" Scatchard (SHE) plot of z/x vs. z (Fig. 8,f), but actually plots z/L vs. z. What will such a plot look like?

To answer this question it is instructive to replot the data of Fig. 10 in the form (but not the substance) of an authentic Scatchard plot, in which the values of z and L (relative to R and K, respectively) are given as z/L vs. z. The results are shown in Fig. 11, along with those for R/K = 0 (omitted from Fig. 10).

It is apparent from Fig. 11 that an attempt to fit a straight line to the data of this plot by linear least-squares techniques might lead to any of several different straight lines and several different conclusions, depending on (a) the value of R/K, (b) the number of points plotted, (c) the accuracy of the data, and (d) the portions of the curve from which the data are taken.

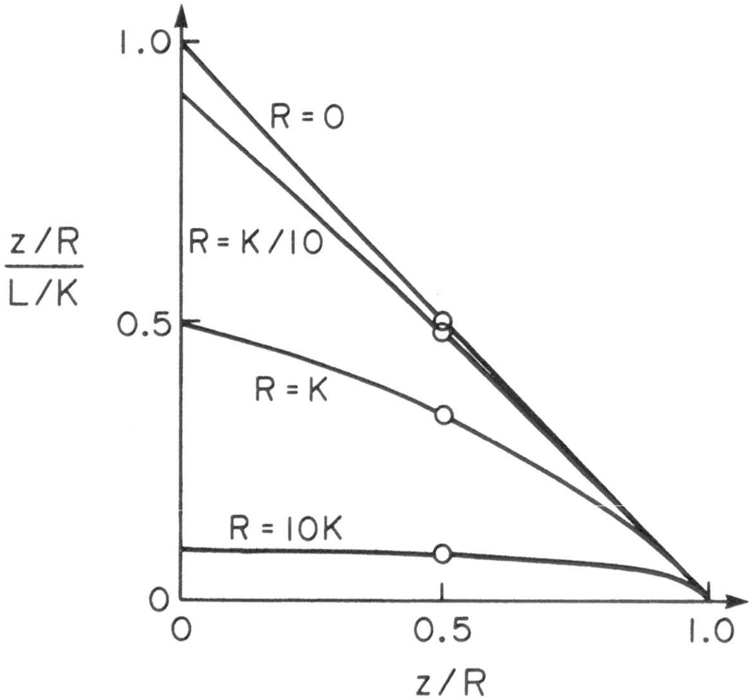

FIG. 11

Effect of substituting L for x in a Scatchard type "linear" plot of binding data. Here the data of Fig. 10 are regraphed in "Scatchard" form, in which z/L, in the dimensionless form (z/R)/(L/K), is plotted against z, in the form z/R. (As in Fig. 10, the dimensionless forms are used here only for scaling purposes.)

6. BINDING EQUILIBRIUM (IV): COMPETING LIGANDS

6.1. Significance of Competition Between Ligands

6.1.1. Tracers as Competing Ligands: Competition between two ligands for the same population of receptor sites is among the most common situations encountered in receptor research. The most obvious example is the competition between a labeled ligand and its unlabeled counterpart. As we shall see below, if the dissociation constants of labeled and unlabeled forms of the same molecule are the same (and this is usually, though not always, at least a reasonably good approximation), and the ratio of their concentrations (specific activity) is uniform throughout the system, it is perfectly acceptable to treat the two species as a single species, and use a simple proportionality to calculate the concentration of either subspecies from the total concentration.

In addition, there may be times when the investigator wishes to alter the concentration of labeled ligand during an experiment without changing the total ligand concentration. An example of this, mentioned in Section 8, is an experiment designed to test for cooperativity of binding by measuring transient association or dissociation of ligand at a fixed level of receptor occupancy or loading. In this case it is logical to consider unlabeled and labeled ligand as distinct species with identical characteristics. So far, such imaginative experimental designs have not been widely employed, but they may become more popular as their potential uses are better understood.

6.1.2. Competitive Inhibition of Binding: In contrast to the non-equilibrium experiments to which I have referred in the preceding paragraph, equilibrium measurements with competing ligands have been very widely utilized for half a century in the study of concentration-response curves, and for a much shorter time in the study of ligand binding. A typical example of the latter is the displacement experiment (see below), in which the binding of a labeled ligand is used to characterize the binding of an unlabeled analog that competes with it for the same site. Such studies can be very valuable in helping us better understand the actions of both the primary and the secondary ligands.

6.2. The Binding Isotherm for Competing Ligands

6.2.1. Description of the System: All the essential features of ligand competition can be seen from examination of a system of two competing ligands, 1 and 2. Equations 8, 9, and 15, which describe the single-ligand system, are replaced by five analogous equations governing the variables x_1, x_2, y, z_1, and z_2:

$$x_1 y = K_1 z_1 \tag{49}$$

$$x_2 y = K_2 z_2 \tag{50}$$

$$x_1 + z_1 = L_1 \tag{51}$$

$$x_2 + z_2 = L_2 \tag{52}$$

$$y + z_1 + z_2 = R \tag{53}$$

It must be emphasized that the competition of the two ligands is expressed entirely by Eq. 53; in all other respects they are absolutely independent.

6.2.2. Dimensionless Form of the Binding Isotherm: The effect of each ligand on the binding of the other is most simply expressed in the dimensionless binding isotherms for the two ligands. We begin by defining the dimensionless variables

$$\alpha_1 = x_1/K_1 \tag{54}$$

$$\alpha_2 = x_2/K_2 \tag{55}$$

$$\phi_1 = z_1/R \tag{56}$$

$$\phi_2 = z_2/R \tag{57}$$

We can then readily obtain separate binding isotherms for each ligand, as in section 3.3, by rearranging Eqs. 49, 50, and 53:

$$z_1 = (x_1/K_1)y = \alpha_1 y \tag{49a}$$

$$z_2 = (x_2/K_2)y = \alpha_2 y \tag{50a}$$

and

$$R = y + \alpha_1 y + \alpha_2 y \tag{53a}$$

and dividing each of the first two expressions by the third to eliminate y:

$$\phi_1 = \alpha_1/(1 + \alpha_1 + \alpha_2) \tag{58}$$

$$\phi_2 = \alpha_2/(1 + \alpha_1 + \alpha_2) \tag{59}$$

Equations 58 and 59 can be expanded to any number of competing ligands. Moreover, dividing Eq. 58 by Eq. 59 we have

$$\phi_1/\phi_2 = z_1/z_2 = \alpha_1/\alpha_2 \tag{60}$$

which likewise is readily generalized to multiple ligands. Notice that Eq. 60 also follows directly from Eqs. 49 and 50. Observe also that, by analogy with Section 3, I have not yet made use of Eqs. 51 and 52; I shall remedy this apparent oversight shortly.

Despite their formal simplicity, Eqs. 58-60 are very powerful tools for understanding and managing systems where two or more ligands compete for a single receptor. Their main practical drawback is that they express bound ligand concentrations in terms of free, rather than total ligand (compare Sections 3-5).

6.2.3. Effects on the Hyperbolic and Sigmoid Curves: Much ingenuity has been devoted to the development of graphic methods for evaluating dissociation constants, especially from linearized forms of the binding curves. I shall therefore briefly review a few of the more important effects of a second ligand on the binding curves for the first ligand.

The effect of ligand 2 on the binding of ligand 1 is shown graphically in Fig. 12. Comparison of Eq. 58 with Eq. 23 shows that the only difference is in the denominator of the right-hand side, where 1 is replaced by $1 + \alpha_2$. As the reader can easily verify, this is equivalent to multiplying K_1 by a factor a_2, where

$$a_2 = (1 + \alpha_2) \tag{61}$$

thus substituting for K_1 the larger value, K_{12}:

$$K_{12} = K_1 a_2 \tag{62}$$

Multiplying K_1 by a_2 is equivalent to dividing x_1 by a_2; thus x_1 must be increased by the same factor to maintain the binding of ligand 1 at a constant level. Of course, ligand 1 has an exactly analogous effect on the binding of ligand 2.

This change in the apparent dissociation constant is the sole effect of one ligand on the binding of the other. In Fig. 12, this effect is reflected in the fact that every point in the isotherm is shifted to the right, i.e., to a higher value. In linear coordinates (Fig. 12,a) this obviously changes the shape of the isotherm. When the curve is plotted in semi-logarithmic

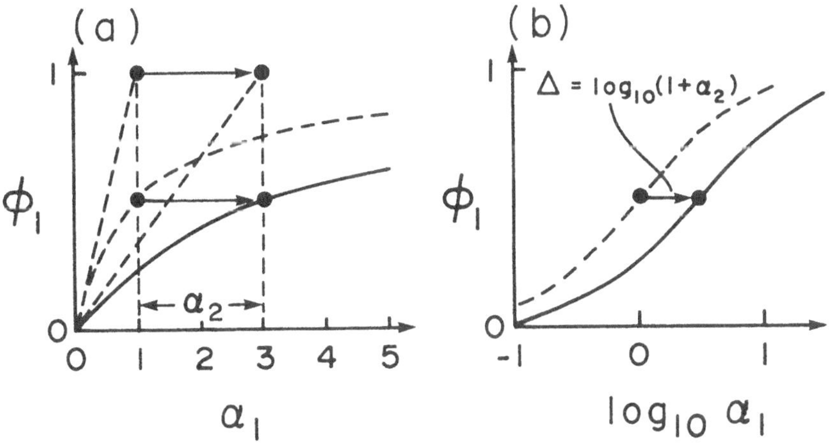

FIG. 12

The effect of ligand 2 on the binding isotherm for ligand 1 (a) in linear coordinates; (b) in semi-logarithmic coordinates. The isotherm is shifted to the right, as explained in the text.

coordinates, on the other hand (Fig. 12,b; compare Fig. 6,b), every point in the curve is shifted to the right by an increment, $\log_{10} a_2$, with the result that in this coordinate system the shape of the sigmoid curve remains unchanged.

6.2.4. Effects on Linearized Isotherms: These effects are reflected in different ways in LIB, HOW, and SHE linearized forms of the isotherm (see Eqs. 37-39a, Section 4.2, and Fig. 8). In LIB (see Fig. 8,a), the slope increases by the factor a_2, but the vertical intercept is not changed. In HOW (see Fig. 8,c), the reverse is true: the intercept is increased by the factor a_2, but the slope remains the same. Since these transforms are much less frequently used in receptor research than SHE, I leave the proof of these statements to the interested reader, and from this point on I shall confine my remarks about linear versions of the binding isotherm to SHE, which I shall henceforth call the "Scatchard" plot in submission to seemingly overwhelming social pressure,

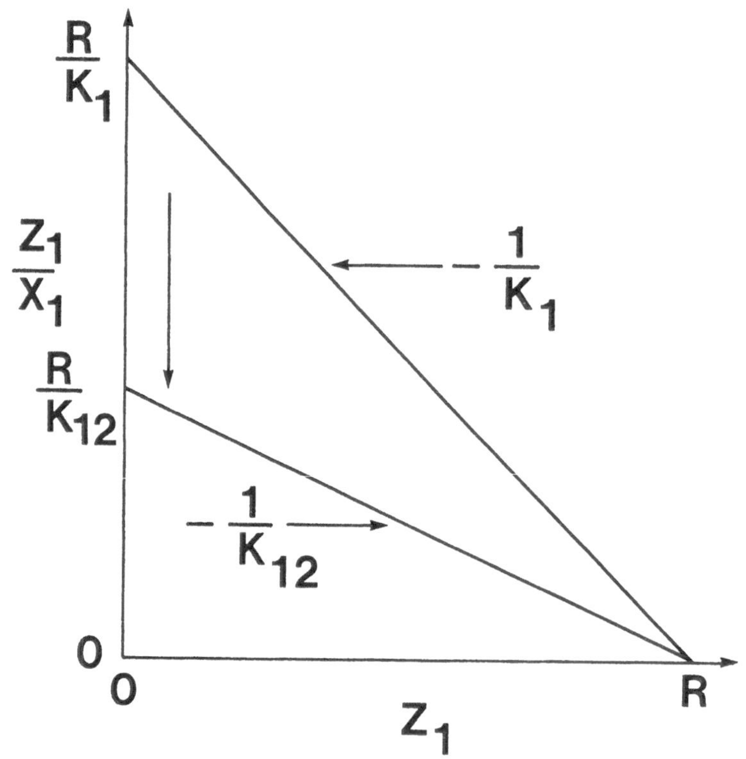

FIG. 13

Scatchard plot of the binding isotherm of ligand 1 in the presence of ligand 2. The apparent K is increased by the factor a_2; correspondingly, the slope and vertical intercept are decreased.

despite Eadie's clear claim to priority (16,61).

The Scatchard plot of the binding isotherm of ligand 1 in the presence and absence of ligand 2 is shown in units of K_1 and R (corresponding to Fig. 8,f) in Fig. 13. Since the maximum value of z_1 is not affected by ligand 2, the horizontal intercept must remain unchanged by it.

On the other hand, the vertical intercept of the Scatchard plot decreases; in this plot the vertical intercept is always the same as the initial slope of the hyperbolic isotherm (R/K in the absence of ligand 2; compare Fig. 7 and Fig. 8,f). Since the presence of ligand 2 decreases this initial slope by the factor a_2 (Fig. 12,a), the vertical intercept of the Scatchard plot, and therefore its slope, must also decrease by the same factor. Thus a careful determination of the slope or vertical intercept of the Scatchard binding plot for ligand 1, in the presence and absence of ligand 2, can be used to estimate α_2, and therefore x_2 or K_2, whichever of the two is unknown.

Detailed discussions of the use of these and other graphic representations to determine kinetic constants may be found in most standard works on enzyme kinetics (27-29). In most cases these discussions may be applied verbatim to ligand binding.

6.3. Displacement Experiments

6.3.1. The Cheng-Prusoff Equation: In studying competitive inhibition of binding, it has become almost de rigeur in recent years to determine something called the "IC_{50}," defined as the concentration of ligand 2 (the inhibitor) that causes a 50% decrease in the binding of ligand 1 (usually labeled). Such an experiment is known as a "displacement" experiment. One reason for the immense popularity of this measurement is the exquisite simplicity of a formula for calculating the IC_{50}, essentially introduced by Gaddum (8) and known to contemporary investigators chiefly through a paper by Cheng and Prusoff (62).

In the terminology of Eq. 58, the formula may be simply derived as follows: As we know, in the absence of inhibitor, the binding of ligand 1 is given by

$$\phi_1 = \alpha_1/(1 + \alpha_1) \tag{23}$$

From Eqs. 23 and 58, it follows that in the presence of ligand 2 the binding of ligand 1 will be reduced to one-half the original amount if

$$2\alpha_1/(1 + \alpha_1 + \alpha_2) = \alpha_1/(1 + \alpha_1) \tag{63}$$

from which we see that the condition for 50% inhibition is

$$\alpha_2 = 1 + \alpha_1 \tag{64}$$

Equation 64 is the celebrated "Cheng-Prusoff" equation. There is nothing mystical about the value of 50% inhibition used in the derivation; in fact, this derivation may instantly be generalized to any level of inhibition (8), as the reader can easily show: the binding of ligand 1 will be reduced to 1/n of the original amount (i.e., the amount in the absence of ligand 2) if

$$\alpha_2 = (n - 1)(1 + \alpha_1) \qquad (65)$$

Some recent articles suggest that the Cheng-Prusoff formula has not always been correctly applied (63,64). The preceding derivation makes clear that the Cheng-Prusoff formula holds if and only if α_1 is the same on both sides of Eq. 63, i.e., before and after the addition of ligand 2. This condition is represented graphically in Fig. 14. The calculation is also illustrated in Table 4 for four points, including the two shown in Fig. 14. For each point the value of α_2 is included, calculated from Eq. 60.

It is no coincidence that α_2 is constant at 1/2; the reader can easily show algebraically that this must be so. The reason lies in the fact that we have reduced the amount of bound ligand by one half while holding constant the concentration of free ligand. Mathematically this is exactly equivalent to reducing

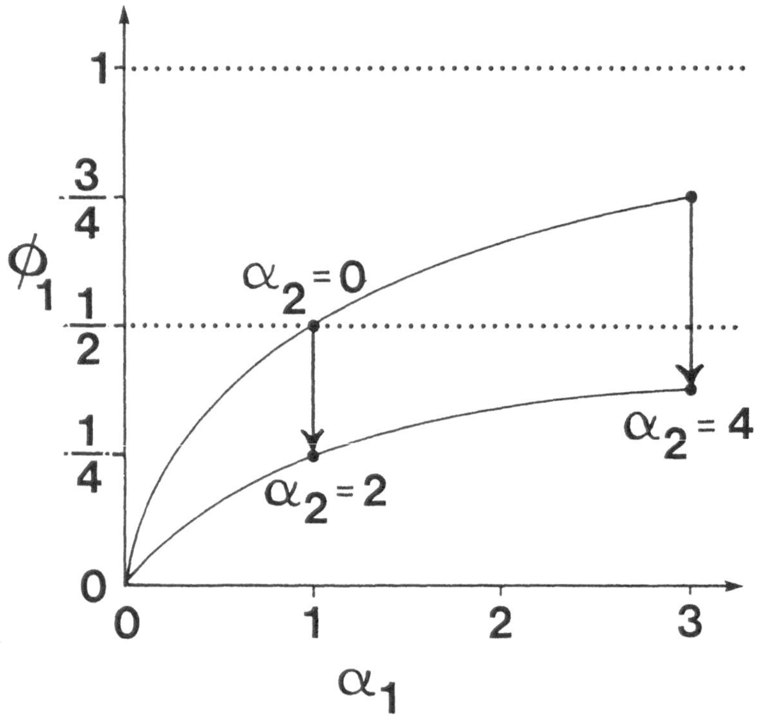

FIG. 14

The "Cheng-Prusoff" relationship (Eq. 64). If the concentration of free ligand 1 is held constant, the binding of ligand 1 is reduced by 50% when $\alpha_2 = 1 + \alpha_1$.

TABLE 4

The Cheng-Prusoff Relationship

α_1	α_2	ϕ_1	ϕ_2
1/2	1 1/2	(1/3→) 1/6	1/2
1	2	(1/2→) 1/4	1/2
2	3	(2/3→) 1/3	1/2
3	4	(3/4→) 3/8	1/2

by one half the total amount of receptor R "seen" by ligand 1 (compare Eqs. 9 and 15). In other words, under these conditions the second ligand in effect "removes" half the receptors, so far as ligand 1 is concerned, by binding to them.

Equation 64 is occasionally confused with another equation to which it bears a superficial resemblance, but which refers to a totally different set of conditions--this is the equation for 50% binding of ligand 1 in the presence of ligand 2:

$$\alpha_1 = 1 + \alpha_2 \qquad (66)$$

It is clear that Eqs. 64 and 66 are mutually contradictory, and can not possibly refer to the same process. Equation 66 describes the case where α_1 retains the same value, 0.5, in the presence and absence of ligand 2 (Fig. 12,a, horizontal arrow). Equation 64, by contrast, refers to a process where α_1 remains constant, while α_1 is reduced by one half in the presence of ligand (the vertical arrows in Fig. 14). These situations are depicted together in Fig. 15. The Cheng-Prusoff equation (Eq. 64) is represented by the vertical arrow (1 + 1 = 2), Eq. 66 by the horizontal arrow (1 + 2 = 3).

6.3.2. The Actual Situation: On further scrutiny, however, it becomes evident that neither Eq. 64 nor Eq. 66 describes what really happens when one ligand is simply added to a system that contains the receptor and another ligand. The reason for this is that the addition of ligand 2 always reduces z_1 and increases x_1 simultaneously; the actual effect of this addition, therefore, will be intermediate between the horizontal and vertical arrows (Fig. 15). Thus it is impossible to change either α_1 or ϕ_1 independently of the other by adding ligand 2, unless ligand 1 is added or withdrawn at the same time, in exactly the right amount necessary to keep z_1 or x_1 constant.

In addition to their formal symmetry Eqs. 61 and 63 share the undeniable virtue of infallibility. The main problem in applying elegant equations such as these is the practical difficulty of performing the experiments. The papers cited above (63,64) offer approaches that would help alleviate the problem, and simplify the determination of IC_{50} and ultimately of K_2.

If, however, determining K_2 is the primary goal of such experiments, as it often is, it may be that the determination of IC_{50} as such can be dispensed with altogether. The approaches set forth in the following sections, mathematically equivalent to others recently suggested (63,64), offer not just one, but two simple alternatives.

6.4. A Practical Stepwise Procedure for Two Ligands

6.4.1. Conceptual Basis: Let us assume that we are able to measure R and K_1 with ligand 1, in separate experiments without ligand 2, following the concepts laid down in previous sections of this chapter. Let us further assume that we are able to conduct one additional experiment in which we control the total ligand concentrations L_1 and L_2, and can measure z_1 as we do in the absence of ligand 2. (Needless to say, I do not recommend performing only one additional experiment, but I want to stress that only one additional set of data would suffice in principle if the receptor is ideal and the data are sufficiently accurate.)

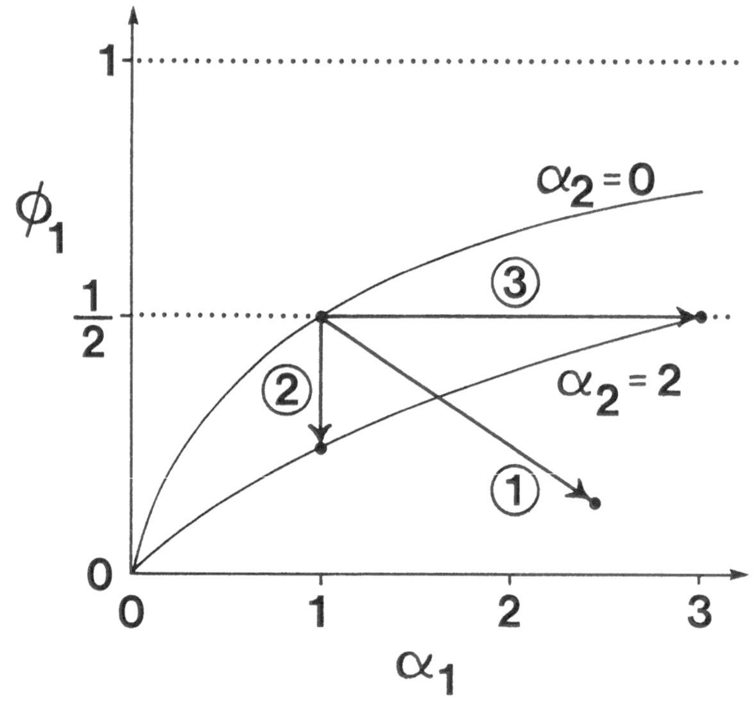

FIG. 15

Effect of adding ligand 2 without changing L_1 (arrow 1); displacement of ligand 1 is not compensated, in contrast to processes described by Eqs. 64 (arrow 2) and 66 (arrow 3). Note that lower curve differs from lower curve in Fig. 14, where α_2 varies continuously.

We know that all the relationships we will need to take into account have already been written down in the form of Eqs. 49-53. From our understanding of these equations we realize intuitively that if R, K_1, L_1, and z_1 are known, y is determined, and we ought to be able to calculate it. We also realize that if R, z_1, and y are known we can calculate z_2. Finally, we somehow feel that if all these variables are determined, and if L_2 is given, we should be able to calculate K_2. I shall offer not just one, but two equivalent ways to proceed.

6.4.2. Stepwise Protocol: Many of us have been trained to seek answers in the form of a general equation. With systems of equations like Eqs. 49-53, however, it is frequently a mistake to look for a single equation for each desired variable, especially since the advent of programmable calculators and computers. In the case of K_2, for example, an algebraic expression in terms of R, K_1, L_1, L_2, and z_1 is utterly horrendous, but if Eqs. 49-53 are solved stepwise each step is extremely simple, even without a programmable calculator. If one is available, all calculations may be programmed and each quantity in turn printed and stored for the remaining calculations.

Here is a suggested stepwise protocol that will yield the values of all variables for a two-ligand system, where ligand 1 is radioactive and ligand 2 is not:

1. In a series of experiments, measure R and K_1 in the absence of ligand 2. (See Sections 3-5 and Section 8.)
2. In an experiment with L_1 and L_2 known, measure z_1.
3. Using Eq. 51, calculate $x_1 = L_1 - z_1$. Print and store.
4. Using Eq. 49, calculate $y = K_1 z_1/x_1$. Print and store.
5. Using Eq. 53, calculate $z_2 = R - z_1 - y$. Print and store.
6. Using Eq. 52, calculate $x_2 = L_2 - z_2$. Print and store.
7. Using Eq. 50, calculate $K_2 = x_2 y/z_2$. Print.

An obvious major advantage of this approach is that it yields not just one number or two, but a complete description of the state of the system in our experiment. Analysis of the extra information can sometimes provide an unexpected clue to the behavior of the system. Some variation of this approach may also be successful in other experimental situations, where different information is available.

6.5. An Alternative Method: Simultaneous Equations

6.5.1. Derivation of the Equations: For those who prefer to work with a minimum number of equations, and more importantly, for solving various kinds of problem where one might not have the same kinds of information as in the hypothetical experiment just described, we can readily derive the analogous equations to Eq. 41. Proceeding exactly as we did in section 5.2.1, except that

$$y = R - z_1 - z_2 \tag{67}$$

we immediately obtain the following equations for z_1 and z_2 in terms of R, L_1, L_2, K_1, and K_2:

$$(z_1)^2 - (L_1 + R + K_1)z_1 + RL_1 = (L_1 - z_1)z_2 \quad (68)$$

$$(z_2)^2 - (L_2 + R + K_2)z_2 + RL_2 = (L_2 - z_2)z_1 \quad (69)$$

It may be reassuring to know that when $K_1 = K_2$, Eqs. 68 and 69 may be added to obtain, after a little rearrangement, Eq. 41 (section 5.2.1). For this, it is not necessary for ligand 1 to be a labeled form of ligand 2, or even a related compound, for that matter, so long as their dissociation constants are equal. Thus in this very special situation one ligand acts as if it were equivalent to the other, and at equilibrium the ratio of their concentrations in both the free and the bound form will be the same as at the beginning of the experiment. If k_a and k_d are different for the two ligands, but their ratio, K, is the same, their non-equilibrium behavior will be different, but they will go to the same equilibrium. I leave the rigorous demonstration of these truths to the energetic reader, and pass on to the more usual case where the dissociation constants are not equal to each other, and Eqs. 68 and 69 are not, in general, reducible.

In both Eq. 68 and Eq. 69, the coupling (competition) between concentrations of the two bound ligands, z_1 and z_2, appears entirely in a single term on the right hand side, of the form

$$(L_m - z_m)z_n = x_m z_n \quad (70)$$

When this term is zero, the competition disappears completely, and the form of the equations again reduces exactly to the form of Eq. 41, as we would expect. Moreover, the form of this term tells us that the concentration of either bound ligand can be written in simple form entirely in terms of values pertaining to the other ligand. For instance, by dividing the left-hand side of Eq. 68 by $L_1 - z_1$ we obtain z_2.

6.5.2. Application of the Equations: In practical terms, what the foregoing remarks tell us, again, is that if we know R and everything about ligand 1 (K_1, L_1, and z_1), we can calculate z_2; and if we also know L_2, we can calculate K_2. These statements are true in principle for all (reasonable) values of L_1 and L_2, and not just those very special values that give, say, 50% inhibition of binding. I reemphasize this point at the risk of seeming redundant (is not redundancy, after all, the key to successful communication?), because I am persuaded that it has not been widely appreciated.

On comparing the preceding discussion of Eqs. 68 and 69 with the stepwise procedure outlined in Section 6.4.2, the reader will notice that to solve Eq. 68 is exactly equivalent to performing steps 3-5 of the stepwise protocol, except that it does not give x_1 and y explicitly; and solving Eq. 69 is exactly equivalent to performing steps 6 and 7, except that it does not yield x_2.

Similarly, it is true that by solving Eq. 68 for z_2 and then inserting the value into Eq. 69 we can obtain an equation for z_1. This clearly starts out as a quartic equation, but it reduces spontaneously to a cubic (A.K. Thakur, personal communication). For such equations, in the majority of cases, it is theoretically possible to find an explicit solution, but practically impossible to read it. In my judgment, for most ordinary purposes there is a good deal more to be lost than gained, in terms of both time and information, from this sort of intriguing moral exercise.

7. THE APPROACH TO EQUILIBRIUM

7.1. Introduction

7.1.1. Rationale: Up to this point, we have confined our attention to equilibrium binding measurements, which give us information about the constants R and K. We remember that the dissociation constant K is the ratio of the rate constant k_d for dissociation to the rate constant k_a for association. A large value of K may be due, for example, to a large k_d or a small k_a, and so on. Thus a complete understanding of observed differences or changes in K requires knowledge of k_a and k_d, which can only be obtained in non-equilibrium experiments.

To be able to interpret non-equilibrium binding experiments quantitatively, we must first solve the differential equation of binding, Eq. 12. The solution will tell us how binding proceeds with time, depending on the properties of the receptor and the concentrations of receptor and ligand. The solution, as it happens, is neither very mysterious nor very difficult.

7.1.2. The Differential Equation of Binding: Proceeding once again by exact analogy with section 5.2, we can readily obtain explicit non-equilibrium expressions for z (and also, by extension, for x and y), in terms of the constant concentrations L and R and the dissociation constant K. From these we can calculate x, y, and z for any known values of L, R, K, and t.

We first rewrite Eq. 12 in terms of L, R, and z, as

$$dz/dt = k_a(L - z)(R - z) - k_d z \quad (71)$$

which expands to

$$dz/dt = k_a z^2 - k_a(L + R)z + k_a RL - k_d z \quad (72)$$

With the substitution $k_d = k_a K$, this is simplified to the form, analogous to Eq. 42, Section 5.2.2,

$$dz/dt = k_a(z^2 - bz + c) \quad (73)$$

where, as before,

$$b = L + R + K$$

and

$$c = LR$$

7.2. Solution of the Differential Equation

7.2.1. The Riccati Equation: In receptor literature Eq. 73 is sometimes referred to as a form of the "Riccati equation," after a Count Riccati who investigated (1724) the equation

$$dz/dt + az^2 = bt^m \quad (74)$$

Ever since the 18th century, the term "generalized Riccati equation" has been used to designate equations of the form

$$dz/dt = p_0(t) + p_1(t)z + p_2(t)z^2 \quad (75)$$

Extended discussion is given to methods of solving such equations in advanced textbooks on differential equations (65).

From the standpoint of practical methodology, however, it is essential to recognize that in Eqs. 74 and 75, dz/dt is a function of both z and t. Such equations may be difficult or impossible to solve explicitly, in terms of trigonometric or algebraic functions. Nowadays it is more common to solve such equations numerically. In general, any equation of the form

$$dz/dt = f(z,t) \quad (76)$$

may be integrated numerically, e.g., by the Runge-Kutta method (66,67), when the initial value of z is known. In fact, many desk-top calculators may be programmed, or are provided with programs, to yield numerical solutions for such equations.

7.2.2. Separation of Variables: Equation 73 is clearly an instance of the generalized Riccati equation, Eq. 75, but it has the far simpler form

$$dz/dt = f(z) \quad (77)$$

in other words, dz/dt does not depend explicitly on t. In the "ideal" case, k_a and k_d are constants (they do not depend on either z or t). Even when they are not, however, Eq. 73 can always be directly integrated, at least in principle, so long as k_a, k_d (or K), x, and y are all either constants or functions of z alone, since in that case the independent variables may be separated, with z one side of the equation and t on the other:

$$dz/f(z) = dt \quad (78)$$

Since the left-hand side of the equation contains only z, and the right-hand side contains only t, the integrations over the two variables can be carried out independently.

7.2.3. Solution of the Equation: The binding equation, Eq. 73, is a particularly straightforward case of Eq. 78; it can be integrated directly from a table of integrals. In the table found in the CRC Handbook (68), for example, formula 110 is the appropriate one. The other similar formulas given there are excluded since, as we have already seen (p. 28), the quantity I have called F (see Eq. 46) is neither zero nor imaginary.

We first rearrange Eq. 73 to separate the variables:

$$dz/(z^2 - bz + c) = k_a dt \tag{73a}$$

Applying Formula 110 to this equation, substituting the values of b and c, and introducing the same symbols as before (Section 5.2), namely,

	$D = L - R$	("Difference")	(44)
	$S = L + R$	("Sum")	(45)
and	$F = (D^2 + 2SK + K^2)^{1/2}$	("Fudge")	(46)
	$P = (S + K - F)/2$	("Physical")	(47)
	$Q = (S + K + F)/2$	("Queer")	(48)

we immediately obtain the solution

$$(1/F)\ln\frac{z - Q}{z - P} + C = k_a t \tag{79}$$

To convert Eq. 79 into a simpler and more practical form, it is convenient to introduce two more definitions:

$$w_0 = e^{FC} \tag{80}$$

and

$$w = w_0 e^{-Fk_a t} \tag{81}$$

With the help of these, and a little more shuffling of terms, we can now solve for w in terms of z,

$$w = \frac{z - P}{z - Q} \tag{82}$$

and finally for z in terms of w:

$$z = \frac{P - wQ}{1 - w} \tag{83}$$

Equation 83 completely describes the time course of binding in the great majority of binding experiments where "ideal" receptors bind single ligands. The parameter w incorporates the time-dependence of z in a familiar form (Eq. 81), and serves as a kind of substitute time variable. The main thing to remember about w is that although z _does not_ follow a simple exponential time course, w _does_, so that we can analyze the behavior of w just as we would that of any other simple exponential function.

7.2.4. Behavior of w and z as Functions of t. In order to apply Eqs. 82 and 83 to a particular case, we must be able to specify z, the concentration of bound ligand, at some particular finite time. Typically we will know the concentration at the beginning of the experiment (t = 0), but the curve will be uniquely defined if the concentration at any time is given. In fact, it is perfectly reasonable to define the time for which the concentration is known as $t = 0$, and simply consider earlier times as negative.

Since the parameter w is an exponential-decay function, its behavior as a function of t is familiar. At $t = 0$,

$$w = w_0 = \frac{z_0 - P}{z_0 - Q} \tag{84}$$

At negative times, the absolute value of w becomes larger without limit. At positive times it becomes smaller, approaching 0 as t increases without limit. It has a characteristic half time, given by $(\ln 2)/k_aF$ (compare Eq. 6).

Notice that from Eq. 82, w may be either positive or negative, depending on whether z is approaching its equilibrium value from above or below. Since z and P are always less than Q, the denominator in Eq. 82 is always negative. In association experiments, when z is less than P and increasing toward it, the numerator in Eq. 82 is also negative, so w is positive. In dissociation experiments, when z is greater than P and decreasing toward it, the numerator is positive, so w is negative.

Of course, what we are most interested in is the behavior of z. Here again there are two cases, according to whether z_0 is greater or less than P. These are illustrated by Fig. 16, which shows how it is possible for a single equation, Eq. 83, to describe either the rising or the falling time course of z.

7.3. Practical Application of the Theory

7.3.1. Basic Procedure: Remember that what we are trying to determine is k_a or k_d. We assume that we have already determined K and R in a separate series of experiments. Since we know K, by determining either rate constant we should be able to calculate the other one (as before, we are still assuming that the behavior of the system is ideal).

A typical protocol for the application of Eqs. 82 and 83 might be the following:

1. For a specific total ligand concentration, L, calculate P, Q, and F, using the values of R, K, and L. Remember that L is the total concentration of ligand, bound and free, included in the experiment to be performed. Whatever ligand, bound or free, is initially present in the system must be taken into account in calculating L.
2. Adding or removing sufficient ligand to or from the system to make up the desired value of L, perform an association or dissociation experiment (depending on whether you expect z to increase or decrease), measuring a series of values of z as a function of time.
3. Calculate a series of values of w as $(z - P)/(z - Q)$.
4. Plot w (for an association experiment) or - w (for a

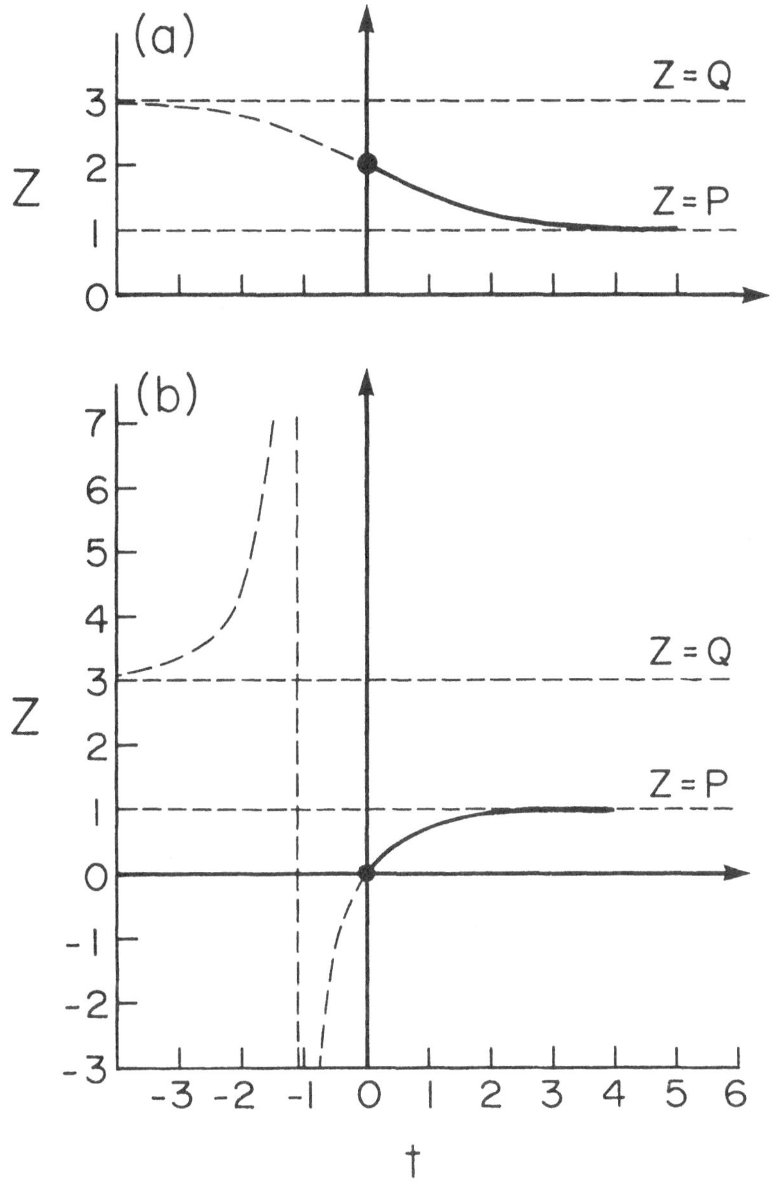

FIG. 16

Variation of z, concentration of bound ligand, with time: (a) in dissociation experiments (z <u>decreasing</u>); (b) in association experiments (z <u>increasing</u>). P and Q, the roots of Eq. 41, are limiting values of z at positive and negative infinite time, respectively. The units of z and t here are arbitrary; Fk_a (see Eq. 81) = 0.5

dissociation experiment) vs. time on semilogarithmic graph paper. From the half life of w in the graph and the calculated value of F, above, calculate k_a.

5. From k_a and K, calculate k_d.

Reported values for k_a are mostly around 10^7-10^8 M^{-1} min^{-1}. Values for k_d vary widely, but fortunately many lie near or below 10^{-2} min^{-1}, thus making it possible to perform a wide range of binding experiments in a conventional manner. Efficient blocking agents have the lowest values. The rate constants are consistent with the generally observed K values of 10^{-6}-10^{-10} M or even less.

7.3.2. Particular Cases: The preceding discussion is valid in general for both association and dissociation reactions. In certain special cases, however, the form of the solution becomes a little simpler. For example, when there is no bound ligand present at the beginning of an association experiment, as is commonly the case, $z_0 = 0$, and the form of Eq. 84 simplifies to

$$w_0 = P/Q \tag{85}$$

In the case of irreversible dissociation, where there is no back formation of bound ligand, Eq. 83 is replaced by a simple exponential decay process,

$$z = z_0 e^{-k_d t} \tag{86}$$

As one would expect, the rate constant k_a does not appear in this expression, in contrast to Eqs. 79 and 81. As was pointed out in Section 2.2.1, the dissociation rate constant k_d is simply a fractional turnover rate, and is independent of the concentration of bound ligand; in practice, therefore, the simplest way to obtain essentially "irreversible" dissociation of the receptor-ligand complex is to allow dissociation to take place at high enough dilution so that the back formation of bound ligand, which depends strongly on concentration, may be neglected. A reasonable approximation to irreversible dissociation (or association) may often be obtained by examining the very early behavior of the system in a dissociation (association) experiment where the product or products are initially absent, so that the reaction proceeds almost entirely in a single direction.

It is evident from the derivation of the binding equation, Eqs. 71-73, that the form of Eq. 83 is not simplified in the case of irreversible association, since setting $k_d = 0$ does not alter the quadratic form of the right-hand side in Eq. 73. (Formally, the solution is different in the highly exceptional case where L = R, but I shall not go into the details here.) Since the rate of association, unlike the rate of dissociation, depends on the concentration of reactants, one would expect the observed time course of association to be different for different values of L and R, but we also expect the calculated value of k_a to be independent of L and R. If L is made very large in an association experiment, it remains essentially constant during binding; in these conditions the time course of binding becomes exponential.

8. FROM THEORY TO PRACTICE: FURTHER CONSIDERATIONS

8.1. Non-Ideal Binding

8.1.1. Introduction: In the preceding seven sections, I have summarized the basic gospel--the "good news"--about the theory and practice of receptor-ligand binding studies. "Now for the bad news," the reader is probably thinking. It is true that the situation is often less simple than one might suppose from the foregoing discussion. Still, the "bad news" is not all that bad; otherwise there would not be so many people in laboratories doing binding studies. In the final section of this chapter I shall give a brief outline of some complications that one is likely to encounter, and some suggestions concerning what to do about them. A complete discussion is clearly beyond the scope of an introductory presentation, so I shall propose some further reading from time to time.

8.1.2. Multiple Ideal Sites: We have so far considered only the possibility that the ligand binds to a single ideal species of receptor or site (in the following discussion I shall use the latter term, to avoid any question of whether the site is really a "receptor" site). But what if two such species are present, or more? And what if they are not ideal? These questions arise out of very real experiences in which the binding of one or another ligand has been found to deviate from the ideal behavior described earlier, e.g., where the Scatchard plot could not be fitted by a straight line. I shall consider the two questions separately.

Clearly, if two ideal sites bind a single ligand with the same values of R and K it will never be possible to tell them apart by equilibrium binding measurements alone; indeed, this will be true even if their R values are different, so long as their K values are the same. For this reason the discussion of multiple sites centers on multiple values of K, and one hears a good deal about the presence of "high-affinity" (low-K) and "low-affinity" (high-K) binding sites in the same system.

The total concentration of bound ligand is simply the sum of the concentrations bound to each species of site. To understand how that sum will look in a given experiment, consider the behavior of the isotherm for a system of two ideal binding sites at low ligand concentrations. When the concentration of free ligand is very low, the slope of the isotherm for each ideal site will be approximately given by R/K for that site. Consequently, the R/K value for each site will be a measure of the quantitative contribution of that site to the total ligand binding.

If the high-K ("low-affinity") site has a low value of R ("low capacity"), or if the low-K ("high-affinity") site has a high value of R ("high capacity"), the contribution of the high-K site may be neglible at low ligand concentrations. In this situation the two sites may be readily distinguished, and the presence of two sites may not present much of a methodological problem.

On the other hand, if the two R/K values are similar, the two sites will make similar contributions, and it may be difficult to separate them. The most troublesome case, clearly, is that in which the low-affinity binding site has high capacity, relative to the high-affinity site. Here the low-affinity site may totally obscure the high-affinity site; on the other hand, if the ratio of R/K for the low-affinity site is not too great it may still be possible in some instances to distinguish the two sites experimentally, e.g., by making a large number of very careful measurements, over a very wide range (many orders of magnitude) of ligand concentrations. The analysis of multiple sites has even been extended to continuous affinity distributions (69).

8.1.3. Non-specific and Non-saturable Binding: In Section 1, two aspects of receptor-ligand binding were mentioned that have not figured prominently in the discussion so far: (a) specificity and (b) association with one or more cellular responses. In most cases where low-affinity binding has been observed, it has sooner or later been found to show (a) little or no specificity for the chemical structure of the ligand (e.g., stereospecificity), and (b) little or no correlation with the level of any interesting physiological response. Deferring further consideration of the concentration-response relationship for the moment, we can say that low-affinity binding is usually nonspecific, and vice versa.

In practice, the phrase "nonspecific binding" is employed to refer to all nonspecific association of ligand with the receptor at the time of measurement (e.g., counting of radioactivity). This may include not only ligand actually bound to the receptor preparation, but also such experimental artifacts as (a) ligand present in the small volume of residual medium left with the receptor (cells or membranes) after washing, or (b) ligand bound to the filter paper used for separation of receptor from medium. Such artefacts generally show no "affinity" whatever, i.e., no observable tendency to saturate; thus the phrase "nonsaturable binding" is also used to describe them. In current practice, then, "nonsaturable" and "nonspecific" binding often refer to the same thing, even though some nonspecific binding is saturable.

Of the methods that have been used to correct for nonspecific binding, two are particularly important. By both methods, specific binding is obtained by subtracting nonspecific binding from total binding, which often means that we calculate a small difference between two comparatively large numbers. The first method uses a high-affinity (low-K) blocking agent, if one is available, to compete successfully with the measured ligand for the receptor site. Some efficient blocking agents may have K values one or more orders of magnitude smaller than the hormone or other ligand under investigation. Under proper conditions specific binding can be reduced to negligible levels by the use of blocking agents (Eq. 60). This method has been used with considerable success, e.g., in the study of neurotransmitters, where a number of high-affinity blocking agents are available.

The second experimental method in common use to correct for nonspecific binding is based on the assumption that such binding is nonsaturable. Instead of blocking the specific binding site, one saturates it with high concentrations of ligand. It does not matter conceptually whether the added ligand is labeled or not;

usually it is unlabeled, to avoid unnecessary expense. Typically a series of concentrations of labeled ligand is added to a series of paired tubes; a 100-fold excess of unlabeled ligand is also added to one tube of each pair, called the "nonspecific" tube. Under these conditions the binding of ligand to any high-affinity saturable sites is expected to be saturated; thus the binding of label to the specific site should be reduced to 1% of saturation. True nonsaturable binding will be unaffected by unlabeled ligand, and will be proportional to the free ligand concentration.

If the labeled and unlabeled ligands have identical binding properties the system will be unable to distinguish between them. Therefore, the "nonspecific" tube is nothing more nor less than a tube containing a high concentration of ligand at low specific activity. We really have only a single binding curve, spread out over several orders of magnitude of ligand concentration. The curve for binding in the "nonspecific" tubes is in fact only a smaller version of the curve for total binding, derived from it, in essence, by the method of similar triangles, as follows: First the "total binding" curve is plotted. Then straight lines are drawn through the origin to each point on the "total binding" curve. Finally, a "nonspecific binding" point is located on each straight line at a fixed fraction of the distance from the origin: in the present example each point would be placed at 1/101 of the distance from the origin to the point on the "total binding" curve. The difference between the measured "total binding" curve and the "nonspecific binding" curve calculated from it is construed as "specific binding."

The saturation method just described is perfectly satisfactory for estimating nonspecific binding in many situations where it can be shown that the nonspecific component is truly nonsaturable. If it is not, however, the method may artificially elevate the calculated curve for specific binding, since the subtracted binding in the "nonspecific" tube will be less than expected. The reason for this, in physical terms, is that the "nonspecific" component will begin to saturate at higher ligand concentrations, whereas the model assumes that it will not. Consequently, the entire "nonspecific" binding curve will be displaced downward.

The reader may want to calculate the magnitudes of these effects from the expected isotherms, using various values of R and K in the specific and nonspecific binding terms for the "total" and "nonspecific" tubes. In any event, one can never be quite certain that only one binding site is being measured unless saturation of binding can be clearly demonstrated over, say, a ten-fold range of ligand concentration. It is always advisable to estimate binding over the widest possible concentration range.

8.1.4. Positive and Negative Cooperativity: Over the past decade a sizeable number of receptor systems have been observed which behave as if the dissociation constant K were a function of the concentration of bound ligand--or, if two or more ligands are present, a function of total "occupancy" of receptor sites, i.e., the sum of the concentrations of all bound ligands. To put the matter in physical terms, when some of the receptor sites are filled in such systems, the apparent dissociation constant of the remaining sites either increases ("negative cooperativity") or decreases ("positive cooperativity"). The classic example of negative cooperativity is the case of the insulin receptor (70).

This change in K is usually apparent from curvature of the Scatchard plot of the data, where the slope is given by -1/K. With negative cooperativity, for example, the increase in K as one moves from lower to higher concentrations causes a decrease in the (negative) slope, i.e., a flattening towards the right end of the curve. With positive cooperativity, the opposite effect is seen: the slope becomes steeper at the higher concentrations.

As I have mentioned in Section 1, the positive cooperativity of oxygen binding to hemoglobin was extensively investigated much earlier by A.V. Hill (12), among others. At one point (11) Hill happened to mention almost casually that what we would now call a "logit-log" plot of the data should yield a line with a slope of 1 in the absence of cooperativity, greater than 1 in the presence of positive cooperativity, and less than 1 when cooperativity is negative. Such was the force of the great man's personality that to this day people persist in using the "Hill plot" for analysis of cooperativity, even though it adds little to our understanding of specific mechanisms of binding cooperativity (71). According to Levitzki (72), Hill himself stated in 1965 that "the equation originally deduced in 1910 from the aggregation theory had been laid decently to rest in the 1920s, its body lay mouldering in the grave, but apparently its soul goes marching on."

The discovery of positive and negative binding cooperativity has generated a sizeable literature, which I shall not attempt to summarize here. In my judgment, a recent succinct and analytical editorial by Rodbard (73) is one of the best entry points into the literature. In this editorial the author briefly summarizes the history of the controversy surrounding the insulin receptor, and endorses a novel approach used by Faguet (74) in the same issue to elucidate negative cooperativity in leukoagglutinin binding to human lymphocytes. Faguet was able to measure both occupancy and dissociation rate directly during dissociation experiments, by using graded concentrations of unlabeled and labeled ligand during the dissociation phase. As the editorial suggests, this method should be useful in the study of cooperativity in other systems.

De Lean and Rodbard (20) have investigated a linear model of cooperative binding of a labeled and unlabeled ligand. Rescigno et al (75) have recently proposed a general mathematical model of receptor occupancy effects on binding parameters.

8.1.5. Statistical Simulation and Analysis: As studies of binding have progressed, interest in the statistical analysis of binding data has increased. Dowd and Riggs (76) were among the first to simulate the effects of measurement errors in enzyme reactions upon the estimation of kinetic parameters by graphical methods. Rodbard adapted the results of this and similar studies to the statistical analysis of receptor-ligand binding (19).

It is one thing to fit data by accepted statistical methods to a mathematical model such as the binding isotherm when one is sure the model is valid; it is something else to analyze the data when both the data and the model are uncertain. Recently Thakur et al. used Monte Carlo techniques to evaluate various methods of graphical analysis in the presence of (a) multiple classes of sites and (b) cooperativity (77). If the investigator wishes, the whole question of graphical methods can now be circumvented by the use of computer programs such as "LIGAND," designed to fit data to models having a wide range of complexity (21,78)--for example, "Case 6" (21), a design including multiple experiments with three ligands, two classes of sites, and nonspecific binding.

8.2. Before and After Ligand Binding

8.2.1. Distribution of Ligand in the Body: A primary goal--many would say the ultimate goal--of *in vitro* studies of receptor-ligand binding is a clearer and more quantitative understanding of the role of such binding in the intact organism. Success in reaching this goal will largely be measured by the ability to explain, predict, and control receptor-related functions, and especially in the diagnosis, prognosis, and therapy of receptor-related diseases (45,55).

In the preceding sections the concentrations of receptor and ligand have been assumed to be under the direct control of the investigator, and uniform within the reaction volume--reasonable assumptions in the test tube, although diffusion through the medium may influence the rates of association and dissociation (79). Thus much of the task of applying binding information from *in vitro* experiments to intact organisms involves the specific application of pharmacokinetic principles to transport of the ligand throughout the organism from the site of administration, and its distribution to the receptor's immediate neighborhood, where local concentrations of receptor and ligand are controlling factors in binding and subsequent events. A major contribution linking *in vitro* binding studies to the whole organism, and specifically integrating such studies with pharmacokinetics of the ligand, is a recent two-volume work edited by Eckelman (80).

A substantial number of recent publications further attest to the growing importance, in whole-body applications, of estrogens and neurotransmitters and various synthetic analogs of these, labeled with ^{3}H, ^{125}I, and such short-lived radionuclides as ^{11}C, ^{75}Br, ^{77}Br, ^{99m}Tc, and ^{18}F, among others (81-103). Because of their ability to deliver a very high-activity label (see Section 1.2.7) to a specific target for a comparatively brief period of time, the short-lived radionuclides especially may be expected to play an essential role in future applications in this field.

8.2.2. Time-Dependent Receptor-Ligand Interactions: Among the important achievements of direct binding studies has been the clear demonstration of a whole class of time-dependent events capable of influencing not only the biological response but the binding reaction itself. They include, e.g., (a) changes in the affinity (1/K) of the receptor; (b) activity cycles within the membrane; (c) internalization of the ligand-receptor complex; (d) degradation of the ligand, the receptor, or both; (e) turnover of the receptor; (f) recycling of the receptor, and (g) cellular regulation of many of these processes. Some of these events are set off by the initial binding reaction. Investigation of such processes is one of the most rapidly developing areas of receptor-ligand research, and I shall not attempt to do more than cite some pertinent references. While it is obvious that several of the effects listed above are concerned primarily or solely with the plasma membrane, it seems likely that others may have counterparts for receptors in other locations.

The regulation of receptor-ligand binding by the cell clearly has important implications for everyone working in the field. It is well established that there is more than one type of receptor regulation; for example, the number of receptors may decrease ("down-regulation") or increase ("up-regulation"), or "coupling" to the biological response may be diminished ("desensitization"). A valuable reference on this subject has been edited by Lefkowitz (104). Recently substantial progress has been made toward understanding the up- and down-regulation of receptors for insulin and epidermal growth factor (EGF) in cell culture (105,106).

The regulation of membrane receptor numbers involves multiple processes of receptor turnover, internalization of ligand-receptor complexes, and degradation, biosynthesis, and intracellular transport of receptors, which are just beginning to be understood (51,107,108,109). Mathematical modeling of these events is in an even more primitive stage; a first-order model, in which the <u>rate</u> of internalization is proportional to the concentration of reversibly bound ligand on the cell surface, appears adequate to describe many processes as diverse as the irreversible binding of cholera toxin by G_{M1} ganglioside (110) and the irreversible binding of intrinsic factor-B_{12} complex by intestinal cells (111). Wiley and Cunningham have recently advanced a simple model based on the concept of the "endocytotic rate constant" (112, 113), and Lloyd and Ascoli have utilized this model with considerable success in describing the regulation of cell-surface receptors for human choriogonadotropin (HCG) and mouse epidermal growth factor (EGF) in cultured Leydig tumor cells (114).

Regulatory processes, which involve negative feedback, may lead to oscillations, especially if there are significant delays in the feedback loop. In some recent unpublished observations, Cook has observed oscillations, presumably due to transport delays, in the concentration of Na^+, K^+-ATPase sites in HeLa cells, and has used a linear model of the regulatory cycle to compare the consequences of regulation by <u>synthesis</u> with those of regulation by <u>turnover</u> (J.S. Cook, personal communication).

<u>8.2.3. The Relation of Ligand Binding to Response</u>: It is now over a century since Langley (1) first advanced his ideas about "receptive substances," and more than half a century since Clark (6,7) suggested that the concentration of a pharmacological agent bears a hyperbolic relationship to the biological response. In view of this comparatively long history of quantitative investigation of biological responses to drugs, it has been of great interest to link observable receptor-ligand binding to such responses quantitatively. As yet, for want of solid information efforts to do so have largely been rather speculative in nature.

It has long been apparent that, in contrast to binding, where different ligands have different affinities (1/K) for a receptor but share the same "capacity" R, with respect to their ability to elicit a response different pharmacological agents not only show different apparent affinities but also display very different maximum responses ("agonists" vs. "partial agonists," etc.). Indeed, with the advent of direct binding studies it has been possible to demonstrate that some ligands with the highest affinities give no response whatever ("antagonists," blockers).

One of the major contributions of direct binding studies, moreover, is the demonstration that some ligands show binding affinities up to one or more orders of magnitude greater than the apparent affinity based on the response. Shifts in the opposite direction are much less common. There has been no lack of imaginative explanations for disparities in either direction, but in most cases it has not yet been possible to determine which explanation is correct. In the common case, where the midpoint concentration of the response curve is less than K, the system is sometimes said to carry "spare receptors," a concept which really just restates the observation. A particularly simple explanation for "spare receptors" has recently been put forward in terms of a chain of binding reactions, in which binding of the primary ligand generates a second ligand ("mediator"), whose binding to a second receptor leads to another response (115). It is easy to show that a hyperbolic function of another hyperbolic function is generally "shifted to the left," i.e., has its half-maximum point at a lower concentration than the first function.

With this I shall leave the important subject of "coupling" of binding to response, and invite the reader to investigate it further in one of the many recent references that discuss it in detail (116-119).

FOOTNOTES

*1 nanogram = 1 ng = 10^{-9} g.

ACKNOWLEDGMENTS

This work was supported by the Medical Research Service of the Veterans Administration and by grant GM-24704 from the National Institutes of Health. I gladly acknowledge countless valuable conversations with my friend and former student, Ajit Thakur. For generous contributions of their own reprints I especially thank M. Ascoli, P. Davis, C. DeLisi, D. Rodbard, and D. Triggle. J.S. Cook supplied unpublished data and helpful information. E. Lerner provided useful comments on statistics. J. Harvey, M.C. Carter, and J.R. Harriett skillfully executed the figures and Greek lettering. M. Schafer gave indispensable assistance with numerical calculations, graphing of functions, and organization of bibliography. G.M. LaScola and F. Bernstein patiently checked and gathered many references.

REFERENCES

1. Langley JN: On the physiology of the salivary secretion. Part II. On the mutual antagonism of atropin and pilocarpin, having especial reference to their relation in the submaxillary gland of the cat. J Physiol (Lond) 1:339-369, 1878

2. Langley JN: On the reaction of cells and of nerve-endings to certain poisons, chiefly as regards the reaction of striated muscle to nicotine and to curare. J Physiol (Lond) 33:374-413, 1905

3. Langley JN: On the contraction of muscle, chiefly in relation to the presence of "receptive" substances. Part I. J Physiol (Lond) 36:347-384, 1907

4. Dale HH: Some physiological actions of ergot. J Physiol (Lond) 34:163-206, 1906

5. Ehrlich P: Ueber den jetzigen Stand der Chemotherapie. Ber Dtsch Chem Ges 42:17-47, 1909

6. Clark AJ: The reaction between acetyl choline and muscle cells. J Physiol (Lond) 61:530-546, 1926

7. Clark AJ: The antagonism of acetyl choline by atropine. J Physiol (Lond) 61:547-556, 1926

8. Gaddum JH: The quantitative effects of antagonistic drugs. J Physiol (Lond) 89:7P-9P, 1937

9. Gaddum JH, Hameed KA, Hathway DE, Stephens FF: Quantitative studies of antagonists for 5-hydroxytryptamine. Quart J Exp Physiol 40:49-74, 1955

10. Cook JS: Turnover and regulation of Na-K-ATPase in HeLa cells. Am J Physiol 241 (Cell Physiol 10):C173-C183, 1981

11. Hill AV: The possible effects of aggregation of the molecules of haemoglobin on its dissociation curves. J Physiol (Lond) 40:iv-vii, 1910

12. Brown WEL, Hill AV: The oxygen-dissociation curve of blood and its thermodynamic basis. Proc Roy Soc (Lond) B94:299-334, 1922

13. Adair GS: The haemoglobin system: VI. The oxygen dissociation curve of haemoglobin. J Biol Chem 63:529-545, 1925

14. Klotz IM: The application of the law of mass action to binding by proteins. Interactions with calcium. Arch Biochem 9:109-116, 1946

15. Klotz IM, Hunston DL: Protein affinities for small molecules: conceptions and misconceptions. Arch Biochem Biophys 193:314-328, 1979

16. Scatchard G: The attractions of proteins for small molecules and ions. Ann NY Acad Sci 51:660-672, 1949

17. Scatchard G: Molecular interactions in protein solutions. Am Sci 40:61-83, 1952

18. Yalow and Berson SA: Topics in radioimmunoassay of peptide hormones. In Margolies M, Ed. Protein and Polypeptide Hormones, Part I (International Congress Series No. 161). Amsterdam, Excerpta Medica, 1968, pp 36-44

19. Rodbard D: Mathematics of hormone-receptor interaction. I. Basic principles. In O'Malley BW and Means AR, Eds. Receptors for Reproductive Hormones (Advances in Experimental Medicine and Biology, vol 36). New York, Plenum Press, 1973, pp 289-326

20. De Lean A, Rodbard D: Kinetics of cooperative binding. In O'Brien RD, Ed. The Receptors: A Comprehensive Treatise. Vol I. General Principles and Procedures. New York, Plenum Press, 1979, pp 143-192

21. Munson PJ, Rodbard D: LIGAND: A versatile computerized approach for characterization of ligand-binding systems. Anal Biochem 107:220-239, 1980

22. Brown AJ: Influence of oxygen and concentration on alcoholic fermentation. J Chem Soc (Trans) 61:369-384, 1892

23. Henri V: Lois générales de l'action des diastases. Ph.D. Dissertation, University of Paris, 1903

24. Michaelis L, Menten ML: Die Kinetik der Invertinwirkung. Biochem Z 49:333-369, 1913

25. Langmuir I: The constitution and fundamental properties of solids and liquids. J Am Chem Soc 38:2221-2295, 1916

26. Haldane JBS, Stern KG: Allgemeine Chemie der Enzyme. Dresden, Verlag von Theodor Steinkopff, 1932

27. Dixon M, Webb EC: Enzymes. New York, Academic Press, Third Edition, 1979

28. Segel IH: Enzyme Kinetics: Behavior and Analysis of Rapid Equilibrium and Steady-State Enzyme Systems. New York, John Wiley & Sons, 1975

29. Wong JT-F: Kinetics of Enzyme Mechanisms. New York, Academic Press, 1975

30. Hevesy G, Hahn L: Kgl Danske Videnskab Selskab, Biol Medd 16:1, 1941. Cited in Kamen MD: Isotopic Tracers in Biology, 3rd edition. New York, Academic Press, 1957, pp 243-244

31. Artom C, Sarzana G, Perrier C, Santangelo M, Segre E: Arch internat physiol 45:32, 1937. Cited in Kamen MD: Isotopic Tracers in Biology, 3rd edition. New York, Academic Press, 1957, pp 243-244

32. Hevesy G: Radioactive Indicators. New York, Interscience, 1948

33. Hoffman JF: The interaction between tritiated ouabain and the Na-K pump in red blood cells. J Gen Physiol 54:343s-350s, 1969

34. Lefkowitz RJ, Roth J, Pricer W, Pastan I: ACTH receptors in the adrenal: specific binding of ACTH-^{125}I and its relation to adenyl cyclase. Proc Natl Acad Sci USA 65:745-752, 1970

35. Lin SY, Goodfriend TL: Angiotensin receptors. Am J Physiol 218:1319-1328, 1970

36. Waud DR: Pharmacological receptors. Pharmacol Rev 20:49-88, 1968

37. Rodbard D, Weiss GH: Mathematical theory of immunoradiometric (labeled antibody) assays. Anal Biochem 52:10-44, 1973

38. Kahn CR: Membrane receptors for polypeptide hormones. In Korn ED, Ed. Methods in Membrane Biology, Vol 3, Plasma Membranes. New York, Plenum Press, 1975, pp 81-146

39. Clark JH, Peck EJ: Steroid hormone receptors: Basic principles and measurement. In O'Malley BW and Birnbaumer L, Eds. Receptors and Hormone Action, Vol 1, New York, Academic Press, 1977, pp 383-410

40. Maguire ME, Ross EM, Gilman AG: β-Adrenergic receptor: Ligand binding properties and the interaction with adenylyl cyclase. Adv Cyclic Nucleotide Res 8:1-83, 1977

41. Williams LT, Lefkowitz RJ: Receptor Binding Studies in Adrenergic Pharmacology. New York, Raven Press, 1978, pp 27-52

42. Gardner JD: Receptors for gastrointestinal hormones. Gastroenterology 76:202-214, 1979

43. Levitzki A: Quantitative aspects of ligand binding to receptors. In Schulster D and Levitzki A, Eds. Cellular Receptors for Hormones and Neurotransmitters. New York, Wiley, 1980, pp 9-28

44. Jones SW: Identification of receptors in vitro. In Eckelman WC, Ed. Receptor-Binding Radiotracers. Boca Raton, FL, CRC Press, 1982, pp 15-36

45. Blecher M, Bar RS: Receptors and Human Disease. Baltimore, Williams and Wilkins, 1981, pp 2-23

46. Cuatrecasas P, Greaves MF, Series Eds: Receptors and Recognition. New York, Chapman and Hall, 1976-

47. Straub L, Bolis RW, Eds: Cell Membrane Receptors for Drugs and Hormones: A Multidisciplinary Approach. New York, Raven Press, 1978

48. Smythies JR, Bradley RJ, Eds: Receptors in Pharmacology. New York, Marcell Dekker, 1978

49. Leavitt WW, Clark JH, Eds: Steroid Hormone Receptor Systems (Advances in Experimental Medicine and Biology, Vol 117). New York, Plenum Press, 1979

50. Jacob J, Ed: Receptors (Advances in Pharmacology and Therapeutics, Vol 1). New York, Pergamon, 1979

51. Middlebrook JL, Kohn LD, Eds: Receptor-Mediated Binding and Internalization of Toxins and Hormones. New York, Academic Press, 1981

52. Kohn LD, Ed: Hormone Receptors (Horizons in Biochemistry and Biophysics, Vol 6). New York, Wiley, 1982

53. Furchgott RF, Way EL, Aronow L, Chairmen: Receptors (Symposium: Sixth FASEB Conference, Federation of American Societies for Experimental Biology). Fed Proc 37:113-178, 1982

54. Czech MP, Chairman: Cellular dynamics of insulin action (Symposium). Fed Proc 41:2717-2741, 1982

55. Wilson JD, Chairman: Receptors and endocrine disease (Symposium). Am J Physiol 243 (Endocrinol Metab 6):E3-47, E81-108, 1982

56. Haldane JBS: Graphical methods in enzyme chemistry. Nature 179:832, 1957

57. Lineweaver H, Burk D: The determination of enzyme dissociation constants. J Am Chem Soc 56:658-666, 1934

58. Hanes CS: Studies on plant amylases. I. The effect of starch concentration upon the velocity of hydrolysis by the amylase of germinated barley. Biochem J 26:1406-1421, 1932

59. Wilkinson GN: Statistical estimations in enzyme kinetics. Biochem J 80:324-332, 1961

60. Hofstee BHJ: Noninverted versus inverted plots in enzyme kinetics. Nature 184:1296-1298, 1959

61. Eadie GS: The inhibition of cholinesterase by physostigmine and prostigmine. J Biol Chem 146:85, 1942

62. Cheng Y-C, Prusoff WH: Relationship between the inhibition constant (K_I) and the concentration of inhibitor which causes 50 per cent inhibition (I_{50}) of an enzymatic reaction. Biochem Pharmacol 22:3099-3108, 1973

63. Jacobs S, Chang K-J, Cuatrecasas P: Estimation of hormone receptor affinity by competitive displacement of labeled ligand: effect of concentration of receptor and of labeled ligand. Biochem Biophys Res Commun 66:687-692, 1975

64. Linden J: Calculating the dissociation constant of an unlabeled compound from the concentration required to displace radiolabel binding by 50%. J Cyclic Nucleotide Res 8:163-172, 1982

65. Ince EL: Ordinary Differential Equations. London, Longmans, Green, 1926 (reprinted New York, Dover Press)

66. Ceschino F, Kuntzmann J: Numerical Solution of Initial Value Problems (D Boynanovitch, Transl). Englewood Cliffs, NJ, Prentice-Hall, 1966, pp 37-77

67. McCalla TR: Introduction to Numerical Methods and FORTRAN Programming. New York, Wiley, 1967, pp 313-321

68. Weast RC, Ed: Handbook of Chemistry and Physics, 52nd edition, Cleveland, Chemical Rubber Co, 1971 (later editions Boca Raton, FL, CRC Press), p. A-120

69. Thakur AK, Munson PJ, Hunston DL, Rodbard D: Characterization of ligand-binding systems by continuous affinity distributions of arbitrary shape. Anal Biochem 103:240-254, 1980

70. De Meyts P, Roth J, Neville DM Jr, Gavin JR III, Lesniak MA: Insulin interactions with its receptors: experimental evidence for negative cooperativity. Biochem Biophys Res Commun 55:143-156, 1973

71. Schafer D, Thakur AK: Quantitative description of the binding of G_{M1} oligosaccharide by cholera enterotoxin. Cell Biophys 4:25-40, 1982

72. Levitzki A: Quantitative Aspects of Allosteric Mechanisms (Molecular Biology, Biochemistry and Biophysics, Vol 28). New York, Springer-Verlag, 1978, p 14

73. Rodbard D: Negative cooperativity: a positive finding? Am J Physiol 237 (Endocrinol Metab Gastrointest Physiol 6):E203-E205, 1979

74. Faguet GB: Leukoagglutinin binding to human lymphocytes: experimental support for negative cooperativity. Am J Physiol 237 (Endocrinol Metab Gastrointest Physiol 6):E207-E213, 1979

75. Rescigno A, Beck JS, Goren HJ: Determination of dependence of binding parameters on receptor occupancy. Bull Math Biol 44:477-489, 1982

76. Dowd JE, Riggs DS: A comparison of estimates of Michaelis-Menten kinetic constants from various linear transformations. J Biol Chem 240:863-869, 1965

77. Thakur AK, Jaffe ML, Rodbard D: Graphical analysis of ligand-binding systems: evaluation by Monte Carlo studies. Anal Biochem 107:279-295, 1980

78. Munson PJ: LIGAND: a computer analysis of ligand-binding data. In Langone JJ and Van Vunakis H, Eds. Immunochemical Techniques (Methods in Enzymology, Vol 92, Pt E). New York, Academic Press, 1983, pp 543-576

79. DeLisi C: The biophysics of ligand-receptor interactions. Q Rev Biophys 13:201-230, 1980

80. Eckelman WC, Ed. Receptor-Binding Radiotracers. Boca Raton, FL, CRC Press, 1982

81. Katzenellenbogen JA, Heiman DF, Senderoff SG, McElvany KD, Landvatter SW, Carlson KE, Goswami R, Lloyd JE: Estrogen receptor-based agents for imaging breast tumors: binding selectivity as a basis for design and optimization. In Lambrecht RM and Marcos N, Eds. Applications of Nuclear and Radiochemistry. New York, Pergamon Press, 1982, pp 311-323

82. McElvany KD, Katzenellenbogen JA, Shafer KE, Siegel BA, Senderoff SG, Welch MJ, the Los Alamos Medical Radioisotope Group. 16α-[^{77}Br]Bromoestradiol: dosimetry and preliminary clinical studies. J Nucl Med 23:425-430, 1982

83. McElvany KD, Carlson KE, Welch MJ, Senderoff SG, Katzenellenbogen JA, the Los Alamos Medical Radioisotope Group. In vivo comparison of 16α-[^{77}Br]bromoestradiol-17β and 16α-[^{125}I]iodoestradiol-17β. J Nucl Med 23:420-424, 1982

84. Katzenellenbogen JA, Senderoff SG, McElvany KD, O'Brien HA Jr, Welch MJ: 16α-[^{77}Br]bromoestradiol-17β: a high specific-activity, gamma-emitting tracer with uptake in rat uterus and induced mammary tumors. J Nucl Med 22:42-47, 1981

85. Katzenellenbogen JA, McElvany KD, Senderoff SG, Carlson KE, Landvatter SW, Welch MJ, the Los Alamos Medical Radioisotope Group. 16α-[^{77}Br]Bromo-11β-methoxyestradiol-17β: a gamma-emitting estrogen imaging agent with high uptake and retention by target organs. J Nucl Med 23:411-419, 1982

86. Katzenellenbogen JA, Carlson KE, Heiman DF, Goswami R: Receptor-binding radiopharmaceuticals for imaging breast tumors: estrogen-receptor interactions and selectivity of tissue uptake of halogenated estrogen analogs. J Nucl Med 21:550-558, 1980

87. Landvatter SW, Mao MK, Katzenellenbogen JA, McElvany KD, Welch MJ: Preparation and properties of halogenated estrogens as imaging agents for breast tumors. In Proc. of the Fourth International Symposium on Radiopharmaceutical Chemistry, Juelich, 1982, p 22

88. Hanson RN, Seitz DE, Botarro JC: E-17α-[^{125}I]Iodovinylestradiol: an estrogen-receptor-seeking radiopharmaceutical. J Nucl Med 23:431-436, 1982

89. Gatley SJ, Shaughnessy WJ, Inhorn L, and Lieberman LM: Studies with 17β(16α-[^{125}I]iodo)-estradiol, an estrogen receptor-binding radiopharmaceutical, in rats bearing mammary tumors. J Nucl Med 22:459-464, 1981

90. Mazaitis JK, Gibson RE, Komai T, Eckelman WC, Francis B, Reba RC: Radioiodinated estrogen derivatives. J Nucl Med 21:142-146, 1980

91. Feenstra A, Nolten GMJ, Vaalburg W, Reiffers S, Woldring MG: Radiotracers binding to estrogen receptors: I: tissue distribution of 17α-ethynylestradiol and moxestrol in normal and tumor-bearing rats. J Nucl Med 23:599-605, 1982

92. Eckelman WC: The development of muscarine cholinergic receptor-binding radiotracers. In Lambrecht RM and Marcos N, Eds. Applications of Nuclear and Radiochemistry. New York, Pergamon Press, 1982, pp 287-297

93. Eckelman WC, Grissom M, Conklin J, Rzeszotarski WJ, Gibson RE, Francis B, Eng R, Reba RC: In vivo displacement by muscarinic acetylcholine receptor (m-AChR) binding ligands. In Proc. of the Fourth International Symposium on Radiopharmaceutical Chemistry, Juelich, 1982, p 19

94. Maziere M, Berger G, Comar D: ^{11}C-radiopharmaceuticals for brain receptor studies in conjunction with positron emission tomography. In Lambrecht RM and Marcos N, Eds. Applications of Nuclear and Radiochemistry. New York, Pergamon Press, 1982, pp 251-270

95. Comar D, Maziere M, Godot JM, Berger G, Soussaline F, Menini Ch, Arfel G, Naquet R: Visualisation of ^{11}C-flunitrazepam displacement in the brain of the live baboon. Nature 280:329-331, 1982

96. Maziere M, Godot JM, Berger G, Baron JC, Comar D, Cepeda C, Menini Ch, Naquet R: Positron tomography. A new method for in vivo brain studies of benzodiazepine, in animal and in man. In Costa E et al, Eds. GABA and Benzodiazepine Receptors. New York, Raven Press, 1981, pp 273-286

97. Maziere M, Comar D, Godot JM, Berger G, Sastre J, Prenant C, Crouzel M, Artola A, Guibert B, Naquet R: Investigation of muscarinic receptors "in vivo" by external detection. In Raynaud C, Ed. Nuclear Medicine and Biology, Proc. of the Third World Congress of Nuclear Medicine and Biology, Paris, 1982, Vol 2, Pergamon Press, pp 2204-2207

98. Mintun M, Wooten GF, Raichle ME: A quantitative model for the measurement of brain receptor binding and number in vivo with positron emission tomography. In Raynaud C, Ed. Nuclear Medicine and Biology, Proc. of the Third World Congress of Nuclear Medicine and Biology, Paris, 1982, Vol 2, Pergamon Press, pp 2208-2211

99. Fowler JS, Arnett CD, Wolf AP, MacGregor RR, Norton EF, Findley AM: [^{11}C]Spiroperidol: synthesis, specific activity determination, and biodistribution in mice. J Nucl Med 23:437-445, 1982

100. Arnett CD, Fowler JS, Wolf AP, MacGregor RR: Specific binding of [^{11}C]spiroperidol in rat brain in vivo. J Neurochem 40:455-459, 1983

101. Eckelman WM, Gibson RE, Vieras F, Rzeszotarski WJ, Francis B, Reba RC: In vivo receptor binding of iodinated beta-adrenoceptor blockers. J Nucl Med 21:436-442, 1980

102. Scholl H, Laufer P, Kloster G, Stoecklin G: A potential benzodiazepine receptor-binding radiopharmaceutical for positron emission tomography: [^{75}Br]-7-bromo-1,3-dihydro-5-(2'-fluorophenyl)-1-methyl-2H-1,4-benzodiazepine-2-one ([^{75}Br]-BFB). In Proc. of the Fourth International Symposium on Radiopharmaceutical Chemistry, Juelich, 1982, pp 24-25

103. Laduron PM: ^{3}H-ligand to label brain receptors in vivo. In Proc. of the Fourth International Symposium on Radiopharmaceutical Chemistry, Juelich, 1982, p 18

104. Lefkowitz RJ, Ed: Receptor Regulation (Receptors and Recognition, Series B, Vol 13). New York, Chapman and Hall, 1981

105. Knutson VP, Ronnett GV, Lane MD: Control of insulin receptor level in 3T3 cells: Effect of insulin-induced down-regulation and dexamethasone-induced up-regulation on rate of receptor inactivation. Proc Natl Acad Sci USA 79:2822-2826, 1982

106. Krupp MN:, Connolly DT, Lane MD: Synthesis, turnover, and down-regulation of epidermal growth factor receptors in human A431 epidermoid carcinoma cells and skin fibroblasts. J Biol Chem 257:11489-11496, 1982

107. Goldstein J, Anderson R, Brown M: Coated pits, coated vesicles, and receptor-mediated endocytosis. Nature 279:679-685, 1979

108. Pastan IH, Willingham MC: Receptor-mediated endocytosis of hormones in cultured cells. Annu Rev Physiol 43:239-250, 1981

109. King AC, Cuatrecasas P: Peptide hormone-induced receptor mobility, aggregation, and internalization. N Engl J Med 305:77-88, 1981

110. Osborne JC Jr, Chang PP, Moss J: Kinetic analysis of agonist-receptor interactions. Model for the "irreversible" binding of choleragen to human fibroblasts. J Biol Chem 257:10210-10214, 1982; J Biol Chem 258:1377, 1983

111. Kapadia CR, Serfilippi D, Voloshin K, Donaldson RM Jr: Intrinsic factor-mediated absorption of cobalamin by guinea pig ileal cells. J Clin Invest 71:(in press), 1983

112. Wiley HS, Cunningham DD: A steady state model for analyzing the cellular binding, internalization and degradation of polypeptide ligands. Cell 25:433-440, 1981

113. Wiley HS, Cunningham DD: The endocytotic rate constant: A cellular parameter for quantitating receptor-mediated endocytosis. J Biol Chem 257:4222-4229, 1982

114. Lloyd CE, Ascoli M: On the mechanisms involved in the regulation of the cell-surface receptors for human choriogonadotropin and mouse epidermal growth factor in cultured Leydig tumor cells. J Cell Biol 96:521-526, 1983

115. Strickland S, Loeb JN: Obligatory separation of hormone binding and biological response curves in systems dependent upon secondary mediators of hormone action. Proc Natl Acad Sci USA 78:1366-1370, 1981

116. Triggle DJ: Receptor theory. In Smythies JR and Bradley RJ, Eds. Receptors in Pharmacology. New York, Marcel Dekker, 1978, pp 1-65

117. Colquhoun D: The link between drug binding and response: theories and observations. In O'Brien RD, Ed. The Receptors: A Comprehensive Treatise. Vol I. General Principles and Procedures. New York, Plenum Press, 1979, pp 93-142

118. Ariëns EJ, Beld AJ, Rodrigues de Miranda JF, Simonis AM: The pharmacon-receptor-effector concept: a basis for understanding the transmission of information in biological systems. In O'Brien RD, Ed. The Receptors: A Comprehensive Treatise. Vol I. General Principles and Procedures. New York, Plenum Press, 1979, pp 33-91

119. Minton AP: Steady-state relations between hormone binding and elicited response: quantitative mechanistic models. In Kohn LD, Ed: Hormone Receptors (Horizons in Biochemistry and Biophysics, Vol 6). New York, Wiley, 1982, pp 43-65

ACKNOWLEDGEMENTS

We thank the lecturers and their collaborators for their enthusiastic cooperation in providing their manuscripts in advance so that it was possible to have this resource material available in print on the day of the seminar. The patience of their respective secretarial staffs was surely challenged by the deadlines required for meeting this goal.

The editors extend their heartfelt expressions of thanks to Ms. Carol Roberts for her conscientious editorial assistance in the deadline preparations of the final camera ready copy for publication. We acknowledge Ms. Laura Kosden and Ms. Karen Schools of the Publications Department at the Society of Nuclear Medicine for their cheerful cooperation as well as staff members of Springer-Verlag, New York and Heidelberg, for their role in publishing this book on schedule.